THE TIMES

COMPLETE

FAMILY

HEALTH

First published in Great Britain in 2001 by
Hamlyn, an imprint of Octopus Publishing Group Ltd
2–4 Heron Quays, London E14 4JP

ISBN 0 600 60236 2

A CIP catalogue record for this book is available from the British Library

The material in this book has previously been published by Hamlyn

Printed and bound in China

Note
This book is not intended as an alternative to personal medical advice.
The reader should consult a physician in all matters relating to health and
particularly in respect of any symptoms which may require diagnosis or
medical attention. While the advice and information are believed to be
accurate and true at the time of going to press, neither the authors nor the
publisher can accept any legal responsibility or liability for any errors or
omissions that may be made.

THE TIMES

COMPLETE

FAMILY

HEALTH

Dr MICHAEL APPLE
BA, MB, ChB, MRCGP

Child Health Consultant:
Dr JANE COLLINS
MSc, MD, FRCP, FRCPCH
Medical Director, Great Ormond
Street Hospital for Children

hamlyn

Contents

Ailments

INTRODUCTION

MODERN MEDICINE continues to develop at an amazing rate, with new ideas and treatments appearing daily. It is hard enough for professionals to keep up to date, let alone the lay public. What is more, today's breakthrough may be tomorrow's discredited theory.

However, now more than ever people want to become informed about and involved in the management of their health. They want to know the latest information about their illnesses, the options for treatment and the side effects of medication. They want to know how to lead a healthy life, what they should do about screening and what the long-term implications are of any illnesses they or their family members do develop.

Most health professionals welcome this trend. A person who is well informed about their illness handles the anxiety of illness more successfully and is better placed to share in decisions on treatment. This is because the practice of medicine is not an exact science. The early symptoms of illness are usually non-specific and do not allow for an immediate diagnosis. Even once an illness is diagnosed, its course may vary from one individual to another and treatments do not always work. The extent of a person's recovery varies enormously, and their attitude to illness will affect this.

This book contains information as up to date as possible on a wide range of illnesses, investigations and treatments. There is a great emphasis on preventive care and in adjusting lifestyles to preserve health from birth to old age. There are also sections on first aid and safety. Scattered throughout the book are special features on major life events such as birth, and important health hazards such as pollution.

The book is written from the viewpoint of conventional Western medicine, but complementary therapies are welcomed. There is advice about complementary remedies throughout, especially about when they may or may not be appropriate.

This book is intended to be informative, but it is not a substitute for professional medical care. If in doubt consult a doctor, although we hope that you will become better informed about illness and take positive steps towards a healthier lifestyle.

HOW TO USE THIS BOOK

THE BOOK IS DIVIDED into a number of sections. Several deal with the prevention of ill-health. There is a major section on common illnesses, including features on important topics (identified in the Contents page and elsewhere by the ☛ symbol), and information about complementary therapies. Other sections cover the process of diagnosis, types of treatment, caring for the sick and first aid. You will also find information about most health hazards a family may face and what to do when illness occurs.

PREVENTION

This section reviews healthy living at all ages in a person's life, from infancy right through to advanced old age. It covers important health measures at each stage such as immunization, screening procedures appropriate to different ages and gender, and physical safety, including accident prevention. This chapter is where you will find information about having cervical smear tests, blood pressure checks and prostate checks among many other topics.

SYMPTOMS

Use the main index for the particular illnesses you are interested in. Use the symptoms index when you are not sure what a symptom means or you wish to know the possible causes.

AILMENTS

Here you will find information about some 200 illnesses and common health problems. The ailments are organized within systems of the body, for example the circulatory system, and infectious illnesses. This is the method doctors use to categorize disease. If you cannot find an illness under the system you expect, check in the index of symptoms or in the main index at the back of the book.

Each system begins with an informative introduction, which explains how that system works and gives an insight into how illnesses begin and are investigated. There is also a special section covering childhood ailments.

Each ailment is organized as follows:

A definition of the ailment

Causes This section examines the typical causes of an illness.

Symptoms Discusses the symptoms you may experience and the signs discovered on examination, plus the tests your doctor may use in diagnosis.

Treatment Both the conventional and complementary treatments are given. Complementary treatments can be easily identified by their coloured icon (see table right).

Questions These are the commonly asked questions about each ailment and will appear when further information is required.

Within some ailments, there will also be cross-references in bold type to other ailments covered elsewhere in the book. At certain points in this section there are special feature articles reviewing an area of medical interest that cuts across conventional classifications, for example diet and weight control, and giving birth. These features include health information, prevention and treatment.

DIAGNOSTIC

Arriving at a diagnosis is a fundamental aim of medicine, with a wide array of techniques available. Within this section you will find explanations of commonly used tests, including some of the latest available such as MRI scans. Here, too, is a description of how doctors examine patients for signs of illness and how they take a comprehensive medical history.

TYPES OF TREATMENT

Treatment is covered at many points in the book, relevant to specific illnesses. This section includes explanations of general techniques such as chemotherapy and drug treatment, with information about how they work and their side effects.

CARING FOR THE SICK

In this section you will find detailed advice about coping with sick children and the elderly and also what to expect when going into hospital.

FIRST AID

This section covers emergency treatment at home and at work and practical advice on preventing accidents. Included are details of performing resuscitation and mouth-to-mouth respiration and how to deal with choking, though these techniques should really be learned at a first aid class.

COMPLEMENTARY THERAPIES

Here you will find an authoritative review of the therapies available together with explanations of how they are thought to work and where their use is most appropriate. This is in addition to the many references to complementary therapies elsewhere in the book.

DRUG GLOSSARY

This section covers the most common generic drugs and drug groups, giving details of how they are used in treating specific ailments and conditions.

DIRECTORY OF ORGANIZATIONS

This section provides a list of useful organizations. International counterparts are also given where possible.

 Acupuncture, Auricular therapy

 Shiatsu-do

 Chinese herbalism

 Ayurveda

 Chakra balancing

 Osteopathy, Cranial osteopathy

 Chiropractic

 Massage

 Reflexology

 Aromatherapy

 Homeopathy

 Nutritional therapy

 Western herbalism

 Naturopathy

 Bach flower remedies

 Alexander technique

 Hypnotherapy

 Yoga

 Tai chi/chi kung

 Autogenic training

 Healing

 Cymatics

 Biodynamics, Hellerwork, Rolfing

 Arts therapies

 Play therapy

THE PREVENTION OF ILL HEALTH can be a worthy but rather dull topic, with its constant repetition of things that we think we already know. The important measures are those that have been known for years, so it is rare that big breakthroughs in prevention hit the headlines.

Risk

Prevention is really about risk and how best to manage it. This is always a balance. Things that prevent ill-health come at some cost – usually of time, personal inconvenience, a challenge to established behaviour or diet. If prevention gave an immediate benefit, surely we would all make changes. But a benefit such as not having a heart attack in 30 years feels like no benefit at all, since we do not feel under an immediate threat. This is why people so often seek advice on prevention only after a colleague has had lung cancer or a heart attack, which brings home the risk of certain behaviours.

Statistics alone can often fail to convey the real level of risk. For example, it has long been known that 25–50% of smokers will die from a smoking-related illness – a threat to stimulate panic on the streets, you might think, but not so. On the other hand, the tiny and still controversial risk of catching BSE from cattle rocked the agricultural industry.

Public health

While everyone has to take decisions about risk in their own lives, there are certain decisions that governments take for the benefit of the population. Childhood vaccination is deemed so important and well proven that pressure is applied by health professionals to have children vaccinated, making it difficult although not impossible for parents to refuse. The risk to the population of a reappearance of diphtheria or whooping cough is judged too high to let individuals choose to opt out easily and there is even less choice about testing milk for TB or having fire exits in buildings.

Thinking prevention

The major threats to health in the developed world are cancers and heart and circulatory disease. Measures that have really big effects on these require dietary and behavioural changes, the benefits of which will not be seen for decades.

Fortunately, there are many strategies for safeguarding health which produce quicker results. For example, accident prevention, control of blood pressure and immunization (see page 260) are all areas where immediate protection from risk is possible, while increased exercise improves a person's fitness within a few weeks.

PREVENTION

Screening

Screening programmes, such as those for cervical cancer (see page 148), cost a great deal of money. This can be expressed as the cost per life saved, taking into account the costs of early treatment and whether this improves survival. There are also, for individuals, the emotional costs produced by the wait for results, or by misleading results and uncertainty as to the accuracy of the screening procedure.

Governments are cautious about introducing new sceening procedures until there is evidence of benefit. For example, a programme to screen for bowel cancer (see page 174) is currently under trial, while much controversy surrounds screening for prostate and ovarian cancer using blood tests.

Screening will probably become more widespread over the next few years, but this should not allow the fundamental preventive strategies to be forgotten.

Right: A doctor vaccinating
a child against smallpox
in an 1820 painting
by Desbordes.

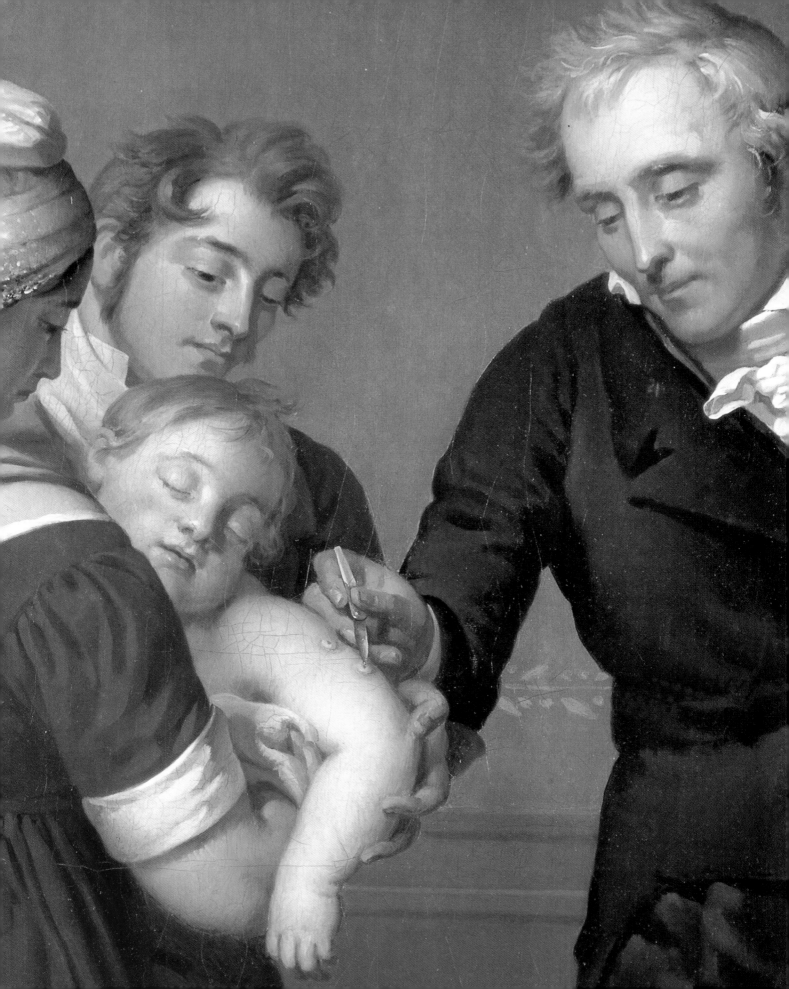

BABIES

Human babies are unique in their helplessness and their reliance on others for feeding, warmth, cleaning and protection. Some argue that this very vulnerability has shaped human development and supported the family system. All parents feel the burden of responsibility that babies put on them.

Physical development

Ninety-eight per cent of newborn babies are physically normal; the two per cent of physical problems are often of a relatively minor or correctable nature such as birthmarks, heart murmurs or undescended testicles. Similarly, most babies grow adequately; only the few who do not grow need monitoring or investigation.

Prevention of problems All babies should be physically checked over after birth (a neonatal check), again a few days after birth, again at between six and eight weeks and every few months thereafter. The purpose is to pick up abnormalities as soon as possible, and to decide which ones require treatment. Neonatal checks are also a baseline for judging later development. For example, a doctor cannot decide if a baby has an abnormally large head without knowing the previous head circumference. Therefore do take full advantage of baby health checks, question the doctor or health professional about any worries and draw their attention to anything that concerns you. After all, you are the person in closest contact with your baby and are therefore more likely to notice possible physical or mental problems.

Minor infections

A newborn baby is a happy hunting ground for all the germs of the world which invade at the moment of birth. This is not all bad; without exposure to infectious challenge the baby will not build his own immunity. It starts with small skin blemishes a day or so after birth and may include infection of the umbilical cord and sticky eyes. It will not be long before the baby has its first cold, especially when eager older children push their faces into the baby's face. Soon the baby will have a cough and most babies can be expected to get mild gastroenteritis, with diarrhoea and vomiting (see page 334).

Prevention If you are bottle feeding, keep all the equipment sterile with a sterilizing solution. Give feeds promptly before they have a chance to go off, and chill or dispose of any milk that is left.

You should keep your baby clean but that does not mean keeping him sterile. Baby soap and water are perfectly adequate for skin hygiene, although spots may require an antiseptic cream. It does, however, make sense for someone with a streaming cold not to breathe over babies. As a parent wash your hands frequently and wear a face mask if you have to get close to your baby while you yourself are not well.

If your baby has a fever, be especially careful not to overwrap him or her. You should bring the baby's temperature down with paracetamol syrup, and if necessary undress the baby and cool it with a fan. It is natural to want medical advice when a baby is unwell until you gain confidence in dealing with your baby's inevitable minor illnesses. Learn your baby's reactions to minor infection so you can judge when he or she seems more than usually unwell and therefore when you need medical help (see When to call a doctor – some important symptoms, in the box opposite).

Feeding

It is increasingly suspected that feeding patterns in infancy may lead to later physical problems such as obesity and heart disease, not to mention faddy eating. An average baby should gain about 200 g/7 oz a week up to three months and about 150 g/5 oz a week thereafter, approximately doubling birth weight by about six months and trebling it by a year.

Prevention of problems Breast feed for as long as possible; the mother's milk contains antibodies to infections she has come across and to which she has immunity. These antibodies give breastfed babies protection, too, quite apart from giving them a perfectly balanced diet. Introducing cows' milk too soon, that is before four months, may predispose a baby to allergies and food intolerances in later life.

Have your baby weighed regularly to ensure adequate weight gain, but do not get too fixated on precise weights since the above are only general guidelines. In the developed world overfeeding is likely to be more of a problem than underfeeding. Be prepared for your health visitor to discuss this if your baby appears to be gaining too much weight.

Many authorities recommend giving vitamin supplements to all babies, breast or bottle fed; these are A, B, D and C.

Introduce different textures and flavours using solid food from about four months. This early experience of variety and 'lumpiness' reduces the likelihood of faddy eating and food refusal later (see page 344).

Major infections

Infectious disease is by far the most dangerous threat to babies worldwide. Serious infections include measles, mumps, polio, tetanus, whooping cough, diphtheria and many localized threats such as malaria.

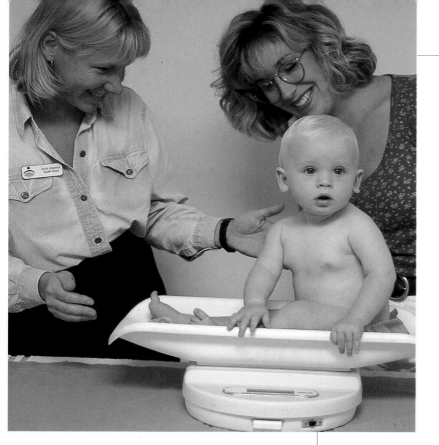

Above: Routine checks are opportunities to judge standards of care and the baby's development and happiness; carers can share pride, worries and frustrations.

Prevention Most developed countries offer immunization against the above-mentioned common childhood diseases and often others with smaller but still serious risk such as haemophilus B, which is a cause of meningitis. So successful has immunization been in reducing the risk of infections that paradoxically there are now valid and understandable worries about the risks of immunization itself (see page 260).

Before embarking upon foreign travel, consider whether you may be needlessly exposing your baby to hazards.

Physical comfort

Babies need warmth, since they cannot maintain their own temperature efficiently. On the other hand they must not be overheated, as this can lead to convulsions and may be a factor in cot death. Newborn babies should be kept in a temperature of about 18°C/65°F and be well wrapped up when going outside. Do not smoke when a baby is in the room. It is well established that children brought up in a smoking environment suffer more coughs, colds and chest infections and are at higher risk of cot death.

Put your baby to sleep on his back; this simple precaution greatly reduces the risk of cot death. (See page 345 for more information on cot death.)

Emotional comfort

Despite a vast amount of literature on the subject it is impossible to be sure how important early emotional experiences are on a baby's later emotional stability. We have to rely on our intuition to give the baby an emotionally healthy environment. It seems sensible to provide a stable family unit where the baby becomes used to being handled by just a few individuals. Handling, even at this stage, should be consistent. For example, if a baby is sometimes comforted when crying and other times neglected it seems likely that the baby's behaviour will become irritable and that he will learn that his environment is always inconsistent. This may have later consequences for discipline, eating and general behaviour.

In truth we just do not know at this stage. We can only guess and do what seems to be the right thing.

Keeping your sanity

A demanding, difficult baby is tremendously stressful; parents may experience resentment, tiredness and depression. It is a short step from these emotions to inflicting physical harm, by shaking, neglecting or worse forms of non-accidental injury. Rather than reach this extreme, talk to friends and health professionals about your feelings, which you will find are common.

TODDLERS

This section covers children from 15 months to about 3 years. The main characteristics of this age are relentless curiosity, combined with an almost complete lack of appreciation of danger. All the things said about babies remain important but there are additional worries as a result of the toddler's mobility.

Immunization

As toddlers increasingly mix in groups as they get older the risks from transmission of infection grow. The great majority of these will be simple colds and minor skin infections; the infectious diseases that are great childhood killers elsewhere – tetanus, gastroenteritis and malaria – are extremely rare in the developed world.

You should continue the immunization process begun in infancy.

Physical safety

External physical dangers are by far the greatest threat to your toddler's wellbeing and you must be constantly aware of them. Some common areas to think about are in the home, in the garden, at play and in the car.

But before you get down to worrying about detail, there is something fundamental about hazards that toddlers have to learn. Until they experience risk they will not know what risk is; until they experience heat they will not know why fire is a hazard; until they fall they will not know what a bump is, or a scratch. These things can and should be taught so that toddlers come to appreciate just why their parents are forever shouting 'careful' or 'put that down'.

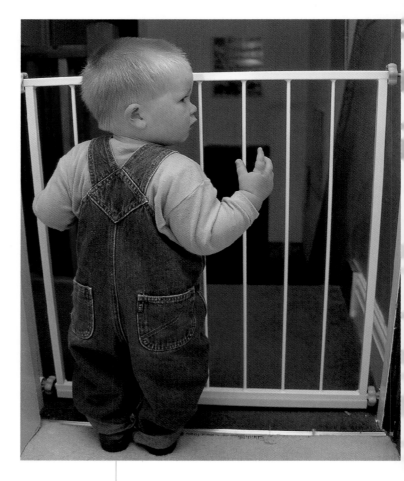

Above: Parents need to allow their children a considered path between gentle risk taking and unreasonable hazards.

Let your toddler touch a radiator to learn what heat is and feel a pen top to know what sharp is. Bumps and scratches will come for free; your child will get them but after the tears, try to turn it into a learning experience. This is how to give toddlers a proper sense of their environment so that they can make judgements for themselves about their personal safety, a lesson they will have to learn for when they are older.

Prevention of accidents

In the home So many things we take for granted can be hazardous for toddlers, looked at from their perspective. Make sure they cannot pull heavy objects on to themselves, for example a plant stand, or a TV resting precariously on a work surface. Toddlers will tug any electrical flex; secure it or hide it and ensure that electrical sockets are guarded so they cannot poke objects inside.

Glass, pointed objects and fires are special risks. Keep such risks out of reach or completely guarded. Remember that small objects such as beads, while a source of endless innocent amusement, can also be shoved into the nearest orifice or inhaled. Keep these for play only under close supervision, or else for a later age when the toddler is better at manipulating objects.

Modern kitchens are less of a hazard than once was the case, with electrical hobs and neat units. Even so, there is plenty of danger for the child who clambers on to a work surface, grabs a pan of hot water or finds where the household cleansers are kept. Make your kitchen safe from waist-height down by having toddler-proof locks on cupboards and by keeping sharp and hot things well above your toddler's reach.

Keep medicines where your toddler cannot see or grasp them – including ones prescribed for them – preferably in a locked cupboard. One commonly overlooked drug is the contraceptive pill, left lying where you won't forget to take it. Keep that out of reach, too.

Stair guards are essential until children are three or four years old. It is not that toddlers are unaware of height. They are, but their sense of curiosity will lead to clumsy and risky attempts to clamber down stairs.

In the garden The pleasures of playing outside are enhanced by a few simple measures. Cover ponds and pools unless you can watch your child constantly – this

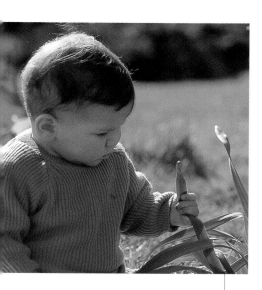

Above: Touching, sniffing and tasting – a toddler's attitude to enjoying gardening.

does mean *constantly*. Do not leave a toddler alone by water even for a few seconds; a child can drown in just inches of water. Teach your child to swim.

Many plants have poisonous berries, thorns or leaves; know what is growing in your garden and what is likely to be hazardous. Keep garden tools and garden chemicals under lock.

At play Toys are generally now designed with safety in mind and are made from non-toxic materials, with no sharp edges and no small parts that can fall off and be swallowed. This is all very worthy but there is another aspect of play that does call for the manipulation of small objects, cutting paper, gluing things or tying them together. Only you can judge when your toddler is ready to learn these skills. The key, of course, is careful supervision while the toddler learns. Do not leave your toddler alone with potentially hazardous objects.

Many toddlers will go to playgrounds or have bikes and swings of their own. No matter how brilliant your toddler is, he or she will not be safe to play alone in such environments; she will not appreciate that a swing that is such fun swung forward will hit her if she stands behind it as it swings back. In these and in so many other ways, the toddler has to be eased into the world of risk.

In the car Just as no adult should be in a car without a safety restraint, nor should any child. There are many well-designed child seats available. Your toddler should not be allowed to roll down windows to stick out his arms or, almost as bad, to throw things out. For some reason people think that it is all right for children to ride in the boot of an estate car and without restraint, although it is one of the most vulnerable parts of a car. If your family needs that amount of space, consider instead a 'people carrier'.

Emotional problems

The remarks about emotional problems in babies apply as much to toddlers, except that toddlers can give feedback. This may be in the form of tantrums, violence, disturbed sleep or sheer awkwardness. Try to provide consistent handling and consistent messages, whether about eating, playing or discipline. This is a goal, not an essential; no parents will ever be completely consistent, any more than adults are in other situations of life. But an upbringing with broad ground rules and broad limits on behaviour is likely to be emotionally healthier than one without bounds, where a toddler is unaware of what is expected of him or her and so cannot make sense of the response from his carers.

Physical health

Regular medical assessments should be continuing. Major congenital problems should have been picked up by now, although some do slip through the net and a few new problems can arise. Hearing loss is probably most common at this age, whether through congenital deafness or acquired through glue ear (see page 204). If you think your toddler has a hearing problem or is rather slow in speaking, trust your judgement and seek professional advice. Likewise, see the doctor if you suspect an undescended testicle or a twist in the spine that may have been missed on previous checks.

Other less specific things that might concern you at this age are difficulty in walking, unusual clumsiness, wild, uncontrollable behaviour or lack of an emotional response. There will often be perfectly innocent reasons for these problems and they may just be a phase in your toddler's development. It is the skill of child development specialists and family doctors to decide whether such behaviour is indeed just a phase or does require further professional help.

CHILDREN

The age from about three to the teenage years scans a period of enormous mental development and increasing physical independence. Accidents are still the major cause of injury, so accident prevention is a top priority. A balance has to be struck between developing independence and coping with the risks of life.

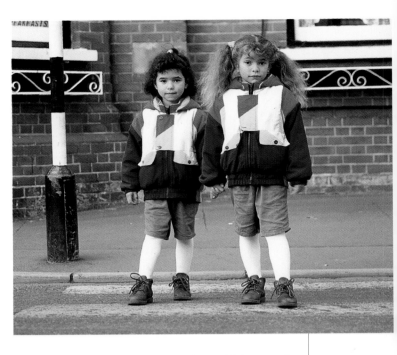

Above: Adults can make the path to independence for children as safe as possible.

Physical safety and accident prevention

Now that the hazards of life as a toddler are a thing of the past, there are other equally worrying causes for concern, although the need for constant parental supervision should be gradually lessening. (See also page 86.)

Road safety Children must be introduced to the realities of roads and traffic. This means learning to:

- *Cross a road only at crossings and in a safe fashion*
- *Not dash into a road in pursuit of anything*
- *Take care not to walk close to the edge of a pavement*

In the author's opinion no child under the age of ten is safe to cross a road alone.

Cycling is enjoyed by most children; there are many organized courses that deal with cycling safety, handling bikes and wearing visible clothing and helmets.

Road safety also includes being safe within a car, wearing seatbelts and not opening a car door without a parent's permission and guidance.

Water and sun Teach your child to swim but remember the hazards of swimming unsupervised – swimming pools should have a lifeguard or a responsible adult who keeps an eye on swimmers. Again, do not let children play unsupervised in gardens with pools or ponds.

Remember sun protection: sunscreens and protective clothing. Do not let kids burn in the sun. (See also page 226.)

Healthy eating

Evidence suggests that healthy eating habits in childhood will provide benefits into adult life. Introduce your children to a varied and healthy diet: fruit and vegetables every day, fibre in wholemeal bread, low-fat foods and lean meat, if they eat meat. Try to encourage them to eat fruit for snacks instead of sweets, crisps or biscuits. Steer them towards water, fruit juices and diet drinks rather than heavily sweetened drinks. Support the children's school in its efforts to provide healthy eating options on its menu, or give your child a healthy packed lunch.

Even though you may fail initially – after all, you are up against tremendous advertising and peer pressures – console yourself with the thought that you are giving your children a variety of experience, some of which will rub off.

Healthy eating in childhood will reduce the chances of later obesity, heart disease from high cholesterol, tooth decay, bowel problems such as diverticulitis and possibly even cancers through improving antioxidant and vitamin E intakes from vegetables and fruit. Obesity in children, as much as in adults, is an increasingly worrying health hazard (see page 98), which bodes poorly for the future health of the nation.

Admittedly, telling your children to eat their greens so they won't get diverticulitis will go down no better than telling them to start saving for their pension scheme. It is probably best not to reason with them; just provide healthy food while they remain under your control.

Exercise

Sport and physical exertion should be a natural part of childhood. Some children have an innate ability and will shine in some area, which is a source of great self-esteem and confidence. All children should learn about the pleasures of sheer

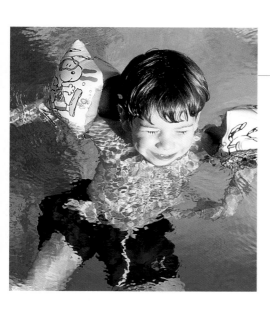

physical exertion, again in the hope that they will carry these healthy habits with them into adult life.

Take your children for walks, let them try all sorts of sports, give them adventure holidays. They will have great fun. At the same time you will be reassured, knowing you are helping them to have healthy bones – which will provide protection against future osteoporosis – and hearts, and to enjoy the more indefinable benefits from playing sport: the winning, the losing and the supporting.

At the same time, do make sure they wear the correct gear, are supervised by properly qualified adults and do not train beyond their reasonable abilities.

Emotional hazards

Your child will soon be faced with the emotional stresses of real life; there may be a younger child who gets more attention or the parents may have relationship problems. At school he has to cope with 'in groups' and 'out groups', with rejection, shifting friendships, bullying and aggression. Incidents trivial to an adult may be devastating for a child. Although you cannot prevent such happenings you can give your child the opportunity to talk about things which are worrying him. Where the emotional distress appears excessive you might need professional help through the school. Warning signs would be reappearance of bed-wetting, nightmares, regression of behaviour, unusually disturbed and aggressive behaviour, depression or withdrawal.

Sexual and physical abuse

Neither of these is new; what is new is the openness with which they are now discussed and a readiness much greater than before to take a child's complaints of abuse seriously. Children at greatest risk are those with parents who were themselves abused or who are splitting up, and those with step-parents or who live in institutions, such as children's homes.

Carers should be aware of the possibility of abuse in children whose behaviour changes dramatically, who become withdrawn, run away from home, show ambivalence and wariness about certain adults (or children) in their lives, have unexplained bruises of varying ages, have unusual burns – especially cigarette burns – show precocious sexual behaviour or, of course, make allegations of abuse.

This is a very difficult area in which unfounded allegations can have devastating consequences. Child protection procedures have become much less heavy-handed in recent years, so if your concerns remain, do discuss them with the school, social services or childcare agencies.

Part of this awareness is to teach your child how to protect their personal safety. Teach them to avoid parks and deserted places if alone and after dark, not to accept lifts from strangers, to be prepared to run away or shout if they feel in danger, and to know they can talk to a trusted adult about things that are troubling them. There are no easy answers as to how to strike a balance between teaching reasonable streetwise behaviour and making childhood lose its innocence.

Abuse of drugs, cigarettes and alcohol

These substances may be dangerous in themselves, lead to criminal behaviour or carry future health hazards. Children who indulge in these usually start by following parental example or peer pressure. The responsibility on parents is to limit such behaviour by not smoking in the presence of children, nor drinking to excess.

Suspect drug abuse if your child's behaviour and school performance alters, if he or she starts to play truant, appears emotionally unstable, has sores around the mouth and nose (from glue sniffing) or if he or she mixes with children known to have these problems. A child who starts to steal money may be doing so to pay for such activities.

It is a parent's responsibility to know where their children are, what they are doing and who they are with. You should be prepared to ask your child about drug use and so on and to speak to other parents, the school or special police units.

In some cases, drug and alcohol abuse may be part of a greater behavioural or personality problem. The child may be generally uncontrollable, indulging in bullying, aggression or petty crime. In such a case you need help from a child psychiatrist to see if anything can be done to channel your child's abilities in a more positive direction.

Rarely, children well below the age of ten can be mentally ill, with depression and psychosis. This has to be considered if their behaviour becomes bizarre.

ADOLESCENTS

The years from puberty to late teenage are widely accepted as being filled with emotional and physical turmoil. Despite the problems, on the whole this is a healthy period of life, the main serious risks still being from accidents.

Physical health

Any significant health problems are likely to have become apparent well before adolescence. It is still worth checking for previously missed undescended testicles; a scoliosis (twist in the spine) may become more prominent (see page 332). In both sexes, failure to enter puberty by 16–17 calls for specialist assessment, looking for one of the unusual hormonal causes of delayed puberty. Growth should take off just before puberty and again, failure to grow requires hormone studies.

Some girls, conscious of their breast development, adopt a hunched, round-shouldered stance. Try suggesting a bra that has good support and encourage your daughter to maintain an upright posture.

Diet

Teenagers grow rapidly and need large quantities of food to keep going. They will shovel in anything at hand, especially fast or junk food. Even so parents should try to keep the faint flame of healthy eating alive during these guzzling years, offering fruit and vegetables and discouraging empty, salt-filled snacks. Poor dietary habits now may lead to later obesity, heart trouble and high blood pressure.

A significant number of adolescents – mainly girls but occasionally boys – become anorexic. The pressure seems to be from a culture where thin is good and

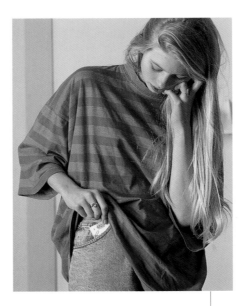

Above: Using a condom greatly reduces the risk of HIV infection.

where anorexic role models abound. Your adolescent may have an eating problem if she loses weight steadily, will not eat at family mealtimes and considers herself overweight despite clearly being normal or thin. Bulimia is compulsive overeating, often followed by self-induced vomiting. Depression and self-mutilation frequently accompany eating disorders. Fortunately most adolescents recover spontaneously but those few who become severely malnourished require psychiatric help.

Sex

Few children now reach adolescence unaware of at least the basic facts of sex and reproduction. While thinking they know it all, however, adolescents are ignorant of the true nature and risks of sexual relationships. It is inevitable that they will experiment. As a responsible parent you should ensure that the risks of pregnancy and sexually transmitted diseases are minimized.

Adolescents should be aware of the legal framework regarding sex with underage children and the consequences.

You should not condone underage sexual activity. However, once your teenagers are of age legally (16 in the United Kingdom) there is little you can do about it if they choose to have sex.

Your adolescent should know about condoms and how to use them, and should regard using them as the norm and not a sign of weakness. Teenagers should also know that condoms prevent the transmission of venereal diseases and are reasonably good at preventing pregnancy.

Girls who take the contraceptive pill should ensure their sexual partners also use condoms for the above hygiene reasons, and especially if they do not know a partner's sexual history. Once a girl starts having regular sex, she should have a smear test; her risk of cervical cancer, although low, increases the earlier she has sex and the more sexual partners she has (see page 148).

HIV/AIDS and sexually transmitted disease

The risk of HIV/AIDS is low for people having heterosexual intercourse in the Western world. High-risk behaviour is having anal intercourse with homosexual men or intercourse with intravenous drug users. HIV can be transmitted by heterosexual intercourse but at present this is a significant risk mainly in parts of Africa and Asia, although it is expected to become important worldwide over the next few decades. Using a condom greatly reduces the risk of transmission and they should be used in addition to other more reliable methods of contraception such as the pill, unless one is entirely certain of a partner's HIV status.

Adolescents should be aware of the symptoms of sexually transmitted diseases such as heavy vaginal discharge, discharge from the penis, painful spots around the genitalia or persistent sores. They should know that confidential help is available at a sexual diseases clinic. (See also pages 122, 162 and 268.)

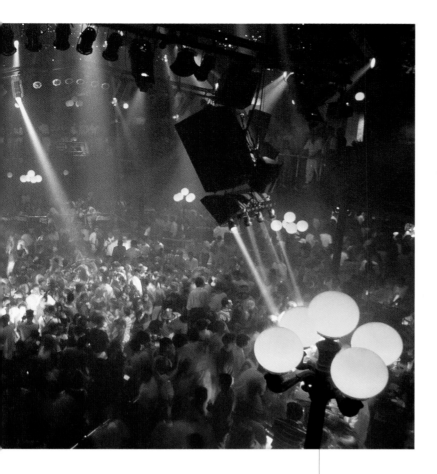

Above: Adolescence features group activities in the guise of individualism.

Emotions

The emotional strain of adolescence leads to apparently irrational attachments and just as irrational abandonment of previously cherished friends. It can be difficult for adult onlookers to detach themselves from these events, which are part of a necessary learning curve. Many adolescents fall foul of emotions too large for them to handle alone and will welcome, albeit reluctantly, a sympathetic non-judgemental ear.

A significant number of teenage girls take an overdose on impulse at a period of emotional turmoil. These teenagers should have a psychiatric assessment as a small number will be in genuine despair and may contemplate suicide. Although the numbers are relatively small, suicide is the most common cause of death in these years after accidents. The same goes for any teenage boy who appears deeply depressed and apathetic. Depression and schizophrenia are not rare in adolescents and are treatable. It takes tact to persuade teenagers that they need help. There are self-referral agencies to which they can go in confidence and without stigma.

Aggression and road accidents

Many teenage boys, and increasingly teenage girls, show aggressive gang behaviour which can be unprovoked and vicious. This competitive nature extends to sports and driving, especially in the first years after learning to drive. Road traffic accidents are the major cause of death in the teenage/early adult age group. In this age group half of all deaths in girls are from road traffic accidents, as are two-thirds of deaths in boys. Stringent driving tests are one way of dealing with risk-taking on the roads. Other methods are driving with probationary (new driver) plates, taking advanced driving tests soon after passing the basic test and driving a safer, less powerful car. Unfortunately, all these measures count for little for the adolescent who is tempted for personal reasons or by peer pressure to show bravado, as the worryingly constant stream of statistics of teenagers killed and injured in car crashes proves.

Drink and drugs

Experimentation and peer pressure extend to alcohol and drugs. Alcohol in particular plays a significant role in aggressive behaviour and in accidents – especially road traffic accidents. Drug-taking appears to have become accepted behaviour by many young people in the teenage social scene, mainly using the so-called soft recreational drugs such as ecstasy and cannabis. Responsible parents cannot condone such addictive behaviour, even though the risks of these drugs may be less than the risks of the acceptable drugs in our society – alcohol and tobacco. The whole topic is blurred by moral and pseudo-scientific considera-tion, but the recurrent reports of drug-related deaths should be enough to dissuade anyone from taking additional risks in what is already a dangerous age for accidents.

Smoking

Smoking is one of the most dangerous activities anyone can voluntarily indulge in. Recent government action in the United Kingdom and in the United States may at last herald a move from the laissez-faire attitude to this. It is difficult to get across to teenagers just how dangerous smoking is, because the conse-quences are a lifetime away. This puts all the greater responsibility on parents and governments to reduce the pressures on teenagers to take up smoking and to make it easier for them to quit.

WOMEN: CHILDBEARING YEARS

As a woman you will enjoy a greater life expectancy than men, even allowing for the common female cancers of breast, ovary and womb. You can enhance this in-built advantage and, by maintaining your physical health, also ensure that you are in peak shape for pregnancy.

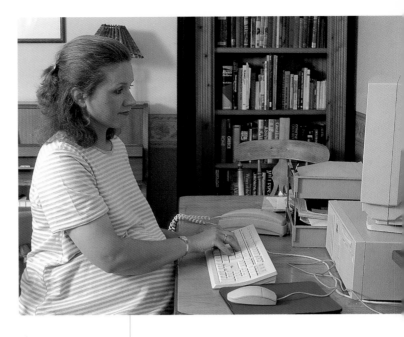

Above: Women today often have to juggle a number of conflicting responsibilities.

Physical wellbeing

During these years women, by virtue of being female and subject to oestrogen, are protected against the heart and circulatory problems to which men are more liable. This protection will ebb away at the menopause; therefore the earlier years are the ones in which to tackle risk factors for later heart disease. Keep to a healthy diet, avoiding hard fats and eating polyunsaturated and low-fat foods. Dietary fibre in fruit and vegetables will avoid constipation, reducing a risk of diverticulitis or cancer of the bowel. These same foods provide vitamin E and other antioxidants, believed to protect against circulatory problems and cancers.

Diet As well as healthy eating, try to keep your weight under control. You should not be more than 10% over a healthy body mass index or you may later develop the problems of obesity (see page 98): early osteoarthritis, tiredness, hiatus hernia or high blood pressure. Furthermore, if you are overweight at the beginning of pregnancy, you will find it very much harder to lose weight and return to fitness after the birth of your baby.

Exercise Keep active and try to build exercise into your weekly routine, be it a walk at lunchtime or going to the gym. As well as the sense of wellbeing this provides, you will maintain healthy bones, protecting against osteoporosis from your 60s onwards.

Sun Bear in mind the guidelines about sun exposure and resist the temptation to use sunbeds for a year-round tan. This is high-risk behaviour for skin cancer 20 years down the line. (See also page 226).

Smoking If you give up smoking now, there is plenty of time for your body to recover from the smoke, tars and nicotine that poison your lungs and affect your blood vessels. Lung cancer is the form of cancer most rapidly increasing in women. Within one year of giving up, your risks are greatly reduced, while by five years they are little more than those of a non-smoker (although the risk is always a little greater than in someone who has never smoked).

If you smoke during pregnancy, you may cause your baby to miscarry or to be born prematurely. Smoking affects the growth of your baby, reducing birth-weight by about 10%, in itself a major health risk. Remember, too, that the children of smokers suffer more upper respiratory infections.

Accidents and road safety

The greatest risk to your health from childhood right through to the age of about 40 is from accidents, of which road traffic accidents are overwhelmingly the greatest risk. Between one-third and one-half of all deaths of women in this period are due to road accidents, quite apart from the many thousands that are left permanently injured. You owe it to yourself and others to drive as carefully as possible, not to drink and drive and not to indulge in 'road rage'. Other causes of serious accidents are sports, recreation such as climbing and, much less in women than in men, industrial accidents.

Whether for sport, recreation or at work, take pride in knowing the right equipment, the right procedures and what to do if something goes wrong. Remember, too, the risks at home and with do-it-yourself projects. (See also pages 86 and 396.)

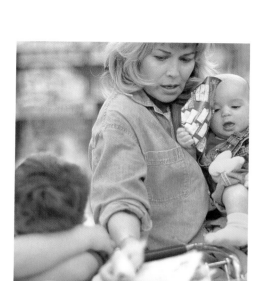

Above: The responsibility for parenting is still mainly a woman's role.

Cervical smears

Sexually active women should have a cervical smear every three years. Twenty per cent of the 1800 deaths from cervical cancer a year occur in women below the age of 45. These may be preventable by regular screening and detection. More often, a smear at this age reveals inflammatory changes that may lead to cancer of the cervix. These changes, called dyskaryosis, are treatable by laser or by cauterizing (burning) the cervix. Women at greater risk are those who have had sexual intercourse from their early teens with multiple partners. (For other female cancers, see pages 146, 149 and 150.)

Breast checks

Check your breasts every few weeks for lumps: nine out of ten are innocent and breast cancer below the age of 30 is extremely rare. There is no scientific evidence to support having mammograms in this age group unless there is a strong family history of breast cancer, in which case you should seek specialist advice.

Sexual health

The advent of HIV/AIDS has made it respectable for women to take the initiative in sexual safety. You should know the sexual background of your partners. If one is bisexual or an intravenous drug user, or comes from a country where AIDS is prevalent, you should take seriously the risk of acquiring HIV through normal intercourse. You should insist that your partner uses a condom, and you should avoid risky behaviour such as oral or anal intercourse. Even if your partner does not appear to fall into a high-risk group, you should still insist on a condom until you are sure of his safe status. Take seriously any symptoms you notice of possible sexually transmitted diseases (see page 162), including such symptoms as genital spots, discharges, cystitis or pelvic pain. Early treatment will help avoid later problems of subfertility.

Anxiety, tension and depression

Increasingly women are having to juggle social, work and family commitments, any of which could demand all their time and which at any one time could be mutually exclusive. Discuss the issues with your partner and friends. It is hard to choose between career progression and economic necessity, or the chance to be there to see your children grow up, and this has to be a personal choice.

One of the few areas in which women are at greater risk than men is in attempting suicide. Tens of thousands of women a year attempt this; many are below the age of 30. However far fewer women than men are successful and actually commit suicide. There are many anonymous and supportive counselling services available to those who are contemplating a suicide attempt. Depression is a common and perfectly treatable condition and one that you need not put up with on your own (see page 70).

Preventive planning for pregnancy

Rubella vaccination In the United Kingdom all babies are immunized against rubella at the age of around 12 months. The vaccine fails to take or to last in a few individuals, so some women are therefore at risk of rubella during their pregnancy (see page 262). This illness affects the baby's heart, ears and brain. Have a blood test to see if you are immune a year before you plan to get pregnant; this allows plenty of time for revaccination and for repeat blood tests (see page 356).

Folic acid and other vitamins By taking just 0.4 mg of folic acid a day, you greatly reduce the chances of having a baby with spina bifida. You should start taking folic acid before you conceive and continue it until 12 weeks after becoming pregnant.

There are not such compelling reasons to take other vitamins, as long as your diet is healthy and includes plenty of fruit and vegetables. However, if you have heavy periods and plan to breastfeed – both of which lead to loss of iron – it makes sense to take iron to avoid anaemia at the start of pregnancy. Do not worry too much about this – blood tests during pregnancy will show whether you really need iron supplements later.

Alcohol Currently, in the United Kingdom, the recommended maximum weekly alcohol intake for women is 21 units – a unit is a glass of wine, 300 ml/½ pint of beer or a measure of spirits. There is controversy about whether drinking is harmful to the foetus during pregnancy; babies born to heavy drinkers have a distorted facial appearance. Most doctors think that moderate drinking is OK; some women feel happier to avoid alcohol altogether during pregnancy, and especially during the first three months.

WOMEN:
THE MENOPAUSE
AND AFTER

These years, when day-to-day family responsibilities generally lessen and financial pressures ease, should be fulfilling and healthy. It should be a time to reap the rewards from previous healthy living and to take steps to ensure an active mind and body for the years up to retirement. A number of female cancers become more common from this age; early detection greatly improves the outlook.

The menopause

Women enter the menopause on average at around 50 years of age, although the range is from the late 30s to mid-50s. The event is characterized by increasingly irregular and infrequent periods until they cease altogether. Flushes may appear a year or so before periods cease. If there is any doubt, a blood test will confirm whether it is indeed the menopause.

With the menopause women lose the protection of their female hormones, which hitherto protected them against heart disease. They also lose bone density rapidly for several years afterwards.

HRT (hormone replacement therapy)

Other than lifestyle changes, the most beneficial preventive strategy at this age is HRT. It reduces flushes, improves skin texture, reduces vaginal dryness and helps mood swings. It protects against heart disease while being taken. HRT maintains bone density and so protects against osteoporosis. These are advantages that

many women find helpful. The most important disadvantages are the return of periods (although newer forms of HRT avoid this), weight gain and a risk of thrombosis. This risk is greatest in the first year on HRT. After eight years or so, HRT increases the risk of breast cancer. Statistical studies favour remaining on HRT indefinitely but even staying on it for just two to five years, as many women do, is a considerable benefit. Women coming off HRT suffer the usual menopausal symptoms for a few weeks, possibly longer, and should continue with a healthy diet and regular exercise.

Osteoporosis

Prevention of osteoporosis involves taking regular active, weight-bearing exercise – either walking or something a little more strenuous. Ensure your diet is rich in calcium and vitamin D by eating dairy products or taking calcium and vitamin D supplements. These measures will help maintain bone density (see page 238). Smoking increases the rate of calcium loss and hastens the onset of osteoporosis.

Certain women run a greater risk of osteoporosis and should have their bone density measured. These include women who have been on steroids, for example for asthma, women who are immobile,

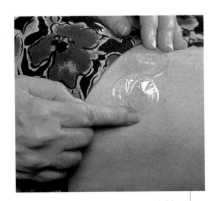

Above: HRT is available in many forms. Here a patch is worn on the skin.

have a poor diet, smoke, have a family history of osteoporosis or who have an early menopause (before the age of 45). Bone density helps decide whether it is worthwhile taking medication to reverse osteoporosis and for how long.

Breast cancer

This is the peak time for this disease (see page 146), in recognition of which there is, in the United Kingdom, a breast-screening service using mammography. Currently this invites women over 50 years of age for screening every three years. Screening is not 100% accurate so continue to check your breasts regularly yourself, reporting any lumps or changes in the nipple, and any bleeding or discharge from the nipple. Even at this age, most breast lumps prove benign.

Cancers of the cervix, womb and ovary

You should continue to have regular cervical smears every three to five years up to the age of 65. About 70% of the 1800 deaths a year from cervical cancer occur in women over the age of 55. Cancer of the womb is more common from this age; post-menopausal vaginal bleeding or lower abdominal pains should be checked out. A smear test also allows an internal examination, which may pick up an abnormality in the womb or ovary before you notice any symptoms, greatly improving the prospects of cure for these cancers (see pages 148, 149 and 150).

Blood pressure, cholesterol and heart disease

Because of the requirements of contra-ception or because of pregnancy, most women will have had their blood pressure checked during their reproductive years and high blood pressure should have been dealt with. As blood pressure tends to increase as you get older, have yours checked every couple of years.

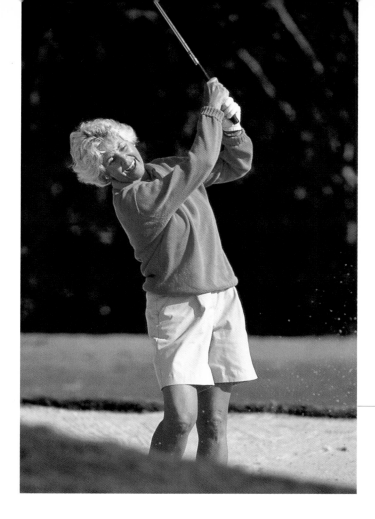

Left: Middle age often coincides with having more time for the pleasures important for your physical and mental health, as well as providing more time to socialize.

If your family has a history of high cholesterol, you should have had a cholesterol blood test well before now. Otherwise, ask your doctor to perform a cholesterol test as a baseline.

From the menopause onwards women are at a similar risk of heart disease as men. You should take seriously any chest pains, unusual breathlessness and tiredness, each of which could be due to heart trouble. Heart disease in women tends to progress more rapidly than in men, so you should expect such symptoms to be taken seriously and be properly investigated.

Diabetes

About 2% of the population are affected (see page 96), and probably 5% of those are over 65 years of age – especially the overweight. Screening for diabetes is very simple: a sample of urine is tested for sugar. If in doubt your doctor may send you to have blood tests. Have a urine test every couple of years.

Alcohol and smoking

Excessive alcohol will have a bad effect on your liver and pancreas. Smoking will affect your heart, which is no longer protected by female hormones. This will vastly increase your risk of heart disease, especially if you also have other high risk factors such as a family history of heart disease, high cholesterol or particularly high blood pressure.

Glaucoma

This condition, characterized by raised pressure within the eyes, affects about 0.5–1% of women of this age group and can lead to blindness in the most extreme cases (see page 194). Have your eyes tested every few years, or more often if a close relative suffers from it.

Diet

It is tempting at this age to let everything go, on the basis of 'what difference can it make now?'. This is a pity; you should be looking forward to another two or three decades of life, so why risk it? It is still important to eat healthily, with a low-fat high-fibre diet. More than ever you should eat high fibre as protection against bowel cancer and diverticular disease. A low-carbohydrate and low-sugar diet will also reduce your chances of diabetes.

Mental health

The menopause often coincides with children leaving home or careers peaking; and it may throw into focus marital and relationship problems hitherto ignored. Certain health problems are almost inevitable, for example arthritis, dry skin and loss of stamina. It is hardly surprising that many women find that their self-confidence takes a knock at this stage and they may get depressed when further contemplatiing their life. HRT helps mood swings and can ease this transition.

Otherwise talk about your worries before they get out of hand and you fall into a deeper state of depression or anxiety. You might share worries with friends or family, seek a counselling service or discuss how you feel with your doctor. The sympathetic listening ear is the only medication most women require, but a few become significantly depressed. You may be one of these if you are waking in the very early morning, take no pleasure in life, keep crying, think only black thoughts or lose your appetite. Help is available with one of the effective modern antidepressants, so discuss it as soon as possible with your doctor.

General body awareness

Be alert to changes in your body which could signal early disease. Important symptoms are weight loss, breathlessness, persistent cough, coughing blood or bleeding from the bowels, bladder or vagina. Recurrent abdominal pains, new lumps and old skin lumps that change colour or bleed should also be checked.

YOUNG AND MIDDLE–AGED MEN

This section covers men from their mid-20s to the age of 65. It is a large age group with very different health risks at either end. If you have always enjoyed a healthy diet and take regular exercise you are unlikely to meet any serious health hazards until you reach your fifties.

Accidents

Until the age of about 40, accidents on the road, at work or from sport pose the greatest risk of death or serious injury for both men and women. Up to the age of 25 road traffic accidents account for nearly two-thirds of all deaths in men. This is partly through inexperience; partly through male aggressive behaviour and irresponsibility; partly it is the statistical consequence of the numbers of men driving and pursuing hazardous sports or jobs. Prevent yourself from becoming one of these statistics by driving carefully. Think of it not just for yourself but to protect others from the consequences of you having a serious accident: the loss of a wage earner, the loss of a husband or son.

In a male environment safety procedures may be skimped on as being wimpish or even unnecessary; if your factory or work-place has a safety policy adhere to it, and if it does not, perhaps it should have. The same goes for sports such as climbing or parachuting. The professionals in these sports take safety seriously because they see the things that go wrong more often than the amateur does. Follow their advice and guidance.

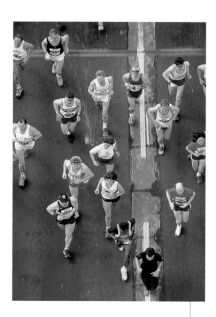

Above: Many sports welcome participants across all ages.

Alcohol

Excess drinking plays a part in many road traffic accidents. It also contributes to industrial and sports accidents and reduces efficiency at work. This is on top of the medical consequences of alcohol excess (see page 93). Currently in the United Kingdom the recommended maximum intake for men is 28 units per week, where a unit is 300 ml/½ pint of beer, a glass of wine or a measure of spirits.

Smoking

Lung cancer is the single most common cancer affecting men (see page 66). The good news is that men have taken on board the message about smoking less; consequently the rates of lung cancer in men are slowly falling. It still remains a fact that 25–50% of men who smoke will die as a consequence of cigarette smoking, of which lung cancer is just one disease, along with heart disease, chronic lung disease and many other conditions.

Heart disease

Men are 20 times more likely than women to develop heart and circulatory problems by their early 50s, a period of time during which women are protected by female hormones. Little wonder then that there is so much emphasis on men trying to improve their lifestyles to reduce this risk. Reducing smoking is the biggest single step you can take. Other important measures are to reduce cholesterol and to have high blood pressure treated.

Cholesterol

If you have followed a healthy diet there is a good chance that your cholesterol levels are reasonably low anyway. You should have a cholesterol check in your mid-40s – and sooner if there is a history of early (pre-60s) heart disease in your close family, that is parents or siblings. Thereafter, it is a good idea to have cholesterol rechecked every three to five years. Modestly raised cholesterol can be treated by adjustments to diet; very high levels may need medication. Such a decision has to take account of your overall risk, including smoking and high blood pressure.

Blood pressure

All men should have a blood pressure check at some time in their 20s, and again in their 30s. By the 40s blood pressure should be checked every three to five years. It may be possible to deal with mildly raised blood pressure by losing weight and decreasing the amount of salt in your diet, for example.

Testicular cancer

Although not common (about 1250 cases a year in the United Kingdom), testicular cancer is the most common cancer for men in their 20s and early 30s (see page 120). It is nearly always curable if caught early. Men should check their testicles regularly for lumps and take notice of persistent pains, seeing a doctor for either.

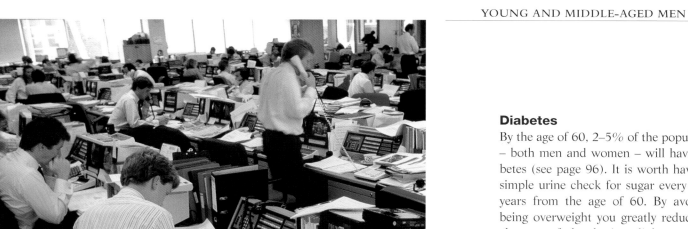

Above: The more stressful your work, the more important it is to find some relaxation.

Prostate cancer

Below the age of 45 prostate cancer is rare and even in men in their 50s it is uncommon, but by their 60s many men will be affected by benign or cancerous prostate problems (see page 118). It is not possible to prevent cancer of the prostate, but it may be possible to screen for it, although this is still a controversial area. Several specialists recommend that men from the age of 50 have an annual rectal examination of their prostate gland, plus a blood test called PSA (Prostate Specific Antigen). At the time of writing it is by no means agreed what is the best course of action on finding an abnormality, so speak to your doctor about the latest opinions and practices.

Suicide and depression

Remarkably, suicide is the second most common cause of death, after accidents, in young men. Although many fewer men than women attempt suicide, those that do seem to have a more serious intent. Men may feel despair caused by work pressures, unemployment or relationship problems. Some men develop a pure depressive illness for no obvious reason or have another psychiatric condition triggering depression, like schizophrenia. There are many agencies to help those in despair – in Britain the Samaritans are the best known. Other sources of help are counselling services, your doctor and psychiatric teams. However, the first step is always to acknowledge that you have a psychological problem that you cannot deal with on your own and for which you need support and help. This is not an admission of weakness, but sensible self-knowledge and self-assessment.

Glaucoma

This is a condition causing raised pressure within the eyes and possibly blindness (see pages 194 and 196). If you have a family history of this, go to your optician for screening before the age of 40. Others should be screened for this common condition regularly after the age of 60.

Diabetes

By the age of 60, 2–5% of the population – both men and women – will have diabetes (see page 96). It is worth having a simple urine check for sugar every three years from the age of 60. By avoiding being overweight you greatly reduce the chances of developing diabetes, quite apart from the other health benefits.

Overweight

Middle-aged spread need not be the inevitability it can appear to be. Try not to let your weight edge more than 10% above your healthy Body Mass Index (see page 98). Otherwise you run the risks of obesity in your later years – arthritis, heart disease, high blood pressure, diabetes and digestive problems. It is better not to gain the weight in the first place than to have to lose it in later life when mobility and exercise tolerance may already be affected by your age.

Exercise

Try to carry the habit of exercise through from childhood right into old age. Although the theme will be the same the melody will vary. Vigorous contact sports and squash in your 20s and 30s will naturally give way to gentler, although not necessarily less competitive, exertion later. Tennis, badminton, dancing, cycling, swimming, walking and jogging can all carry on into late middle age and beyond, as long as you wear the right clothing and footwear and take notice of any unusual chest and joint pains and breathlessness that occur.

Being aware of your body

The warning symptoms for men in these years are weight loss, persistent coughs, especially if you cough up blood, bleeding from the bowel or bladder, difficulty when passing urine, chest pains on physical exertion and unusual breathlessness. If any of these occur, contact your doctor.

RETIREMENT

The age of retirement from full-time work is no longer the sudden definite event at a predetermined age that it once was. Where many men used to work until 65 and women until 60, it is increasingly common to reduce working hours from the 50s onwards while many people plan to retire at no later than 60, if not before. Whatever the age of your retirement, you will be faced with similar transitional problems.

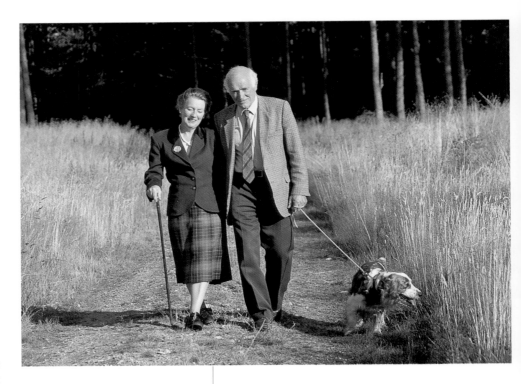

Above: With careful planning, this scene need not be an unrealistically idyllic goal.

Maintaining a routine

Those adults who go out to work have to fit leisure time around it: the time they get up, leave the house and return home are largely determined by the demands of work. Irksome as this may be, it does give a structure to the day, which is all too easily lost after retirement. Unless you have activities planned, those free hours are no longer a great opportunity but become filled with boredom and worse, as you brood over the loss of status and loss of self-respect. Ideally, increase the time devoted to an interest that you may have taken up well before you retire. It may be bridge, model-making, walking or bingo – it does not matter as long as it gives a pattern to your week and events for you to look forward to.

Keeping active

You would be surprised at how much activity even an apparently sedentary job involves: walking to get there, walking around an office or up and down stairs. Therefore it is as important as ever after retirement to take exercise. Many sports are suitable for older people; particularly ideal ones are swimming, walking, bowls, golf and badminton. But if you feel up to it there is every reason to continue tennis, riding, running, climbing and so on. Regular daily exercise keeps your heart and muscles in shape and adds to the structure of your day.

There is nothing like idleness to breed idleness. Have you noticed that it is the people who always seem to be on the go who do not run out of energy, whereas those who will not make an effort become tired in front of your eyes?

Diet

Working people need about 2500 calories per day, even in sedentary jobs. After retirement your need for food should decrease unless you continue particularly vigorous exercise. Yet you will be finding it easier than ever to snack and graze in a way that you may not have done since you were a teenager. Again, it helps to have a routine of regular meals at specific times to avoid overeating all day long. If you need a snack, try to keep to fruit. In this way you will avoid obesity and its effects on your heart, lungs, joints and blood pressure. You will also have the fibre to keep your bowels open naturally without having to turn to laxatives.

Empty calories are as bad for you at this age as at any other. Avoid sugar and fatty foods; in this way you will reduce your risk of diabetes.

Osteoporosis

Both men and women are at risk of this disease. Keeping active, not smoking and taking calcium are important preventive measures. Women can consider starting HRT or continuing on it, although there is a small risk of breast cancer (see page 20). Men or women with established osteoporosis can take drug therapy such as alendronate or etidronate to reverse the effects of osteoporosis (see page 238).

Blood pressure

Have this checked every couple of years. Accept treatment if recommended as well as the regular checks every few months that are part of monitoring treatment. The main benefit is in reducing the risk of a stroke or heart disease. Some 40% of the population in this age group have high blood pressure so there is really nothing unusual about this.

Cholesterol

It is not necessary to be obsessive about cholesterol as minor changes at this age will have little effect on health. Very high levels should still be dealt with, but it is not worth worrying about modestly raised cholesterol unless you have heart disease, in which case it is beneficial to get it under control. However, everyone should follow a prudent low-fat diet of fibres, fruit, lean meat and low salt.

Smoking and alcohol

It is still not too late to give up smoking, although the benefits will be relatively small. However, you should drop it in earnest if you develop heart or circulatory problems which nicotine makes worse.

Drinking three or four units a day of alcohol appears to offer continuing protection against heart disease (but see also pages 19 and 22). This is probably the first time in your life when you can view a health message with pleasure, without worrying about whether you have to get a column of figures to add up after lunch!

Accidents

Although still an important threat to your wellbeing you probably need take no more precautions than any other prudent adult in order to avoid, for example, household, car or pedestrian accidents.

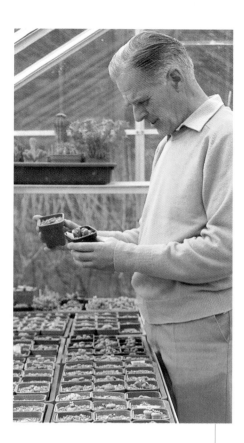

Above: Once the novelty of leisure time wears off, pursuing enjoyable hobbies will provide a structure to your day.

General health screening

Every couple of years it is a good idea to have a basic physical check-up. This should include tests for raised blood pressure, abnormal functioning of the heart and lungs and the presence of diabetes or glaucoma. Now is also the time to have minor but annoying health problems sorted out, for example a hernia, a mole which keeps snagging, a painful hip or prostate symptoms. The reason is starkly simple: you may not be fit enough for surgery if you delay too long.

An aspirin a day

There is good evidence that an aspirin a day helps prevent strokes and heart trouble. Between 75 and 150 mg a day seems effective – ask your doctor about the latest recommended dosage.

Mental health

If you enter retirement without forward planning you may suffer depression through the sudden loss of status, a structure to your day and companionship. This holds true for women as well as men. It is all too common to find that retirement is less financially comfortable than expected so money worries limit your horizons, which makes for a bitter end to a working lifetime.

It is usually a mistake to move house immediately after retirement, leaving behind the memories and networks of previous times. If you do intend to move try to plan it well before retirement, preferably building up a circle of friends in the area where you plan to go. Think very carefully about how you will manage physically – not just now but when your mobility worsens later, as it inevitably will. That short walk to the shops which seems so easy now may be a nightmare if you have angina.

Older people who get depressed get very depressed indeed. If you see this in yourself or your partner get help or try to persuade them to do so. Warning signs are poor sleep, morbid thoughts, loss of appetite and constant anxiety. Take particularly seriously any hint of suicidal intent – when an older person says this they mean it. People especially vulnerable are those who are living alone, recently bereaved, in poor social circumstances, drinkers and those with other serious health problems.

General health awareness

Without being obsessional about your health you should take seriously any new and persistent symptoms. The most important ones include weight loss, loss of appetite, passing blood in urine, bowel or the vagina, coughing blood, skin changes in moles, ulcers, chest pain, bone pains, difficulty passing urine, profound tiredness or lumps in the breast or elsewhere.

ADVANCED OLD AGE

After the age of 75 you must expect to have a number of health problems, with heart disease and arthritic disorders high on the list. Some general preventive measures can help you preserve your mobility, mental alertness and safety.

Accident prevention

The older you get the more you must anticipate accidents, as eyesight fails and agility diminishes. In women 60% of all accidental deaths are the result of falls, especially following a fractured hip; the figure for men is 40%.

In the home Make your home safe. Have good lighting in the most hazardous areas – stairs, front and back steps and kitchen. Look at the risks of tripping: have carpets properly fitted, run electrical flexes by walls and not across a room, secure rugs so as not to catch your foot. Make spaces easy to navigate, placing tables and chairs so you do not keep bumping into them.

It may no longer be wise to cook on gas or to have a gas heater; electrical cooking and heating reduces the risk of fire. Food and cooking utensils should be within easy reach so step-ladders are not needed. Cigarette smoking is a common cause of accidental fires. Never smoke in bed.

In the bathroom, have grab handles to assist getting in and out of a bath, or else a shower seat, with safety handles within the shower. Run a bath in a safe way, letting cold water in first, then adding hot, so reducing the risk of scalding.

Wear well-fitting footwear – get rid of those old loose slippers, while outdoors wear shoes with non-slip heels, which

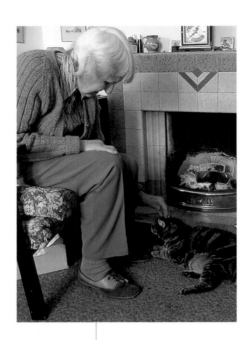

Above: However reduced your horizons, find room for warmth, entertainment and companionship.

remain non-slip in wet conditions. Many elderly people feel dizzy when they stand up as a result of changes in blood pressure. Get up slowly, holding something for support for a few moments until you feel ready to walk.

Outside When you go out be sure you know what you want to do. Write a checklist of what you need to buy and the places you have to visit – this way you should not find yourself confused and uncertain of where to go next. In bad weather consider whether your journey is really essential; this is especially prudent in winter when the risk of a fall on ice or snow is very high.

On the road Most insurance companies insist on a medical check if you continue to drive past the age of 75: your doctor will pay special attention to your eyesight,

alertness and mobility. If a time comes when you fail to meet the required standard, accept that driving is no longer in your best interests.

Road safety also includes safety as a pedestrian, which is why it is important for you still to have regular eye checks, to wear your glasses and to wear a hearing aid, if appropriate. Cross the road only at a designated crossing.

The figures reinforce the importance of these measures. In the over-75 age group, 20% of accidental deaths in men and 10% of those in women are the result of road traffic accidents, the bulk of them as pedestrians.

Activity

Reading the above you may think you should pass these years cocooned in cotton wool; this is not so. It is important to take as much exercise as you feel capable of. Exercise keeps joints mobile – even those affected by osteoarthritis – and keeps up muscle tone. Gentle exercise will reduce the chances of osteoporosis. There is a psychological benefit from keeping everything moving as well as a social benefit from meeting people and from them expecting to meet you. If you fail to appear for a regular walk, this might trigger legitimate concern for your safety, a morbid but realistic thought.

Even if your exercise consists of simply walking to a corner shop, you should keep it up. Increasingly there are exercise classes and activities for the elderly: swimming or perhaps gentle aerobics and stretching exercises. You will know what level of activity is comfortable for you. Many people in their 80s and 90s can still walk briskly, do the gardening and visit places. Others are confined to their home, but they can still do some exercise – stretching the neck, swinging the arms, bending, lifting their legs. These keep joints mobile and can be done even if you have osteoarthritis.

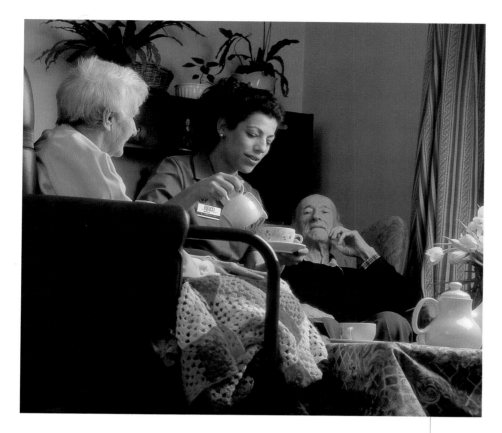

Above: There is often a good network of social support, which allows safe independence well into advanced years.

Diet

The older you get, the less you need to eat as your body's metabolism slows down. The principles of a healthy diet remain: avoid empty calories in bread and cakes, eat fruit, vegetables and fibre, eat dairy products for calcium. The days of worrying about cholesterol are behind you unless you have serious heart disease.

Physical comfort

Because you cannot get out so easily, make sure your home is always well stocked with drinks and easily prepared convenience foods.

Warmth The elderly cannot control temperature as well as they once did; being less active affects temperature too. Have efficient heating and use it if you feel cold.

Walking aids However much you may resist it, there comes a point for walking sticks or a walking frame. It is far better to use these than, in mistaken pride, to go it alone and fracture your hip.

Mental agility

Keep your mind as active as possible, since evidence confirms that this delays the onset of memory and confusional problems. Read a daily newspaper and watch the news; this orientates you for time and place. Read books, magazines, racing tips – the subject does not matter as long as something is making you think, plan, remember and anticipate. Your mental stimulation may come from meeting friends and family, from going to bingo, from a day class, theatre trips or the cinema – the more the better.

Do not worry unduly about developing Alzheimer's disease. Even by their 80s about 80% of people do not have any serious memory problems, certainly none that interferes with their daily activities.

Medication

Almost inevitably an elderly person will be on medication for blood pressure, heart disease, diabetes, glaucoma, arthritis or chest problems. It is all too easy for doctors to prescribe one medication after another, any of which may cause you inconvenient side effects. The common ones to look out for are drowsiness, dizziness, constipation, urinary problems and indigestion. If you think your medication may be to blame discuss it with your doctor. Do not discontinue medication without discussion – especially for high blood pressure, the control of which is effective in reducing the risk of a stroke.

Depression

Depression is common because of all the losses of old age – loss of partner, family, independence and health. Maintaining as active a life as possible is the preferable way of dealing with this. However, persistent depression is dangerous because of a high risk of suicide and should be taken as seriously as depression in a younger person. Depression in the elderly is less likely to be characterized by crying and morbid thoughts, but more likely by self-neglect, loss of appetite, weight loss and anxiety.

Alertness to symptoms

It is a mistake to think that symptoms should be ignored simply because of your age, while recognizing that there are many symptoms of age that doctors can do little for, such as dizziness, arthritis, poor vision and tiredness. You should still report to your doctor any symptoms that are new or that are worrying you – particularly weight loss, persistent pains, bleeding from the bowel, bladder or vagina, and palpitations.

faeces	Gallstones	180
	Jaundice in children	342
	Liver problems	178–9
and itching	Gallstones	180
	Liver problems	178–9
Jaw, stiff	Tetanus	263
Joints, painful/swollen	Gout	104
	Menopause	154–5
	Osteoarthritis	234
	Rheumatoid arthritis	235
	Systemic lupus erythematosus	255
Kidney infection		
and back pain and fever	Cystitis	109
	Urinary problems in children	331
and painful urination	Cystitis	109
and stones	Kidney stones	111
Knee, painful/swollen	Knee pain	245
	Osteoarthritis	234
	Rheumatoid arthritis	241
Laryngitis	Laryngitis	209
Leg *painful*	Atherosclerosis	40
	Cramp	237
	Deep vein thrombosis	51
	Osteoarthritis	234
	Sciatica	240
	Varicose veins	42
restless	Cramp	237
Ligaments, strained	Soft tissue damage	237
Lumps *breast*	Breast problems	145
eye	Styes	193
neck	Glandular fever	248
	Hodgkin's disease	250
	Lymphoma	253
penis	Cancer of the penis	120
scrotum	Cancer of the testicles	120
skin	Boils, spots and abscesses	221
	Skin lumps, bumps and moles	225
	Warts	222
Lung infection	Lung cancer	66
	see also **Chest infection**	
Miscarriage	Miscarriage	144
	Pregnancy problems	134–5
Mood swings	Behavioural problems in children	344
	Brain tumour	92
	Depression	70–1
	Head injury	85
	Pregnancy problems	134–5
	Premenstrual syndrome	151
	Pregnancy problems	134–5
Morning sickness	Hand, foot and mouth disease	341
Mouth *infection*	Oral thrush	209
sore	Mouth ulcers	211
	Oral thrush	209
Muscle strain, with back pain	Backache	236
Muscle weakness	Muscular dystrophy	241
	RSD	242
Nappy rash	Nappy rash	329
Nausea	Indigestion	173
	Vertigo and dizziness	206
	see also **Vomiting**	
in pregnancy	Pregnancy problems	134–5
Neck, painful/stiff		
and numbness/tingling	Osteoarthritis	234
and infection	Viral meningitis	266
Nose *bleeding*	Nose bleeds	207
runny/blocked	Colds	54
	Hay fever	64
	Nasal polyps	207
	Sinus problems	208
Numbness/tingling	Multiple sclerosis	82
	Neuralgia	77
	RSD	242
	Sciatica	240
Overweight	Obesity	98–9
	Thyroid problems	105
	see also Diet and weight control	100–3
and coronary heart disease	Angina	41
	High blood pressure	38–9
Palpitations	Palpitations	49
Panic attacks	Anxiety	72
	Stress	74–5
Penis *lumps and swellings*	Cancer of the penis	120
painful	Balanitis	330
	Urethritis and NSU	110
painful urination	Cystitis	109
	Urethritis and NSU	110
Periods *absent*	Period problems	152–3
heavy, painful or irregular	Endometriosis	157
	Fibroids	158
	Menopause	154–5
	Pelvic inflammatory disease	156
	Period problems	152–3
Phlegm	Catarrh	56
	Chronic bronchitis	57
Phobias	Anxiety	72
	Phobias	91
Pins and needles	*see* **Numbness/tingling**	
PMS	*see* **Premenstrual syndrome**	
Pneumonia	Pneumonia	65
	see also **Chest infection**	
Post-menopausal bleeding	Cervical cancer	148
	Menopause	154–5
	Uterine cancer	149
Postnatal depression	Post-delivery problems	140–1
	see also Birth	136–9
Pregnancy	*see also* Conception, pregnancy and genetics	126–33
and ankle swelling	Pregnancy problems	134–5
and back pain	Pregnancy problems	134–5
and haemorrhoids	Haemorrhoids	183
	Pregnancy problems	134–5
and heartburn	Pregnancy problems	134–5

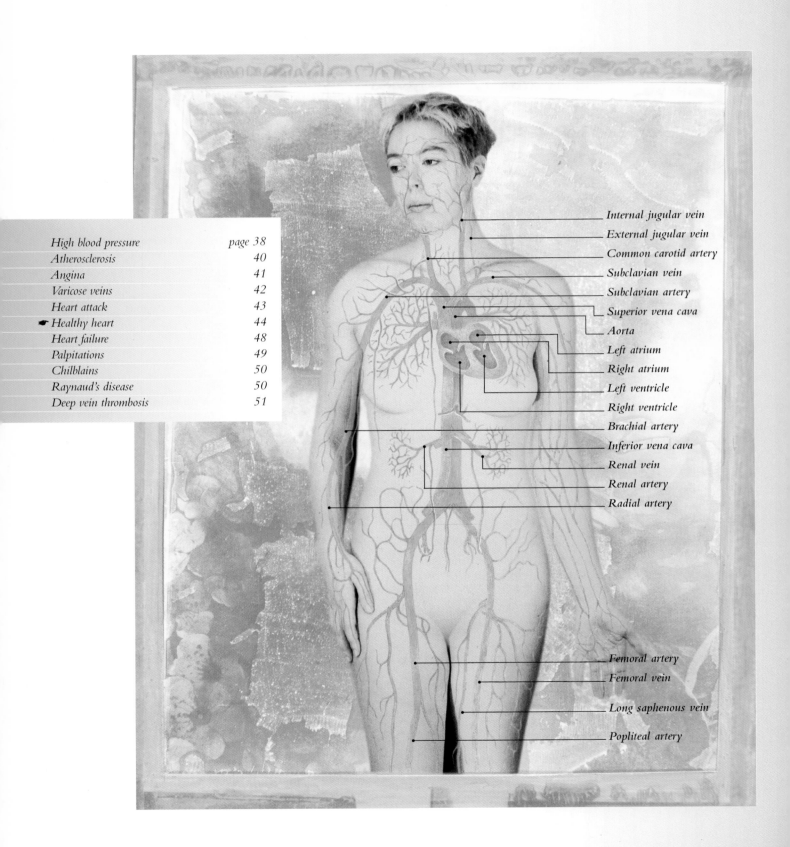

Internal jugular vein

External jugular vein

Common carotid artery

Subclavian vein

Subclavian artery

Superior vena cava

Aorta

Left atrium

Right atrium

Left ventricle

Right ventricle

Brachial artery

Inferior vena cava

Renal vein

Renal artery

Radial artery

Femoral artery

Femoral vein

Long saphenous vein

Popliteal artery

It could be said that the circulatory system, also known as the cardiovascular system, is all a matter of plumbing – but what plumbing! It consists of a pump, the heart, which keeps going for upward of 70 years and which anticipates the body's demands for output, and a system of pipework which is self-sealing and which continues to operate efficiently despite all degrees of cold, heat and posture.

CIRCULATORY SYSTEM

WE NEED A CIRCULATORY system in order to carry essential nutrients to every cell of the body: oxygen to keep energy production going; glucose, which is the basic fuel of the body; and all the chemicals and hormones essential to the regulation of our metabolism. In addition blood carries away waste products from the cells – carbon dioxide to be exhaled by the lungs, and other substances to be handled by the kidneys or by the liver.

The human heart is a four-chambered pump which maintains a steady blood pressure and flow of blood. It has two sides: the left and the right. Each side has a chamber where blood arrives – the atrium – and a powerful ventricle that pumps the blood. The circulation begins with the arrival in the left atrium of blood fresh from the lungs. This blood is carrying maximum amounts of oxygen and is therefore bright red – typical of arterial blood. With each beat of the left ventricle about 70 ml of blood is squeezed into the circulation. It enters the aorta, the great main artery 2.5 cm/1 in in diameter, from which blood flows into ever smaller arteries which eventually become microscopic in size.

The blood now enters the capillary system of blood vessels. These microscopic channels are so narrow that blood can flow through them only one cell at a time, finally reaching the furthermost cells of the body in the fingers and toes. It is at this stage in the system that oxygen is swapped for carbon dioxide and fuel is exchanged for waste products. This ends the arterial side of the circulation. The blood now begins its homeward journey. Having lost its oxygen, its colour changes to the dark red typical of venous blood, such as we see after a minor cut. The blood returns via the system of veins, channel joining channel until eventually it flows through the great vena cava back to the heart.

Blood enters the right atrium. From here it passes into the right ventricle, from where it is pumped into the lungs. In the lungs carbon dioxide is given up, to be breathed out, and oxygen is picked up. The blood is once again fresh and red, fit to be sent around the body.

How the system is regulated

The whole system of heart, lungs, arteries and veins is carefully regulated by complex controls. There are nerves that open and close blood vessels and that make the heart beat faster or stronger. There are chemicals that have the same effect. The best known is adrenaline, a surge of which sets our pulses racing and our hearts thumping when we are exposed to stress. There are many other subtle mechanisms which fine tune the efficiency of the circulation, including pressure detectors in the neck and within the heart itself.

Clearly there are many possible ways in which the complex circulatory system can go wrong. This section discusses some of the most common problems that arise.

Left: The heart pumps oxygen-rich blood through arteries and capillaries; stale blood returns to the heart via the veins.

HIGH BLOOD PRESSURE

◆

The condition of abnormally raised pressure within the arterial system, also called hypertension. It is one of the most common chronic health problems there is.

CAUSES

◆

Overall 10–20% of the Western adult population has high blood pressure, depending on what definition is used. Most cases remain unexplained; it is not known why one person develops it and another does not. There is a suspicion that something in the Western way of life predisposes us to high blood pressure, be it **stress**, diet, being overweight or high alcohol intake. High blood pressure also runs in families.

About 5% of people with high blood pressure do have a specific identifiable cause – most often kidney disease, as blood pressure is partly controlled by a hormone system involving the kidneys called the renin/angiotensin system. Other rare hormonal causes include hyper-aldosteronism and a disease of the adrenal glands called Cushing's syndrome. Both of these produce changes in blood chemistry detectable in blood tests. In other uncommon disorders, for example phaeochromocytoma, there is a sudden release of hormones which increase blood pressure. These would be considered in a young person who has unusually high blood pressure.

High blood pressure may also be the result of high blood calcium. This, in turn, is caused by other diseases so needs to be investigated. Finally, certain anatomical abnormalities cause high blood pressure, for example coarctation of the aorta, which is a congenital narrowing of that great artery and which is suspected if there are weak pulses in the legs.

SYMPTOMS

◆

Contrary to popular view, high blood pressure rarely causes any symptoms. Although some say they feel headachy or unwell with high blood pressure, objective studies do not bear this out, except in cases of extremely high pressure where there might be a very severe headache plus blurred vision.

How blood pressure is measured

Blood pressure is measured with a sphygmomanometer – a cuff, which is wrapped around the upper arm, connected to either a column of mercury or an electronic gauge.

There is an artery just below the surface at the bend of the elbow and the cuff is inflated to the point at which it closes the artery beneath it. The doctor then places a stethoscope over the artery and listens to its sound reappear. This is the

point of systolic blood pressure and is the maximum pressure. It corresponds to the pressure as the heart gives a beat. Then the cuff is relaxed; as blood flows again there are characteristic changes in the sounds until a point is reached called diastolic blood pressure. This is taken to be the lower level of pressure and corresponds to blood pressure in between beats, that is, while the heart is momentarily at rest. Both figures are important and are given equal priority. Ideally, one should have a systolic no higher than 140 mmHg (millimetres of mercury) and a diastolic no more than 90 mmHg; the exact figures aimed at depend on age and associated risk factors.

The doctor will probably take blood tests to check for kidney trouble or any of the rarer causes of high blood pressure mentioned earlier. Blood tests also help decide which drugs to use, for example someone with a biochemical tendency to **gout** should not be put on a diuretic (commonly known as a water tablet) since this can raise the uric acid responsible for gout. Cholesterol is checked and an electrocardiogram (ECG) and possibly a chest X-ray taken. These show whether the high blood pressure is putting a strain on the heart.

It is usual to check the pressure several times over a few weeks before deciding whether it is truly raised. This is because a single high reading can be a 'one-off' event.

TREATMENT

◆

Why are doctors so keen to treat high blood pressure? Many trials have now shown that the higher the blood pressure the greater the risk of a **stroke**. This is understandable; put any liquid system under pressure and leaks are bound to occur. So it is with the arterial system. If an artery leaks it can cause paralysis and affects sight and thinking. In addition, sustained high blood pressure puts strain on the heart which, in time, can lead to **heart failure**. Lastly, really high blood pressure can damage the kidneys (see KIDNEY FAILURE).

Even a modest reduction in blood pressure lessens these risks, especially the risk of having a stroke. This holds across all ages – even hypertension in the elderly is worth treating to greatly reduce the risk of a stroke.

Self-help measures

Modern medicine has a wide range of drugs available, but before reaching for drugs there are some simple and extremely worthwhile self-help measures you can take. The most important one is to reduce an excessive intake of salt. Next, maintain an ideal weight: your doctor will tell you what to aim for. Relaxation through meditation, yoga or whatever

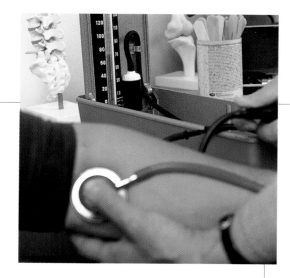

Above: Measuring blood pressure using a mercury-filled sphygmomanometer. Testing blood pressure is one of the most useful health checks.

else suits you has also been shown to help in lowering blood pressure. These simple measures can make all the difference to blood pressure which is just above borderline, making drugs unnecessary.

Assessing risk

There are other factors to be considered in the treatment of high blood pressure, all of which increase the risk from even mild cases. These include smoking, a family history of heart trouble, raised cholesterol and diabetes. Having any of these risk factors makes it more important to treat even mild high blood pressure.

Drugs

If drug treatment is needed, the choice is large. Two classes of drugs stand out above the others. Thiazide diuretics act on the kidney and, in low doses, are a tried and tested remedy for high blood pressure. Commonly used ones are bendrofluazide and hydrochlorothiazide. Then there are beta-blockers such as atenolol or propranolol. These drugs work on the heart and kidney and have more side effects than the diuretics, such as causing cold hands, tiredness and breathlessness. They are very effective drugs and would be a first or second choice.

Newer agents

Angiotensin-converting enzyme (ACE) inhibitors are a fairly new class of drugs, used at all ages and especially in diabetes. They work on a subtle hormonal aspect of the kidney and also have a strengthening effect on the heart. Their main side effect is that they cause coughing. Common names are lisinopril and captopril. Another widely used class of drugs are the calcium-channel blockers which affect cell metabolism. These include

nifedipine and amlodipine. Many of the drugs mentioned can be used in combination; in fact 40% of people with high blood pressure need two or more drugs to control it. It often takes time to find drugs that suit the individual. Thereafter reviews are needed three or four times a year, with occasional checks on blood chemistry and an ECG.

See also PROBLEMS IN PREGNANCY.

QUESTIONS

Is treatment forever?
Usually, high blood pressure will require lifelong treatment. However, some people's blood pressure does return to normal, typically on retirement, reduction of stress levels or loss of weight. In recognition of this fact, doctors might try reducing the patient's medication every few years.

Can nervousness increase blood pressure?
Certainly; doctors call this the 'white coat' effect. Measuring blood pressure continuously over 24 hours shows that blood pressure varies remarkably at different times and in different situations and especially when with a doctor. Twenty-four hour monitoring of blood pressure is becoming more common as the cost of the recording equipment falls.

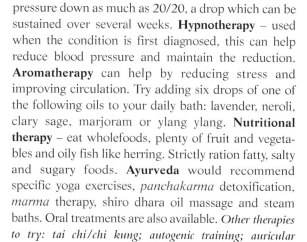

Complementary treatment

If you are on medication, you should maintain it. **Chakra balancing** – deep relaxation can bring blood pressure down as much as 20/20, a drop which can be sustained over several weeks. **Hypnotherapy** – used when the condition is first diagnosed, this can help reduce blood pressure and maintain the reduction. **Aromatherapy** can help by reducing stress and improving circulation. Try adding six drops of one of the following oils to your daily bath: lavender, neroli, clary sage, marjoram or ylang ylang. **Nutritional therapy** – eat wholefoods, plenty of fruit and vegetables and oily fish like herring. Strictly ration fatty, salty and sugary foods. **Ayurveda** would recommend specific yoga exercises, *panchakarma* detoxification, *marma* therapy, shiro dhara oil massage and steam baths. Oral treatments are also available. *Other therapies to try: tai chi/chi kung; autogenic training; auricular therapy; shiatsu do; yoga; cymatics; Western herbalism.*

ATHEROSCLEROSIS

The accumulation of a fatty material within blood vessels which underlies much heart and arterial disease.

CAUSES

In childhood the linings of the major arteries are smooth and clean. By late adulthood many people have atherosclerosis of the walls of their blood vessels – from atheroma, a mixture of fat and the breakdown products from blood clots. Cholesterol is one major cause of atheroma, deposits gradually building up on the lining of the arteries in the same way that water pipes become furred up with calcium salts. The abnormal layer of cholesterol affects the walls of the artery so that blood is likely to clot on it, something that should not normally occur. Over many years the original patch of cholesterol becomes overlaid and entwined with fibres of old blood cells. Eventually there is a significant obstruction to the flow of blood; symptoms begin to show. The arteries most liable to atheroma are those around the heart, the legs and the brain.

SYMPTOMS

Symptoms only appear when the blood flow is obstructed. If the arteries to the heart are affected, the earliest symptoms are **angina** – pain in the chest on exertion. Often the very first symptom may be an actual **heart attack**, with chest pain and breathlessness. Frequently, there is simply a general reduction in the efficiency of the heart, causing breathlessness and an inability to exert oneself. Some patients will go on to develop **heart failure**.

If the obstruction is in the arteries to the legs, the resulting symptoms are pains in the legs, which begin on exertion and go after a few minutes' rest – termed intermittent claudication. Typically the pain is felt in the calf; the leg may feel constantly cold. In severe cases the toes may even start to decay from a form of gangrene. This is called peripheral vascular disease.

Atherosclerosis of the blood vessels in the brain leads to **stroke** or to a slow decline of mental function.

TREATMENT

Cigarette smoking makes atherosclerosis worse by increasing the tendency of the blood to clot, so it is essential to stop smoking. Similarly, **high blood pressure** and **diabetes** make it worse and should be dealt with. Established obstruction can often be remedied by replacing or bypassing the diseased artery. For the heart this is coronary artery bypass grafting

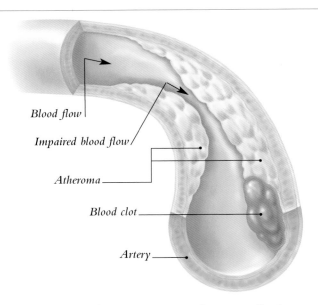

Blood flow

Impaired blood flow

Atheroma

Blood clot

Artery

Above: A cross-section of an artery affected by atherosclerosis, potentially causing pain, death of surrounding tissue and stroke.

(see ANGINA). The arteries to the legs can also often be either replaced or bypassed using artificial tubing. In most cases, however, obstruction to the blood flow in the legs can be significantly bypassed simply through regular exercise over a period of time. This encourages small new blood vessels to find a way round the diseased area. Only if this does not occur is surgery called for.

At present there are no proven treatments to improve blood flow to the brain (except surgery on the carotid arteries in the neck if narrowed by atheroma). Medication to improve blood flow to the brain remains experimental.

Raised cholesterol is widely recognized as underlying these problems. Ideally, diets should be adjusted to reduce cholesterol, otherwise a number of drugs can do this effectively.

Complementary treatment

Autogenic training improves blood circulation via the relaxation response, allowing greater flow and reducing auto-aggression. The warmth from exercise is helpful, slightly raising skin temperature. A **nutritional therapist** will advise on good and bad dietary fats. Eat fresh wholefoods containing plenty of dietary fibre, B vitamins, and antioxidants – vitamins A, C and E, and selenium. **Ayurveda** would focus on cleansing, detoxification and diet. *Other therapies to try: tai chi/chi kung; cymatics; hypnotherapy.*

ANGINA

Chest pain due to poor flow in the heart's own blood supply, the coronary arteries.

CAUSES

The heart is a highly specialized muscle which, like any other muscle in the body, relies on a steady supply of oxygen-rich blood to function efficiently. Anything that interferes with the blood supply will starve the heart of oxygen and cause angina.

The heart is supplied by four major arteries which are especially prone to blockage with atheroma, a mixture of cholesterol and blood (see ATHEROSCLEROSIS). Blockage builds up over many years until eventually the restriction of blood flow is critical and angina starts.

Occasionally, other conditions cause angina in an otherwise healthy heart, for example severe **anaemia** or disorders of the valves controlling blood flow within the heart.

SYMPTOMS

The cardinal symptom is pain over the heart on exertion; this means pain over the central and left side of the chest. Angina pain also typically radiates away from the heart, so people with angina feel the pain rising up their chest towards the jaw and often down their left arm as well. There can be odd variants on this such as pain in one hand on exertion.

The other typical feature of angina is that it is relieved by a short rest. Unlike the pain of a **heart attack**, which it can closely resemble, angina pains last only as long as you exercise and disappear after a couple of minutes of rest.

TREATMENT

All people with angina need checking for **high blood pressure**, raised cholesterol and anaemia. Smokers should quit as smoking makes atherosclerosis worse, and those who are obese should lose weight to reduce strain on the heart.

The simplest treatment is with a class of drugs called nitrates, which are related to tri-nitro-toluene – also known as TNT. These work by opening up the arteries to the heart just enough to bring extra blood flow and relief. They can be taken as single tablets, allowed to dissolve under the tongue, or a spray at the time of need. If angina is more frequent, they are given in longer-acting tablet forms, such as iso-sorbide mononitrate. Nitrates are available as patches worn on the skin which release nitrates slowly over 24 hours. Other drugs used to treat angina are beta-blockers and calcium-channel blockers (see HIGH BLOOD PRESSURE). Angina can be further investigated using a stress test, an ECG taken during exercise. This helps confirm the diagnosis and indicates the severity of the condition. If appropriate, the next step is coronary artery angiography: a catheter is guided to the heart from the femoral artery in the groin. A dye is then injected to show how blood flows around the heart. If this reveals serious blockage in the vessels, coronary artery bypass grafting (CABG) may be required to replace the obstructed portion of artery with a vein graft. Other options are to dilate the narrowed section of artery via angioplasty (see page 47) or to insert a small tube called a stent. The decision to employ surgical, as opposed to medical, treatment depends on the individual's age and overall state of health and on how many coronary arteries are narrowed and how severly.

QUESTIONS

How safe is coronary artery bypass grafting?
Roughly 95–98% of operations are successful in relieving angina and in improving the quality of life. The main risk is having a stroke during surgery, which happens in about 1% of cases.

Why is low-dose aspirin useful in angina?
This remarkable drug reduces the blood's tendency to clot. Thus it decreases the chances of worsening arterial blockage in the coronary arteries, and is recommended for individuals with angina.

Does angina lead on to a heart attack?
Although it is a warning of heart circulatory problems, angina is a fairly safe condition to have. Only 2–4% of cases a year progress to a heart attack. For many people angina can be managed by modest adjustments to lifestyle and simple medication.

Complementary treatment

Acupuncture – a typical point is Pericardium 4, on the arm, plus points on the chest and upper back. **Homeopathy** – possible remedies, depending on circumstances, include cactus, spigelia and naja. **Chakra balancing** can help prevent attacks by reducing blood pressure. Diet is important for prevention; a **nutritional therapist** will be able to advise. **Hellerwork** improves circulation and reduces tension around the heart. *Other therapies to try: Chinese herbalism; shiatsu do; autogenic training; biodynamics.*

VARICOSE VEINS

Unsightly and uncomfortable dilation of veins in the legs.

CAUSES

Varicose veins are one of the prices that human beings pay for standing upright. Being part of a low-pressure system for returning stale blood to the heart, veins are not sturdy structures and do not cope well with the higher pressure of a column of blood when upright. Their walls stretch and distort and form the familiar worm-like varicosities. This is why people who spend a lot of time on their feet are at risk of varicose veins.

Anything that interferes with the return of blood through the veins will also increase pressure and predisposition to varicose veins. The most common reason is pregnancy, since the enlarged womb obstructs blood flow from the legs back into the abdomen. For similar reasons, a large growth within the abdomen may show itself as varicose veins. They may also follow years after a **deep vein thrombosis**. However, many people have simply inherited the tendency from their parents.

Varicose veins lead to stagnation of blood flow. There is a tiny but significant leakage of blood from the veins, eventually leading to a brownish discoloration of the lower limb.

SYMPTOMS

There are soft, blue, dilated blood vessels in the legs, usually around the ankles, calf and in the groin. They may ache. As time passes they become more prominent and irregular in shape and are there all the time and not only while the individual is standing. Most people have only cosmetic problems but some develop swelling, scaling and irritation with discoloration of the leg and eventually extensive, chronic ulceration around the ankle.

Phlebitis is a blood clot within the varicose vein, which then looks red, feels painful and is hard. Although uncomfortable, it is not a dangerous condition, as opposed to deep vein thrombosis.

TREATMENT

The varicose veins of pregnancy can be expected to go after delivery. Losing weight reduces pressure within the abdomen and this, too, will relieve mild varicose veins.

Wearing a support stocking helps the return of blood and is a sensible alternative to surgery, but many people do eventually need surgery, either because of the aching in their legs or through unhappiness with their appearance.

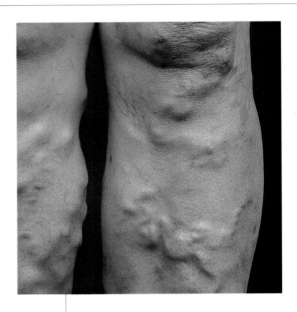

Above: Typical dilated and distorted varicose veins below the knee – one of the most common sites for this condition. Surgical treatment is the only cure for such severe and established varicose veins.

There are two types of surgery. One is to strip out the whole varicose vein from the groin to the ankle. This is rather brutal surgery; moreover this vein may be useful one day for coronary artery bypass grafting (see ANGINA). The other method is to tie off the deeper veins which feed the surface veins. This calls for a series of cuts down the leg to reveal the feeder veins, which are then tied with surgical thread.

Whatever the surgery, varicose veins tend to recur unless lifestyle changes are made to avoid standing or to lose weight.

See also ULCERS.

Complementary treatment

Homeopathy – the treatment depends on the case, for example if the varicose veins worsen with warmth and swinging the legs, pulsatilla might be appropriate. **Aromatherapy** can strengthen the circulatory system and improve the tone of the veins. Try adding six drops of one of the following oils to your bath: cypress, geranium or lemon. Inverted **yoga** positions can reduce swelling. **Ayurveda** would recommend *panchakarma* detoxification and *marma* therapy.

HEART ATTACK

◆

Sudden severe chest pain due to blockage of blood flow to the heart. Medically called myocardial infarction (MI).

CAUSES

◆

Most heart attacks are the result of a blood clot suddenly forming in coronary arteries diseased with **atherosclerosis**, thus blocking blood flow to part of the heart. The heart reacts to the drop in blood supply, as any other muscle does, with pain and loss of function. This means that the heart fails to beat efficiently, leading to sudden **heart failure**. It may go into chaotic rhythms or stop altogether.

Sometimes heart attacks happen in the absence of atherosclerosis, and the cause is unclear. The heart might suddenly go into an abnormal pattern of beating for some reason. Sometimes there is disease of the heart muscle itself, a cardiomyopathy, which carries an increased risk of heart attack. Other causes are electrical shocks or blows to the chest.

SYMPTOMS

◆

The first symptom is severe pain over the breast bone or the left side of the chest. The pain feels like it is deep inside the chest as if something is squeezing or crushing internally. Unlike **angina**, the pain persists for many minutes or hours. There is sweating from the pain and the sufferer looks grey.

Severe heart attacks cause heart failure, with breathlessness; the victim may turn blue from poor blood flow, fall unconscious or collapse. It can happen that the first symptom is when the individual cries out with a sudden chest pain and collapses immediately. Even in this apparently hopeless situation victims should still have cardiopulmonary resuscitation (see page 392) as there is a chance of recovery.

Not all heart attacks are painful. In the elderly especially a heart attack may be suspected because of rapidly appearing heart failure or sudden vague tiredness or **stroke**.

Besides the clinical picture, the diagnosis depends on finding characteristic changes in the ECG or on detecting enzymes released by the damaged heart into the blood stream.

TREATMENT

◆

In recent years there have been some great advances in the treatment of heart attacks, thanks to drugs popularly called 'clot-busters'. These dissolve the abnormal blood clot within the coronary arteries. They should be given by drip immediately, although it is still worth giving them within 24 hours of the heart attack. Drug names are streptokinase and urokinase. Even before this treatment, a heart attack victim should swallow an aspirin because this humble drug actually reduces the stickiness of the blood and so reduces the size of the blood clot in the arteries. Together, these measures have led to a remarkable 30% drop in the immediate death rate.

Long-term treatment

A low daily dose of aspirin (75–150 mg) reduces the chances of a further blood clot and should be taken lifelong. Drugs called ACE inhibitors and beta-blockers strengthen the heart and help prevent abnormal heart rhythms. Cholesterol should be reduced to low levels by diet or drugs if necessary and, of course, you must stop smoking. Some people may need coronary artery bypass grafting (see ANGINA).

QUESTIONS

Can shock bring on a heart attack?
Sudden emotional shocks set the heart racing and may start an abnormal heart rhythm. This does increase the risk of a heart attack in those people whose coronary arteries are already diseased with atherosclerosis.

How dangerous is a heart attack?
Despite recent medical advances it is always dangerous. About 30% of all heart attacks lead to death within 24 hours. Another 10% of victims die within the next month from complications. Thereafter there is a 5–10% lifelong annual risk of death.

How important is it to reduce cholesterol?
Latest research shows that reducing cholesterol cuts the risk of further heart trouble by up to 40%. This can be achieved by rigorous dieting or, increasingly, by cholesterol-lowering drugs.

Complementary treatment

This is a medical emergency and no complementary therapy can help in the immediate short term. Many therapies, however, are excellent in the rehabilitation stage. **Yoga** and **tai chi/chi kung** are gentle forms of exercise that can be very beneficial during recovery. Diet is very important; a registered **naturopath** or **nutritional therapist** will be able to make suggestions tailored to you, your condition and your constitution. *Other therapies to try: see STRESS.*

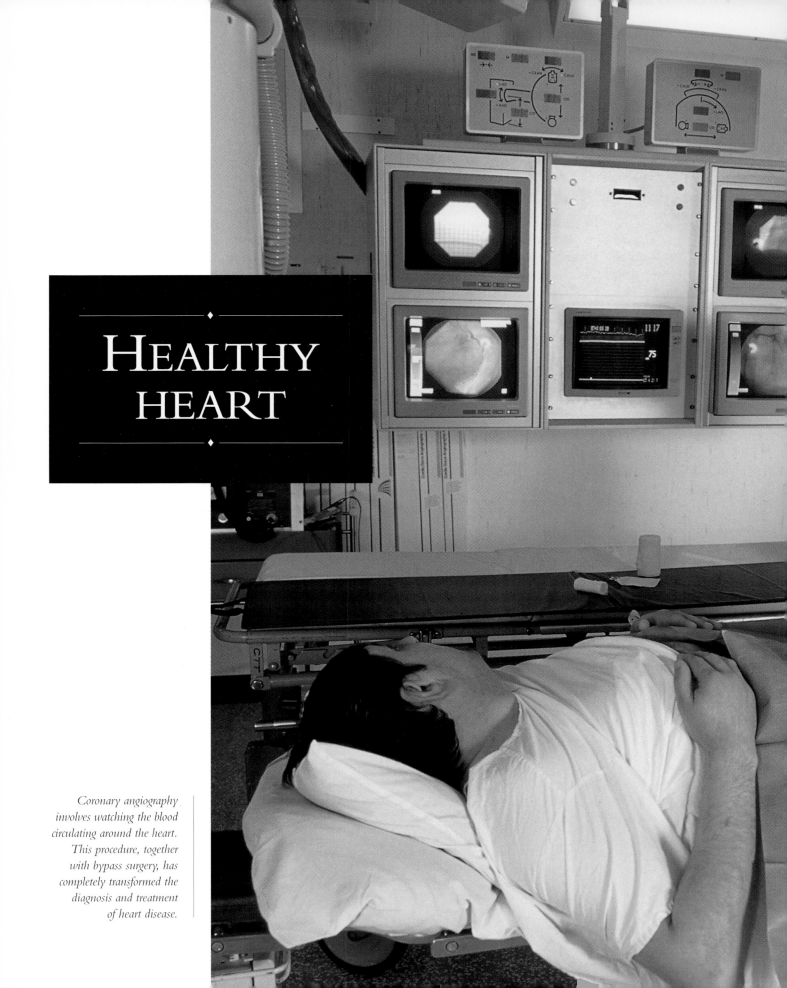

HEALTHY HEART

Coronary angiography involves watching the blood circulating around the heart. This procedure, together with bypass surgery, has completely transformed the diagnosis and treatment of heart disease.

R ISK FACTORS FOR HEART DISEASE can be divided into those you may have some control over and those you do not (see below right). The two sets interlink. For example, if you have a family history of heart disease, it is even more advisable to do something about those things you can control. Moreover, risks do not just add up as in 2 + 2 + 2 = 6; rather they multiply as in 2 × 2 × 2 = 8. Depressing? Not necessarily. It means that reducing smoking or cholesterol intake has an even greater benefit than you might think.

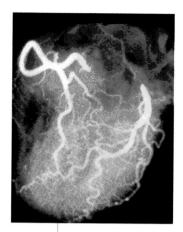

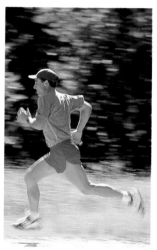

Above: Coronary angiograph showing blood flow through the heart's own arteries. Right: Regular exercise can provide pleasure as well as promoting health.

Your heart must last a lifetime

Smoking and poor nutrition during pregnancy increase the chances of having a low birthweight baby. It would appear that such children have an increased risk of heart disease as adults. Although the link is as yet controversial and unexplained, it is sensible not to smoke during pregnancy and to eat a properly balanced diet right the way through from conception to birth.

Childhood   Evidence suggests that obese and overfed children grow into overweight adults who are more at risk of heart disease than slimmer people. Set a pattern of sensible eating habits and regular, healthy meals from an early age. It is also important to encourage your children to get plenty of exercise and play sports.

Adult life   Continue the habits of eating healthily and taking exercise. Check your cholesterol and blood pressure from time to time to make sure that levels are as they should be. Do not smoke.

Old age   Now is the time to pay more attention to your blood pressure and to concern yourself less about cholesterol. An active life promotes good health. **Diabetes** is an important risk factor for heart trouble and if it is present it should be carefully controlled.

Early recognition of heart trouble

You do not want your first symptom of heart trouble to be a **heart attack**. Rather, you should take note of the early warning symptoms.

High cholesterol may cause changes in the eye area of some people. You may notice a white ring around the iris (the coloured part) of the eye – the medical name for this is an arcus senilis. This is normal in people over the age of 60, but

RISK FACTORS FOR HEART DISEASE

These can be divided into those you may have some control over and those you do not:

No control

♦ *Being male*
♦ *Adverse family history*
♦ *Age (risk increases with age)*
♦ *Congenital heart disease*
♦ *Infections such as rheumatic fever or diphtheria*

Some control

♦ *High cholesterol*
♦ *High blood pressure*
♦ *Smoking*
♦ *Obesity*
♦ *Lack of exercise*

MISCELLANEOUS FACTORS LINKED WITH HEART DISEASE

◆

These are factors where research suggests a link to heart disease, but the weight to be attached to them is debatable:

Protective factors

◆ *Alcohol – drinking 2 or 3 units a day (a couple of glasses of wine)*
◆ *Hard water, high in calcium salts*
◆ *Warm climate*
◆ *Higher socio-economic class*
◆ *Vegetarian and vegan diets – people following these diets probably benefit from an improvement in their harmful/beneficial blood-fat ratio*
◆ *Fruit and vegetables – these appear protective thanks to vitamin E and other antioxidants*
◆ *Other trace minerals may be relevant, for example selenium – an area of vigorous current research*
◆ *Taking HRT after the menopause*

Harmful factors

◆ *Stress – people who make their own stress and are hard- driven appear at greater risk*
◆ *The cold – unaccustomed exertion in cold weather is risky, for example shovelling snow*
◆ *Salt intake is probably significant. Do not add salt to food*

Modern investigations

Modern technology allows the clinical impression of heart disease to be objectively proven. The basic tests are harmless and straightforward: first, an exercise ECG, an electrical recording of the heart while running or walking briskly on a treadmill. This shows whether there is a blood flow problem even in people whose resting ECG is normal, and detects about 75% of such cases. If there is still doubt, you might have a radioactive scan of the heart. If that is normal, it is highly unlikely that you have significant heart disease.

Another important investigation is an echocardiogram, to show the valves of the heart beating and to give an idea of how efficiently the heart is working.

A number of people can be diagnosed only by coronary artery angiography (see page 348), where a dye is injected into the circulation around the heart to check for narrowing of the coronary arteries. This carries a one in 2500–5000 risk of death, so it is used only in order to plan surgery or, rarely, to exclude heart disease in someone getting pains suggestive of heart disease but where all other investigations are normal.

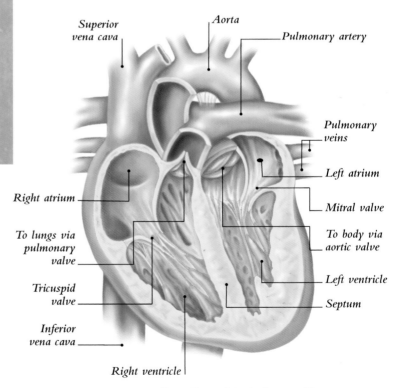

Above: So much in the heart could go wrong, yet it usually remains impressively reliable for many decades.

if you are younger it is advisable to have a cholesterol check. Another warning sign is yellow plaques on the skin beneath the lower eyelids – the medical term is xanthelasma.

Chest pain on exertion This is **angina**, the classic warning sign of heart trouble. It indictaes that the coronary arteries cannot deliver an adequate blood supply to the heart muscle when under exertion. Not all chest discomfort is from angina by any means, but it is the most important possibility to exclude. Get it checked by your doctor.

Breathlessness A heart with a poor blood supply will be inefficient at pumping blood, and breathlessness may be a consequence. Again, there are many more innocent reasons possible, so do get a medical opinion.

Angioplasty This means opening up coronary arteries narrowed by **atherosclerosis**. It is an important alternative to coronary artery surgery. A thin tube is guided to the heart from the large femoral artery in the groin. Once it reaches its destination, instruments are inserted through the tube to clear the blockage.

Coronary artery surgery This involves replacing diseased arteries with a vein graft from the leg or from the chest. It is highly effective and can be repeated if the grafts block up, which happens in 5–10% of people each year.

Heart transplantation This amazing technology has, in 35 years, moved from experiment to routine. It is reserved for people who have no other hope of survival and who are otherwise healthy. There is now the very real prospect of an artificial heart that can be inserted more easily than those currently available, or even of using hearts taken from specially bred pigs. Such developments would transform the prospects for people with **heart failure** which is treatable by no other means.

Treatment of a heart attack

If you experience a sudden constant central chest pain and breathlessness, assume you have a heart attack until proven otherwise. Early treatment greatly improves the outlook, so ring for an ambulance. Take an aspirin immediately, as this reduces the size of the clot forming in the heart.

Once in hospital, you will be given an injection of a clot-busting drug such as streptokinase, unless you are one of the small number who should not have it, for example if you have had recent surgery or a history of abnormal bleeding, especially from the gastrointestinal tract.

For at least six months after recovery you should take a beta-blocking drug such as atenolol to prevent abnormal heart rhythms. You will probably have to take an ACE inhibitor such as ramipril to reduce the chances of subsequent heart failure. These modern measures have lowered the risk of death from a heart attack by some 40%.

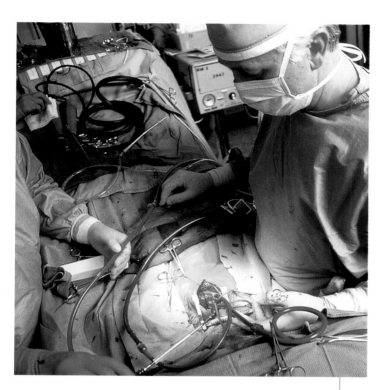

Above: A child has received a new heart. The surgeon inspects his handiwork before removing the pipes that have kept circulation going.

Effective therapy

Never has there been such a wide range of treatment for heart trouble and it should be possible to find something that suits you. Medical treatment is the preferred option, pending exact diagnosis of the state of blood flow in the heart. It may be as simple as taking an aspirin every day. This reduces the tendency of the blood to clot and thereby lessens the risks of a heart attack. It has side effects, especially bleeding from the stomach, so cannot be recommended to everyone, but for those who either have angina or have had a heart attack it is a lifelong option.

HEART FAILURE

An inefficiency of the pumping action of the heart because of some underlying disease or problem.

CAUSES

The heart is made of tough, durable, specialized muscle which beats with impressive reliability for a lifetime. It follows that most cases of heart failure result from a **heart attack** or **atherosclerosis** of the blood supply to the heart. These both diminish the amount of blood flowing through the heart and so reduce how well the muscle can pump, as well as leaving areas of damaged muscle which pump less efficiently.

Other common causes are **high blood pressure** and irregular heart rhythm outside the normal 60–90 beats per minute. This rhythm allows for efficient flow of blood around the body. This efficiency is reduced if the heart beats very fast (above about 120 bpm), very slowly (below about 40 bpm), or irregularly (see PALPITATIONS). There are other uncommon causes of heart failure. Heart failure affects about 1% of those over the age of 65. It used to carry a grim outlook but this has changed in recent years thanks to the latest medication.

SYMPTOMS

The earliest symptoms of gradual heart failure are tiredness, breathlessness and swelling of the ankles. These result from the sluggish flow of blood, which is poorly supplied with oxygen. The body responds to the failing heart by retaining salt and water, and a back-pressure effect swells the legs. Eventually fluid also builds up in the lungs, leading to increased breathlessness especially when lying flat, which is why people with heart failure find they need to sleep propped upright and wake breathless during the night if they roll off the pillows. Certain basic investigations should be done, for example chest X-ray, blood count and ECG.

Acute heart failure

This usually follows a heart attack; there is breathlessness and coughing of frothy phlegm. The victim often turns blue because of poorly oxygenated blood. Heart failure can often be diagnosed on examination. The doctor hears characteristic sounds of fluid on the lungs and notices neck veins distended with blood returning from the head that the heart cannot pump away fast enough. There are also signs of fluid on a chest X-ray and of heart strain on an ECG. The most reliable method of diagnosis is an echocardiogram; this also detects otherwise unsuspected disease of the valves of the heart.

TREATMENT

For immediate treatment of heart failure, diuretic drugs are taken by mouth or, in urgent cases, injection is used to force fluid out of the lungs and cause a high output of urine. This reduces the volume of blood to be pumped around the body and also reduces blood pressure, relieving strain on the heart. These are life-saving measures.

For long-term treatment many people with heart failure need continuous low dosages of diuretics such as frusemide or bumetanide. A class of drugs called ACE inhibitors has also emerged as being highly effective in improving heart function; these drugs are increasingly used to treat heart failure in all age groups.

Several other less common causes are eminently treatable, for example severe **anaemia**, thyrotoxicosis (see THYROID PROBLEMS) or problems in the valves of the heart. Diseased coronary arteries can be treated by CABG (see ANGINA).

QUESTIONS

Can heart failure be cured?
It cannot really be cured but it can be controlled. Common measures to control it are to treat high blood pressure, to lose weight and to reduce salt intake.

What is the role of a heart transplant?
This is reserved for otherwise healthy people, including those who have suffered heart attacks in the past for whom all other measures have failed. It is a marvellous treatment with a steadily rising success rate, despite the need to stay on powerful anti-rejection medication (see page 363).

Complementary treatment

Do not abandon conventional approaches. **Western herbalism** – treatments for water retention might be useful. **Chinese herbalism** remedies can strengthen the heart and circulatory system. Diet – a registered **naturopath** or **nutritional therapist** will be able to advise on how you can switch to a balanced diet, low in saturated fats. **Healing** can be effective in promoting circulatory function. **Yoga** and **tai chi/chi kung** are gentle forms of exercise with much to offer.

PALPITATIONS

An unusual heart rhythm, often entirely harmless.

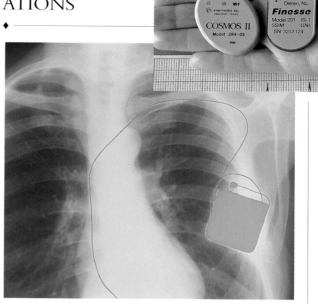

Top: Electronic pacemakers.
Above: X-ray showing a pacemaker
implanted below the skin near the armpit;
the wire carries electrical signals to the heart.

CAUSES

The heart beats regularly thanks to a remarkable electrical system that sends the signal to beat along nerves that form electrical pathways from a 'pacemaker centre' to the rest of the heart. This system ensures that the muscle of the heart beats in an orderly and efficient way; problems with it, however, are extremely common. Everyone at some time experiences harmless, innocent variations of rate and rhythm.

There are innumerable causes of unusual heart rhythms, including **stress**, caffeine, alcohol and inhalers for **asthma**. The diagnosis is often difficult to confirm. Modern devices can record all heartbeats for 24 hours, which can then be computer-analysed in search of abnormalities.

Rapid rhythms

A heart rate above 100 beats per minute causes palpitations and is abnormal. Likely causes are atrial fibrillation, where the rate is rapid and irregular, or thyrotoxicosis (see THYROID PROBLEMS). It is common to have bursts of rapid heartbeats between perfectly normal rates. This may occur in fit young people with no underlying heart abnormality but may also be a feature of underlying heart disease such as **atherosclerosis**.

Slow rhythms

If the heart misses a beat, as it often does, the catch-up beat is unusually hard and will be felt as a thump in the chest. Another common cause is heart block. In this condition there is interference with the electrical flow, so that the heart beats at its own natural rhythm which can be as low as 20 beats per minute. Slow rates can be due to a severely underactive thyroid gland (see THYROID PROBLEMS).

SYMPTOMS

Palpitations are common so take note only if they are a nuisance or accompany breathlessness, chest pain or tiredness, which suggests they are putting a strain on the heart.

TREATMENT

Many cases prove wholly free from disease and need no treatment other than reassuring the patient the heart is basically healthy. Such cases are helped by reducing heart stimulants such as coffee, alcohol, smoking or certain medications.

Rapid rhythms

Several drugs can control these rhythms; the best known is digoxin – most commonly used to treat atrial fibrillation, a rapid and chaotic beating of the heart. Other drugs include amiodarone and verapamil. In atrial fibrillation, specialists increasingly recommend taking anticoagulants to reduce the risk of a stroke. Beta-blockers are used to slow the heart and also have a mild antianxiety effect. The treatment for fast rates unresponsive to drugs is to shock the heart into a normal rhythm.

Slow rhythms

Heart block is treated with a pacemaker. This fires a regular electrical signal so that the heart beats steadily (see page 362).

Complementary treatment

     Chakra balancing – the therapist can help by working over the whole heart. **Nutritional therapy** – deficiencies may be to blame, especially deficiency of B vitamins or magnesium. **Healing** can bring an irregular heartbeat into balance. **Hypnotherapy** calms and lowers heartbeat, and stabilizes palpitations. **Ayurvedic** yoga and oil massages would be recommended, possibly with *panchakarma* detoxification as well. *Other therapies to try: tai chi/chi kung; acupuncture; autogenic training; cymatics; auricular therapy; homeopathy.*

CHILBLAINS

Areas of skin that have been damaged by the cold.

CAUSES

Chilblains are a mild form of frostbite. The final stage in the circulation of blood around the body is via the capillaries, minute channels that reach into the furthermost parts of the body – generally the fingertips, toes and skin. In very cold conditions some of those capillaries can be damaged, which in turn reduces blood flow to that small patch of skin. The result is that a few skin cells die, the skin surface breaks and a small ulcer forms. Anyone can be affected by chilblains if their skin becomes chilled enough.

SYMPTOMS

The most commonly affected sites are fingers, toes and the nose. The initial cold injury is painless and often overlooked unless you happen to notice a small patch of white flesh.

There then follows intense irritation due to the release of breakdown products from the cells that have died. After a day or two a small ulcer appears as a red spot.

TREATMENT

Protection against the cold is the basic precaution – wearing gloves, thick socks and face protectors. If you notice a white chilled area of skin warm it gently by rubbing. Established ulcers should have a smear of antiseptic cream. Drugs are available that increase blood flow to the skin, for example calcium antagonists such as nifedipine, but are used only in the most severe cases.

 Complementary treatment
Aromatherapy – make up three drops of lemon oil in 10 ml of carrier oil. Massaged daily over the toes, this should aid prevention of chilblains. *Other therapies to try: Western herbalism.*

RAYNAUD'S DISEASE

Fingers and toes that go cold and numb unusually readily.

CAUSES

This is a problem with the tiny blood vessels in the fingers and toes. In people with Raynaud's disease these blood vessels are oversensitive to cold; they narrow in response to very minor changes in temperature and are slow to relax again on rewarming. The disorder is more common in women and often other family members are affected.

Occasionally there is some other underlying condition that attacks the blood vessels, such as **systemic lupus erythematosus**, but this would give other symptoms as well. In such cases the condition is called Raynaud's phenomenon. It can also result from using vibrating machinery for long periods of time, and from taking beta-blockers for **high blood pressure**.

SYMPTOMS

When the fingers or toes get even slightly chilled they go first white, because of constriction of the tiniest arteries in the digits, and then blue, because of the resulting poor and stagnant blood flow. They feel numb; as they warm up they gradually

regain normal colour, and often ache until fully recovered. In severe cases the skin becomes fragile, possibly breaking down into small **ulcers**. The whole cycle can last minutes or hours.

TREATMENT

Use common sense; dress warmly and avoid exposure to the cold. Avoid smoking, too, since nicotine causes blood vessels to constrict. Those with severe symptoms can use electrically heated gloves and specially insulated footwear.

There are safety regulations about the use of vibrating equipment in factories. If beta-blockers are the cause, there are many alternatives. Drugs called calcium-channel blockers can help by opening up the blood vessels, but are used only for extreme cases. You may need blood tests to check on the rare illnesses that can underlie severe cases.

 Complementary treatment
Nutritional therapy – try supplements of fatty acids. **Ayurveda** would use detoxification, oil massage and steam baths with oral circulatory stimulants. *Other therapies to try: cymatics; tai chi/chi kung; chakra balancing; autogenic training; Western and Chinese herbalism.*

DEEP VEIN THROMBOSIS

The result of blood clotting, usually in the veins of the legs.

CAUSES

Blood flow through the veins is a more leisurely affair than the urgent rush of blood through arteries. This increases the risk of blood clotting – a risk that is increased by any factors that further reduce blood flow such as bed rest, especially after a **stroke** or **heart attack**, immobility as on long flights and, most commonly, immobility during operations. There are also tiny risks from taking oestrogen in the contraceptive pill and hormone replacement therapy (HRT).

The veins in the legs, deep within the calves and thighs, are the ones most at risk of thrombosis. A further risk is that a small clot in the calf later extends up the leg and even into the major veins within the abdomen. The greatest worry from a deep vein thrombosis is that a portion of the blood clot may fly off and lodge in the lungs, causing a **pulmonary embolism**.

SYMPTOMS

There may be no symptoms at all but often the affected limb suddenly swells up and feels painful. It is usually the calf that swells but it can be the whole leg. The calf looks red and is extremely tender to pressure. Without tests it is frequently impossible to tell whether the cause of a red swollen calf is infection or thrombosis. One test is an ultrasound scan of the veins in the leg, which is good at detecting large clots. The other test is a venogram. This involves injecting a dye into a vein in the foot in order to reveal on X-ray the whole system of veins in the limb. This can detect much smaller clots.

TREATMENT

The aim is to prevent further clot formation, which is done by taking warfarin, a drug that reduces the 'clottability' of the blood. A course of 8–12 weeks is usual. If there is a major blood clot extending into the abdomen, surgery may be a possibility to remove it, but this is a dangerous procedure. Small clots are left alone; the body gradually dissolves them.

Deep vein thrombosis is such a hazard of surgery that great effort has gone into finding ways of preventing it. One method is to inject heparin at and around the time of surgery. This drug reduces the clottability of the blood but not so much that it increases bleeding during surgery. Another technique is for the patient to wear compression stockings during the operation; these increase the rate of blood flow and so reduce the

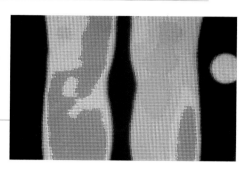

Right: Thermography (heat measurement) revealing thrombosis in the right calf.

chances of stagnation. Finally, all patients are encouraged to become mobile as soon as possible after surgery, in order to reduce the risk of thrombosis. A woman who has had a thrombosis must not take the ordinary contraceptive pill.

QUESTIONS

How does phlebitis differ from deep vein thrombosis?
Phlebitis is a blood clot within a surface vein, causing a tender, firm, inflamed area. This is not dangerous and responds to anti-inflammatory drugs such as ibuprofen.

How big a risk is deep vein thrombosis?
It is extremely common after a stroke or heart attack, abdominal surgery or hip replacement. The associated pulmonary embolus is one of the major complications after these types of surgery.

Can deep vein thrombosis recur?
Having one increases the chances of having another, so always inform a surgeon if you have had a thrombosis. You should also avoid anything which increases the risk such as the contraceptive pill and prolonged bed rest. On long journeys, especially long flights, try to walk around regularly or move your legs about.

Complementary treatment

If you suspect a deep vein thrombosis, you should seek a conventional medical opinion immediately. **Yoga** and **tai chi/chi kung** are gentle forms of exercise which can be beneficial after recovery. Diet is also important in preventing recurrence. A **naturopath** or **nutritional therapist** could help you switch to a balanced diet, containing plenty of wholefoods. Eat plenty of fish, not just white fish, and take fish oil supplements. Also supplement your vitamin E intake, and take garlic supplements.

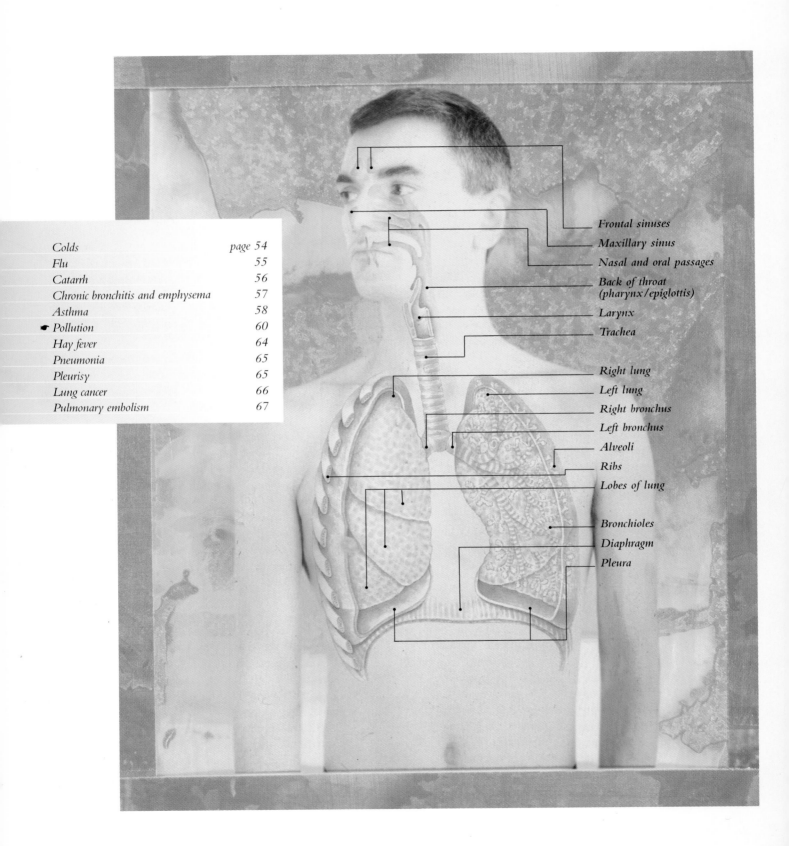

Frontal sinuses

Maxillary sinus

Nasal and oral passages

Back of throat
(pharynx/epiglottis)

Larynx

Trachea

Right lung

Left lung

Right bronchus

Left bronchus

Alveoli

Ribs

Lobes of lung

Bronchioles

Diaphragm

Pleura

*Like any engine, the body needs oxygen to burn fuel.
It also needs a means of disposing of carbon dioxide, which is a
byproduct of the process of generating energy. The respiratory
system performs both of these roles efficiently.*

RESPIRATORY SYSTEM

THE FUNCTION OF THE respiratory system is to bring fresh air into as close contact as possible with blood within the lungs. This is achieved at air sacs, called alveoli, which form the bulk of the sponge-like lungs. In the alveoli air is separated from blood by the thickness of just two cells. This allows oxygen to permeate into the blood, where it is snatched up by the haemoglobin molecules. At the same time carbon dioxide also diffuses across the membrane from the blood stream into the air sacs. When you breathe out, carbon dioxide is released into the atmosphere; when you breathe in, oxygen-rich air rushes into the lungs.

The pathway to the alveoli is via tubes of ever-narrowing diameter – the bronchi and bronchioles. The great airway is the trachea; this splits into left and right main bronchi, which further subdivide in a branching pattern down into the lungs. The smaller airways, the bronchioles, have a muscle layer which can constrict or dilate them and so adjust the amount of air passing through the lungs.

An adult's lungs have some 300 million alveoli with a total surface area of 60–80 sq m/645–860 sq ft. The lungs are designed to filter out dust particles from the inhaled air by trapping them in a layer of mucus; specialized cells then sweep the dust up and out of the lungs. By the time air reaches the alveoli it has become warmed or cooled to body temperature and made just moist enough to optimize gas exchange.

The breathing process

The actual process of breathing is mainly the result of the diaphragm descending, as well as the muscles between the ribs lifting them. The net result is to expand the volume of the chest – and the lungs expand into that volume. Expiration follows through relaxation of the diaphragm and the muscles between the ribs, plus the elastic recoil of the lungs.

Breathing is mainly an unconscious activity that is controlled by the brain, but you can take control of your own breathing to some degree. The depth and rate of breathing responds to the acidity of the blood, which, in turn, is a reflection of how much carbon dioxide it contains. This is detected by specialized cells within the brain and major arteries, which also detect oxygen concentration. You can force yourself to breathe slower or faster but you cannot will yourself to stop breathing, nor can you breathe rapidly for more than a few minutes without causing chemical changes in the acidity of the blood, which trigger the brain to take back control.

The human respiratory system is a very flexible one. Whereas at rest the lungs will be shifting 5–8 litres of air a minute they can increase this 20–30 fold to up to about 200 litres a minute.

Breathing disorders can arise in many different ways – some are caused by environmental problems – and they are extremely common in people of all ages.

Left: Within the myriad air sacs of the lungs, blood exchanges waste carbon dioxide for fresh oxygen.

COLDS

◆

A viral infection of the nose and upper airways.

CAUSES

◆

There are over 120 different viruses that may cause colds. The first time you meet such a virus it is likely to cause a cold because you have no natural immunity. This is why children get so many colds and adults, who have acquired immunity to some viruses, get far fewer. Even so, three or four a year is common. People in offices or areas with poor ventilation are more at risk because of their exposure to others with colds.

SYMPTOMS

◆

The first symptoms are a sore throat, a feeling of tiredness and aching muscles. You may have a fever, even though you feel cold and shivery. This lasts for two or three days, then the nose begins to run. You start sneezing and coughing and feel pretty miserable for two to three days. Most colds take seven to ten days from start to finish, although it is normal to cough for a week or two afterwards.

In children, complications often occur, especially **ear infection** with pain and perhaps a discharging ear, or a chest infection with coughing and wheezing. Adults can get these secondary infections, but far less often than children. More common in adults are inflamed sinuses, giving pain over the front of the face and a feeling of pressure above or below the eyes on bending forward.

TREATMENT

◆

In the early stages stay warm, take plenty of fluids (to relieve pain in the throat) and paracetamol to reduce temperature and aching. Adults can take aspirin if they prefer, but children under 12 should not have aspirin as it can cause Reye's syndrome, with convulsions and liver damage. Although Reye's syndrome is rare, it is usually fatal. Paracetamol (Calpol) is safe for children, or an alternative called ibuprofen.

Antibiotics are of no value at this stage. They usually make no difference to the illness and there is the chance of side effects, such as rashes, diarrhoea and thrush in the mouth or vagina. Only if you develop a complication such as a painful ear or a mild bronchitis might an antibiotic be advisable. Even then antibiotics hasten recovery only by a couple of days. Other helpful measures are taking aromatic sweets, which help unblock congested passages, and avoiding smoky or fume-filled atmospheres, which set off sneezing or coughing.

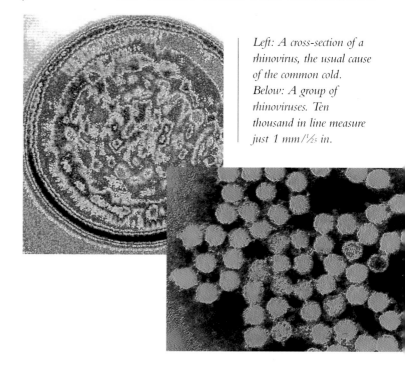

Left: A cross-section of a rhinovirus, the usual cause of the common cold. Below: A group of rhinoviruses. Ten thousand in line measure just 1 mm/¹⁄₂₅ in.

There are many cold cures available at the chemist. These contain a combination of a painkiller, such as paracetamol, and caffeine which gives a 'lift' to your spirits. Some contain a drug which narrows the blood vessels in the nose and thus relieves the runny nose for a few hours (this is also how nasal sprays for colds work). Remedies may also contain an antihistamine, which also relieves the stuffiness and helps you sleep. These remedies are helpful, but should only be used for a few days and only if they do not interact with any regular medication you are taking (your pharmacist will advise if in doubt).

The common cold is usually easily recognizable and does not need medical attention unless you or your child seem to be suffering more than you might expect.

  Complementary Treatment

Aromatherapy – see FLU. **Nutritional therapy** – at the first symptoms take a level teaspoon of pure vitamin C dissolved in water or juice. Repeat every two hours until symptoms subside, then tail off slowly, reducing the dosage and increasing the time interval between doses. If any bowel discomfort occurs, reduce the dosage. Continue to take vitamin C and a cod liver oil capsule daily as a preventive measure. *Other therapies to try: most have something to offer.*

FLU

A viral illness causing sweats, aches and high fever.

CAUSES

Flu, or influenza to be precise, is an infectious illness caused by a number of viruses. Every two or three years a new strain of flu virus emerges from the Far East, works its way across Asia and eventually arrives in Europe. There are always large numbers of otherwise healthy people who catch the illness simply by chance, especially those working or living in institutions, old age homes or offices, where the virus can spread easily. Vulnerable people, for example the elderly and people with chronic illnesses such as heart disease, **chronic bronchitis** and **diabetes**, do not catch the virus more easily but are much more prone to develop serious consequences from the infection such as **pneumonia**.

Unfortunately, resistance to any one strain of the flu virus is only short-lived; in addition, the virus changes from year to year which is why flu is an annual problem. About once every decade the virus becomes particularly aggressive for some reason and causes a serious epidemic.

SYMPTOMS

Flu typically begins abruptly with high **fever**, intense shivering and aching in all and any of the muscles. Backache is a common feature, as are headaches. There is usually a sore throat and often a cough develops after a couple of days. Unlike the common cold, there is no sneezing or running nose. However, in the early stages it can be impossible to decide whether someone is going down with flu or whether they are in the early stages of a common cold. Occasionally people deteriorate rapidly with a serious chest infection and confusion. For most people, however, the illness lasts for five to seven days and gradually goes. Post-flu tiredness is common and can last for several weeks after the original infection.

TREATMENT

Because flu is a viral illness there is no specific treatment that will cure the infection. Instead doctors concentrate on treating any complications that arise. These are most commonly chest infections, which would be treated with antibiotics. Otherwise the patient should stay warm and drink lots of fluids. Fever should be treated with aspirin (but not for children under 12 years old – see COLDS) or paracetamol. This also relieves the muscular aches and pains. In some cases

hospital treatment may be needed, for example if the patient is becoming dehydrated or has a serious chest complication. Flu vaccination is a good idea if you fall into one of the higher risk groups such as diabetics. The single vaccination is given in late autumn, in time to allow a build-up of immunity before the peak flu season, which is late December/January in the northern hemisphere. Vaccination is now offered to everyone over 65 because flu hits the elderly hardest and carries a risk of death in severe cases. Flu vaccination should also be considered by people working in institutions for the elderly and sick, where flu may spread very rapidly.

QUESTIONS

Why do I get flu several times a year?
You are probably getting a flu-like illness, with fever, aches and pains. Any viral illness causes these symptoms in the early stages. Many people call the common cold flu, which drives doctors to distraction. People are surprised at how much more severe true flu is.

Is flu vaccination harmful?
There is no serious risk associated with this vaccine. As it is made from egg protein anyone allergic to eggs must not have it. Also, as with any vaccine, it should not be given if you are already ill with another infection.

Is any other treatment helpful?
A drug called amantadine, originally used for Parkinson's disease, reduces the severity of flu. It is an under-used treatment. Vaccination against the bacterium pneumococcus gives long-term resistance to infection from this germ, which causes many of the complications of flu. Antiviral drugs that relieve flu are still controversial, but are likely to be available soon.

Complementary Treatment

Western herbalism – ginger and cinnamon tea will provide warmth; infusions of elderflower, yarrow and peppermint will help regulate temperature. The following **aromatherapy** oils are helpful: eucalyptus, cajeput, tea tree, sage, thyme. Use them as chest rubs (three drops to 10 ml of carrier oil), inhalations (two to four drops in a bowl of hot water or on a warm handkerchief) or in the bath (six drops). **Nutritional therapy** – see COLDS. *Other therapies to try: most have something to offer.*

CATARRH

Sticky mucus that builds up in the nose or throat.

CAUSES

Mucus is a natural product of the body and protects against infection by trapping germs. In the nose, throat and airways of the lungs there is an elegant system which produces a thin layer of mucus on those linings. The mucus is cleared from the lungs and sinuses by specialized cells with minute hairs which beat it away. When infection occurs, the lining responds by increasing its production of mucus; in addition it sends in large numbers of white cells to attack invading germs. This turns the normally clear mucus into mucus that is stained yellow or green by the debris of invaders and defenders and this is the discoloured mucus that people call catarrh when they cough it up, blow it out or feel it dripping down the back of their throat.

Some people complain that the flow of mucus is constant or is excessive, although what one person finds excessive is normal to another.

SYMPTOMS

Catarrh usually begins after a cold or cough. Those affected have to keep clearing their throat or blowing their nose and are aware of thick secretions at the back of the throat. They may lose their sense of smell and have bad breath and a nasal twang to their voice. There is often a dull ache in the front of the face over the sinuses. People with chronic catarrh lead their lives within reach of handkerchiefs and boxes of tissues.

TREATMENT

Mucus is a natural defence mechanism of the body and it is by no means necessary to have treatment for temporary increases in the flow of mucus where the body is simply doing its job. If the mucus is very heavy, persistent and yellow or green it is reasonable to have an antibiotic. The exact choice of antibiotic depends on where the catarrh is coming from. Decongestant sweets clear sinuses through their aromatic oils. Most cases of catarrh will settle naturally over a few weeks. For chronic cases the path is less straightforward. Doctors will search for chronic infection in the sinuses or lungs by taking X-rays and culturing the mucus to see if a specific antibiotic is required. A child with persistent mucus from one nostril may have pushed a toy up his nose; this can be found by inspection and is a satisfying diagnosis.

Catarrh is more common in smokers and those working in dusty atmospheres. Excessive alcohol and constant emotional stress also contribute to chronic catarrh by affecting the lining that secretes the mucus, causing overproduction. However, this leaves many people in whom no obvious cause can be found. Steroid nasal sprays can help by reducing swelling of the lining of the nose, as do antihistamines as given for hay fever. As a last resort an ENT (ear, nose and throat) specialist might cut out the mucus-secreting lining of the nose.

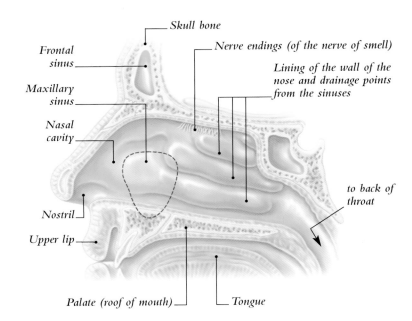

Frontal sinus — Skull bone — Nerve endings (of the nerve of smell) — Lining of the wall of the nose and drainage points from the sinuses — Maxillary sinus — Nasal cavity — to back of throat — Nostril — Upper lip — Palate (roof of mouth) — Tongue

Above: Catarrh comes from the lining of the nose and the sinuses, which drain into the nose. The quantity increases in response to infections and allergies.

Complementary Treatment

In **auricular therapy** mucus is held to be a by-product of a weak digestion, so the treatment aims to strengthen the function of both the digestive system and the lungs. In **aromatherapy** the following are excellent as inhalations (two to four drops in a bowl of hot water or on a handkerchief): cajeput, eucalyptus or ravensara. **Nutritional therapy** – recommends avoiding dairy produce for a week. **Ayurveda** offers nasal inhalations, alongside dietary advice.

CHRONIC BRONCHITIS AND EMPHYSEMA

Two closely related lung diseases, both associated with coughing, wheezing and breathlessness.

CAUSES

Underlying both of these common conditions is the chronic irritation of the lungs. This irritation is most often caused by cigarette smoke and its associated tars; other sources are air pollution, dust from industrial processes and coal mining. These irritating pollutants stimulate the lining of the small airways of the lungs to produce large quantities of mucus. Mucus is the sticky material that traps dust particles; specialized cells then sweep the mucus away from the narrowest parts of the lungs to the larger airways and ultimately the gullet, where the mucus can be swallowed or spat out.

Over time – meaning decades – the irritated lungs produce ever greater quantities of mucus, leading to a persistent cough. In addition, the airways narrow, leading to wheezing and breathlessness. In emphysema a further complication is that the tiny sacs at the ends of the lungs decay into large cavities. These are inefficient for gas exchange and add to the feeling of breathlessness.

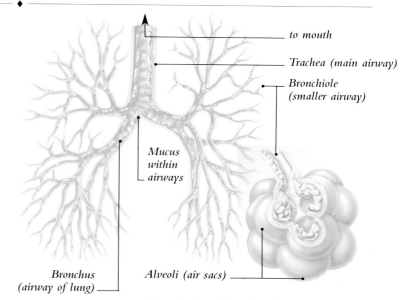

to mouth

Trachea (main airway)

Bronchiole (smaller airway)

Mucus within airways

Bronchus (airway of lung)

Alveoli (air sacs)

Above: In chronic bronchitis the airways of the lungs over-produce mucus. In emphysema, the alveoli break down into large cavities, where air stagnates.

SYMPTOMS

The earliest features of bronchitis are persistent cough and the constant bringing up of mucus. The cough gradually lasts longer until the individual is coughing all year round. **Colds** keep going to the chest, causing increased amounts of mucus and worsening breathlessness. People with emphysema have similar symptoms with, additionally, an over-inflated chest, giving a barrel-chested appearance. However, there is much overlap between bronchitis and emphysema and the exact diagnosis may not be clear without tests of lung efficiency. Eventually sufferers of both diseases can become constantly breathless even when walking a few steps and are effectively housebound. Severe cases also put a strain on the heart.

TREATMENT

At the earliest signs, it is essential to stop smoking and avoid irritating dusts. Although this will not repair the damage done, it reduces the chances of further deterioration. Medical treatment is with a gas inhaler, of which there are many types. These contain drugs called bronchodilators, which relax the muscles that otherwise tend to squeeze the already narrow airways even narrower. Those affected need to use these inhalers several times a day, often in combination. Examples of drugs used are terbutaline and salbutamol. Steroids given via inhalers are very helpful in reducing inflammation within the airways; the most commonly used is beclomethasone.

As well as being used in an inhaler, all these drugs can be given via a nebulizer, which produces a cloud of gas easily breathed in from a face mask. During flare-ups it may be necessary to take high doses of steroids by mouth.

Infections have to be treated aggressively with antibiotics because each infection can damage more of the lung. Many patients need to have oxygen available at home or in portable cylinders for when they go out. Very recently there has been interest in performing operations to remove the part of the lung damaged by emphysema, allowing the other parts to expand and so work more efficiently.

Complementary Treatment

A **Chinese herbalism** remedy would be *Quing Qi Hua Tan Wan* (clean air and transform phlegm). **Acupuncture** points for the lungs include Bladder 13 on the upper back and Lung 5 on the arm. **Nutritional therapy** – ensure your diet is rich in vitamin C and other nutrients. **Ayurveda** offers dietary advice and yoga breathing exercises. *Other therapies to try: auricular therapy; Alexander Technique.*

ASTHMA

◆

Wheezing and breathlessness caused by reversible narrowing of the airways in the lungs.

CAUSES

◆

For oxygen to enter the blood stream and carbon dioxide to leave it, blood has to come into close contact with inhaled air. Within the lungs this takes place in innumerable tiny sacs reached by ever narrower tubes. Here inhaled air passes over blood vessels and the exchange of gases takes place – the stale carbon dioxide passes out of the blood stream and oxygen passes in. The walls of these tubes contain muscle, which, if it contracts, squeezes the tube narrow and conversely lets it widen as it relaxes. In asthma, this muscle is abnormally sensitive and so the walls can be squeezed narrow unusually easily, thereby obstructing the free flow of air. Often, these small airways are also oversensitive to irritants in general, so asthmatics frequently also suffer from **hay fever** and **eczema**.

The easiest way to gauge this obstruction to airflow is called PEFR (peak expiratory flow rate). This is measured by blowing hard into a meter that shows how much air you can shift in litres per minute. This measurement is useful in deciding the diagnosis and in monitoring treatment.

Just why certain individuals are affected by asthma is not known. However, about 10–15% of children get asthma and a high percentage of adults, too. These numbers are increasing as a result, it is believed, of worsening air pollution as well as commonly found irritants such as cigarette smoke and the house dust mite. It may also be that mild asthma is now being recognized more readily by doctors.

SYMPTOMS

◆

During an asthmatic attack, people become increasingly wheezy and feel breathless; their rate of breathing rises and they literally have to force their lungs hard to get air in and out, which can be exhausting. An asthma attack is a dramatic event but fortunately is relatively rare as a first sign of asthma.

A common early symptom of asthma is a persistent cough with a little wheezing, especially during the night – frequently the first symptom in children. They may feel fine until they exert themselves, which brings on the wheezing. These symptoms are made worse by anything that irritates the lungs; this includes dust, fumes, emotional excitement, temperature changes, furry pets and pollen. Certain drugs can also bring on attacks in susceptible people, for example beta-blockers (for high blood pressure) and anti-inflammatory drugs.

In babies with asthma simple **colds** will always 'go to their chest' and any cough is complicated by accompanying wheeziness. If the baby also has eczema it is highly likely that the child is susceptible to these allergic ailments and will develop true asthma as he or she gets older.

There is often a period of uncertainty before the diagnosis is definite. The key to making the diagnosis is to show that the obstruction to airflow – the wheezing – can be reversed quickly by treatment. This is where the peak flow test is useful. During even mild asthma there will be a measurable reduction in peak flow. For example, an adult woman who should have a peak flow of around 550 litres per minute may achieve only 350 but after a couple of puffs of an inhaler the peak flow rises back to normal. Thus both the doctors and the individual can keep a record of how effective treatment is. It is frequently a question of trying out various antiasthmatic treatments to see how the individual responds.

TREATMENT

◆

The modern treatment of asthma has three strands. These are removing irritants, reducing the sensitivity of the lungs and treating acute problems.

Removing irritants

All asthmatics should stop smoking. It is more difficult to control household dust but measures can include fitting special bags to vacuum cleaners to filter dust and wiping surfaces frequently so dust does not build up. Many people worry about the house dust mite, an insect found in enormous quantities in even the cleanest home. Asthma is made worse by sensitivity to its droppings. It is impossible to eliminate these mites but regular cleaning helps and very sensitive individuals can cover pillows with polythene before placing them in pillowcases. Think carefully before you buy a furry pet as people with asthma may develop sensitivities to animals, especially cats, and it is hard to remove a much-loved pet.

Prevention

Preventive treatments consist mainly of inhaled steroid drugs, which have revolutionized the treatment of asthma in the last 20 years. They deliver very small quantities of steroids straight into the lungs, where they reduce the sensitivity of the lining of the lungs. Understandably, people worry about the side effects of steroids, such as weight gain, **diabetes** and poor growth. These are possible only where large quantities are taken by mouth over many months. Inhaled steroids are very

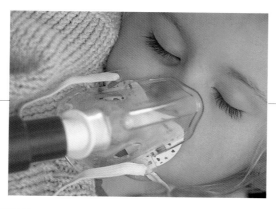

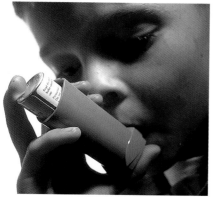

Above and left: Asthma treatment works best as a gas. Older children can handle self-triggered inhalers; young children need a mask.

safe and have not been shown to carry any significant risk. Drugs include beclomethasone and budesonide. There are many devices to deliver these drugs – all rely on producing a fine spray of gas to be breathed deep inside the lungs.

Cromoglycate is an alternative non-steroid preventive drug, very effective in some people. Again, it works by reducing the irritability of the linings of the lungs.

Acute treatment

Drugs called bronchodilators are used to treat acute attacks. They have a direct action on the muscles in the walls of the airways, forcing them to relax, allowing the airway to open up and so ease the flow of air. Drug names include salbutamol and terbutaline. These drugs are given by inhaler, injection, nebulized fine spray or tablet. Long-acting forms relieve night cough, such as salmeterol. New drugs called leukotrienes can further reduce symptoms in children and adults.

In severe attacks it is normal to add a steroid by mouth; this delivers a very high dose with the aim of reducing inflammation rapidly. Typically this would be given for five to ten days. Even young children can benefit from a short course of steroids during a severe attack.

In-hospital treatment might include oxygen and bronchodilating drugs given directly into the blood stream via a drip.

The most difficult to treat are young children, because their lungs do not respond to treatments in the same way as the lungs of older people. Even so, nebulized bronchodilators can help from about nine months of age. Syrups are also available.

Measuring the effectiveness of treatment

Treatment should allow the individual to follow a normal life, which includes exercise and sport. This may not be achieved in the most severe cases, but it is the goal for the great majority and if their treatment does not achieve this then it needs reviewing. Regular PEFR measurement helps show how good treatment is and also warns of any deterioration.

People with severe asthma may have to adjust their lives by giving up jobs involving dust or fumes and giving away pets.

QUESTIONS

Is allergy testing useful?
Generally it is not, because most asthmatics will prove to be sensitive to predictable things such as the house dust mite or pollen. It can be useful if asthma occurs in certain settings or is of recent severe onset, which suggests something very specific is responsible. Allergy testing might help establish whether or not to keep a pet.

Do people grow out of asthma?
A large percentage of mildly wheezy children grow out of it by late childhood. People who still have asthma by late childhood or who develop it as adults are likely to have it lifelong.

Complementary Treatment

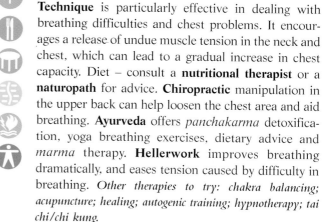

Do not abandon conventional approaches. **Chinese** and **Western herbalism** both offer herbs to reduce the oversensitivity of the airways – experienced practitioners will advise. **Homeopathy** can be extremely effective, but it is impossible to generalize about treatment, which depends on many variables. The **Alexander Technique** is particularly effective in dealing with breathing difficulties and chest problems. It encourages a release of undue muscle tension in the neck and chest, which can lead to a gradual increase in chest capacity. Diet – consult a **nutritional therapist** or a **naturopath** for advice. **Chiropractic** manipulation in the upper back can help loosen the chest area and aid breathing. **Ayurveda** offers *panchakarma* detoxification, yoga breathing exercises, dietary advice and *marma* therapy. **Hellerwork** improves breathing dramatically, and eases tension caused by difficulty in breathing. *Other therapies to try: chakra balancing; acupuncture; healing; autogenic training; hypnotherapy; tai chi/chi kung.*

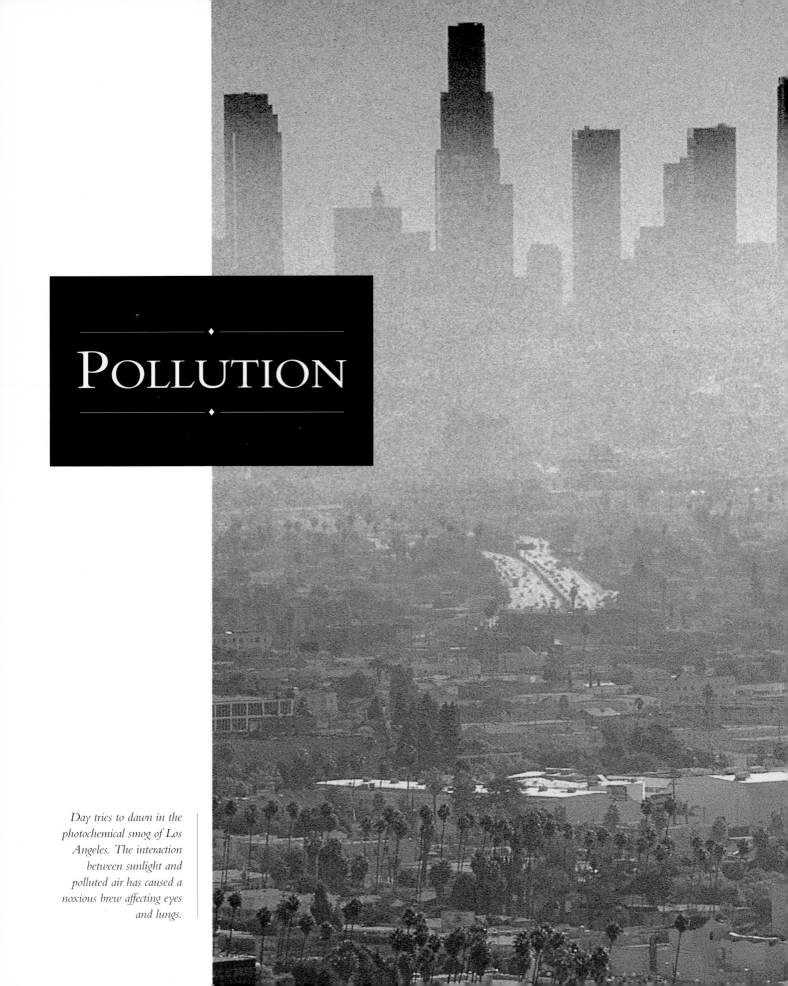

POLLUTION

Day tries to dawn in the photochemical smog of Los Angeles. The interaction between sunlight and polluted air has caused a noxious brew affecting eyes and lungs.

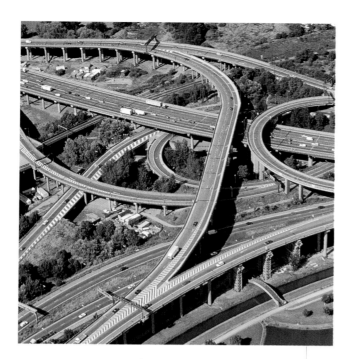

Above: Fumes from vehicles (shown here at a busy interchange in the United Kingdom) are potentially controllable causes of air pollution.

W HILE OUR HIGHLY INDUSTRIALIZED, technological society has many benefits in terms of advanced medical care, economic growth and improved living standards, the Earth is paying a price that is already impacting upon our lives and will do so even more in the future. The 200 years of the Industrial Revolution have introduced waste products of an unprecedented nature and scale that threaten the stability of the whole Earth's environment.

It was probably the photographs taken of the Earth from space that first made us realize that ours is really quite a small planet, limited in its capacity to absorb pollution. The composition of the whole atmosphere is endangered by destruction of the ozone layer, global warming and acid rain.

Ozone depletion

Ozone is a molecule of three oxygen atoms, formed by ultraviolet radiation splitting oxygen molecules in the upper atmosphere. The 'ozone layer' refers to a concentration of ozone in the stratosphere about 15–50 km/9–31 miles above the surface of the Earth. This is a beneficial shield protecting life from the damaging effect of ultraviolet radiation emitted by the sun. In contrast, the ozone formed lower down in the atmosphere by sunlight reacting with pollution such as that from car exhausts, industry and the burning of fossil fuels is harmful to animal and plant life.

It is believed that the ozone layer formed some 400 million years ago as plants emitted oxygen, a byproduct of photosynthesis, the conversion of carbon dioxide and water into organic chemicals. By reducing the intensity of ultraviolet radiation, the ozone layer allowed life to venture out safely on to dry land from the protective waters.

The ozone layer has always been affected by environmental influences such as volcanic eruptions and solar flares. Now there is evidence that it is being reduced by human activity, mainly by the use of chemicals called CFCs (chlorofluorocarbons) in refrigeration, solvents and aerosols.

What happens? Increased ultraviolet light multiplies the risk of **skin cancer**, **cataracts** and possibly genetic damage. It may damage micro-organisms, affecting fish populations and food production. However, much of this is still theory.

What can be done? In 1992 more than 70 countries signed the Montreal Protocol, an agreement that CFCs would be phased out. However, because they remain in the atmosphere for decades, it will be many years before regeneration of the ozone layer is possible; a reduction in the speed of its decline is the most that can be achieved in the short term.

Global warming

The temperature of the world has always fluctuated and has been a major factor driving evolution. The Earth's temperature depends largely on the insulating properties of the atmosphere and the balance between heat gained from the sun and heat lost by radiation from the earth. This balance is threatened by gases given off by industry, especially carbon dioxide, largely from burning coal and wood and from car exhausts; methane, from agriculture and rubbish tips; nitrous oxide, from burning coal and oil, and from nitrogen fertilizers; and CFCs.

What will happen? These gases trap more heat in the atmosphere leading, in theory, to global warming. The concentrations of these gases have risen as a consequence of the 100-fold increases in global energy use in the last 200 years. As the world emerged from the last ice age, global temperatures rose by about 5°C/9°F over several thousand years. Now, computer models used by the Intergovernmental Panel on Climate Change predict a rise in temperature of 1.5–4.5°C/2.7–8.1°F by the end of the 21st century – an astoundingly rapid and worrying rise. This rate of change is 2–5 times faster than that to which natural ecosystems are able to adapt.

It is believed that the result of global warming will be much more unstable weather, with more droughts, cyclones and floods, bringing increased susceptibility to disease and to heat-related deaths. Tropical diseases such as **malaria** may spread to previously temperate zones. Some low-lying islands may be lost altogether as polar icecaps melt and the sea levels rise.

What can be done? The way ahead is not at all clear. Experts do not agree whether global warming is a true phenomenon or just a temporary blip in climate. There is not any worldwide agreement on the threat, let alone coordinated action to counter it. Many developing countries continue to rely on coal and wood burning, while in the developed world people remain wedded to their cars. Scientists fear that these pollutant gases will actually increase as a consequence of escalating industrialization.

Acid rain

This phrase is not a new invention of the modern Green movement but was first used in the 1850s in Manchester. Acid rain is mostly from sulphur dioxide dissolved in water, forming sulphuric or sulphurous acid. Some is from nitrogen oxides, from vehicle exhausts. These gases are given off in vast quantities by industrial processes that burn wood or coal; the worldwide output into the atmosphere has increased from 7 million tons per annum in 1860 to over 150 million tons by the late 1980s.

What does it do? By increasing the acidity of rivers and lakes, acid rain kills fish, damages forests and so indirectly affects human wellbeing. However, studies so far show that drinking slightly acidified water appears not to have any direct effect on human health.

What can be done? Stringent environmental industrial controls in the developed world are reducing the output of sulphur dioxide gases, albeit slowly. However, these are still major pollutants in the developing world, especially in newly industrial countries such as China and India.

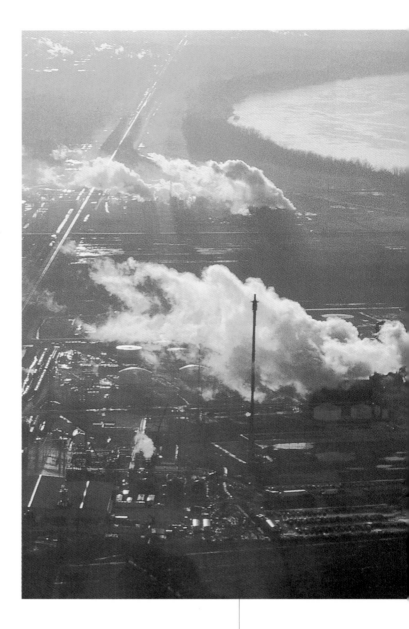

Above: Fumes drift from chemical plants in the United States. The developed countries have the technology to reduce such emissions, if they have the will.

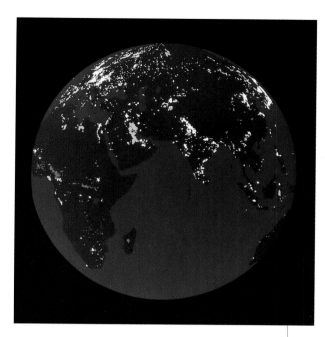

Above: Europe (upper left), Africa (lower left) and Asia (right) at night. City lights glow white, forest fires red, burning gas yellow.

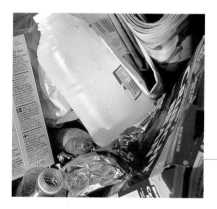

Left: Another day's trash: plastics, metal, chemicals, paper. Life is unimaginable without them, but becoming unbearable with such refuse.

Pollution – localized issues

Our economy depends on thousands of industrial processes using thousands of chemicals, many of which are toxic if they escape into the air, food and water.

Air Our air is contaminated by gases, dusts and tiny particles called particulates. It appears not so much that one single component causes damage, but rather a cocktail of pollutants if they are further degraded by ultraviolet light. This can cause photochemical smog, as in Los Angeles.

The effect on health of the output of a single factory or power station is hard to measure except in the case of unusual accidents, for example the release of toxic fumes at Bhopal in

India, which killed 2500 people in 1984. However, general atmospheric pollution is responsible for a great increase in **asthma**, chest conditions and eye irritation, particularly among children. Carbon monoxide is emitted by vehicles, cookers and heating devices; an excess causies headaches, drowsiness and even coma and death.

Lead pollution was much greater in previous centuries than now; output has more than halved in the last 25 years thanks to control of lead in petrol, paints, toys and plumbing. The effect of lead in the air is controversial but it does appear to reduce IQ in children. If eaten, lead can cause **anaemia**, abdominal pains and nausea.

Dust is another serious pollutant. Its effects are linked with asthma and chronic chest diseases such as **bronchitis**. There is increasing concern about dust produced by diesel fumes.

Water The negligent disposal of waste – chemical residues, pesticides and metals such as lead, copper and mercury – almost inevitably ends in pollution of rivers, lakes or seas, thereby reducing fish stocks and aquatic life in general. Specific examples of toxic effects on humans are harder to come by. The worst documented example was in Japan in the 1950s, where the discharge of mercury wastes into Minamata Bay was linked to hundreds of deaths and deformities.

Otherwise, evidence is more circumstantial, for example inhabitants of polluted areas of the former USSR have worse infant mortality, lower life expectancy and greater incidence of cancers, although socio-economic factors do complicate the picture.

Food From contamination of water it is a short step to the contamination of food, again with heavy metals such as lead, mercury and other organic compounds. It is hard to show examples of definite general harm except where a single food is involved. However, much current concern revolves around organophosphate pesticides, which may contaminate via air or skin, causing nausea, muscle weakness, breathing difficulty and **depression**.

The future

Many lessons have been learnt about the safe disposal of chemicals and control of industrial gases and dust, although the controls set in place are not totally effective. The biggest questions remain unanswered regarding the future of the ozone layer and global warming, the effects of which may transform climatic conditions in ways that still cannot be accurately predicted.

HAY FEVER

◆

For many a seasonal annoyance, for some a year-round nuisance. Also known as allergic rhinitis.

CAUSES
◆

Flowers, trees and grasses release pollen or spores in vast numbers. Each has its own protein fingerprint, which causes an allergic reaction in the nose, throat and lungs. They are called allergens – something that provokes allergy. Animals are another source of allergens, whether hairs or fragments of skin (dander). In hot weather, car fumes and pollution may combine to cause a chemical effect that irritates the eyes and noses of those who do not normally suffer from hay fever. Different people are sensitive to different allergens: some have a general hypersensitivity to all allergens and thus have symptoms all year round – termed perennial rhinitis.

SYMPTOMS
◆

The most common symptoms are itchy eyes and sneezing. The red eyes stream with tears; the nose runs. There is often a tickle in the throat. In severe cases the lungs are affected; there is a persistent cough or wheezing, like **asthma**.

There are all degrees of severity from mild nuisance to fighting a battle each summer against breathlessness and discomfort. Fortunately, there is a tendency to grow out of hay fever during adult life. After years of hay fever one nostril may feel constantly blocked. This may be due to a polyp, which is a harmless fleshy growth that can be surgically removed.

TREATMENT
◆

A selection of modern remedies is available for hay fever. Antihistamines are, for most people, the mainstay of treatment. They reduce the severity of the allergic response and a single tablet helps all the symptoms. Modern antihistamines such as astemizole or loratidine are taken just once or twice a day and rarely cause the drowsiness which the older types do. They are available in liquid form suitable for children.

Antiallergy eye drops contain substances that block the allergic response, for example cromoglycate. Extremely safe, they have to be applied several times a day for full effect.

Nasal sprays contain either low doses of steroids, for example beclomethasone, or the same antiallergy substances used in eye drops. They are safe for long-term use because the steroids are absorbed within the nose itself and only negligible amounts are absorbed into the body as a whole. Nevertheless,

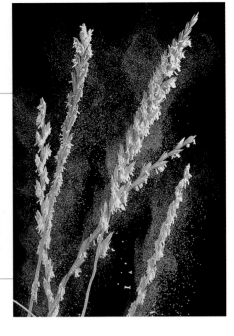

Right: The swirling clouds of pollen that surround even a few ears of rye grass.

do not be tempted to exceed the recommended dose. The whole range of drugs used in asthma may also be used in severe hay fever, for example steroid sprays and substances to dilate the airways such as salbutamol and cromoglycate.

General measures and surgery

To reduce the impact of hay fever avoid bright sunlight; drive with car windows closed and try to keep windows at home shut in the heat of the day. Avoid animals you know you react against. While inconvenient, these measures are unavoidable if symptoms are not fully controlled by other methods.

Surgery is a possibility for those who are not helped by standard remedies. The lining of the nose is removed, relieving the persistent stuffiness and discharge.

Desensitization and allergy testing

In practice allergy testing is rarely useful (see ASTHMA).

Desensitization is done by giving stronger and stronger injections of whatever the individual is allergic to. There is a risk of provoking a serious allergic response, sudden collapse or even death, however, so it is no longer recommended, except in specialized clinics with full resuscitation facilities.

Complementary Treatment

Bach flower remedies – Rescue Remedy and crab apple diluted in water to bathe sore eyes. **Shiatsu-do** can help reduce sensitivity to allergens. Diet – allergy to food and to pollen may be linked; consult a **nutritional therapist** or a **naturopath** for advice. **Hypnotherapy** can be used in conjunction with a desensitizing programme. *Other therapies to try: Chinese and Western herbalism; tai chi/chi kung; chakra balancing; healing; homeopathy.*

PNEUMONIA

A chest infection involving the whole of one lobe of a lung.

CAUSES

Pneumonia can be caused by any of the bacteria or viruses that cause milder chest infections. These infections usually cause mild inflammation of both lungs. Pneumonia occurs when the infection is concentrated in one lobe of the lung, which carries a higher risk of complications. Pneumonia is common in the elderly, in patients following operations and in people who are run down for other reasons.

SYMPTOMS

At first the symptoms of pneumonia are non-specific – a **fever**, feeling cold and a cough. These symptoms then rapidly worsen with high fever, shivering, a harsh cough and aching over the affected part of the chest. Phlegm may contain blood streaks. In the elderly, pneumonia is often less dramatic. On examination the doctor hears characteristic noises over one section of the lung. Occasionally, a number of germs cause pneumonia in younger people but they do not manifest the classic symptoms; instead there is just a vague feeling of ill health, sweating and a mild cough. These germs include mycoplasma and legionella.

TREATMENT

Most cases respond to high doses of an antibiotic, rest and recuperation. Hospital admission might be needed in severe cases, especially if the individual cannot take antibiotics by mouth and needs a drip. Chest X-rays taken afterwards check for complete recovery of the lung and see if there is any underlying lung problem that allowed pneumonia to set in.

Pneumonia has some possible complications. Often fluid accumulates at the base of one lung, called a pleural effusion, and can take several weeks to go. An abscess may form in the lung, although modern antibiotics have made this a rare event.

Complementary Treatment
There is no substitute for antibiotics. **Chakra balancing** reduces pain and loosens sputum. **Naturopathy** – large dosages of vitamin C can shorten recovery time. The **Alexander Technique** can help after recovery.

PLEURISY

A knife-like chest pain, worse when breathing deeply.

CAUSES

The pleura are thin layers of tissue forming an insulating layer between the lungs and the chest wall. Pleurisy is inflammation of the pleura. The most common cause is infection of the lung, which spreads to the adjacent pleura; this often happens with **pneumonia** but can accompany even a minor chest infection. Sometimes the pleura become inflamed without other lung disease.

SYMPTOMS

Pleurisy gives rise to a sharp pain in the chest, which feels like a knife sticking into the side. The pain is worse on breathing in as this stretches the pleura. There may be a cough and **fever**, too, if there is a lung infection. On listening to the lungs through a stethoscope, the doctor may be able to hear a characteristic creaking sound over the area of pleurisy as the patient breathes in, which is called a rub. Pleurisy itself is not dangerous but pleurisy associated with pain in the calf or with coughing blood could mean **pulmonary embolism**, which is dangerous.

TREATMENT

All cases benefit from painkillers; the best type is an anti-inflammatory such as ibuprofen. As well as letting you feel more comfortable, painkillers allow you to breathe deeply, which is important in getting over a chest infection. If there are signs of infection, then you will need an antibiotic. Pleurisy settles over a few days.

Complementary Treatment
Chakra balancing reduces pain, relaxes the whole body, including the thorax, and loosens sputum. The **Alexander Technique** can help after recovery. Diet is important for prevention – a **nutritional therapist** will be able to advise you on this.

LUNG CANCER

A common tumour that grows within the airways of the lungs.

CAUSES

The evidence is overwhelming that the main cause of lung cancer is cigarette smoking. Cigarette smoke contains hundreds of different components and tars, so just which component is actually to blame is unclear. None the less, reputable research has shown beyond all reasonable doubt that the more cigarettes people smoke and the longer they smoke, the higher their chances are of getting lung cancer. The chances become even higher if the individual is also exposed to other irritant atmospheres such as coal mining or to asbestos. It appears that constant exposure to these substances irritates the lining of the main breathing tubes (bronchi), eventually turning cells malignant.

About 15% of cases of lung cancer occur in non-smokers, a percentage of which can be attributed to passive exposure to cigarette smoke.

SYMPTOMS

Most cases begin in an undramatic way as a persistent cough or with dull aching over part of the chest. Other suspicious features are coughing up blood and recurrent chest infections that are slow to improve. As the disease progresses there may be other features of cancer, for example weight loss, a vague feeling of ill health or loss of appetite. Lung cancer commonly spreads elsewhere in the body and so can produce symptoms in bone (with pain), within the brain (epileptic fits, confusion) and the liver (jaundice). When faced with such symptoms in smokers doctors will think immediately of lung cancer and order a chest X-ray.

If the X-ray shows a tumour, the diagnosis has to be checked by obtaining a sample of it. This is commonly done by a technique called a bronchoscopy (see page 355) where a flexible fibreoptic tube is guided to the tumour so that a sample can be taken for analysis.

TREATMENT

Unfortunately, lung cancer can rarely be cured. However, it is possible to give worthwhile relief by cutting out the affected part of the lung. Also, radiotherapy (see page 370) will shrink the tumour for a while, so relieving a cough or breathlessness. Radiotherapy is also used in treating the spread from the tumour, for example secondary cancer in the brain or in bone.

There have been many attempts at developing chemotherapy (see page 371) for lung cancer but so far without finding a cure. At present chemotherapy may halt progress of the disease by about a year at the cost of side effects such as nausea and hair loss.

Why wait to get lung cancer? Stopping smoking results in a steady reduction in risk; even two years after quitting the risks of getting lung cancer are much lower and carry on falling for many years thereafter.

QUESTIONS

Why don't all smokers get lung cancer?
Not all mountaineers fall, but if you're not a mountaineer you can't fall off a mountain . . . Smokers often comfort themselves by arguing that many smokers do not get lung cancer. About 25% of all smokers will die from a disease caused by smoking, be it heart disease, chronic bronchitis or lung cancer.

Is there any way of screening for lung cancer?
Not as yet. Trials have shown that while regular X-ray screening will detect early cancers it does not improve survival. It is important to report to your doctor any of the early symptoms mentioned previously.

Are low-tar cigarettes safer?
They are. Part of the fall in the numbers of cases of lung cancer in men in recent years is thought to be due to a switch to these types of cigarettes, athough there is always the danger that smokers who switch to low-tar cigarettes will compensate by inhaling more deeply. Low tar is safer, but it is not safe.

Complementary Treatment

Complementary therapies cannot cure cancer, and they should be used only alongside conventional approaches; in this way they can offer much support. **Chakra balancing** is a deep relaxation technique, which will help with symptom control and energy balance. **Hypnotherapy** can help you visualize your tumour being attacked by drugs. **Aromatherapy**, especially combined with gentle **massage**, is excellent for reducing the stress and tension of coping with cancer. **Reflexology** can encourage a positive attitude during treatment. *Other therapies to try: see STRESS.*

PULMONARY EMBOLISM

The dangerous condition of a blood clot lodging in the lungs.

CAUSES

Pulmonary embolism poses a risk after major surgery and in individuals who are bed-bound with illnesses such as a **heart attack**, **stroke** or **pneumonia**. It is an important cause of post-operative illness and much research has gone into trying to reduce the risks after surgery.

The problem begins when blood clots within the veins in the calves and thighs. This is the condition of a **deep vein thrombosis**. Fortunately, most of the clots remain within the leg. However, there is a risk that a portion of the blood clot, called an embolus, might become detached and be carried off in the bloodstream to the lungs. The clot then becomes stuck in the blood vessels, causing the symptoms below.

For unknown reasons the risk of pulmonary embolism is higher with certain general illness, especially cancer. This is probably due to some effect that makes blood clot abnormally easily. There is also a very small increased risk of pulmonary embolism in women taking oestrogen in the contraceptive pill or hormone replacement therapy (HRT). The risk depends on the type of pill; those containing hormones called gestodene or desogestrel pose a higher risk. Recent research suggests the period of highest risk from HRT is in the first year of treatment.

SYMPTOMS

There may be the symptoms of a deep vein thrombosis, for example a painful swollen calf, but often there is no warning and the legs appear normal. A small embolus may cause **pleurisy** or slight breathlessness. Doctors will consider a pulmonary embolus if these symptoms occur after a high-risk procedure such as hip replacement or in someone who has just had a heart attack or been bed-bound for some reason.

A large pulmonary embolus blocks off a major portion of one lung, with resulting sudden severe breathlessness, faintness, chest pain and often coughing of blood.

An embolus can also be detected by the absence of sounds over part of the lung and changes on the ECG (an electrical recording of the heart). Ordinary chest X-rays are not especially helpful in making the diagnosis. It is better to have a lung scan. Here a radioactive injection is given, which should spread evenly through the lungs (see page 352). Failure to spread suggests a large embolus.

If the embolus is big enough it will completely block blood flow through the lungs, resulting in sudden death.

TREATMENT

Treatment aims to reduce the risk of abnormal blood clotting after surgery and to prevent a deep vein thrombosis. One way to reduce the chances of thrombosis is for the patient to wear compression stockings during surgery. Drugs, for example heparin, are given to make the blood less likely to clot. If there has been a small embolus, therapy is started with heparin by injection or warfarin by mouth.

Treatment of a large clot can be successful if immediate skilled chest surgery is available to remove the blood clot from the blood vessels of the lungs. This is only possible in a few centres, which emphasizes how important it is to reduce the risks in the first place.

QUESTIONS

How can I reduce my risks of pulmonary embolism?
If you need surgery, see what steps the hospital takes to reduce risk. This might include wearing compression stockings and being given heparin during surgery. Start walking as soon as possible after surgery, a heart attack or stroke. Stop smoking and stop taking the contraceptive pill before major surgery.

What risk of pulmonary embolus does the contraceptive pill carry?
About double the natural risk – less than a one in a hundred thousand chance per annum. This is still less than the health risks from pregnancy.

Can a pulmonary embolism recur?
There is an increased risk in anyone who has had one before. Frequent emboli may result from unusual auto-immune disorders, a source of blood clots within the heart or a hidden cancer.

    ### Complementary Treatment

This is a medical emergency and needs urgent treatment in hospital. Postoperatively, a number of complementary therapies can help the body to heal, for example **chakra balancing**. **Yoga** and **tai chi/chi kung** are gentle forms of exercise which could help after recovery. Diet – to prevent recurrence, a **nutritional therapist** would probably recommend you switch to a diet rich in fish oils and take supplements of vitamin E and garlic.

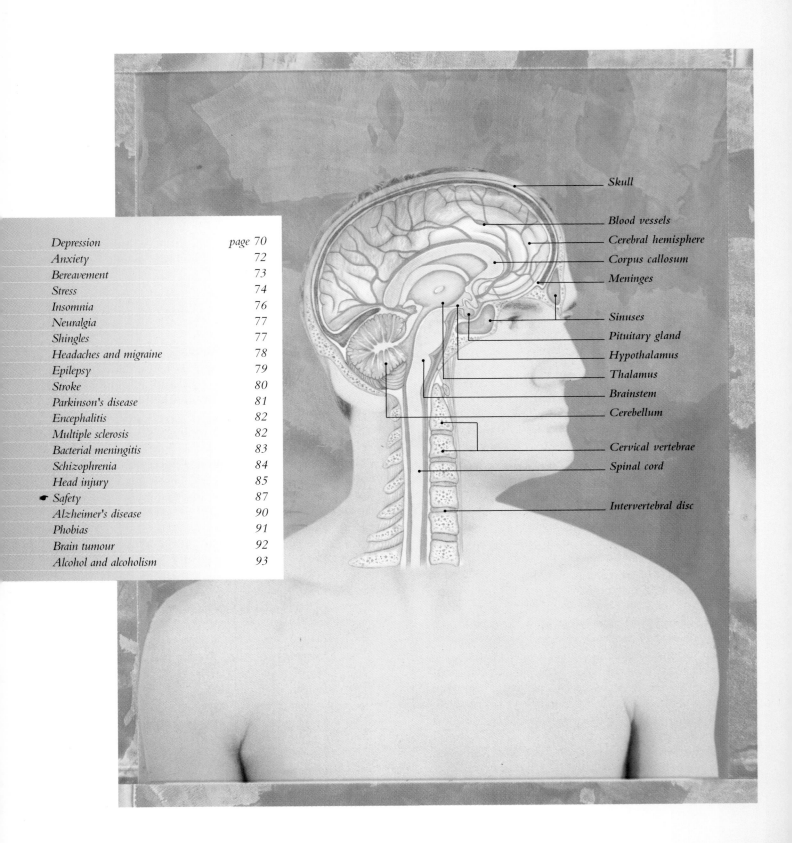

Skull

Blood vessels

Cerebral hemisphere

Corpus callosum

Meninges

Sinuses

Pituitary gland

Hypothalamus

Thalamus

Brainstem

Cerebellum

Cervical vertebrae

Spinal cord

Intervertebral disc

Next time you use your personal computer, spare a thought for the amazing components within your skull. Always 'on-line', it needs no plug and runs on sugar.

MIND, BRAIN AND NERVOUS SYSTEM

THE BRAIN HAS TWO halves (hemispheres) and is a structure of some hundred thousand million nerve cells, supported by billions of additional cells. Each nerve cell, or neurone, has a thin extension called an axon, along which electrical signals pass. Axons of nerve cells within the brain can be just a fraction of a millimetre long, whereas the nerve cells in the spinal cord that control the muscles of the legs have axons 1 m/3¼ ft long. Each axon makes contact with thousands of other neurones at junctions called synapses. The electrical signal cannot jump this synapse; instead the signal is normally carried by chemicals called neurotransmitters to the next cell, setting off an electrical signal for further transmission.

Somewhere within this dance of electrochemical interconnections are the fountains of memory, thought, foresight, emotion, imagination, speech and activity. Although our vocal cords make sound it is the brain that gives speech meaning; although muscles score a goal, control is within the head; and the most agile fingers are only channels through which the brain expresses itself. It is possible to locate quite precisely the parts of the brain that control these activities. However, the location within the brain of personality, consciousness and all the things we call 'higher human functions' is still a mystery.

Much is known about the anatomy and chemistry of the brain; there are many specialized areas responsible for definite activities such as speech or controlling temperature and breathing. Surrounding these areas there are millions of less specialized cells that seem to relate to the function in a diffused way. For this reason it is possible to injure large parts of the brain with little apparent effect on function; conversely there are some areas so critical that damage to just a few square millimetres causes paralysis, arrests breathing or destroys speech.

Messages and signals

Messages get into the brain through the sense organs. The well-known ones are, of course, vision, touch, hearing, smell and taste. However, there are many other less obvious senses, too: detectors in the aorta tell how much oxygen is in the blood, the cells in the brain stem monitor carbon dioxide concentrations in the blood and messages from the inner ear to the cerebellum enable it to maintain balance.

Signals leave the brain via nerves that end in muscles or glands; hence we speak and move, and also regulate body temperature, appetite and thirst. These pathways leave via the spinal cord and via special nerves called the cranial nerves to the structures around the face.

Hard at work

The brain works flat out and demands a staggering percentage of the body's total energy. Twenty per cent of the heart's output goes to the brain. Even brief interruptions in blood flow lead to confusion or unconsciousness, as does a lack of sugar, the fuel of the brain.

Brain diseases are most commonly the result of problems with blood flow (clots or bleeds), tumours or brain cell degeneration. Head injuries are a major cause of disability in all communities.

Left: The brain's electrical networks control and interpret movement, the senses, speech, thought and imagination.

DEPRESSION

◆

A feeling of sadness that can range from occasional low spirits to constant and overpowering despair.

CAUSES

◆

Depression is commonly a natural response of the individual to life, with its disappointments, relationship problems and stresses, for example serious illness, **bereavement**, divorce or money worries. Psychiatrists call this type reactive depression and, in general, both the reason and the degree of depression are understandable to an onlooker sharing the same culture.

Biochemical reasons

Depression beyond these understandable limits is thought to have a largely biochemical cause. Within the brain, nerves communicate by means of biochemical messengers called neurotransmitters. There are hundreds of types, several of which are thought to be linked to moderate and severe depression – these include noradrenaline, dopamine and serotonin.

Depression considered mainly biochemical in origin is called endogenous or psychotic depression. There is no hard cut off between endogenous and reactive types of depression; rather they merge into each other and overlap, although extremes of each type are clearly of a different order of magnitude.

Other causes

Depression is sometimes the expression of an underlying problem – commonly alcoholism (see ALCOHOL AND ALCOHOLISM). The elderly, especially if suffering from early dementia, become depressed probably in reaction to awareness of their deteriorating health and memory. Depression after childbirth affects up to 20% of women and can fast become very severe. Depression in young people can occur because of early **schizophrenia**, where the individual is struggling to cope with disordered thought. Rarely, depression can result from brain disease, although there are usually additional features more specific to brain disease, such as paralysis or **epilepsy**.

Depression runs in families, as do other serious psychological illnesses such as schizophrenia. The close relatives of severe depressives are therefore two or three times more likely to become severely depressed than the general population.

SYMPTOMS

◆

Depressed individuals get no enjoyment out of life; they feel sad and may tell others how sad they feel. They dwell on the things that go wrong at the exclusion of things going right. As depression deepens they cry more easily and are increasingly preoccupied by thoughts of death, decay or bad events. They suffer sleep disturbance and often wake in the early hours of the morning, worrying (see INSOMNIA). This is the common pattern of reactive depression of one degree or other.

If symptoms go beyond this point, the depression is more endogenous in nature. Often great agitation accompanies the depression while some sufferers become withdrawn and apathetic. Eventually, they think of suicide or even attempt it. In the most depressed state, the individual may end up mute and unresponsive, shut away in a world where they feel themselves rotting from within and where suicide is not awful but a logical release. Clearly such profound psychotic depression goes way beyond our normal experience of depression, and is not something out of which one can 'pull oneself together'.

Physical symptoms and investigations

Beyond the recognizable look of sadness, severely depressed people neglect themselves and lose their appetite. Often they suffer from constipation and complain of generalized pains for which no physical cause can be found. Except in the most obvious cases, doctors will do a physical examination and basic blood tests. The conditions most often confused with depression are an underactive thyroid gland (see THYROID PROBLEMS) and, much less commonly, brain disease such as a **brain tumour** or dementia. An underlying cause may be discovered, such as alcohol abuse, which needs specific handling.

TREATMENT

◆

It is common human experience that sharing problems is comforting. Psychological treatment of depression is based on this, although the actual theories may vary. The best known, psychoanalysis, holds that many psychological problems are the result of unconscious conflicts between repressed desires, conflicts influenced in turn by childhood experiences. Psychoanalysis aims to uncover and come to terms with conflicts, and can take years of therapy.

Classic psychoanalysis is too time-consuming for most people and so is less available than counselling, of which there are many varieties with differing theoretical frameworks. Counselling lets people talk about what underlies their depression (or many other emotions), while the counsellor gently tries to guide their thoughts towards a positive outcome. Counselling does not have to be given by a professional to be effective and there are undoubtedly people who are naturally 'good listeners', who can help others simply by psychological

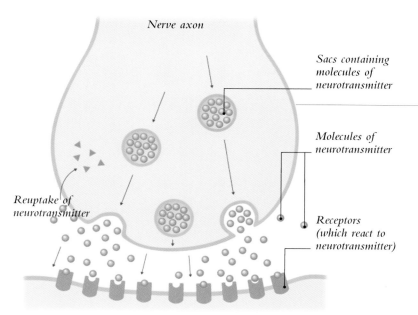

Nerve axon

Sacs containing molecules of neurotransmitter

Molecules of neurotransmitter

Reuptake of neurotransmitter

Receptors (which react to neurotransmitter)

Above: A synapse – where nerves meet, chemical transmitters relay electrical activity from nerve to nerve.

support, although it is difficult to prove this scientifically. Psychological approaches are most useful in mild to moderate depression, which appears to be a reaction to sad life events but where the individual can still cope with life.

Drug therapy

Serious depression that is long lasting or profound needs treatment in addition to psychological support. It is a dangerous condition since 5–10% of sufferers will attempt suicide. (This is why everyone treating them has to be constantly judging the risks and deciding if they should be referred to a psychiatric unit – for enforced treatment if necessary.) Drug treatment reduces depression and this suicide risk rapidly. It also brings the individual to a point at which he can look more rationally at his problems and so get more out of psychological support. Drug treatment is continued for six to twelve months on average.

It is controversial whether antidepressants are of any benefit for people with mild depression but psychiatrists increasingly believe that they are useful in people whose depression, although mild to an outsider, is significantly affecting their quality of life.

Tricyclic antidepressants used to be the drugs most widely used. They work by altering the levels of neurotransmitters in the brain, taking two to three weeks to do so. Drug names include imipramine, amitriptyline and dothiepin.

Each drug varies a little in its type of action and side effects, but they all share the common side effects of drowsiness, dry mouth, blurred vision and, in overdose, dangerous heart rhythm irregularities. The danger of overdose is critical, because of the constant risk that a depressed person may attempt suicide. Nevertheless, tricyclic drugs remain extremely useful and effective in treating serious depression.

SSRIs (selective serotonin reuptake inhibitors) are increasingly popular. The name refers to levels of a neurotransmitter in the brain – serotonin. These drugs have fewer side effects and, crucially, are much safer in overdose than tricyclics and are therefore used for anyone posing a serious suicide risk. As they do not generally cause drowsiness they are useful in treating people who are working or having to cope with family responsibilities. Drug names include fluoxetine and paroxetine. New classes of antidepressants such as venlafaxine combine the benefits of SSRIs and tricyclic antidepressants.

Other treatments

There are many other drugs for selected cases. In particular, lithium is useful for people who swing between depression and excitement – bipolar affective disorder (manic depressive psychosis). Electroconvulsive therapy (ECT) is a controversial option for the most severe and resistant cases of depression where there is a major suicide risk. For some reason, passing a high voltage across the brain cures depression, so ECT may be the only therapy left for someone in the deepest depression.

     ## Complementary Treatment

Western herbalism – St John's wort can be helpful for mild depression. **Bach flower remedies** – try mustard if the depression comes for no apparent reason, gentian if you know the cause, gorse for a sense of hopelessness, sweet chestnut for utter despair, willow for bitterness and self-pity. **Art, dance movement, drama or music therapists** can help you become aware of the underlying unconscious causes by enabling you to express feelings through the arts. Greater understanding leads to improved self-esteem and motivation. **Shiatsu-do** calms the nervous system and has positive benefits on the emotions. Useful **aromatherapy** oils include neroli, rose, jasmine and bergamot. Use as inhalations (two to four drops in a bowl of hot water, or on a handkerchief) or in the bath (six drops). **Nutritional therapy** – try supplementing B vitamins. *Other therapies to try: healing; cymatics; yoga; hypnotherapy; tai chi/chi kung; acupuncture; auricular therapy; Alexander Technique; homeopathy; Ayurveda; chakra balancing; autogenic training; biodynamics.*

ANXIETY

A feeling of generalized worry and apprehension out of proportion to the objective stresses in someone's life.

CAUSES

Humanity is distinguished by its capacity for thought. With thought comes imagination, with imagination comes apprehension and with apprehension comes anxiety. It is normal for human beings to try to look ahead and to plan for that which has yet to happen, or to try to work out how to deal with an immediate problem. Until the problem is resolved there will be a feeling of tension mingled with worry – the 'what if' or 'suppose that' feeling. This we recognize as anxiety; a mild degree is a part of normal existence and may be helpful as a stimulus to action.

Abnormal anxiety – anxiety that dominates thought – happens to ordinary people who find themselves in constantly stressful environments. It may also happen to those who develop **depression** or who are faced with such an array of stressful events that they see no way out of the situation. Severe anxiety is a debilitating, destructive emotion and is in no way simply an inability to cope. Illnesses which can mimic anxiety are thyrotoxicosis (see THYROID PROBLEMS) and depression.

SYMPTOMS

Mild anxiety leads to preoccupation with the problem at hand; there may be disturbed sleep and an inability to relax but on the whole the individual still copes with life. As anxiety gets more severe, however, it starts to interfere with normal activity. The mind cannot be turned to rational thought and it becomes ever more difficult to cope with day-to-day responsibilities, which become neglected. There may be irritability and a short temper. The person might turn to drink or drugs to relieve the anxiety.

In even more severe cases there is a constant tremor of the hands, crying and a complete inability to think normally.

TREATMENT

The mild anxieties of life generally resolve with time and thought. Support from outsiders is helpful in guiding the individual to a solution of her immediate problems. More severe anxiety, by blocking productive thought, feeds on itself. Here tranquillizers are helpful if only to allow the individual to start thinking productively about her problems. Useful drugs are the benzodiazepines (diazepam, lorazepam). These give

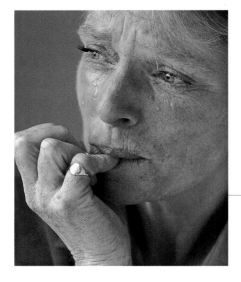

Left: Mild anxiety is common in everyday life. Severe anxiety is harmful, interfering with normal activity and leading to physical and psychological problems.

immediate relief but there is a risk of addiction if taken on a regular basis for more than a few weeks – not in the sense of craving more, but from the withdrawal effects of increased anxiety and tremors, among others.

Beta-blockers, which in much higher dosage are used to treat high blood pressure, are good for reducing tremor and relieving the vague sense of being on edge. These are not addictive and can be taken as needed. Stronger again, there are major sedatives such as chlorpromazine and antidepressants such as amitriptyline.

Many doctors recommend trying relaxation techniques, learning how to structure your day and avoiding drugs or alcohol for relief. Changes that can be made to your life or work should, of course, be followed up, especially as excessive stress on employees is coming to be seen as something that employers have a legal responsibility to control.

Complementary Treatment

Bach flower remedies – the remedy depends on the cause, for example red chestnut for anxiety about loved ones. **Acupuncture** – see STRESS. **Arts therapies** help you become aware of the unconscious causes of anxiety by enabling you to express your feelings through dance, art, music or drama. Gaining insight with the therapist's help can enable you to feel emotionally stronger. **Aromatherapy** – see DEPRESSION. **Nutritional therapy** – try supplementing B vitamins, magnesium and calcium. **Hypnotherapy** changes unwanted patterns of behaviour produced by anxiety. *Other therapies to try: most have something to offer.*

BEREAVEMENT

The loss of a close relative or friend, which has an emotional impact and can lead to months or even years of mourning.

CAUSES

Bereavement usually means loss through death but the same reaction can follow divorce or the disappearance of a friend or relative, the permanent loss of someone who was central in the lives of others. It does not matter whether the person was deeply loved or not; simply to lose someone whom you were used to living with can be enough to provoke problems.

It was really only in the 20th century and in the developed world that bereavement became a relatively unusual event. This is because the illnesses that used to cause high child mortality and poor life expectancy have been greatly reduced. Whereas even 75 years ago most people would have come across early deaths almost routinely, now death occurs mainly among the elderly. This means that the first bereavement experienced at close hand could be the death of a parent when the son or daughter is themself well into middle age.

Ironically, we are surrounded by death in newspapers and films and on television but these are absolutely no preparation for the reality of the death of someone close to us.

SYMPTOMS

There are three well-recognized phases to bereavement. Initially, there is often disbelief, especially if the death is unexpected. Although the person may have been ill and expected to die, the actual event comes as a psychological blow which we seek to reject. This phase lasts a day or two.

Frequently, there then follows a reaction of anger mingled with bewilderment. Questions tumble out. Why this person? Why now? Why in this way? The circumstances are picked over. Were they on the right treatment? Could this have been prevented? If they had taken a different route would they have avoided an accident? This phase can last many weeks and may never be entirely resolved.

Most bereaved people eventually reach the third stage of acceptance and reconciliation; things get back into context: the elderly do die, accidents do happen, tragedies do occur.

TREATMENT

Bereavement rarely needs medical treatment except, possibly, the short-term help provided by sedatives or sleeping tablets. Even medication such as this is probably best avoided for

what, after all, is a fundamental human experience. Someone experiencing profound sadness that lasts for longer than a few weeks may be slipping into a depressive illness, especially if there are other symptoms of **depression** such as disturbed sleep, self-neglect and morbid thoughts. In these cases an antidepressant is often helpful.

Prolonged grieving can suggest unresolved emotions towards the person who has died. One of the most common emotions is guilt for something that had not been sorted out by the time of death – 'unfinished business' as it were. These feelings, which are actually very common, are best handled by specialized counselling.

QUESTIONS

What assists mourning and acceptance?
The process of mourning should include recalling as much as possible of the relationship, difficult memories as well as happy ones. This way each emotion can be dealt with and not left to engender guilt or resentment.

How can friends and relatives help?
Their immediate support is essential, especially in handling the administrative matters. They can help guide mourners through the process of remembering, putting an emphasis on the best memories. After the funeral they should keep in touch regularly because that is when grief can grow.

Should children be told about a death?
They will find out eventually so why conceal things? Young children, below eight years old or so, will not take it in, unless by relating the emotions to those they felt on, for example, the death of a pet. Older children follow the same pattern of mourning as adults but will need more help to express their emotions.

Complementary Treatment

Bach flower remedies – star of Bethlehem for the shock and grief of sudden loss, sweet chestnut for utter dejection, pine to relieve feelings of guilt, willow if there is inclination to bitterness. **Acupuncture** – see STRESS. **Aromatherapy** – see DEPRESSION. **Autogenic training** is a self-administered psychotherapy that can help. *Other therapies to try: yoga; hypnotherapy; tai chi/chi kung; biodynamics; healing; shiatsu-do; auricular therapy; homeopathy; massage; chakra balancing.*

STRESS

◆

A form of pressure that leads to the associated psychological feelings of tension and anxiety.

CAUSES

◆

It might be said that everyday life is all about stress: the stress of dealing with family; the stresses of personal growth and development; stresses of study, of job finding and job keeping. In the modern developed world the most primeval sources of stress are usually taken care of, that is, the stresses of finding food, shelter and security. Far from this fact relieving stress, we find other things to get stressed about. It might not be immediately clear what is stressful about having to wear up-to-date fashions, but millions of people find it so. Nor is it clear why, having a superabundance of food in the local supermarket, the act of going there to shop should provoke stress; but it does, and so on.

These might seem frivolous examples but they do make a serious point. What is benign to one person is stressful to another and this is what makes dealing with stress so difficult. People who are struggling to make ends meet will probably show little sympathy towards someone obsessed with keeping up with the latest fashion. But everyone lives within a particular environment and the stresses are no less real for being bizarre to another person in another environment.

That said, the stresses imposed by life in a modern complex society are heavy and demanding. Increasingly, it is recognized that unreasonable stress leads to poor performance, which is ultimately counterproductive to society in general and to employers in particular.

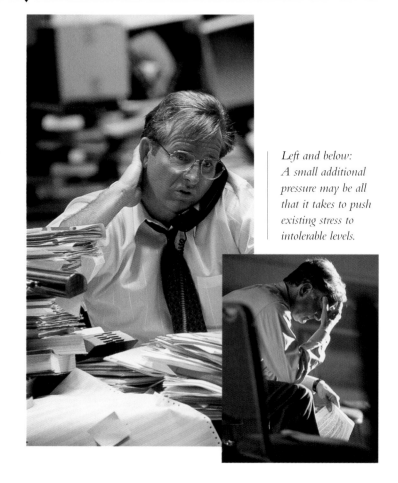

Left and below: A small additional pressure may be all that it takes to push existing stress to intolerable levels.

SYMPTOMS

◆

Stress produces **anxiety**. This is a feeling of general worry plus poor concentration and a range of physical symptoms from headaches, tremors and sweating to abdominal pains and **indigestion**. As stress increases, anxiety can become more prominent with a constant fear of doing something wrong and worrying about your performance. Family life suffers; the individual becomes irritable and snappy; he loses interest in sex and may turn to drink. As stress builds up further, individual tasks are neglected because of the need to turn attention to some other more pressing problem. This poor performance ultimately leads to even more stress in a self-perpetuating vicious cycle. It is fairly easy to see how things can then deteriorate into a state of **depression**. The type of depression most likely is called agitated depression: the

individual is on edge, appears hyperactive and talks freely – unlike classic depression where thought and activity slow down. However, outsiders will notice that the activity is empty and that it achieves little. Tasks that are quickly begun are just as quickly abandoned unfinished, causing yet more stress. Finally there may be a complete breakdown in the person's ability to cope; all the stresses build up into one apparently insoluble threat; the individual collapses in tears and bewilderment. This is what is commonly known as a nervous breakdown.

Evidence suggests that stress lasting over months or years increases the risks of developing a peptic ulcer and may increase the risk of heart disease. The condition called 'burn out' may result from years of stress; it is characterized by lack of enthusiasm, neglect of responsibilities, delaying even important tasks, chronic irritability and a feeling of utter worthlessness in one's job or life generally.

TREATMENT

A degree of stress is not in itself unreasonable and is indeed a necessary stimulus to high performance. We all recognize the benefits of having a deadline, while juggling priorities is simply a fact of life. There may be times when these stresses build up and seem overwhelming, even though each itself is not excessive. This is where counselling is helpful, together with time management and setting priorities.

The aim is rarely to transform your life, which would be unrealistic. Rather the counsellor guides you towards agreeing your own agenda for dealing with demands, sorting out what is essential and what can be delayed. Time management helps by organizing your week and devoting time in a preplanned manner instead of reacting to the latest demand. Where excessive stress is leading to anxiety, treatment may include further counselling or sedatives. In extreme cases the individual needs complete rest in a tranquil environment before being gradually encouraged to resume responsibilities.

Constant stress is not healthy. Try to arrange your schedules so that it includes time not subject to demands, perhaps for developing hobbies. Talking problems over is worthwhile and helps put stresses into perspective. In the end, people may be faced with choices about their lifestyle or jobs and may simply have to opt for alternatives if they cannot negotiate changes or cope with what is expected. Increasingly, people are using litigation to force changes to unreasonable stress at work.

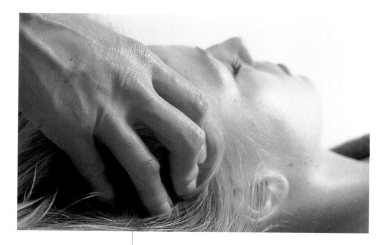

Above: Aromatherapy head massage is one of several complementary therapies that can help you defuse stress without resorting to conventional tranquillizing medication.

QUESTIONS

Surely some people just cannot cope with stress?
People do vary in how well they handle stress and so there is self-selection in the lifestyles that people choose. For example, you do not become a test pilot if you cannot deal with multiple demands. However, for any individual there will be a point at which stress becomes unreasonable.

What can be done if severe stress is unavoidable?
People do cope under extraordinary stresses but the question is for how long. If there really are no changes possible to a person's lifestyle, he or she will eventually develop an anxiety state. Whether this progression takes a matter of weeks or years will depend on the individual.

What about using drugs to cope?
Most societies have found certain drugs to alleviate stress: alcohol, tobacco and coca, for example. Although they are helpful in the short term, excessive use simply adds to stress, quite apart from providing their own health hazards.

Complementary Treatment

Bach flower remedies – Rescue Remedy is a stand-by for stressful situations; otherwise the remedy depends on the cause. For example, vervain suits people who get stressed by injustice. **Acupuncture** is good at calming and strengthening the spirit. Typical points include Heart 7, whose name is *Shenmen*, gate of the spirit, and Pericardium 6. **Chakra balancing** can help suppress the body's biochemical responses to stress, thus boosting the immune system. **Arts therapies** – therapists can help you to become aware of the underlying, unconscious factors contributing to stress by helping you to express your feelings through the arts media. Increased understanding allows you to make informed decisions about your life. **Reflexology** – your practitioner will concentrate on areas that correspond to the zones in the head. **Ayurveda** would recommend meditation, breathing mediation and yoga, along with *panchakarma* detoxification. **Osteopathy** can help if stress causes pain in the musculo-skeletal tissues, particularly the neck and shoulders, but also the lower back. *Other therapies to try: most have something to offer.*

INSOMNIA

Strictly speaking, insomnia means complete loss of sleep, but is usually taken to mean sleep disturbances varying from poor quality of sleep to an inability to sleep.

CAUSES

Insomnia is defined in relation to one's normal pattern of sleep. As people grow older their need for sleep decreases. Whereas babies naturally sleep for upwards of 16 hours a day, adults need on average 7–8 hours and the elderly just 5–6 hours. It is when the pattern of sleep deviates from what is usual for the individual that there may be a problem.

By far and away the most common cause is worry, including worry about getting to sleep itself, so that a run of bad nights can be self-perpetuating. Although worry leads to difficulty in getting to sleep there is a reasonable night's sleep once asleep.

Depression, by contrast, is not associated with difficulty in getting to sleep. Instead the sufferer wakes and worries in the early hours of the morning.

Environmental disturbances might include noisy neighbours or hot nights. Eating or drinking to excess disturbs sleep through discomfort or the need to pass urine during the night. Many people find that stimulants, especially tea and coffee, keep them awake. In older people illness often leads to insomnia – the pain from **osteoarthritis**, a chronic cough or the need to pass urine associated with prostate trouble.

SYMPTOMS

There may be constant tiredness and daytime drowsiness. Losing sleep on a regular basis will lead to poor concentration, tension and irritability. A complete lack of sleep even for just one night results in a serious fall in performance at skilled tasks or tasks involving judgement.

TREATMENT

Short periods of insomnia are self-limiting: eventually the need for sleep catches up on you and you return to your normal pattern. Firstly, do something about whatever is disturbing sleep, be it noise, excess alcohol or pain. Then adjust eating or drinking patterns to avoid stimulants and reduce the amount of fluid you drink for a few hours before going to bed.

It often helps to make a ritual for going to bed: preparing the bed, having a warm bath and a small warm drink. This sets up the mind for sleep psychologically. Avoid daytime snoozes since this time will be lost from nighttime sleep.

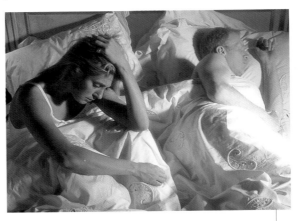

Above: When sleep escapes you, nothing seems longer than the night hours.

Once you are awake, the usual advice to get up and do something useful until you feel drowsy is rarely practical. It is better to make a warm drink, read and go back to bed. If you regularly wake, delay going to bed until you feel drowsy even if that is in the early hours of the morning.

It is difficult to treat the effects of **stress** and **anxiety**; a short course of sleeping tablets (see below) may be unavoidable.

Drug treatment

So-called hypnotic drugs are used in the short-term treatment of serious insomnia. Modern sleeping tablets are very safe unless taken with alcohol. People can get used to them within a couple of weeks of regular use, so they should be kept for occasional use only. The drugs most commonly used are short-acting benzodiazepines, such as temazepam. Even so, these may have a hangover effect the next day. Some newer drugs such as zopiclone are claimed to avoid this. Depression should be treated specifically.

Complementary Treatment

Bach flower remedies – the remedy depends on the cause, for example agrimony for sleeplessness caused by hidden worries behind a cheerful facade. **Acupuncture** – see STRESS. **Massage** fosters calm, especially if given by your partner last thing at night. **Aromatherapy** – try adding six drops of lavender or chamomile oil to your bath, or sprinkle them on to your pillow. **Nutritional therapy** – cut out coffee; try taking supplements of B vitamins and magnesium. *Other therapies to try: most have something to offer.*

Neuralgia

◆

Pain in a nerve of a recurrent and persistent nature.

Causes

Any irritation of a nerve through pressure or inflammation will cause neuralgia, although often no definite disease is found. This is particularly so with nerve pains around the face and upper body. Even though they are severe and upsetting exhaustive investigation may reveal nothing, leaving a simple diagnosis of 'neuralgia'.

States of **anxiety** and **depression** are associated with neuralgia. It is unclear whether they cause pain through muscular tension, such as clenching of teeth, or through lowering the tolerance threshold for the minor pains everyone experiences.

Symptoms

The most common symptoms of neuralgia are pain around the face, shooting from the jaw to the ear, or pain across the lower chest. Neuralgia together with altered sensation in the fingers and muscle weakness suggests causes such as **multiple sclerosis** or other nerve damage.

Treatment

It can be curative simply to know that all investigations are negative. In the case of facial pain, adjustments to the dental bite can help by relieving stress on the joints in the jaw. A painkilling injection into the tempero-mandibular joint, between the upper and lower jaws, will relieve this common source of facial neuralgia. Always mention facial pain or headaches to your dentist. He or she might be able to offer some other useful suggestions to ease the pain of neuralgia.

Where no definite cause is apparent, treatment with a low dose of an antidepressant or an antiepileptic drug is often effective although it takes several weeks to work. If pain is specific to one nerve, for example pain below one rib, it is worth trying a nerve block, which is done by injecting an anaesthetic into the nerve.

Complementary Treatment

Acupuncture achieves excellent results. **Chiropractic** helps if neuralgia is triggered by nerves in the neck. *Other therapies to try: healing; tai chi/chi kung; shiatsu-do; hypnotherapy; Ayurveda; chakra balancing.*

Shingles

◆

A painful skin rash caused by the herpes zoster virus.

Causes

On first contact with this virus you develop **chickenpox**. Afterwards the virus does not completely disappear from the body. It lives on in a dormant state within collections of nerve cells called ganglia, which are found along the spinal cord. For reasons not well understood, the virus can become active again decades later, this time causing shingles.

You cannot catch shingles from shingles – but you may catch chickenpox from shingles if you have not had it before. The virus is spread by skin-to-skin contact.

Symptoms

At first there is an uncomfortable sensation over an area of skin. This may be facial pain, pain across the ribs or down one limb, and appears to be **neuralgia**. After seven to ten days a blistery rash appears over the site of pain. In cases of chest or abdominal pain the rash spreads around one half of the trunk only, which is unique to shingles. The rash takes about three weeks to fade. Afterwards pain is common where the rash was, which in some cases can last months or years.

Treatment

During the puzzling neuralgia stage the treatment is with painkillers. Once the typical rash appears, treatment is with an antiviral drug such as acyclovir or famciclovir. These reduce the severity of the illness and the chances of persistent pain afterwards. Shingles on the upper part of the face needs more specialized treatment to avoid ulceration of the eye.

Complementary Treatment

Nutritional therapy – supplement vitamins C, B_{12} and E. **Homeopathy** – if you have been exposed to the shingles virus, try taking variolinum as a preventive measure. *Other therapies to try: Western herbalism; acupuncture; chakra balancing; healing; hypnotherapy.*

HEADACHES AND MIGRAINE

Extremely common conditions that affect everyone occasionally and some people more often than others.

CAUSES

The causes of most headaches are uncertain, although many are clearly the result of muscular tension arising from the muscles of the neck and spreading across the scalp. Migraine is caused by abnormal dilation (widening) of blood vessels within the skull and around the brain. This can be provoked by tension, certain foods, the menstrual cycle, overtiredness, eye strain, overuse of painkillers and excitement.

Many people fear more serious causes of headaches or migraine but in practice sinister causes are rare. The box (right) shows features that would suggest a more serious cause. It is a myth that high blood pressure causes headaches, unless it is exceptionally high. Headaches and migraines affect all ages and are surprisingly common in children, when the child often also gets stomach ache.

SYMPTOMS

Headaches are described as a pressure on the top of the head, a band drawn across the skull, or a constant throbbing pain.

Classic migraine follows a pattern: at first there is a fore-boding of something happening within the head, often with nausea; there may be a shimmering in the field of vision, called a fortification spectrum, and, more dramatically, some people go blind in one eye, develop slurred speech or get an odd sensation in one limb. There then follows a severe headache, affecting one side of the skull ('migraine' means half of the skull), more nausea and vomiting.

Headaches and migraines can last hours or a few days.

TREATMENT

Most headaches and migraines respond to simple painkillers such as aspirin or paracetamol. Often these are combined with an antisickness drug such as prochlorperazine. It is important to take these early in the attack because once the nausea sets in painkillers are poorly absorbed from the stomach. There is a temptation to take stronger and stronger painkillers but these can actually make headaches worse.

Drugs called triptans are effective at cutting short severe migraine. Examples are sumatriptan and rizatriptan. People having frequent attacks may find it worth taking preventive treatment; the most widely used are beta-blockers, which also

have a mild calming effect, or pizotifen. Both of these have to be taken every day for full benefit. It is worth keeping a diary to see if headaches or migraines link up with certain foods, days of the week and so on. Foods commonly provoking migraines are cheese, chocolate, red wine, oranges, bananas and nuts. Certain drugs can cause migraines, especially the contraceptive pill and calcium-channel blockers (for high blood pressure), and may have to be stopped. A constant dull headache may be caused by **depression** and may respond to a low dose of sedative or antidepressant. It is difficult to control **stress** underlying headaches but relaxation techniques help.

Investigations are rarely necessary unless the headaches or migraines include the features in the box below.

SYMPTOMS THAT MAY POINT TO SERIOUS CAUSES OF HEADACHE

- ◆ *Sudden onset over seconds or minutes (bleeding around the brain)*
- ◆ *A fever, neck stiffness and aversion to bright lights (meningitis or encephalitis)*
- ◆ *Loss of use or clumsiness in a limb (brain tumour or blood clot on the brain)*
- ◆ *Following a head injury (blood clot on the brain)*
- ◆ *Worse in the mornings and with nausea or change of personality; the new onset of epileptic fits (brain tumour)*
- ◆ *Migraine for the first time or worsening after beginning the contraceptive pill (sensitivity to the hormones)*

Along with these, doctors would look for irregular pupils, disturbed thought or behaviour, weakness in limbs and raised pressure within the skull as seen by examining the back of the eyes.

Complementary Treatment

The **Alexander Technique** encourages the release of muscle tension in the neck. **Chiropractic and osteopathy** – loss of joint movement and flexibility in the neck with associated muscle spasm contribute to headache and migraine. These manipulative therapies can help, although they work on different principles. Diet – a **naturopath** or **nutritional therapist** could offer dietary advice which would help reduce the severity and frequency of headaches. *Other therapies to try: most have something to offer.*

EPILEPSY

An electrical disturbance within the brain, leading to bizarre behaviour or sensations.

CAUSES

Like a computer, the brain relies on an orderly flow of electrical current to work efficiently. Epilepsy is the result of a major electrical storm within the brain. Any scarring or area of tissue damage is a likely focus for the disorder. This may accompany **cerebral palsy** or follow a **head injury**, a **stroke**, brain surgery, drugs or excess alcohol (see ALCOHOL AND ALCOHOLISM).

High **fever**, especially in children, is an extremely common cause of fits, fortunately with no long-term consequences. Other causes are heat stroke, **brain tumour** and disorders of body chemistry such as **diabetes** and lack of oxygen. After all these have been excluded there remain about 75% of epileptics for whom no cause can be found despite investigation.

SYMPTOMS

The classic epileptic fit begins with a sense of something about to happen, called an aura. Auras may consist of an odd sensation, an emotion or a smell. They come from electrical activity in the part of the brain where the fit is beginning. Then there is a phase of generalized muscle activity, first stiffening up, followed after a few seconds by regular jerking of limbs, often with frothing at the mouth and incontinence of urine. This is the time when epileptics may come to harm through falls. After a few minutes most fits end, followed by a period of drowsiness that can last several hours. There are many variations on this classic fit. The fit may consist of unusual behaviour or a momentary lapse of consciousness.

A reliable eyewitness account is a good way to make the diagnosis; otherwise an EEG may show characteristic electrical wave forms from the brain. Most cases nowadays would be investigated with a brain scan (see pages 350 and 351).

TREATMENT

Treatment is not always essential for single or very infrequent fits, as in a feverish child. Treatment aims to stabilize electrical activity in the brain and so reduce, if not stop, further fits. Drugs in general use include phenytoin, valproate, vigabatrin, carbamazepine and several others. Each one suits different people. The correct dosage is found by experience and by monitoring blood levels of the drug. Any precipitating causes such as alcoholism or high fever need to be dealt with.

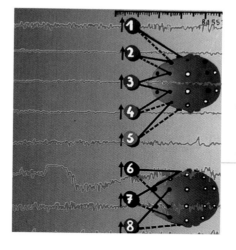

Left: An EEG, which shows disordered electrical activity throughout the brain during an epileptic fit.

If someone is having an epileptic fit, the only action to take is to put him into a safe position on his front so that he will not choke. After the fit has ended he should be allowed to recover from the ensuing drowsiness. Only if a fit is prolonged might active treatment be necessary, such as the injection of a sedative like diazepam.

It is possible to perform brain surgery for certain highly localized types of epilepsy, with the aim of cutting off the part of the brain where the abnormal electrical impulses begin.

Providing an epileptic remains fit-free for a number of years, he can lead a completely normal life, including driving a car, although some occupations are forbidden such as driving public service vehicles or flying a plane. Deciding whether medication can be stopped is difficult, depending on the consequences if fits recurred. It is helpful to show first that brain activity is normal with an EEG, then the dosage of drugs is slowly reduced. Withdrawing medication is often done for children. Adults may be reluctant to stop medication despite years of being fit-free because of the implications for their job or driving licence if fits restarted.

Complementary Treatment

There is no substitute for orthodox treatment; however, any of the relaxational therapies will be useful on a day-to-day basis. **Bach flower remedies** – try taking Rescue Remedy immediately after a fit. **Nutritional therapy** can offer some long-term help; recommendations might include supplementing vitamin B_6 and magnesium, zinc and selenium. Through **healing** the frequency and severity of attacks can be reduced, as this therapy has a calming effect on the whole being. *Other therapies to try: see STRESS.*

STROKE

A brain injury occurring as the result of some kind of interference with blood flow within the brain.

CAUSES

The brain relies on a constant flow of oxygen-rich blood via the carotid arteries in the sides of the neck and the vertebral arteries up the back of the neck. Disruption, even for seconds, leads to giddiness and blackouts; loss of blood flow for more than a couple of minutes leads to death of nerve cells and a resulting stroke. Nerve cells cannot regrow so any loss is permanent but recovery is possible by other cells taking over the functions of the dead cells.

Some strokes follow a leakage of blood from one of the arteries in the brain; most result from blockage of arteries with a blood clot. Least common are strokes due to **brain tumour** or brain injury. The risks of a stroke are increased by anything that increases the risks of diseased blood vessels. This includes, most importantly, **high blood pressure**, raised cholesterol and smoking. Strokes become much more common with age, due to a general deterioration in the otherwise remarkable reliability of the circulation in the brain. They are a major cause of disability in old age and a common reason for death in the elderly.

SYMPTOMS

The symptoms can range from momentary to permanent. The most obvious symptoms are paralysis of muscles, for example sudden loss of use of an arm or a leg or both, drooping of half the face, slurred speech and difficulty in swallowing. There are more subtle changes in the senses, for example blindness for part of the field of vision, inability to feel part of the body, loss of balance and giddiness.

There is loss in the so-called higher brain functions: an inability to read or articulate correct words, loss of emotional control and confusion – in fact a complete change of personality. The most serious strokes cause sudden unconsciousness then death; others lead to chronic ill health with immobility, incontinence and the increased risk of chest infections.

TREATMENT

After a stroke, the treatment is to provide skilled nursing care while time does its healing. About 25% of stroke victims will recover rapidly and completely. A brain scan (see pages 350 and 351) will localize the site of damage and confirm the type of stroke: bleeding, obstruction or unexpected disease. It is important to control blood pressure and to stop smoking. Aspirin, in a dose of 75–150 mg a day, reduces the tendency of the blood to clot and so lessens the risks of a future stroke by up to 30%. Investigations may reveal that a blood clot has come from deposits of cholesterol in the carotid arteries; surgery can reopen these vessels (carotid endarterectomy).

Rehabilitation ideally involves a team of physiotherapists, speech and occupational therapists as well as relatives, all pushing the individual to make the best use of her remaining abilities. It can be a long, demanding business because of the changes in personality produced by strokes. Many practical problems need addressing such as learning to transfer in and out of chairs or beds, help with swallowing and with feeding.

QUESTIONS

What is a TIA?
A transient ischaemic attack, or mini-stroke. By definition a TIA has all the features of a stroke but complete recovery occurs within 24 hours. They are caused by small blood clots and should lead to as full an investigation as a complete stroke. Aspirin is a very effective treatment for a TIA.

How long can recovery take after a stroke?
Most recovery occurs within three days but still worthwhile improvement happens for at least 12 and possibly 24 months. During this period the brain 'reprogrammes' itself to overcome the damaged area of permanently lost nerve cells.

Is it worth treating blood pressure in the elderly?
Yes, even in the very old. However, doctors do not look for such tight control as they do in younger people.

Complementary Treatment
Stroke requires prompt hospital treatment. Complementary therapies have a role in prevention and rehabilitation. **Nutritional therapy** – a high intake of oily fish and vitamin E with a wholefood diet helps prevent small clots in the brain, which cause strokes. **Western herbalism** – ginkgo promotes cerebral circulation. **Acupuncture** is excellent when used in conjunction with physiotherapy, as is **chiropractic**. **Ayurveda** – regular treatment helps restore muscular strength. *Other therapies to try: shiatsu-do; reflexology; tai chi/chi kung.*

PARKINSON'S DISEASE

A degeneration of the brain marked by shaking of limbs and a generalized stiffness of movement.

CAUSES

For reasons not understood, there is an abnormally rapid loss of certain specialized cells within the brain in individuals with Parkinson's disease. These cells produce a chemical called dopamine, which is involved in the fine control of muscle activity. Dopamine is one of a number of neurotransmitters in the body, which are the chemicals through which one nerve cell communicates with another.

Parkinson's disease is mainly a disease of ageing, affecting about 2% of those over 80, but it is not unknown in younger age groups. A few cases are caused by drugs that have reversible Parkinsonian side effects, for example sedatives such as chlorpromazine. There are a number of other rare neurological diseases that mimic Parkinson's disease but are differentiated on investigation. In this case the condition is called Parkinsonism.

SYMPTOMS

The early symptoms are easily mistaken for the general effects of ageing: lack of mobility, dizziness, slow speech and a mild tremor of the hands. The diagnosis becomes more obvious once the more typical symptoms appear, for example a tremor of the hands in a pattern where the thumb keeps rubbing against the index and middle fingers – a so-called pill-rolling movement. There is a general rigidity of the limbs. For example, walking is with a stiff gait with the arms held rigidly at the sides and the whole body bent over. As the condition worsens patients have an immobile, expressionless face. They have difficulty in starting to walk, making a few shuffling paces before getting into their stride. In addition, there is frequently **depression** and **constipation**.

Interestingly, handwriting becomes small and cramped and the diagnosis can be suspected on this evidence alone.

TREATMENT

The drugs available work by boosting the levels of dopamine in the brain. Probably the best known is L-Dopa, given alone or in combination with other drugs, such as carbidopa, which improve the brain uptake of L-Dopa. Side effects such as nausea, low blood pressure and confusion are common. Unfortunately, most patients develop resistance to these drugs

after a few years. There are a few alternative drugs, such as selegiline, which can relieve symptoms and put off the need to go on to L-Dopa. Newer drugs such as cabergoline or entacapone enhance the effect of L-Dopa.

Physiotherapists and occupational therapists are useful to many sufferers, helping people with Parkinson's to make their home environment as safe and convenient as possible.

Surgery is occasionally performed, cutting certain nerve pathways in the brain to relieve disturbances of movement. There is also the possibility of implanting brain cells taken from a foetus to replace the dopamine-producing cells in the brain. This is still an experimental and controversial method of treatment with unpredictable results but may lead to an eventual cure of this common and distressing condition.

QUESTIONS

Is there anything other than drug treatment?
Physical aids are important, such as something as simple as slip-on shoes that don't need lacing up. Enthusiastic physiotherapy encourages people to make the best use of their remaining mobility.

Does it affect the mind?
Parkinsonism does not cause dementia; it can be difficult to accept this when faced with a severely disabled individual, but the mind does remain intact. Having a normal mind in a diseased body is one reason why people with Parkinson's frequently get depressed.

What is the long-term outlook?
Many people have mild symptoms with little progression even over several years. A few people deteriorate rapidly. For the majority there is a gradual decline over 10–20 years; life expectancy is little affected.

Complementary Treatment

WARNING: Vitamin B_6 should only be administered by a doctor to Parkinson's patients. **Biodynamics** can help in the early stages of the disease. Regular exercise via **tai chi/chi kung** can help delay the progress of the disease in its earliest stages, as can the **Alexander Technique**. Diet – **nutritional therapy** can be helpful. Ask your therapist about a low-protein diet. Various vitamin and mineral supplements could help, for example vitamins B_1, C and E – but note the warning above with regard to vitamin B_6.

ENCEPHALITIS

Inflammation of the brain leading to confusion and drowsiness.

CAUSES

Any infection that irritates the brain can result in encephalitis. The most common cause is a non-specific viral infection although it can accompany **mumps** and **chickenpox**. Probably the headache so common with these viral illnesses is a mild form. Certain biochemical disorders can cause encephalitis, for example alcoholic poisoning. Infection with the herpes virus is one potentially treatable cause. There is a rare and incurable form caused by **measles**, one reason for offering vaccination against this disease. There are several tropical insect-borne diseases which also cause encephalitis.

SYMPTOMS

It begins as a typical viral illness with widespread muscular aches and headache. After a day or two the sufferer becomes drowsy, the headache worsens and the sufferer may lapse into a coma. There may be epileptic fits and paralysis of certain facial muscles. The coma can become profound. The diagnosis is confirmed by detecting viruses on a lumbar puncture, showing brain inflammation on a brain scan and, occasionally, taking a biopsy of the brain to detect the herpes virus.

TREATMENT

Most cases of encephalitis can be treated only with nursing care and steroids to reduce inflammation within the brain. A brain scan may show some treatable cause such as a brain abscess. If caused by herpes, the treatment is with high doses of antiviral drugs. Although most victims do recover, encephalitis is always a serious condition with a risk of death or of permanent neurological damage.

Complementary Treatment

Complementary therapies are not an appropriate response to encephalitis. During recovery any of the relaxational techniques could help – see STRESS.

MULTIPLE SCLEROSIS

Degeneration of the central nervous system leading to widespread weakness and changes in sensation; commonly called MS.

CAUSES

The cause of MS remains unproven, but wide international variations in frequency suggest an environmental cause, possibly a virus. It is the most common serious neurological condition in young adults. It is caused by degeneration of the cells that surround the nerve cells as a form of insulation.

SYMPTOMS

In a first attack there is blurred vision or loss of vision, numbness in various parts of the body, weakness of a limb or difficulty controlling urination. The symptoms appear rapidly and disappear within weeks. It may be years before further problems develop. A pattern eventually emerges of recurrent neurological symptoms affecting different parts of the body at different times. An MRI scan (see page 351) will reveal abnormal nerve structures scattered throughout the brain. The disease does not affect thought processes or intelligence.

TREATMENT

For a first attack, nature is left to take its course. Occasionally steroid tablets are used to control symptoms and help acute flare-ups. Interferon-B reduces the frequency and severity of flare-ups in the relapsing form of MS but not in other types and not by very much. It remains a controversial treatment.

In first attacks the pattern of the disease is unpredictable. It is likely to progress, but many people with MS find that their disability is manageable and only a minority deteriorate to the point of needing intensive nursing.

Complementary Treatment

Complementary approaches cannot cure MS. **Chakra balancing** relaxes spasms and eases aching muscles and pain from bladder infections. **Chiropractic** is useful as part of an overall treatment regime, helping the individual to keep mobile, using manipulation and soft tissue massage of the spine and other joints. **Ayurveda** can help in the early stages. Oil **massage** is given, along with *marma* puncture. *Other therapies to try: biodynamics; tai chi/chi kung; naturopathy.*

BACTERIAL MENINGITIS

◆

An infection of the brain with potentially very serious effects.

CAUSES

◆

The brain is surrounded by delicate layers of specialized tissue called the meninges; meningitis means infection of this tissue. Most cases arise from viral infections that reach the brain via the blood stream. Fewer cases are caused by bacterial infection but these are always more serious. Meningitis is actually rather difficult to catch but the risks are higher in institutions where many people are close together. This is why outbreaks often spread through schools and colleges. Meningitis can follow any penetrating injury of the skull such as may occur in a road accident. The peak time for meningitis is winter.

SYMPTOMS

◆

The illness begins as an unremarkable infection with **fever**, mild headache, muscle aching and possibly a cold. Over a few hours or a couple of days the severity of the illness becomes rapidly worse. The headache becomes intense, bright lights hurt the eyes and there is pain on attempting to bend the neck. Eventually, features of **encephalitis** occur, such as drowsiness, irritability, epileptic fits and possibly coma. These symptoms are caused by irritation of the meninges over the brain, which is made worse by anything that stretches them such as bending the neck.

If the cause is bacterial, for example meningococcal meningitis, then there may be a widespread purple rash in the skin which consists of tiny bruises. This rash appears over just a few minutes and is a sign that the infection has spread into the blood stream (septicaemia) and is destroying the blood's ability to clot.

In babies the disease is often much less dramatic and more difficult to recognize. The baby may be simply irritable, drowsy, possibly vomiting and possibly with a bulging fontanelle – caused by pressure within the skull.

TREATMENT

◆

If bacterial meningitis is even suspected, the first essential is to give an injection of penicillin. The diagnosis is confirmed by lumbar puncture – this means withdrawing fluid from around the spinal cord and analysing it for the bacteria responsible. If the cause is bacterial, the patient is maintained on high doses of the appropriate antibiotic. If the cause is viral, the illness will settle with just nursing care. The terrible

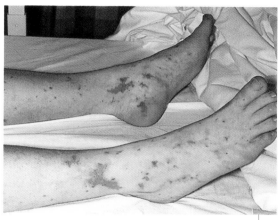

Above: The sinister scattered purple rash of meningococcal meningitis, which signals septicaemia. Get medical help immediately.

effects of septicaemia lead to bleeding not only in the skin but in internal organs. Patients are desperately ill and require intensive care, blood transfusion, artificial respiration and control of epileptic fits.

With bacterial meningitis, people who have been in close contact should have antibiotics to reduce the likelihood of contracting it. Ninety-nine per cent of people who contract **viral meningitis** make a full recovery; unfortunately, bacterial meningitis is more dangerous with a 10% risk of death. After-effects such as **epilepsy** and partial paralysis are common.

A vaccination against haemophilus B is now offered in childhood. This bacterium causes about 50% of all cases of bacterial meningitis. Even though this vaccination has been used for only a few years, the number of cases caused by haemophilus B has plummeted to one-third of previous levels.

See also VIRAL MENINGITIS.

       Complementary Treatment
Complementary therapies are not appropriate in response to the medical emergency of meningitis. However, many therapies will be able to offer help during the recovery stages. Any of the relaxational therapies mentioned under STRESS will help with the tensions of illness. There are many therapies that can help boost the immune system, including **Western** and **Chinese herbalism**, **homeopathy** and **acupuncture**. The gentle arts of **tai chi/chi kung** and **yoga** can also help restore the battered system.

SCHIZOPHRENIA

A disturbance of thought often marked by delusions, hallucinations, self-neglect and paranoia.

CAUSES

Schizophrenia is considered a disorder of brain chemistry. Probably there is disease in the system of neurotransmitters – chemicals through which one nerve communicates with another. Of these, the dopamine system is most suspected.

It has a strong hereditary tendency, with a chance of about one in seven to ten of the offspring of a schizophrenic parent developing it – a much greater than average risk. There are similarly increased risks if a sibling has the condition.

Although most psychiatrists accept that environment and upbringing also play a role in schizophrenia, it has been hard to prove scientifically and many such theories have largely been abandoned for lack of evidence.

SYMPTOMS

In its mild form the individual simply seems a little eccentric: a loner, poor at socializing, reticent and wary of eye contact. This is the schizoid personality and may progress no further; such individuals often find solitary occupations and lead a quiet, withdrawn life.

If the condition worsens schizophrenics start to experience bizarre events, voices commenting on their behaviour and hallucinations. Thinking becomes disordered: certain ideas become absolute certainties resistant to any reasoning. For example, a schizophrenic may be convinced that radio waves are being emitted by a light switch and influencing his mind

and that his own thoughts are being broadcast to the world at large. These are termed delusions, unshakeable beliefs based on no objective evidence. There is a strong feeling of being under the control of others, be it voices from the television or a central heating unit or just vague, menacing 'others'.

This paranoia is a common feature of schizophrenia, as is **depression** and extreme **anxiety**. These symptoms increase the chances of schizophrenics becoming aggressive towards their supposed persecutors or harming themselves, and suicide is a risk. As the disease deteriorates there is disintegration of the personality and increasing self-neglect.

TREATMENT

Drug therapy has revolutionized treatment since chlorpromazine was first discovered 40 years ago. Various drugs control symptoms in individuals who would otherwise languish in institutions or drift on to the streets. These drugs are given by mouth or injection to ensure reliability of dosage. New drugs such as olanzapine are freer of side effects. Schizophrenics cannot cope with normal stresses of life; calm, orderly and careful handling is important, at home or in hostels.

Up to 40% of schizophrenics have just one episode of schizophrenia and return to normal life eventually. Pointers to eventual full recovery are if the condition came on rapidly and was accompanied by minimal hallucinations or delusions, and the patient had a previous reliable personality within a stable family. About 10% of schizophrenics remain seriously disturbed despite treatment. The rest will experience relapses from time to time. Severely paranoid schizophrenics may pose a major risk to the safety of others and may remain so dangerous that they have to stay in special secure psychiatric prisons.

Families need much support in caring for schizophrenics, whose bizarre, unpredictable behaviour strains family loyalty.

Complementary Treatment

WARNING: Visualization, hypnotherapy and deep relaxation techniques, including chakra balancing, are extremely dangerous for schizophrenics and should never be used *except* by people trained in psychiatry. They bring about altered states of consciousness and schizophrenics have reported seeing lights and disturbing visions during treatment. Complementary approaches cannot cure schizophrenia. **Yoga** and **tai chi/chi kung** are calming forms of exercise which might benefit schizophrenics. **Reflexology**, **massage** and **aromatherapy** are generally supportive.

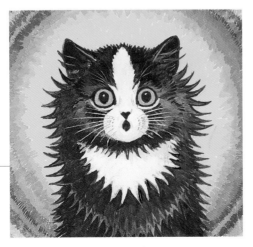

Right: A drawing by Louis Wain, a well-known schizophrenic who drew cats. The drawings became more bizarre whenever he relapsed.

HEAD INJURY

Any blow to the skull is serious, potentially risking brain damage.

CAUSES

The brain is a soft structure with a filigree of delicate blood vessels entering and leaving it. It is protected from hard blows and shaking by the strength of the skull all around it.

Head injuries may have a direct impact on the brain by fracturing the skull and damaging the brain beneath, or a less obvious effect by shaking the brain. Any injury causes the brain to swell within the rigid skull, which compresses the base of the brain against the skull. The base of the brain controls certain vital functions, in particular breathing and regulation of the heart, so it is pressure on this structure that often causes more problems than the head injury alone.

Common reasons for head injuries are falls, road traffic accidents and deliberate blows to the skull, especially boxing.

SYMPTOMS

A severe head injury has effects similar to those of a **stroke**, the exact effect depending on which part of the brain is damaged. There may be paralysis, loss of speech and variable consciousness, if not coma. Less severe effects, such as those caused by shaking, lead to confusion and loss of memory. Injuries that cause bleeding or swelling around the brain may not result in any immediate symptoms until the blood clot or swelling has become large enough to put pressure on the underlying brain. The effects of this pressure can be confusion, double vision, nausea and vomiting, progressive drowsiness, coma or simply a rapid change in personality. If not treated this situation may lead to death through further pressure on the brain's vital centres.

Brain scans (see pages 350 and 351) have greatly increased the accuracy of diagnosis of head injuries and especially in detecting blood clots (subdural haemorrhage, extradural haemorrhage) – previously confirmed only by exploratory surgery in which a tap hole was driven through the skull.

TREATMENT

A serious head injury requires immediate stabilization of breathing and circulation, both of which are controlled by the brain, while removing debris and dealing with the other injuries that so often accompany a severe head injury. Once stable, patients may have to be maintained on a respirator until they regain consciousness. Where the injury appears milder and there is no obvious damage, it is still important to be vigilant over the next 24–48 hours for any symptoms that might reveal that damage is taking place and is causing increased pressure within the brain.

Rehabilitation follows similar lines to those given to stroke victims, pushing individuals to use their remaining faculties. Head injuries are most common in the young but fortunately, younger brains have a better chances of recovery than older brains; even so, rehabilitiation may take years.

WARNING

Even though someone may appear perfectly well straight after the injury, there are features to look out for afterwards which may indicate underlying brain damage:

Short-term symptoms *(appearing within hours or days of the injury)*
♦ *Unusual drowsiness*
♦ *Severe persistent headache*
♦ *Double vision*
♦ *Difficulty in using a limb, walking unsteadily or slurred speech*
♦ *Vomiting for no apparent reason*
♦ *An epileptic fit*

Longer-term changes *(appearing over the following weeks after the injury)*
♦ *Alteration in personality*
♦ *Unusual drowsiness*
♦ *Progressive paralysis of a limb*

Mild confusion and drowsiness are common signs of simple concussion, which should improve over 24–48 hours.

Complementary Treatment

Chakra balancing can help with relaxation during rehabilitation, as can the **Alexander Technique**. **Chiropractic** treatment or **osteopathy** can help patients with head injuries, as often they will have also suffered neck and back injuries. Treatment aims to restore spinal joint function and mobility, as part of an overall treatment regime. Any treatment listed under STRESS can help relieve tension during rehabilitation.

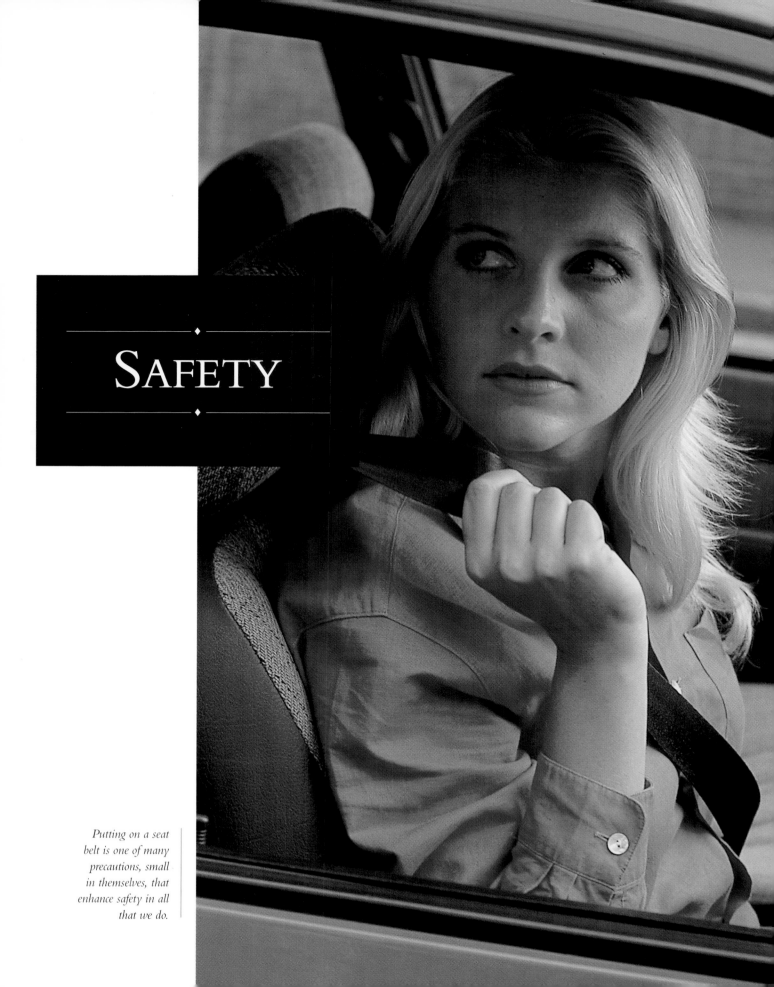

SAFETY

Putting on a seat belt is one of many precautions, small in themselves, that enhance safety in all that we do.

IN DEVELOPED COUNTRIES, as advances in medicine and surgical techniques have reduced the threat from fatal birth injury, malnutrition and infections, so health promotion and accident prevention have been given greater resources. Physical danger has always taken its toll on human society; archaeological remains often show old injuries, such as fractures and other signs of violent injury or death. There are great differences in the safety and accident rates between different countries. This discussion is based on experience in the United Kingdom.

An overview

While accidents account for approximately 2% of all deaths, between the ages of one and 35 they are the single greatest cause of death. Above 35 they are steadily overtaken by illnesses related to advanced age such as heart disease, cancer and strokes.

While most accidents occur at home, since this is where we spend the greatest part of our time, the majority of accidental deaths occur not surprisingly on the road. Domestic accidents,

particularly falls, can be fatal, however, as can accidents that take place in the workplace or sportsfield. The consumption of alcohol plays a part in at least 30% of all accidents.

What are accidents?

In this context an accident can be defined as an unforeseeable event leading to injury. In practice, and with the benefit of hindsight, many accidents are predictable although not necessarily preventable. It is an important goal of public health to try to reduce the incidence of accidents, while realizing that some accidents are, by their very nature, unavoidable. The risk and nature of accidents vary greatly at different ages.

The lure of the familiar The more often we perform a familiar task the more likely we are to take risks, for example when going up a ladder to clean windows or remembering not to tread on a loose floorboard. It is better to do something about a hazard now than to be saying in hospital, 'I always knew I ought to do something about those slippery stairs.'

Safety and children

The aim is to encourage exploration in a safe environment. The onus is on carers to anticipate hazards, especially those that adults take for granted, such as being careful with pointed objects. Checklists can be tedious – just about anything can be a hazard if misused – and common sense should guide you.

The home Secure objects which children might pull on to themselves; fit guards to the top and bottom of stairs; remove trailing electrical flexes, sharp objects and poisonous substances such as bleach, medicines and garden chemicals. Fit socket guards; lock doors leading to hazardous areas such as the garage. Do not leave children unattended near fires, hot pans or other hot objects.

Always test the temperature of baths, food and drinks meant for children. Keep only safe domestic pets and avoid leaving children alone in a room with a dog, no matter how well behaved it normally is. Secure the area around garden ponds or swimming pools and never allow young children to go near them without close adult supervision.

Transport Fit safety seats in your car and use them, making sure they are the right size for the child and in good condition; always strap children in the car and do not let them hang out of an open window. Children love bikes but make

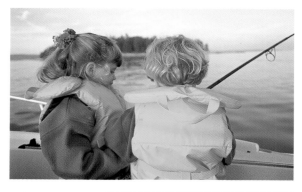

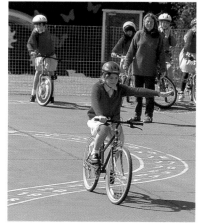

Above and right: Life involves balancing adventure and risk against sensible although possibly boring precautions.

sure they get into the habit of wearing safety helmets and reflective clothing, even during daylight hours. Teach road safety from the earliest age, while remembering that no child under the age of 10 is safe alone on a road.

Other risks Satisfy yourself about the safety of playgrounds and the degree of supervision on trips and special outings.

Unless you are going to cocoon your child in an unrealistic world, however, accidents in childhood are unavoidable. But you can make sure that accidents are as minor as possible.

Safety from the age of 13 to 35
The aim is to enjoy life without endangering someone else's. Adolescence is a period of flexing all the muscles and trying everything. So, not surprisingly, this is the period where accidental deaths peak, mainly through road traffic accidents.

Road safety Nearly half of all male deaths in this age group are through road traffic accidents. The means to reduce risk are simple: wearing seat belts whether you are a driver or a passenger, driving at a safe speed, not drinking and driving. Pedestrian safety is equally important; many accidents occur to inebriated pedestrians.

Sports and workplace safety Although far less important numerically, workplace accidents and sporting injuries account for significant numbers of deaths and disabilities

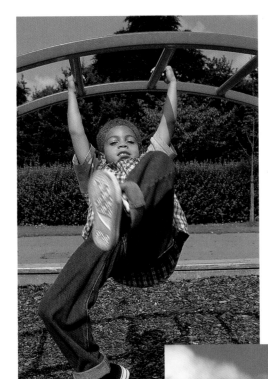

Above: Soft ground covering in a playground will protect against injury while allowing uninhibited play. Right: Safety measures can be made attractive and even desirable.

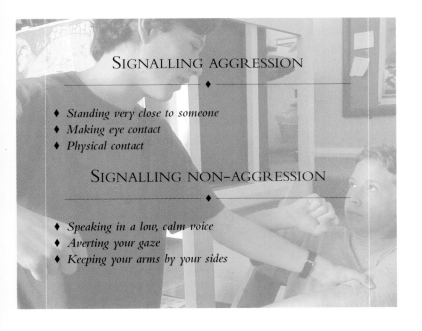

SIGNALLING AGGRESSION
♦

♦ *Standing very close to someone*
♦ *Making eye contact*
♦ *Physical contact*

SIGNALLING NON-AGGRESSION
♦

♦ *Speaking in a low, calm voice*
♦ *Averting your gaze*
♦ *Keeping your arms by your sides*

each year. Young people may feel they jeopardize a macho image if they use safety equipment, but office and factory personnel and sports instructors should keep emphasizing the safe way of doing things.

Aggression Violent assaults make a small but important contribution to injuries in teenage years and early adulthood. Most societies find youth aggression a difficult problem, with no simple answers. It is tied to socio-economic disadvantage, unemployment, alcohol and drugs, but, at root, young people

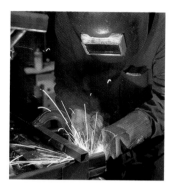

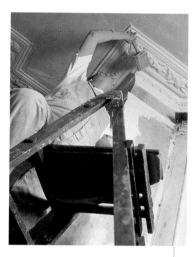

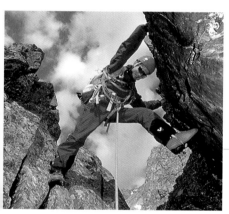

Above left: In certain occupations, safety cannot be left to individual choice.
Above: In other activities the responsibility is ours.

Left: Many hazardous sports recommend safety standards that you would be foolish to ignore.

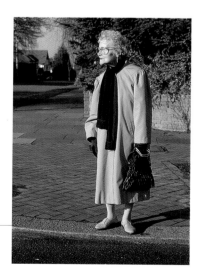

Right: Accidents to elderly pedestrians are a common cause of injury and death.

are aggressive and large groups are aggressive towards each other. Those wishing to avoid confrontation must keep away from troublespots and learn to recognize anger in themselves so they can alter their body language and walk away from tense or hostile situations.

Safety from the age of 36 to 64

The aim for this age group should be to benefit from wisdom and experience! Road traffic accidents are still the major hazard, less so workplace, home and sports injuries. Alcohol still continues to play an important role.

Safety beyond the age of 65

The aim for older people is to maintain independence despite deteriorating senses and balance. Accidents become increasingly prevalent the older you get, although as a percentage of death and disability they appear less important. Falls alone account for 60% of all deaths due to accidents in women above the age of 75, and 40% in men. Road traffic accidents account for 10–20% of deaths through accidents, most of which relate to elderly pedestrians rather than elderly drivers.

General Make sure your glasses and hearing aid, if worn, are as efficient as possible because you will be relying on your eyes and ears for your safety.

The home Look at the potential hazards in the home. The simplest things are the most important to fix. Secure loose rugs, fit handrails on stairs and tidy up trailing flexes. Do not lift things beyond your capability. Try not to have open flames or candles, which could start a fire. Have bright lighting, especially in dangerous areas like the stairs.

Many elderly people feel giddy on standing up or turning their head; allow for this by taking your time moving around. Consider getting a personal alarm, especially if you have fallen before, and let neighbours have a key for an emergency.

Outside Wear well-fitting shoes with non-slip heels. Think twice about going out in the ice or snow – just a minor fall can fracture your wrist or thigh. Take advantage of handrails and support from a friend or partner and if the time has come for a walking stick do not let pride stop you from using one.

Crossing the road is a potential hazard for the elderly: you should choose your spot with care at a proper marked crossing and cross with the lights. Do not assume that being elderly suspends the laws of motion, so give traffic time to stop.

ALZHEIMER'S DISEASE

A progressive brain disease with loss of recent memory, confusion and eventually dementia.

CAUSES

Personality, thought, emotion and foresight reside somewhere within the billions of cells of the brain and their complex intertwinings. Alzheimer's disease is the result of the degeneration of these interconnections. Instead of being orderly the connections become tangled; as the tangling increases so personality decreases. Evidence is growing that there is a defect in the acetylcholine system, one of the neurotransmitter chemicals in the brain.

A number of sub-variants of dementia are recognized, for example Lewy body dementia, but, as yet, they can only be differentiated post-mortem. Premature dementia – before the age of 60 – should be investigated for the uncommon but treatable disorders which can cause a similar picture such as a blood clot on the brain or a slow-growing **brain tumour**.

There is a very small hereditary risk factor in people with dementia which begins before the age of 60. However, even among the elderly only a minority are affected; about 80% of the over 80s have no particular problems. Alzheimer's affects 2–3% of people aged between 65 and 75.

SYMPTOMS

The basic symptom is loss of recent memory; individuals still maintain clear recollections of events that occurred decades earlier. Early symptoms mimic the benign forgetfulness of age, such as mislaid glasses and people not recognized. Soon it becomes clear that there is more of a problem: even offspring go unrecognized, the individual starts wandering from her home and her life drifts into a permanent gloom of confusion. At some point there is **incontinence**, and often aggression shown towards family, as a result of complete confusion as to what carers are trying to do.

TREATMENT

It is important to exclude treatable causes by blood tests, used to detect severe **anaemia**, thyroid disease and syphilis. A brain scan may exclude blood clots or brain tumours (see pages 350 and 351). Otherwise the diagnosis rests on showing loss of short-term memory plus confusion, but all in clear consciousness, that is the sufferer is not drowsy or comatose. Drugs should be reviewed in case they are adding to confusion.

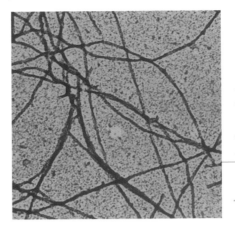

Left: A micrograph of brain tissue, showing the tangle of fibres characteristic of Alzheimer's disease.

As yet, there is no recognized treatment for Alzheimer's disease. A couple of drugs claim to delay deterioration in patients but there is little supportive evidence for this so far.

What can be done?

People with Alzheimer's should be kept stimulated by talking, reading and going out. It is important to keep them aware of time and place by talking about where they live and what they do each day. A regular schedule helps to root people in whatever remains of their appreciation of events. Many people get by, despite being quietly demented, while there is a routine and someone to keep an eye on them. This precarious hold on reality can be broken by moving into unfamiliar surroundings, loss of a companion who looked after them or other illness. Ultimately, people may need constant nursing care to help with all aspects of daily life. Agitation and physically wandering can be major problems, often treatable only by sedation.

People suffering Alzheimer's can live long after the onset of their illness, and usually die of an unrelated illness although chest infections are a common cause of death.

Complementary Treatment

Complementary approaches cannot reverse Alzheimer's disease. A **Western herbalist** might be able to help alleviate symptoms of the disease through the controlled use of ginkgo. **Massage**, especially when combined with **aromatherapy**, can offer support. An experienced **reflexologist** might be able to delay the progression of the disease. **Ayurveda** can offer oral preparations, along with oil baths to the head. Carers must ensure detoxification programmes are followed. **Tai chi/chi kung** can be beneficial in the earliest stages of the disease.

PHOBIAS

An abnormal degree of anxiety and fear provoked by one situation or object, leading to excessive steps to avoid that object or situation.

CAUSES

Mild phobias are common but about one in a hundred people has a phobia serious enough to cause them significant **anxiety**. There is no one agreed cause but there are some theories.

Certain things are common subjects of phobias: spiders, heights and by extension a fear of flying, and fear of open or crowded spaces. One theory is that these phobias derive from our prehistoric forebears, for whom poisonous insects were a real hazard; heights carried the risk of falling and open or crowded spaces the risk of being some other animal's lunch.

The psychological theory is that a phobia is a conditioned reflex. Through pure chance something provoked an episode of severe fear and thereafter the thing and the emotion it caused have become firmly entwined. A large friendly dog jumping up and scaring a toddler, for example, can become the source of a lifelong phobia of dogs. This theory has been extremely useful in planning treatment. Psychoanalytic theories, on the other hand, view objects of phobia as symbolic, stirring deeply buried emotions. Thus fear of open spaces is a

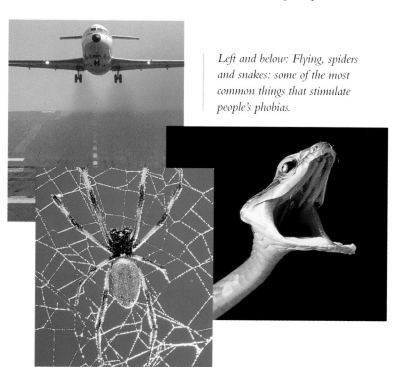

Left and below: Flying, spiders and snakes: some of the most common things that stimulate people's phobias.

mourning for loss of the womb and the mother; and the fear of snakes is a fear of male sexuality. Although thought provoking, such interpretations have not led to successful treatment.

SYMPTOMS

The prime symptom is anxiety at the sight or thought of the feared thing. For arachnophobes the mere thought, let alone sight, of a spider is enough to set them sweating and their heart racing. Severe phobias dominate one's life, turning it into a constant enterprise, for example, to root out spiders and to avoid anywhere that spiders might lurk. Clearly, such phobias become personally destructive.

Mild phobias can often be laughed off by people whose mental health is otherwise good. Severe phobias are socially disabling; the more bizarre they are, for example a fear of electricity leaking out of plugs, the more they might be symptomatic of other problems like alcoholism or **schizophrenia**.

TREATMENT

Mild phobias respond to sympathetic support plus sometimes a mild sedative, as experienced by those whose slight phobia of flying is overcome by encouragement and a glass of wine. Certain antidepressants help relieve severe phobias.

Severe phobias are also successfully treated using desensitization techniques. With spiders, for example, arachnophobes first visualize one until they can cope with the emotion. They move on to looking at pictures of spiders, then observe real spiders in glass tanks and perhaps eventually handle one.

This slow process uncouples the anxiety from the object by the process of deconditioning and is now the preferred treatment for most phobias. There will be cases resistant to even this, for whom sedatives are the only answer. Any underlying mental illness of course needs treatment, too.

Complementary Treatment

   Bach flower remedies – mimulus for known fears, aspen for inexplicable fears, rock rose for absolute terror, cherry plum for a fear of losing control and crab apple for a phobia relating to cleanliness. **Hypnotherapy** is also excellent for changing unwanted patterns of behaviour. **Autogenic training** is self-administered psychotherapy which can help. **Ayurveda** might include *panchakarma* detoxification, meditation and *marma* therapy. *Other therapies to try: homeopathy; healing; Alexander Technique.*

BRAIN TUMOUR

A growth originating in the brain itself or a growth that has spread from a cancer elsewhere in the body.

CAUSES

Brain tumours can be malignant (cancerous) or benign. The benign ones, called meningiomas, are very slow growing and cause symptoms not through destruction of tissue but by placing pressure on the brain.

Malignant growths within the brain are actually relatively uncommon, despite the enormous numbers of cells that make up the brain and its supporting structures. There are a hundred thousand million nerve cells alone. In theory, any one of these could turn malignant but in fact such primary tumours are unusual. It is far more likely that a brain tumour has spread from a cancer elsewhere, for example the breast or the lung. (Cancers similarly often spread into the bones, lungs and liver, which also have exceptionally good blood supply.)

Brain tumours in children may follow from the abnormal development of the foetus' nervous system.

SYMPTOMS

These depend on where the tumour is growing. There are parts of the brain where tumours can grow large without obvious problems, as in the frontal lobes. Yet even a tiny tumour in the pituitary gland produces symptoms. More destructive tumours lead to the loss of various functions, similar to the effects of a **stroke** but happening over weeks rather than instantly. So there may be progressive loss of use of an arm, giddiness, slurred speech or epileptic fits.

Most brain tumours eventually cause headaches. The particular features of these headaches are that they are worse in the morning and awaken you during the night. Often there is nausea and, if more advanced, abrupt vomiting without any warning. These are effects from pressure on the brain.

A particular feature of tumours in the frontal lobes is a change in personality: the individual tends to become moody and irritable. Tumours in the pituitary gland can cause unusual hormone disturbance leading to, for example, acromegaly, which is excessive bone growth.

Examination involves testing tendon reflexes, looking for weakness or unusual briskness. By examining the back of the eye through an ophthalmoscope it may be possible to detect signs of increased pressure within the brain called papilloedema. The diagnosis of brain tumours has been revolutionized by CT and MRI scanning (see pages 350 and 351).

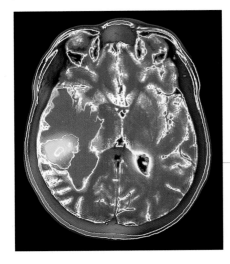

Left: An MRI scan clearly showing a large tumour in the left half of the brain.

TREATMENT

Some brain tumours can be successfully cut out – this is so with meningiomas and can lead to complete recovery. Even malignant tumours can sometimes be removed to give sufferers some relief of symptoms.

Unfortunately, most cannot be dealt with so directly. In this case the main option is radiotherapy (see page 370) to try to shrink the tumour. Steroid drugs also relieve the swelling around the tumour. The decision on treatment depends on the precise type of brain tumour, since some are more sensitive than others to radiotherapy.

Chemotherapy (see page 371) has not proved helpful in most cases, although some tumours do respond.

For all these reasons, the outlook for an adult with a malignant brain tumour is very poor. Although brain tumours are especially aggressive in children, they are often more sensitive to radiotherapy than in adults and are therefore more likely to be curable.

Complementary Treatment

Complementary therapies will not be able to kill the tumour itself; however, many can help postoperatively. **Chakra balancing** will help with symptom control and energy balance, and also aid relaxation during orthodox treatment. **Hypnotherapy** can encourage a positive attitude. **Aromatherapy**, **massage** and **reflexology** are generally supportive. Any of the therapies listed under STRESS will be able to help ease the tensions associated with this disease.

ALCOHOL AND ALCOHOLISM

Alcoholism means compulsive drinking taking precedence over other activities, with withdrawal effects if alcohol is unavailable.

CAUSES

Alcohol is really a brain sedative: the pleasure comes from a mild degree of sedation of the brain, the pain comes from oversedation. A small amount of alcohol just slightly inhibits the brain's higher functions – thought, emotion and social inhibition. The shy become more extrovert, the anxious relax, the tongue-tied find unexpected eloquence.

With more drink the brain becomes more sedated, releasing controls on behaviour on which we can usually rely. We take a sharp comment as an insult; we stop noticing social cues such as the expression that says 'OK, stop there'; but we still imagine we are in control. As drinking continues muscle control becomes poor, with staggering and slurred speech; there is difficulty concentrating, then a slide into unconsciousness.

SYMPTOMS

Alcohol makes the blood vessels dilate, causing a flushed face and heat loss. (This is why it is a bad idea to give people too much alcohol to warm them up – they will experience an initial flush, followed by a feeling of cold as they lose heat.)

Alcoholism is basically a dependence on alcohol. This means craving a drink even in the morning, drinking a lot each day, drinking so much the drinker loses track of time. Drink or drunkenness begins to interfere with work and with the drinker's relationships.

Chronic alcohol abuse is associated with poor nutrition, because the energy derived from alcohol reduces appetite, leaving the drinker short of protein and vitamins. This can give rise to a permanently abnormal gait and tingling in the fingers. There is an increased risk of heart disease in drinkers, through a direct effect of alcohol on the muscle of the heart. In time the brain deteriorates, too, with a loss of memory and possibly even epileptic fits.

Heavy drinkers are at risk of **pancreatitis**, a painful inflammation of the pancreas. This gives rise to recurrent abdominal pain and **diabetes**. Cirrhosis of the liver is another long-term risk: the liver becomes hard and inefficient, with jaundice, easy bruising and potentially life-threatening bleeding from enlarged veins in the gullet (see LIVER PROBLEMS).

In addition to causing harm to the drinker, alcohol in excess is involved in much crime and violence and is still a major contributor to road traffic accidents and other accidents.

TREATMENT

Acceptance by the drinker that they have a drink problem is a major step in the treatment of alcohol abuse. When people are given evidence as to how their health is being affected as well as guidance on sensible levels of alcohol, many people manage to pull back from alcoholism. Those people with a serious drink problem often need skilled support to reinforce their own will power. Sometimes drugs are given to aid rapid withdrawal of alcohol. This is called detoxification, but must be given under medical supervision.

STEPS TO COPING WITH A DRINK PROBLEM

♦ *Accept that there is a problem*
♦ *Recognize the effects on health, work and family*
♦ *Adopt safe limits*
♦ *Use medication short term to aid withdrawal*

There are many support groups that offer drinkers help: Alcoholics Anonymous is the best known.

Safe alcohol intake
The current British recommendations of maximum alcohol intake for men are 28 units a week and for women 21 units a week (see below).

The consumption of alcohol is measured in units:
♦ *A glass of wine = 1 unit*
♦ *A measure of spirits = 1 unit*
♦ *A pint of beer = 2 units*

Complementary Treatment

Massage promotes feelings of self-esteem and fosters a positive body image. **Auricular therapy** can help reduce harm during periods of alcohol abuse, ease the detoxification process when you come off, and help maintain abstinence. **Hypnotherapy** is excellent at changing unwanted patterns of behaviour and reducing cravings. Diet – seek help from a **nutritional therapist** or **naturopath**: you may well be malnourished because alcohol provides empty calories that suppress appetite. *Other therapies to try: healing; acupuncture; Hellerwork; Ayurveda; chakra balancing.*

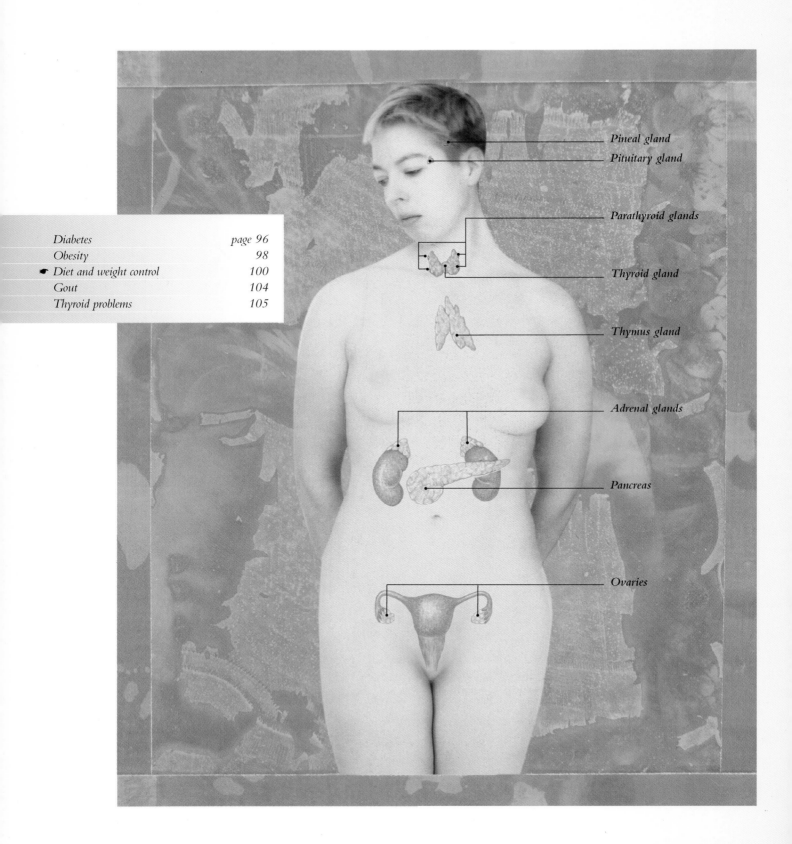

Pineal gland

Pituitary gland

Parathyroid glands

Thyroid gland

Thymus gland

Adrenal glands

Pancreas

Ovaries

*All living organisms need to exert control over their more distant components —
the most well-known control system is the nervous system with its pathways of
muscle-controlling nerves. The endocrine system is less obvious and relies on glands.*

ENDOCRINE SYSTEM AND METABOLISM

THE GLANDS OF THE endocrine system are really specialized tissues, which release biochemically active substances called hormones. Hormones move around the body in the body fluids. The cells on which hormones act detect them by means of receptors on their surface, which latch on to the hormone molecule and trigger a desired effect within the cell. Most hormones, such as adrenaline, are small molecules; some, like insulin, are much larger and more complex molecules.

Insulin and thyroid hormones are well known; less well recognized but vitally important are calcitonin and parathormone, involved in the calcium balance needed for muscle activity and bone density. These hormomes are produced in the parathyroid glands which are in the neck. The ovaries and womb produce progesterone and oestrogen, which control the menstrual cycle and pregnancy. The adrenal glands secrete adrenaline, noradrenaline and cortisol, which enhance the body's reaction to stress. Yet more hormones stimulate growth, sperm formation and blood pressure. There is also a whole array of hormones that help control the intestinal tract and they play a crucial role in regulating metabolism.

Metabolism refers to all the biochemical processes within the body by which it survives and grows. It includes especially the digestion of food, and how it is used to create proteins and the innumerable other biochemical ingredients of life. Metabolic disorders include **gout**, which involves abnormal handling of protein, and **obesity**, due to excess food intake.

Many hormones are regulated by elegant feedback loops, involving the hypothalamus and pituitary gland. This pea-sized gland located beneath the brain is the origin of some hormones, called releasing factors, that regulate the concentration of other hormones. The hypothalamic/pituitary unit

*Left: Hormones from glands affect digestion,
energy use, emotion and menstruation, among
many other aspects of metabolism.*

monitors the blood levels of these other hormones and increases or decreases their production accordingly by sending releasing factors to stimulate the endocrine glands. This is why disease of the pituitary gland can have widespread effects on health. Examples are growth deficiency, gigantism (acromegaly), **subfertility** and collapse of blood pressure.

How the system can go wrong

Endocrine disorders are often the result of an auto-immune condition. In such illnesses the body turns against its own tissues and destroys them with antibodies, which can be detected in blood samples. Examples of auto-immune hormone disorders are thyroid disease and adrenal insufficiency. Growths (usually benign) in endocrine glands are a common cause of excess secretion of hormones. The critical hypothalamus/pituitary complex is most often affected by benign tumours or by deterioration of blood flow to the gland.

Detecting and treating disorders

Fortunately many deficient hormones can be replaced or, if the problem is an excess of hormone, the output of the gland responsible can be biochemically blocked. For this reason many hormone disorders can be successfully treated.

Hormone disorders are detected by measuring the amount of hormones in the blood. The interpretation of these tests is complex because hormone levels are affected by the time of day, stress, medication and even how long it takes to analyse the blood sample. Additional investigation of hormone disorders may call for brain scans to detect disease of the hypothalamus or pituitary gland, or scans of the neck or abdomen to detect disease of important glands such as the pancreas, the thyroid and the adrenal glands.

This section concentrates on four conditions that are linked with hormones. Many other parts of this book deal with other hormonal problems, such as menstruation, **pregnancy problems**, subfertility and **osteoporosis**.

DIABETES

◆

An abnormality in the body's handling of sugar.

CAUSES

◆

Sugar, in the form of glucose, is the basic fuel of the body, obtained from carbohydrates (bread and starch) in the diet or made within the body by a complex biochemical pathway. It circulates within the blood stream to all body cells; close bio-chemical control ensures the quantity of sugar in the blood matches the body's needs. Too little blood sugar leads to light-headedness and tiredness; too much blood sugar is diabetes.

A constant high sugar intake in the diet takes its toll on this control system, which eventually can no longer control the blood sugar accurately. Blood sugar then remains persistently high and the individual becomes diabetic – known as Type II, maturity-onset or non-insulin dependent diabetes.

Insulin

Without insulin little sugar would be absorbed by most cells (the brain is an exception since it absorbs sugar regardless of insulin levels). Insulin is the hormone switch that tells cells to let sugar in. It is produced by the pancreas gland and released into the blood stream in response to the body's needs for energy. Any disease of the pancreas causing a deficiency of insulin will lead to high levels of blood glucose. This insulin deficiency is the other major cause of diabetes, called Type I, or insulin-dependent diabetes.

Just why the pancreas fails to produce insulin is not well understood. Certain illnesses, such as **pancreatitis**, cause damage to the pancreas, but this is not the case for most diabetes; yet something causes the insulin cells to switch off. This switching off can be a dramatic event in young people in whom diabetes can develop over a few weeks.

SYMPTOMS

◆

Diabetes causes both immediate and long-term problems. The immediate problems are the direct chemical consequences of high blood sugar while the long-term problems are the result of damage to cells after years of exposure to high blood sugar.

Short-term effects

Excess urine output/increased thirst: High sugar levels present the kidneys with too much sugar to be properly reabsorbed, so sugar leaks out with the urine. Large amounts of fluid leave with the sugar, thus one of the early symptoms of diabetes is passing a lot of urine. Because of the fluid loss, the diabetic feels thirsty and drinks much more than usual. In extreme cases the individual cannot keep pace with the fluid loss and becomes seriously dehydrated, with confusion and weakness, ultimately lapsing into a coma. Before insulin was discovered, this was how many young diabetics died.

Tiredness: Despite a superabundance of sugar in the blood stream, without adequate insulin the body cannot transport it into the cells where it is needed as fuel.

Weight loss: Unable to use sugar, the body turns to making its energy from fat and even protein from muscle, hence the weight loss. This presentation is especially dramatic in diabetics whose pancreas has failed – the younger diabetics. They become rapidly ill with weight loss and dehydration.

Infections: Bacteria feed on sugar. Diabetics have masses of the stuff in their urine and blood. This makes them walking banquets for bacteria, leading to **thrush** (a fungal infection of the groins, armpits and vagina), boils and abscesses.

Long-term effects

Over years the high blood sugar levels damage blood vessels all around the body permanently. In the retina blood vessels leak and overgrow and may lead to **blindness** – diabetes is the most common cause of acquired blindness. Small blood vessels in the legs become diseased, thus diabetics are prone to leg **ulcers** and poor blood flow to the legs. Disease of the kidneys reduces their efficiency and can lead to **kidney failure**. Disease of the circulation of the heart and brain explains why diabetics are at greater risk of heart disease and **stroke**. It is therefore very important to detect and to treat diabetes.

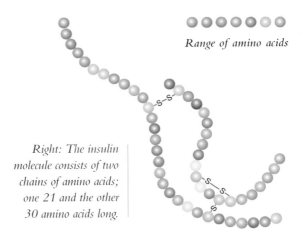

Range of amino acids

Right: The insulin molecule consists of two chains of amino acids; one 21 and the other 30 amino acids long.

Detection

Urine can be checked for sugar using a biochemical testing strip. If sugar is present then a blood test is taken to see whether blood sugar really is high. If there is still doubt then a glucose tolerance test might be required: you drink a very sweet drink and have half-hourly measurements of blood sugar for the next two hours.

TREATMENT
◆

The aim of treatment is to keep blood sugar levels close to normal. This is done by reducing sugar intake with a balanced diet and by using drugs or insulin or, recently, both in combination.

Diet

A diet with balanced amounts of fat, protein and sugar is important for diabetics. The sugar should be in a natural, unrefined form, as in fruit and vegetables. Diabetics should aim to lose excess weight. Most people with maturity-onset diabetes find that diet alone will give good control.

Drugs

These are used where diet is insufficient but they are not a substitute for a diet. The sulphonylurea drugs stimulate the pancreas to release more insulin and are best for those who are not overweight and who therefore have some reserve of insulin. Drug names include gliclazide and glibenclamide.

Biguanide drugs help sugar to be absorbed by cells as well as reducing the absorption of carbohydrates from the intestinal system. A kind of insulin substitute, they are used in diabetics who are overweight. The best known is metformin.

Insulin

There is no substitute for insulin for severe diabetics and especially for young people with acute diabetes. Modern devices allow diabetics a high degree of control of their insulin dosage – for example discreet syringes, which look like pens, are used to give a boost of insulin when needed, on top of a regular dose once or twice a day. Almost anyone can learn to self-inject with these user-friendly devices. Because insulin is a protein it is not possible to take it by mouth – the body would just digest it. Research is aiming to overcome this.

Quality of control

The aim is to keep blood sugar levels within a fairly narrow normal band; it is checked by taking finger-prick samples of blood for analysis in glucose meters. Testing urine for sugar is a more rough-and-ready check but adequate for non insulin-dependent diabetics. Diabetics need regular medical checks so complications can be detected and treated early. They should check their feet for ulcers and have chiropody to avoid injuries ulcerating. Annual eye checks will reveal disease in the retina or **cataracts**, which are more treatable at an early stage. Kidney function is monitored by testing urine for protein. Since they have a high risk of heart and circulation trouble, diabetics should avoid other risk factors, including **high blood pressure** and smoking.

QUESTIONS

Who needs insulin?

Most young diabetics with disease of sudden severe onset require insulin. Otherwise, it is considered when diet and drugs have failed to gain control and the individual is running into complications.

What are the hazards from drugs or insulin?

An excessive dosage will send blood sugar below normal, called hypoglycaemia. This starts with light-headedness; severe hypoglycaemia causes confusion, sweating and then unconsciousness, including a risk of epileptic fits. Diabetics, especially those on insulin, and their companions should learn to recognize the early signs of hypoglycaemia. Treatment is to take a sweet drink or an injection of glucagon, a hormone which raises blood sugar rapidly.

Complementary Treatment

Diabetes becomes a medical emergency if it is not properly controlled, so do not abandon conventional treatment. **Autogenic training** allows mind and body to rebalance themselves; hormone levels may rise and fall according to the system's needs. Severe insulin-controlled diabetes will probably not respond but, in combination with dietary control, good results can be achieved for late-onset diabetes. Diet – changing to a wholefood, even vegan, diet can help all diabetics. Nutritional deficiencies can be implicated in adult-onset diabetes, for example zinc, chromium, magnesium and B vitamins. Consult a **nutritional therapist** about supplementation. Increased vitamin E may be needed. **Ayurveda** can help if diabetes is linked to diet, when a number of preparations are available; **yoga** and *marma* puncture also help. **Tai chi/chi kung** is a gentle form of exercise which may benefit diabetics.

OBESITY

◆

Carrying a great excess of weight in relation to your build and height.

CAUSES

◆

In the developed world the days are gone when eating was purely and simply for survival. The 1500–3000 calories that most people need are there in plenty.

Eating has become a focus for many other things: a social affair, a business event, even a fashion statement. Food is marketed in appealing and convenient ways. It is cheap, abundant and desirable, ready to eat at the flick of a switch. It is little wonder that babies are overfed, becoming children who graze all day, then adults who eat instant convenience foods containing sugar and large quantities of fat and salt.

It is important not to overfeed babies as there is evidence that fat children grow into fat adults, and obesity is an increasingly serious problem in childhood. The fat child will experience ridicule quite apart from future health problems.

A slow route to obesity
The obese are rarely relentless gluttons who have guzzled themselves into fatness. It takes just a small but regular excess intake of food over many years to accumulate into obesity.

Whatever calories are not needed each day the body turns into fat and puts by for a 'rainy day': a bit on the hips, a bit on the belly until eventually there is more than a bit everywhere and the rainy day never comes.

Physical causes or inherited from parents?
There is some truth that obesity is all to do with glands or genes, or parents or **depression**. Underactivity, however, is a more likely cause. People who do not walk or exercise but eat as much as an athlete are heading straight for trouble. Comfort eating is universal. Never has it been so easy, nor the comfort so dangerous, with salt-, sugar- and fat-enriched cakes and biscuits rather than fruit or vegetables.

There are a few gland problems that lead to overweight. The most probable is an underactive thyroid gland, but this is less common than many believe (see THYROID PROBLEMS).

There is some evidence that obesity is partly inherited. Doctors do not yet know how significant the 'obesity gene' is. It may explain obesity in some individuals who are apparently resistant to normal dietary control, but it is inconceivable that the gene has spread in a generation or two to cause the widespread obesity that is now seen across the developed world. (See also page 100.)

SYMPTOMS

◆

After being weighed and measured, you can be compared to a table of 'normal' height and weight. But what if everyone is already overweight? If you weigh an 'average' weight the table will tell you that you are average even if, objectively, you are overweight. A more meaningful statistic overcomes this problem with averages; it is called the body mass index (BMI) (see below).

The formula for BMI is:

$$BMI = \frac{Weight\ (in\ kilograms)}{Height\ (in\ metres)\ squared}$$

For example, for a woman weighing 90 kg/14 st who is 1.75 m/5 ft 9 in tall, the calculation is:

$$BMI = \frac{90}{1.75 \times 1.75}$$

which gives a BMI of 29.39. A BMI between 19 and 24 is normal for a woman, and between 20 and 25 for men. A BMI above 30 is obese. Clearly, there are degrees of overweight short of obesity.

General effects
Imagine a large sack of potting compost weighing 25 kg/ 55 lb. This is equivalent to a modest degree of overweight. Mentally place that across your shoulders and stand up. You would experience pressure on your hips while sitting; as you stand your knee joints will groan and your hips twinge. Although you have only stood up, already a thin film of sweat coats your brow. You walk, feeling clunks in your ankles, knees and hips on each step and that is just on the level. You plod up a gentle slope that feels like a mountain; by now your heart is racing, your breathing is short, your shoulders ache, you feel tired. You are experiencing obesity.

Your joints, heart and lungs are under strain and you face early **osteoarthritis** and **high blood pressure**, increasing the risks of **heart disease** and **stroke**. In terms of specific effects, the overweight are prone to skin infections, especially in warm moist areas beneath the breasts and between the upper thighs. **Diabetes** is a likelihood. The sheer enjoyment of life is reduced because of awkwardness and self-consciousness.

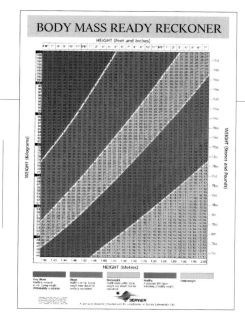

BODY MASS READY RECKONER

Right: Very high and very low BMIs are abnormal, as shown on this chart.

TREATMENT

Overweight people have to take the mental step of accepting that the control of the problem is in their own hands. It is unproductive and too easy to blame the food industry, **stress** of work or depression, although these may all play a part.

Targets and diets

Using the BMI, calculate your target range of healthy weights – you may feel more comfortable a little heavier or lighter within that band. Then calculate how long it will take to reach that weight on the basis of losing 0.5–1 kg/1–2 lb a week. This may seem a surprisingly long time, but it has taken you a lifetime to reach your current weight. By losing weight slowly you lose true excess fat. Crash diets appear successful but it is mainly fluid that is lost, which reaccumulates rapidly.

All diets share one property: eating less, although the details vary. The aim is to eat 1000–1200 calories a day. This must include all snacks and nibbles, which are so easily 'overlooked'. Most people lose weight steadily on such a regime. Some people are truly more resistant and need an 800–1000 calorie diet; these must be specially designed for the individual to be nutritionally sound, balancing fat, carbohydrate, protein and vitamins. There is a weight-loss diet for everyone, although for some it will be uncomfortably low in calories.

Exercise and other manoeuvres . . .

As well as reducing energy intake, you should increase your energy output to really make a difference. Walking just 1.5 km/ 1 mile as briskly as possible three times a week is a target that everyone should be able to incorporate into their lifestyle. Appetite-suppressant drugs are frowned on, because their effects are temporary and they can be addictive. Several appetite-suppressing drugs are now banned because of concerns about side effects on the heart. Orlistat is a more recent drug that causes the body to excrete fat.

Surgery for obesity fluctuates in popularity. It is possible to staple the stomach, clamp the jaws or even remove part of the intestine. These drastic measures are resorted to only after careful psychological assessment.

QUESTIONS

How dangerous is overweight?
Modest overweight, i.e. a BMI of 25–30, is not necessarily a significant health risk. True obesity – a BMI above 30 – carries significant hazards for the heart and joints.

How should I choose a diet?
Healthy diets should include fat, carbohydrate, minerals and vitamins – it is unhealthy to exclude one thing, such as fat, completely. Do check the nutritional content of dietary drinks and foods. You will lose weight on any crash diet in a week, but it is not good for long-term results.

Can I lose weight without following a particular diet?
Aim to eat less and exercise more. Strategies include using smaller plates (which still look satisfyingly full), eat only at meal times, eat slowly. Don't snack; if desperate nibble on fruit or vegetables.

Complementary Treatment
Complementary therapists are likely to recommend gentle exercise, reducing calories and healthy eating, as well as specific treatments. Be wary of any tablets for weight loss, no matter how natural the ingredients appear. No diet should make you feel ill or involve bizarre foods. **Aromatherapy** is excellent for raising self-esteem; try one of the following oils in the bath (six drops) or as inhalations (two to four drops in a bowl of water or on a handkerchief): cypress, fennel, rosemary, lemon, juniper or black pepper. Diet – it is vital to get sound advice from a **nutritional therapist** or a **naturopath**. **Hypnotherapy** can identify and release emotional or psychological causes; suggestion is used to change eating and lifestyle habits. **Ayurveda** – some preparations restore metabolism and eliminate toxins. *Other therapies to try: homeopathy; tai chi/chi kung; autogenic training; healing; chakra balancing.*

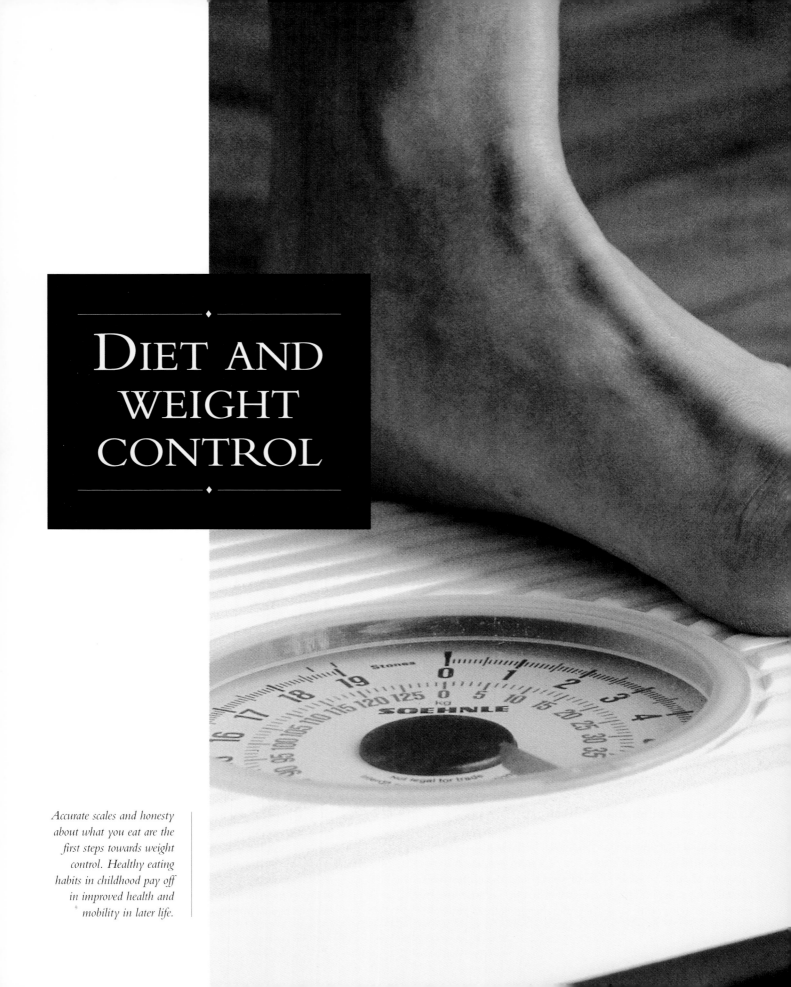

DIET AND WEIGHT CONTROL

Accurate scales and honesty about what you eat are the first steps towards weight control. Healthy eating habits in childhood pay off in improved health and mobility in later life.

Ours is probably the first century in which large numbers of people in some countries have had more food than they need. This welcome change from widespread starvation and malnutrition, still so common in much of the world, has however brought its own problems in the form of diseases of affluence. There are health consequences from the sheer fact of being overweight, and from the types of food we eat.

Diseases of affluence

The consequences of overeating include heart disease, **diabetes** and the physical effects of **obesity**. What is the route to this? Why have **heart attacks** moved from being rare to being the most common cause of sudden death?

It appears that the affluent diet leads to high levels of cholesterol, and thus to **atherosclerosis** and heart attacks. Saturated fats (hard fats) are ubiquitous in our Western diet – in cakes, biscuits and chocolate especially – and these are thought to be a major factor in cholesterol levels.

Fat, fibre and physical exertion

In some ways the 20th century was an enormous experiment with regard to what the human body can get away with. Can we eat more saturated fat and get away with it? The answer appears to be no. We develop high cholesterol, followed by atherosclerosis and then **high blood pressure**, **strokes** and heart disease. The experimental conclusion? 'Nice but nasty.'

Can we safely eat less fibre? We do not go out of our way to eat less fibre – it is just that it seems so boring to eat all those breads and grains. As for brown rice . . . Instead, we have turned to high protein/low fibre food – essentially meats and fewer green vegetables and potatoes. The experimental conclusion? Increased **constipation**, **diverticular diseases**, possibly **irritable bowel syndrome** and probably an increased risk of **bowel cancer**.

As well as changes in diet there have been profound changes in our physical activity: we walk less, move less and exert ourselves less. Lack of activity, by leaving our cardio-vascular system unchallenged, compounds the effects of diet, increasing our susceptibility to circulation problems. Increasing obesity is linked to decreasing general fitness.

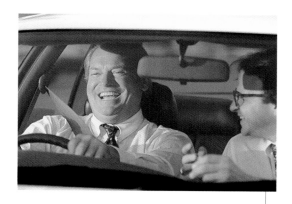

Above: Our increasingly sedentary lifestyles can result in health problems.

Other factors

There are a number of other dietary factors that affect health and weight control.

Salt Salt is a ubiquitous flavour enhancer, particularly in processed food where it is used in everything from custard to cakes. It is clear that high salt levels increase high blood pressure and therefore heart disease. Some evidence suggests that salt may also play a role in **stomach cancer**. The World Health Organization recommends no more than 5 g/¼ oz a day. Avoid crisps, biscuits and instant foods.

Sugar Sugar in all its forms is an answer to a human dream. We cannot get enough of it. In ancient civilizations people risked their lives to get honey, so deeply was sweetness craved. Now that we can get it out of a vending machine our desire knows no bounds. Why is it bad for us? Refined sugar predisposes to obesity and exhausts the pancreas, leading to diabetes. It contains no supplementary health benefits and blunts our appetite for more health-giving foods. This is over and above **tooth decay**, once a rarity but now common.

Vitamins These chemicals play vital roles in the body's metabolism but the body cannot make them for itself. Though they are required in only small quantities, deficiency can cause many illnesses. Vitamin deficiency is uncommon in affluent societies among those who eat a broad and balanced diet. Strict vegetarians may become deficient in Vitamin B_{12} if they eat no animal or dairy products and pregnant women may become deficient in folic acid, otherwise vitamin deficiency is most likely to result from deliberate self-neglect, for example in alcoholics, or diseases such as pernicious anaemia.

Minerals The body requires many simple elements such as iron, zinc, copper, selenium, calcium, sodium and potassium. All play more or less vital roles in metabolism. Excess is more likely than deficiency, most notably in the case of sodium, in salt. In large parts of the world iodine is naturally deficient in food, leading to **thyroid problems** and goitre. It is therefore often added to salt and dairy products. Iron deficiency is very common, especially in women, who lose it in pregnancy and through menstruation, and in children coping with the demands of growth.

Vitamin and mineral supplements There is little need for these in adults who eat a normal healthy diet. They may be advisable for the elderly if they eat little fresh fruit or for rapidly growing children, whose eating habits are also picky.

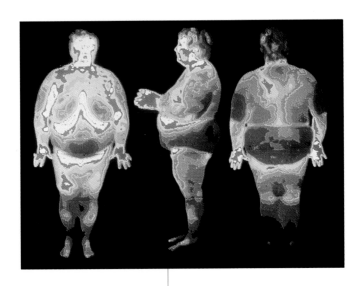

Above: Heat radiation in an obese person; the lighter coloured areas are mainly over the warm fatty parts.

A STRATEGY FOR HEALTHY EATING

♦

- ♦ *Try to eat something from each food group (see Food Values table on opposite page) every day*
- ♦ *Eat more carbohydrates in the form of pasta, potatoes, rice, pulses and bread*
- ♦ *Eat more fibre from fruit, vegetables and wholemeal bread. You need at least 25–30 g/1 oz a day*
- ♦ *Eat more fruit and vegetables – as well as providing fibre and vitamins these contribute antioxidants, which may be important in preventing cancer of the stomach or lung by scavenging free radicals – naturally occurring biochemicals, which are believed to have a role in causing disease. Green leafy vegetables are particularly good for you. Eat three helpings of vegetables and two of fruit a day. It makes no difference whether these are fresh or frozen; salads and fruit juices can be counted as helpings*
- ♦ *Select processed foods that are low in salt, sugar and saturated fat*
- ♦ *Eat less fat – reduce your intake to 77–87 g/3 oz a day. Select sources of non-saturated fat, e.g. fish. Select milk and dairy products low in fat and eat only lean meat*

Children and the elderly equally benefit from healthy eating, but if you plan to make wide-ranging changes to your children's diet take your health visitor's advice first.

Obesity

The physical effects of obesity are those to be expected from carrying more than your recommended body weight: arthritic pains, breathlessness and **gallstones**, which are common in affluent countries but rare elsewhere. **Breast cancer** shows an association with high-energy and high-fat diets.

Being obese means having a body mass index (BMI) of at least 30 – implying at least one-third over ideal weight (see page 98). This index has been steadily creeping up: in 1980 7% of the population of the United Kingdom had a BMI over 30. By 1995 this figure had more than doubled: 15% of men and 16.5% of women were obese.

Dieting

Most sensible diets restrict fat and empty calories (sugar) while maintaining the necessary amounts of protein, minerals, complex carbohydrates and vitamins. The amount of carbohydrate you need depends on your activity levels. Most people will lose weight if they restrict total calorie intake to about 1100 calories a day. Do this by restricting fat and simple carbohydrates – sweets, biscuits and cake. A healthy daily calorie intake for men and women aged 19–60 is 2550 and 1940 calories respectively, assuming average physical activity and that there is no need to lose weight.

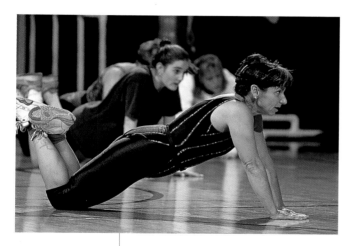

Above: Exercise is complementary to sensible eating for a healthy life style.

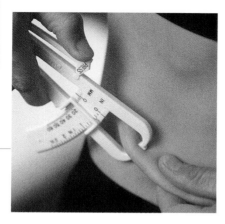

Right: Skin fold thickness reliably indicates total body fat.

LOSING WEIGHT – THE PRINCIPLES

◆

◆ *Work out a target weight*

◆ *Review your food intake, especially empty calories from alcohol, sweet drinks, snacks, crisps, sweets and chocolate*

◆ *Remember you still need some carbohydrate and fat*

◆ *Choose a balanced diet – you're more likely to stick to it, preferably forever*

◆ *Diet with a friend*

◆ *Aim to lose slowly but certainly (250–500 g/½–1 lb a week), not 'dash and crash'*

◆ *Eat slowly, from small plates and only at meal times*

◆ *Combine dieting with increased exercise – three half-hour walks a week will do*

◆ *Reward yourself for success – but not with food!*

Always take professional advice before beginning strict dieting or greatly increased activity.

FOOD VALUES

◆

This simple table gives some idea of what each type of food provides. Clearly a vegetarian diet can be perfectly healthy, although one lacking dairy products and eggs could lead to vitamin and mineral deficiencies.

Food	Provides
Meat, fish, eggs, pulses, nuts	Protein Carbohydrates Fat Minerals (iron, potassium, copper, selenium, zinc, phosphorus) Vitamins (B_{12}, thiamine, niacin)
Dairy products	Protein Carbohydrates Fat (especially saturated fat) Minerals (calcium, phosphorus, zinc) Vitamins (especially A and B_{12})
Fruit and vegetables	Carbohydrates and fibre Vitamins (folic acid, A, C) Minerals (potassium, magnesium)
Cereals (includes bread, pasta, rice)	Protein Carbohydrates and fibre Minerals (iron, calcium, zinc) Vitamins (B complex and E)

GOUT

A disease of the joints due to an excess of uric acid in the blood.

CAUSES

Somewhat unfairly, gout has the image of a self-inflicted disease, the result of overindulgence on heavy wines and red meat. In fact, most cases have little to do with lifestyle.

The condition is due to excess uric acid within the body. Uric acid is produced by the digestion of protein and is usually excreted in urine. If the blood contains too much uric acid, it can crystallize inside the joints, the earlobes and the kidneys.

People who have gout nearly always have an inherited tendency to high blood levels of uric acid. There are certain drugs that can increase uric acid levels, notably thiazide diuretics used to treat **high blood pressure** such as bendroflu-azide. A much less common cause is anything that increases cell turnover, and therefore protein load; this includes certain forms of **leukaemia**.

Those with a tendency to gout may indeed find that overindulgence in rich foods or alcohol brings on an attack, probably by giving a little more protein than the body can handle. The disease is very unusual in women. It is most common in middle-aged men; finding it in a young person should prompt a search for an underlying blood disorder.

SYMPTOMS

The most common initial symptom is sudden and extreme pain in one joint – most often the big toe, although any joint can be affected including the knees, elbows and shoulders. The pain is a result of crystallization of uric acid within the joint, which becomes swollen, hot and reddened, and tender to the slightest movement. Pain lasts for several days.

After repeated attacks the joints become misshapen and stiff. Crystals also precipitate in the ear lobes and the tissues around joints. Crystals may form within the kidneys, affecting kidney efficiency. These complications are unusual nowadays because the disease is recognized early and treatment is straightforward. The diagnosis is confirmed by finding high blood levels of uric acid, or by showing that fluid from an affected joint contains crystals of uric acid.

TREATMENT

Immediate relief is the first priority in the treatment of gout and this is effectively given by an anti-inflammatory drug such as ibuprofen, indomethacin or diclofenac but *not* aspirin.

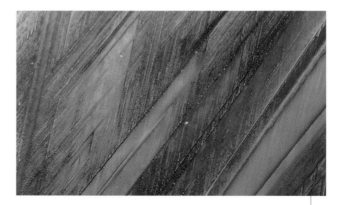

Above: These crystals of uric acid, seen here glowing under polarized light, are the cause of gout.

Failing that, one old remedy for gout is colchicine, although this does tend to cause **diarrhoea** as a side effect. It is important to review any medication people with gout may be taking in case certain drugs are to blame and, if so, to stop or alter their dosage. A blood count will detect the rare blood disorders that can cause gout. Some adjustments to lifestyle may be sensible, especially reducing alcohol intake and being cautious about rich foods.

Many people with gout have only occasional attacks, which are adequately handled by pain relief alone. However, if attacks are frequent, if there is kidney damage or if the blood uric acid is persistently very high, then long-term treatment usually becomes advisable. Allopurinol is the mainstay. This is a drug that increases the output of uric acid in the urine by making it into a more water-soluble form. Taken just once a day and with few side effects, allopurinol now makes the complications of gout a thing of the past for the great majority of sufferers.

 Complementary Treatment

Western herbalism remedies containing celery seed can speed up uric acid excretion, helping to reduce pain and inflammation. Celery seed is particularly useful in cases of recurrent gout. **Chakra balancing** can be used for pain control. **Hypnotherapy** can be used for pain relief, and to change unwanted patterns of behaviour. Possible **Ayurvedic** treatments include *panchakarma* detoxification, oral medications and diet. *Other therapies to try: Chinese herbalism; homeopathy; cymatics; autogenic training.*

THYROID PROBLEMS

Disease of the thyroid gland is a common cause of vague ill health, weight loss or weight gain.

CAUSES

If there is one switch that controls the body's activity it is the thyroid gland. This shield-shaped gland lies in the neck on either side of the windpipe. Thyroid hormone regulates the level of metabolic activity of the cells of the body: too much and they go into overdrive (hyperthyroidism); too little and there is a sluggish underactivity (hypothyroidism).

Thyroid disease is usually the result of an auto-immune condition, where the body treats its own tissues as a foreign invader. It sends in white cells and other immune factors which destroy the thyroid gland. This holds both for over- and underactive glands. Underactive glands can also result from treatment of a previous overactive gland. Iodine is essential to the formation of thyroid hormone and iodine deficiency leads to underactivity of the gland.

SYMPTOMS

Both under- and overactivity of the thyroid begin in a slow way and are often overlooked by family, friends and doctors.

Overactivity

The body's rate of activity is speeded up. People feel on edge and notice a fine tremor of their hands. They sweat, feel hot and seem in a rush. The heart rate is raised well above the normal 60–90 beats per minute and they feel **palpitations**. Weight loss is common as the body burns energy at a rapid rate; the appetite is good to ravenous. In Graves' disease a

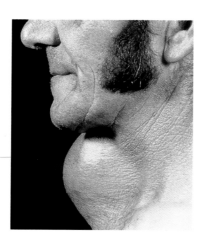

Right: Graves' disease (hyperthyroidism) has here caused an enormous goitre. Underactivity (hypothyroidism) can also cause goitres.

staring eye appearance is due to abnormal tissue deposited behind the eyes. Left untreated, hyperthyroidism (thyrotoxicosis) ends in exhaustion and, ultimately, **heart failure**. It is most common in women between 20 and 50.

Underactivity

The picture is in reverse: people feel sluggish and tired and might gain weight despite a normal appetite. Their skin feels cool and rough and their features look coarse and puffy. The heart rate is below 60. There is sometimes **constipation** and **depression**. Hypothyroidism can lead to severe hypothermia (very low body temperature), apathy, self-neglect and heart failure. It is common in middle age and very common in the elderly. Underactivity is rare in children. It is detectable by a blood test which is done routinely in many countries at birth.

TREATMENT

The diagnosis is confirmed by blood tests of the exact level of thyroid hormone. These tests can also monitor treatment.

Overactivity

Two drugs are used to bring the gland under control: carbimazole and propylthiouracil. Both take several weeks to work, during which time a beta-blocker helps relieve the sense of agitation and palpitations. Treatment continues for several months. Many cases settle like this. If the illness recurs the options are to remove part of the gland (a thyroidectomy) or destroy it with a radioactive, but harmless, form of iodine.

Underactivity

Replacement hormone is given as a daily tablet of thyroxine. It is initially used as a very low dose – as the hypothyroid heart is very sensitive to it – and guided by blood tests as to the right dose. Once stable, the patient remains on thyroxine for life, requiring regular blood tests to check control.

  ### Complementary Treatment

Complementary approaches should not replace conventional treatment. **Autogenic training** allows mind and body to rebalance themselves; hormone levels may rise and fall according to the system's needs. Nutritional deficiencies may be implicated in some thyroid problems, for example zinc, vitamin A, selenium and iron – a **nutritional therapist** will be able to advise on supplementation. *Other therapies to try: cymatics; yoga; tai chi/chi kung; reflexology.*

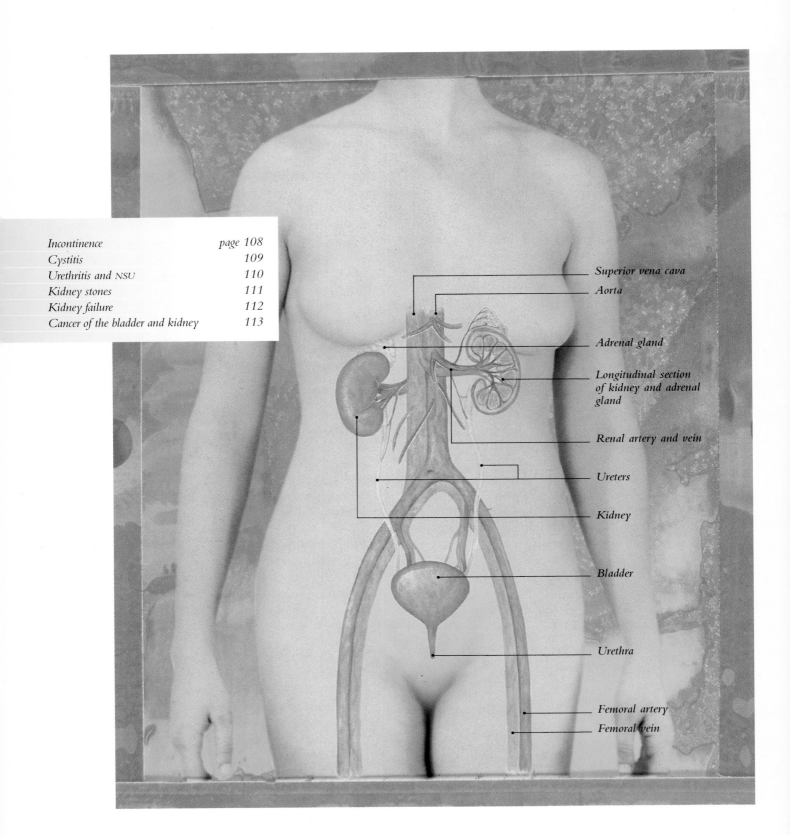

Superior vena cava

Aorta

Adrenal gland

Longitudinal section
of kidney and adrenal
gland

Renal artery and vein

Ureters

Kidney

Bladder

Urethra

Femoral artery

Femoral vein

The urinary system is one of the body's mechanisms for disposing of waste products, especially urea, a breakdown product from the metabolism of protein. The system comprises the kidneys, ureters, bladder and the urethra by which urine empties from the bladder.

URINARY SYSTEM

THE KIDNEYS ARE INCREDIBLY sophisticated filtration units, which process about 1.3 litres/2¼ pints of blood per minute to make urine at about 1 ml per minute. This urine drains through the ureters – muscular tubes that descend down the back of the abdomen, ending in the bladder. Contractions in their walls help propel the urine and prevent it from stagnating. The kidneys and ureters are under automatic control and they function unobtrusively.

The bladder is a storage vessel capable of holding 1 litre/ 1¾ pints or more of fluid. The outlet from the bladder is under more conscious control; we can decide when to hold and when to expel urine. Thus far this system is exactly the same in both men and women and is subject to similar disorders with similar symptoms.

Male and female urinary systems

The differences begin from the bladder onward. The urine empties via the urethra, a narrow tube ending just inside the vagina or at the tip of the penis. The female urethra is very short, so bacteria can easily ascend from the perineum. This is why women are far more likely than men to get a urinary infection or **cystitis**. In addition, the bladder and urethra are supported by the muscles of the perineum, which are often weakened by childbirth. Women are therefore more prone to prolapse leading to urinary problems such as **incontinence**, which is mainly, although not exclusively, a female problem.

The male urethra is much longer, so it is far more difficult for bacteria to ascend. This is why urinary infections in men are unusual and need more investigation than in women. The male urinary system, from the bladder on, joins with the reproductive system to allow sperm to be ejected through the urethra and penis. The male system experiences fewer problems than the female system because changes in supporting muscle structures are less likely and less critical to its efficiency. On the other hand men can expect to get trouble eventually from the prostate gland through which the urethra passes and which obstructs the urethra in about 30% of men by late middle age (see DISORDERS OF THE PROSTATE GLAND).

Potential problems

The urinary system is fundamental for health. In recognition of this there is great overcapacity in the system. It is possible to enjoy normal, and often reasonable, health with only one kidney, even if the remaining kidney is working at half capacity. This fact – that we can survive perfectly well with one kidney – makes kidney donation possible for transplantation.

Primary kidney disease is uncommon. Disease is more often due to infections, **kidney stones**, one of the many drugs that affect kidney function or simply through deterioration in the efficiency of the kidneys with age. Other than congenital disease, the main reasons for acquired kidney trouble are **diabetes**, **high blood pressure** or very low blood pressure after major blood loss or septicaemia.

Left: The kidneys continually filter blood to make urine, which the bladder stores until a convenient moment.

INCONTINENCE

The inability to hold urine, resulting in leakage or wetting.

CAUSES

As the bladder fills, its muscular walls involuntarily contract. This would lead to urination except that a sphincter of muscle around the outlet from the bladder remains closed under voluntary control until the desired time to release urine.

Urge incontinence

The natural tendency of the sphincter is to relax once the bladder is moderately full, as happens in infants. Children and adults gain voluntary control over the sphincter so that they can hold and release urine at will. However, ageing, dementia and disease of the nerves, such as **multiple sclerosis**, can weaken this voluntary control, so that once again the bladder empties automatically when it is only partially full. Urge incontinence can also be as a result of nerve damage caused during bowel and prostate surgery.

Stress incontinence

In stress incontinence anything that increases abdominal pressure, for example sneezing, coughing, laughing or simply standing, causes leakage of urine through the inefficient sphincter. This is a major cause of adult incontinence.

The anatomy of the neck of the bladder is critical to the control of urine. In women childbirth often results in changes to this anatomy and weakens the muscles of the pelvic floor. These factors commonly lead to prolapse (descent) of the womb and stress incontinence.

Incontinence may be made worse by minor infections; this is more common in women, particularly after the menopause.

SYMPTOMS

Urine leaks occur. If leaking follows straining, the likelihood is stress incontinence, that is, weakness of the sphincter. If there is an urge to pass small, frequent amounts of urine there is probably a nerve problem or a chronic irritation of the bladder neck. There may also be signs of dementia such as memory loss and breakdown of personality. There may be a previous history of **stroke** or abdominal surgery.

It is important to detect infections or **diabetes** by testing the urine. The diagnosis of the type of incontinence is aided by very precise tests of urine flow and bladder pressure, called cystometric studies. These help predict the value of treatment with drugs as opposed to physiotherapy or surgery.

TREATMENT

Assuming any infection has been treated, incontinence in women is helped by hormone replacement therapy (HRT), which restores the health of the sphincter muscle. The drugs which decrease unwanted bladder muscle contractions, for example flavoxate and oxybutinin, work best for women. Newer drugs include tolterodine and tamsuldsin.

For stress incontinence, pelvic floor exercises strengthen the muscles around the bladder that assist continence, and are recommended after childbirth. In cases of severe stress incontinence, surgery can restore the anatomy around the bladder neck (repair of prolapse).

For incontinence with brain disease, the above-mentioned drugs can reduce the frequency of incontinence, as does restricting fluid intake before bed and taking the person to the toilet regularly. In the worst cases it may be best to drain urine with a catheter. Modern catheters are non-irritant and designed to stay in place for several weeks.

Lastly, it is possible to divert urine into the bowel or into a bag on the abdomen, called a urostomy. Such operations are done for incontinence after bowel surgery.

QUESTIONS

How common is incontinence?

Exact figures are not available; by the age of 70 probably at least 10% of women and 2–5% of men experience incontinence. The figure rises rapidly above that age.

Why do so many people simply put up with it?

Incontinence has a bad public image with overtones of self-neglect and dementia. Evidently, this is quite unjustified. Also there is a lack of knowledge about treatments available for both men and women, regardless of age.

Complementary Treatment

Shiatsu-do techniques calm the nervous system and have positive benefits on the emotions; they also boost immunity – all factors in combating incontinence. Some **yoga** positions can help, in conjunction with specific exercises to strengthen the pelvic floor. **Hypnotherapy** – the therapist will use visualization, suggestion and regression to strengthen the bladder and uncover the origin of the incontinence.

CYSTITIS

Discomfort on passing urine, often the result of infection.

CAUSES

This very common condition is often caused by infection around the outlet from the bladder or within the bladder itself. Women suffer far more than men, because it is a shorter journey for germs to spread from the anus across the perineum (the area between the legs) up the short urethra and into the bladder. In women, this journey is only 3–4 cm/1¼–1¾ in, while in men it is 15–20 cm/6–8 in.

Often, in women, infection may not be found despite repeated urine tests. Such cystitis is thought to be a chronic inflammation of the bladder neck, making it irritable and giving rise to a burning sensation and a need to pass urine frequently. This inflammation could be caused by a mild infection not detectable on samples. It could be provoked by vaginal douches or wipes, or even bubble baths. Cystitis often follows sexual intercourse through sheer mechanical irritation. If a man has cystitis it points to a urethritis (see URETHRITIS AND NSU).

People who suffer recurrent infections may have an abnormality either within the bladder, such as a bladder stone or a tumour, or further up the system in the ureters. Some people find that certain fruits or acidic foods provoke cystitis.

SYMPTOMS

In women there is an urgent need to pass urine and the urine feels hot and stings. Within minutes the urgent desire returns; this cycle goes on for hours, passing just small amounts each time. There is often a trace of blood in the urine, which may smell fishy and look cloudy because of infection.

Men have similar symptoms, often with an additional aching in the perineum. If a man has a discharge with cystitis, NSU is a possibility. Both men and women may have a dull ache in the lower abdomen over the bladder.

Right: The E. coli *bacterium, which commonly causes cystitis and other urinary infections.*

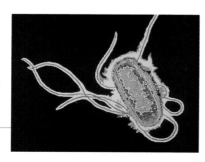

Testing urine reveals protein from pus in the urine, and blood from the inflammation of the bladder and urethra. An MSU is a test to grow the causative organism, which is frequently a bowel organism called *E. coli*.

TREATMENT

The body deals with minor episodes of cystitis naturally over a few days. It is helpful to drink extra fluids to keep washing out the bladder. The MSU result will dictate the appropriate antibiotic to be used. Commonly used drugs are trimethoprim and cephalexin. Any blood in the urine has to be treated seriously.

People with recurrent infections will need a cystoscopy, a procedure to look inside the bladder with a light source, or X-rays (see page 348) to outline the ureters.

Post-menopausal women are particularly prone to cystitis, and are helped by hormone replacement therapy (HRT). It is sensible to avoid vaginal deodorants and douches, which remove natural lubricants, to pass urine before and after intercourse and to wash carefully after opening the bowels.

QUESTIONS

How do over-the-counter remedies help?
These contain salts that make the urine more alkaline. This relieves the stinging and also hampers the growth of the infection responsible. A teaspoon of ordinary sodium bicarbonate dissolved in water may be just as effective.

What if no infection is found?
Even so a regular low daily dose of an antibiotic can help. The doctor will consider irritability in the bladder, which requires cystoscopy to prove. Treatment is often a matter of trial of agents including drugs used for urinary incontinence such as oxybutinin.

Complementary Treatment

Chinese and **Western herbalism** – many antiseptic herbs act on the urinary system to reduce irritation and increase urine output. **Nutritional therapy** – drink plenty of water. Cranberry juice and extracts prevent bacteria from adhering to the bladder walls. **Aromatherapy** – tea tree oil improves even chronic cystitis, take sitz baths daily (six drops). **Shiatsu-do** boosts immunity. **Healing** rebalances internal ecology. *Other treatments to try: acupuncture; homeopathy; Ayurveda.*

URETHRITIS AND NSU

Infection of the urethra, with inflammation and possible discharge.

CAUSES

Infection of the urethra, the narrow outlet tube through which urine leaves the bladder, leads to inflammation and often a thin clear discharge. Women may mistake the discharge for their usual vaginal secretions, whereas in men a discharge from the penis is obvious and always abnormal.

NSU means non-specific urethritis. It is considered a sexually transmitted condition but, by definition, no organism can actually be identified as responsible. The most common identifiable infective causes of urethritis are gonorrhoea and chlamydia, which may also cause **pelvic inflammatory disease** and affect a woman's fertility.

As with **cystitis**, women are affected more often than men as it is easier for bacteria to ascend the urethra. In women, urethritis is often due to infection from the perineum or irritation from bubble baths, vaginal deodorants or sexual intercourse. In a particularly troubling type of post-menopausal urethritis the walls of the urethra become thin and dry.

Strictly speaking, the term cystitis means inflammation of the bladder wall but it is often used to include both urethritis, where no definite infection can be found, and a true urinary tract infection with an identifiable bacterium. The terms are thus used interchangeably.

In about one-third of cases of chronic urethritis no cause is found and it is possible that psychological factors play a part.

SYMPTOMS

A burning of the walls of the urethra causes stinging on passing urine plus the urgency to pass small amounts of urine repeatedly. Often in NSU there is also a clear or cloudy discharge. Urine analysis fails to find an infection in the urine itself, which differentiates the condition from urinary infection. Many cases of NSU are asymptomatic and can be detected only by tracing the sexual contacts of people with known NSU.

TREATMENT

The first step is to take swabs from the urethra to try and identify the germ responsible. It is particularly important to detect gonorrhoea, which causes a heavy discharge in men but may cause no early symptoms at all in a female partner, yet lives on within her reproductive system to cause problems of chronic infection later. It is usual to test for other **sexually**

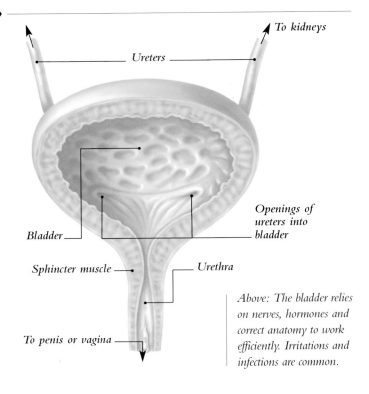

To kidneys

Ureters

Openings of
ureters into
bladder

Bladder

Sphincter muscle

Urethra

To penis or vagina

Above: The bladder relies on nerves, hormones and correct anatomy to work efficiently. Irritations and infections are common.

transmitted diseases with appropriate blood tests and swabs. If an organism is identified the appropriate antibiotic is given. Where none is identified – truly non-specific urethritis – it is usual to give a 'best-guess' antibiotic such as oxytetracycline or doxycycline. Again, it is important to trace sexual contacts who may be infected but symptom-free themselves.

It is difficult to cure chronic urethritis in women. One method is to dilate the urethra under anaesthetic, a procedure performed during cystoscopy. Post-menopausal urethritis responds well to hormone replacement therapy (HRT) or to oestrogen cream rubbed into the urethra. Careful hygiene is sensible and passing urine before and after intercourse.

Complementary Treatment

Chinese and **Western herbalism**, **nutritional therapy** and **shiatsu-do** – see CYSTITIS. **Ayurveda** – a therapist will recommend *panchakarma* detoxification and specific oral preparations to prevent recurring attacks. In **reflexology** the heels reflect zones on the urinary system. **Homeopathy** – many remedies are available, depending on specific symptoms. **Aromatherapy** – try sitz baths with tea tree oil (six drops). **Hypnotherapy** – cell command therapy could have a beneficial effect. *Other therapies to try: acupuncture; chakra balancing.*

KIDNEY STONES

Common abnormalities that are a source of pain and infection.

CAUSES

Kidney stones, in common with stalagmites and furred-up water systems, are formed by deposits of salts precipitating out from filtered fluid. Kidney stones are made of calcium salts and can be tiny or fill the whole kidney.

Some people are prone to kidney stones, having a constantly high level of calcium in the blood. Any abnormality in the kidney's anatomy increases the risk. Another reason is low urine output, which is why stones are more common in hot countries and in summer, as a result of dehydration. Bladder stones form for much the same reasons as kidney stones.

SYMPTOMS

Curiously, the larger stones cause fewer symptoms than the small ones, remaining stable within the kidney. There may be a vague ache over the kidney and an increased risk of urinary infections but, because of their size, the large stones cannot migrate. Small stones, however, eventually begin a journey from the kidney down the ureter to the bladder, with excruciating pain each time one moves, called renal colic. The pain is from spasm in the muscular walls of the ureter plus back pressure from obstruction to the flow of urine down that ureter.

The sickening pain (see also GALLSTONES) radiates from over the kidney across the abdomen down to the vagina or tip of the penis. During an attack the individual is sweating, nauseated and in true agony. There is always some blood in the urine. Most stones make this painful journey to the bladder successfully over a few days or weeks, punctuated by several episodes of renal colic. The passage out from the bladder is also uncomfortable but less than that previously experienced.

Classic renal colic is unmistakable. Minor colic is easily misinterpreted as lumbago or non-specific abdominal pain.

TREATMENT

For immediate relief, only the strongest painkillers dull the pain. Pethidine is widely used and diclofenac by injection is as effective and less sedating. Drinking copiously helps flush the stone through. As 90% of stones show on an abdominal X-ray, it is easy to follow their progress.

Long term, an ultrasound scan (see page 349) of the urinary system is a reliable way to detect and monitor stones. Otherwise sufferers have an IVP, an injection of a dye which is

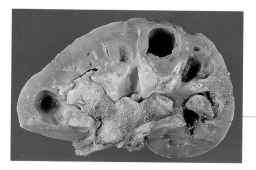

Left: Despite filling the base of the kidney, large stones cause remarkably few symptoms.

concentrated in the kidneys, so outlining the urinary tract. With patience, fluids and ample painkillers the stones pass.

If a stone sticks the preferred treatment is to shatter it using lithotripsy (see page 369) and the smaller fragments pass out without trouble. Thanks to this, surgery is now uncommon. If necessary, it involves opening the kidney to remove a large stone or passing a clever basket-type trap up the ureter to snare and pull out the stone. Stones are analysed to investigate their composition and blood tests are taken, seeking any biochemical disorder that increases the risks of further stones.

QUESTIONS

Do kidney stones recur?
Unfortunately they do. There is a high probability of a second kidney stone within a few years of the first one.

Do stones do any permanent damage?
In theory a stone completely obstructing a ureter could cause permanent damage to that kidney. In practice the stone is surgically removed before this. A large stone within the kidney does interfere with the efficiency of that kidney but only rarely is this significant.

Complementary Treatment
Chinese and **Western herbalism** – anti-inflammatory herbs and herbal diuretics might help. **Shiatsu-do** boosts immunity. **Nutritional therapy** – avoid calcium-rich foods, including dairy produce. Stone formation has been linked with vitamin B_6 and magnesium deficiencies, so consider supplementation. Drink plenty of hot, sweet drinks. **Hypnotherapy** – there are cases of kidney stones shrinking and being passed, possibly in response to hypnotic suggestion. *Other therapies to try: homeopathy; healing; tai chi/chi kung; reflexology.*

KIDNEY FAILURE

Failure of the kidneys to function efficiently for various reasons.

CAUSES

The kidneys filter about 180 litres/40 gallons of blood daily, extracting the waste products of metabolism, especially urea – a breakdown product from protein. Besides filtration, they also regulate blood pressure (via the renin/angiotensin system), blood volume, vitamin D and calcium balance and red blood cell production.

Filtration takes place at a delicate membrane layer, which is the usual site for chronic kidney disease. Damage to this membrane is caused mostly by inflammation of the filtration apparatus or blockage with protein complexes, from an immunological cause. **High blood pressure** damages circulation within the kidneys, while kidney disease itself leads to high blood pressure. The other common cause of kidney failure is **diabetes**, which damages the filtration surface and the blood flow. Less common but still serious causes of kidney failure are infections, large **kidney stones**, obstruction to urine flow, serious falls in blood pressure, certain drugs, tumours and congenital abnormalities of the kidneys.

SYMPTOMS

These are rarely dramatic at the onset; you pass urine that is a little more dilute than usual, blood pressure creeps up. If things deteriorate you feel tired and nauseous as waste products accumulate within the blood. Blood pressure may reach high levels, there is **anaemia** and swelling of limbs. Eventually there is profound tiredness, nausea, itching, bone pain and ultimately confusion or convulsions.

Kidney failure is confirmed by blood tests showing raised levels of the breakdown products urea and creatinine, and specialized measures of the efficiency of the kidneys. Often a kidney biopsy (see page 353) is required to establish the cause. Abrupt kidney failure is usually the result of either low blood pressure, for example after haemorrhage in an accident or major surgery, or acute infection.

TREATMENT

Clearly, blood pressure, obstruction or diabetes must be controlled or eliminated. Special diets control a number of salts poorly handled in kidney failure, such as sodium, potassium, calcium and phosphate. A low-protein diet reduces the load on the kidneys and may slow progression of the disease.

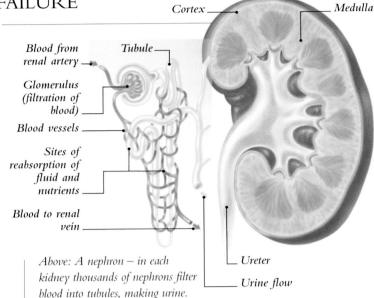

Cortex Medulla
Blood from renal artery Tubule
Glomerulus (filtration of blood)
Blood vessels
Sites of reabsorption of fluid and nutrients
Blood to renal vein
Ureter
Urine flow

Above: A nephron – in each kidney thousands of nephrons filter blood into tubules, making urine.

Anaemia used to be untreatable but can now be helped by injections of synthetic erythropoietin, which the kidneys normally produce to maintain red blood cell numbers.

Eventually the kidney patient may require kidney dialysis (see page 367) or a kidney transplant (see page 363).

QUESTIONS

How common is kidney failure?

Chronic failure resistant to all but transplant affects about one person in ten thousand per year. Many more people have a more modest degree of kidney failure requiring dialysis or special diets.

Can it be avoided?

Most cases are unavoidable, the cause being some as yet unknown immune condition. However, good control of blood pressure and diabetes reduces the chances of kidney failure.

Complementary Treatment

Kidney failure is a medical emergency and needs to be treated in hospital. However, many complementary therapies can aid recuperation. Those listed under STRESS could all help ease the tension associated with being ill and in hospital. See DIABETES and GASTRO-INTESTINAL ALLERGY for kidney disease linked to these conditions. Depending on the cause of the disease, traditional Chinese medicine (**acupuncture**, **herbalism**, **tai chi/chi kung**) may offer help, as may **Ayurveda**.

CANCER OF THE BLADDER AND KIDNEY

Cancer within the kidney, the ureter or the lining of the bladder.

CAUSES

There is evidence that suggests that half of the bladder cancers in both the United States and the United Kingdom are caused by cigarette smoking. Exposure to certain chemicals called amines, which are concentrated in the bladder and which are found in the rubber and chemical industries, probably account for another 10% of bladder cancer cases. In addition, schistosomiasis, a parasitic tropical disease, is an important cause of cancer of the bladder in Africa, South America and Southeast Asia.

Bladder cancer can extend into the urethra, the narrow outlet that leads from the bladder, and the ureters, the tubes that drain urine from the kidneys.

In children cancer of the kidney is usually caused by cells that have been left over from the embryonic development process. (This is also the case with most of the other rare childhood cancers.) Kidney cancer in children is treated much more successfully than it is in adults, in whom kidney cancer develops from normal cells that turn malignant.

In adults there is some weak evidence linking kidney cancer to smoking or chemicals at work. Some cases are due to taking the painkiller phenacetin, now banned in most parts of the world. The majority, however, are of unknown origin.

SYMPTOMS

The prime symptom in both cancers is blood in the urine. Unlike infection, where there is stinging as well as blood, this is normally painless. Even so doctors are cautious if someone with apparent **cystitis** has blood as well. It is a sensible precaution to test urine samples after antibiotic treatment in case microscopic amounts of blood are still present. The same goes for recurrent urinary infections. At some point a specialist must further investigate the urinary tract.

The diagnosis of bladder cancer is made by cystoscopy, looking inside the bladder and sampling any suspicious-looking areas on the walls of the bladder, urethra or ureters.

In cancer of the kidney, pain over the kidney is likely, as well as the general cancer effects of weight loss and loss of appetite. This cancer is an unusual but well-recognized cause of persistent **fever** and sweats. It may be possible to feel an abnormal mass in the abdomen, which is the way in which it is often detected in children. Diagnostic aids are scanning with ultrasound, CT or MRI (see pages 349, 350 and 351).

TREATMENT

Treatment of bladder cancer depends on the stage of the tumour. If the tumour is just on the surface it can be burnt away, with a very high probability of cure. However, you will need to have check cystoscopy for several years to deal with any recurrence of the cancer.

If the tumour is growing deeper into the bladder the options include removing the bladder, radiotherapy (see page 370), chemotherapy given into the bladder or general chemotherapy (see page 371). However, the outlook is much less good.

A kidney affected by cancer nearly always needs removing, after which radiotherapy or chemotherapy may be tried, although results are not good. The tumour may respond to hormones and more recently interferon has proved useful. If the cancer is confined to the kidney there is a 60–70% 5-year survival, which drops if it spreads to the liver, bones or lungs.

QUESTIONS

How common are these tumours?
Growths in the bladder are quite common (nearly 5% of all cancers) and can usually be treated successfully. Kidney cancer (1–2% of all cancers) causes vaguer symptoms so tends to be more advanced by the time of diagnosis.

And in children?
Kidney cancer affects about one in a hundred thousand children up to three years of age, then becomes extremely uncommon until late adult life. In children it is called a nephroblastoma or Wilm's tumour and is much more likely to be curable than in an adult.

How serious is blood in the urine?
It should never be ignored even though the great majority of cases will be due to infection or no detectable serious reason.

Complementary Treatment

Always have blood in urine checked by a doctor. Complementary therapies can play a valuable supportive role, although they cannot cure cancer. Deep relaxation techniques, such as **chakra balancing**, can be helpful. **Aromatherapy** with **massage** can help bring about a sense of wellbeing. **Reflexology** is also recommended. Check that your chosen practitioner is experienced in working with cancer. See also STRESS.

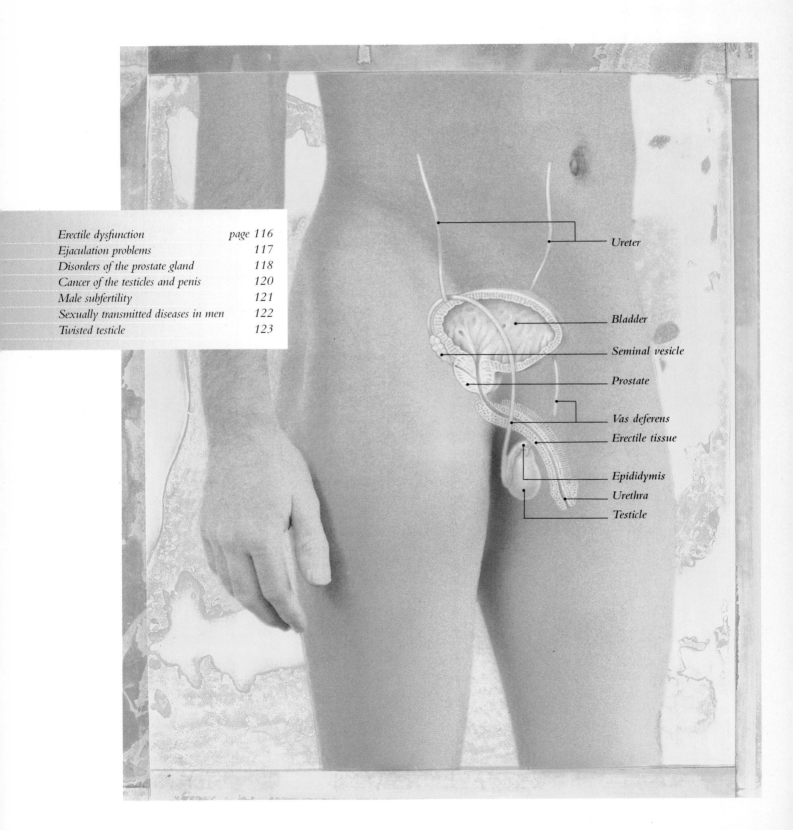

Ureter

Bladder

Seminal vesicle

Prostate

Vas deferens

Erectile tissue

Epididymis

Urethra

Testicle

Although this complex system works reliably in the main, sexual problems affect all men occasionally, while prostate trouble annoys many by late middle age.

MALE REPRODUCTIVE SYSTEM

THE MALE REPRODUCTIVE system shares structures with the urinary system to deal with the tasks of releasing urine and delivering sperm. Urine is stored in the bladder and leaves through the urethra, which runs through the penis. Sperm mature within the testicle and the epididymis – a small structure behind the testicle. They are given nutrition by secretions from the seminal vesicles and the prostate gland, then also leave via the urethra and penis. Sperm and urine do not normally mix thanks to a valve system, which prevents back-flow of urine from the urethra to the seminal vesicles and epididymis. At the time of ejaculation this same system ensures sperm go forward out of the penis and not backward into the bladder.

Most of the male reproductive system is visible, comprising the penis, testicles and scrotum. The prostate gland is hidden in the perineum – that part of the anatomy between the legs – and can only be examined via the rectum or with ultrasound. This visibility is a source of both pride and concern for men, as much male literature testifies. Men worry about size, performance and potency. As far as nature is concerned, however, all that is required is for large quantities of healthy sperm to be delivered into a female reasonably efficiently. Although it is tempting to dismiss all else as vanity, evolutionary theory teaches that there are genetic advantages favouring the potent and aggressive male.

What are sperm?

Sperm are packets of genetic material, each containing 23 chromosomes. Fertilization occurs when the 23 chromosomes from a sperm merge with the 23 chromosomes in the female egg in order to produce the normal human cell of 46 chromosomes. It is the shuffling of these chromosomes and the chance assortment within the fertilizing sperm that underlies and maintains the genetic variations of humanity. Sperm are programmed to swim as fast as possible to deliver that genetic material to the egg (see page 127).

Male hormones

This section concentrates on disorders of the genitalia themselves. However, the overall system of male sexual maturity and fertility relies on complicated hormonal control from the pituitary and hypothalamic glands within the brain, plus hormones from the testicles themselves. These hormonal influences are less noticeable than those of women, because there are not the obvious hormonal cycles of menstruation and pregnancy. They are no less vital for all that but disorders of those factors are not included in these pages because of their rarity and complexity.

An important difference between men and women with regard to the reproductive system is that men's sexual performance is affected by psychological factors and illness, plus a range of depressants of which alcohol is the most common. More controversial is the 'male menopause', a fall in testosterone levels with age, which is yet to be accepted as being an abnormality that requires treatment.

Changing attitudes

Men have been traditionally reluctant to talk about problems of sexuality and the prostate gland, despite the fact that these are exceedingly common. Such attitudes are changing, coinciding with research offering a better understanding of impotence, **subfertility** and **disorders of the prostate gland**.

Left: Several glands and elaborate pipework let the male system work both for sex and passing urine.

ERECTILE DYSFUNCTION

An inability to have or maintain an erection sufficient for satisfactory sexual intercourse – commonly known as impotence.

CAUSES

Erection of the penis occurs when blood flows into large sponge-like chambers along the length of the penis. The blood vessels involved are controlled by the autonomic nervous system, which works largely at an unconscious level but which can be stimulated by conscious will. When those blood vessels dilate blood rushes in and erection occurs; when they contract blood flows out and is not replaced so the penis shrinks. Men with poor blood flow to the lower body or with spinal cord or brain damage are liable to impotence, and research suggests that these factors are the most likely causes in older men.

Psychological factors are also important. **Anxiety** and **depression** in general, and attitudes to sex in particular, frequently cause impotence. Less important, although still significant, are abnormal levels of male hormone – testosterone.

Many drugs affect potency, for example alcohol, which, as Shakespeare said, raises the desire but decreases the ability. Other culprits are drugs for **high blood pressure** such as beta-blockers and diuretics.

Diabetes is very often accompanied by impotence through damage to the nerves and interference with blood flow.

SYMPTOMS

As a general rule, in men who are unable to get an erection at all there is probably a physical cause, whereas men who are impotent but get a nocturnal erection or wake with an erection are more likely to have a psychological cause for their impotence. Other symptoms suggesting a psychological cause are if impotence occurs with certain partners but not with others, or if there is a background of anxiety or depression.

It is important to have a general physical check-up, looking especially for normal blood flow and testing for diabetes.

TREATMENT

Occasionally, blood flow can be improved by microsurgery to dilate the arteries or veins of the penis. Steps are taken to reduce progression of circulatory problems by controlling blood pressure, cholesterol and diabetes, if detected.

Sildenafil (Viagra) is the first of a new class of drugs that induce erection. It is a tablet that works in about 50% of men after an hour. Men with heart disease should use it with caution, otherwise it is well tolerated. MUSE is a pellet of alprostadil which has to be inserted within the urethra (tip of the penis). This is instead of injecting the same drug into the penis. These drugs are replacing older treatments such as self-injection, penile rings and vacuum devices, although these are still used in some cases.

Penile rings fit around the base of the penis, keeping blood within it, and vacuum devices fit over the penis and draw blood in. Another treatment possibility is to implant mechanical devices that are inflated at will; these are becoming more sophisticated and reliable. Proven lack of male hormone can respond to testosterone.

Treating psychological impotence is a specialized area. It involves exploring the couple's attitudes to sex (such as thinking it is 'dirty', or past bad experiences), learning to give mutual sexual pleasure short of intercourse with stroking and stimulation, and de-emphasizing penetrative intercourse as the only goal of each sexual encounter.

QUESTIONS

How important are psychological factors?
Psychological factors were long thought to account for the great majority of cases of impotence. However, research is increasingly showing that it is in fact physical factors that cause well over 50% of cases of impotence. This has obviously led to marked changes in treatments offered.

Is impotence an inevitable consequence of ageing?
Only in that blood flow problems and other physical disease are more common with increasing age. Although levels of the hormone testosterone do decline with age, this plays a relatively minor part in impotence.

Complementary Treatment

Auricular therapy can increase blood flow to the genitals. **Aromatherapy** stimulant oils include jasmine, ginger and black pepper. Try three drops of one of these in 10 ml of carrier oil, to make and use as a **massage** oil. **Hypnotherapy** – sex therapists sometimes use hypnotic suggestion and regression as part of a treatment plan. Many **Ayurvedic** preparations are available to improve sexual potency. **Homeopathy** – see MALE SUBFERTILITY. *Other therapies to try: tai chi/chi kung; acupuncture; healing; chakra balancing; homeopathy.*

EJACULATION PROBLEMS

◆

Common problems with the expulsion of sperm and seminal fluid at the time of orgasm.

CAUSES

◆

The mechanics of ejaculation are quite well understood. It begins with the release of sperm from the testicles, which mixes with seminal fluid from the prostate gland and seminal vesicles. Reflex contractions of muscles at the base of the penis then pump out the 2–5 ml of a normal ejaculate. An internal valve closes to prevent back-flow of semen into the bladder. These reflexes are under unconscious control by the nervous system. Accompanying this is the intense sexual sensation of an orgasm, which is the response of the brain to sexual stimulation. Orgasm includes additional reflex consequences such as rapid heart rate and breathing and a rise in blood pressure.

After orgasm the penis goes limp and there is a feeling of relaxation lasting a half hour or more. There is also a period during which it is not possible to have another full erection or orgasm. This period depends greatly on age, ranging from minutes in a young man to 24 hours or more in the elderly.

The main ejaculation problems are complete failure, usually because of disorder of the nervous system, retrograde ejaculation and premature ejaculation. Retrograde ejaculation is often an inevitable and permanent consequence of surgery on the bladder or prostate gland, which damages the valve mechanism that normally prevents it. Premature ejaculation is so common that it is probably normal, especially in young men.

SYMPTOMS

◆

Failure of ejaculation means little or no semen appears at orgasm. In retrograde ejaculation little appears at orgasm but the urine is clouded with semen that has flowed backwards (retrograde) into the bladder.

In premature ejaculation orgasm occurs rapidly after sexual activity begins, whether during manual stimulation or within a brief time of inserting the penis into the vagina. There are usually feelings of guilt or shame at failing to prolong the sexual act or failing to bring the partner to sexual satisfaction.

TREATMENT

◆

In terms of treatment there is little that can be done about retrograde ejaculation, but it is worth realizing that it is harmless – although it does reduce fertility. Nor can anything be done for failure of ejaculation that follows nerve damage.

Although common, premature ejaculation has become so entangled with sexual mythology, notions of potency and of giving sexual satisfaction to partners that few men will admit to experiencing it. The first step for treatment is therefore to acknowledge the problem.

The treatment is similar to that used for treating impotence (see ERECTILE DYSFUNCTION). The focus is moved away from penetration and orgasm and on to wider sexual gratification, such as gratification by stroking and mutual stimulation. In addition, the man lets his partner know when he feels orgasm is approaching. His partner can then squeeze the base of the man's penis, which very effectively inhibits the reflex. Over time the urgency of the sexual act is modified so that premature ejaculation becomes less likely.

Other treatments for premature ejaculation involve taking relaxants, including alcohol (but see ERECTILE DYSFUNCTION). The latest antidepressants, selective serotonin reuptake inhibitors (SSRIs), appear helpful in retarding ejaculation (see DEPRESSION). There is also an older antidepressant called clomipramine. However, a quick non-psychological answer for treating premature ejaculation has yet to be established.

QUESTIONS

Is premature ejaculation necessarily abnormal?
Premature ejaculation is only a problem if the couple finds it so. If the man's partner is not bothered by him ejaculating quickly, then there is no need to seek medical help.

Are erection and ejaculation necessarily linked?
They involve different nervous mechanisms, although there is great overlap. This is why it is possible and common to have an orgasm with a limp penis, especially during 'wet dreams'.

Complementary Treatment

Auricular therapy – if the problem is emotional, treatment can be weekly; if physical, it should be more frequent, to increase blood flow to the genitals. **Aromatherapy** and **hypnotherapy** – see ERECTILE DYSFUNCTION. **Healing** helps to dispel negative feelings which can manifest in physical problems. Many **Ayurvedic** preparations are available to delay orgasm. If the cause is emotional and not physical, **chakra balancing** can help by balancing energies. *Other therapies to try: homeopathy; acupuncture.*

DISORDERS OF THE PROSTATE GLAND

Benign and malignant disease of the gland that encircles the urethra, the tube which runs from the bladder to the penis.

CAUSES

The function of the prostate gland is not entirely clear. It does, however, produce secretions that mix with the sperm and help to transport and nourish them.

Benign enlargement

By the age of about 60 most men will have some enlargement of the prostate gland – this can be double the usual size. The reason is thought to do with changing concentrations of oestrogen and testosterone as men get older. Benign (non-cancerous) enlargement appears to be a pure function of age and evidence suggests that every man will get it if he lives long enough. The enlarged gland squeezes the urethra, obstructing urine flow to a greater or lesser degree.

Cancer of the prostate

In the United Kingdom cancer of the prostate accounts for about 7% of all cancers. After lung and bowel cancer it is the next most common cause of death from cancer in men and is increasing in frequency. Male sex hormones are part of the cause of prostate cancer but these are by no means entirely to blame since heredity and diet also have a role to play.

Small nests of malignant cells in the prostate gland are extremely widespread in older men, being found in about 80% of men by their 80s. However, only a small percentage of these cells develop into symptomatic prostate cancer.

SYMPTOMS

Both benign and malignant disease of the prostate gland cause similar symptoms so that investigation is needed to differentiate between the two. Both cause pressure on the urethra, constricting it and thereby weakening the flow of urine and causing difficulty in beginning to pass urine, which may just dribble out. There is an irritability to the bladder, with a need to pass urine frequently but, unlike **cystitis**, there is no stinging on passing urine.

The pressure on the urethra causes stagnation of urine in the bladder and a risk of bladder infections. Because of incomplete emptying of urine the bladder enlarges and can reach as high as the belly button. This back pressure can be transmitted to the kidneys, causing aching in the loins. There is always the risk of urinary retention, which is complete obstruction to outflow, with pain and further distension of the bladder. This is a medical emergency treated by passing a catheter into the bladder in order to drain the urine.

Cancer of the prostate can cause all of the above symptoms. In addition, there may be symptoms from the spread of cancer into bones. For this reason doctors suspect prostate cancer in any older man who presents for the first time with back or hip pain and who also has prostatic symptoms.

Examination of the prostate gland

All cases need examination of the prostate gland, which is done by passing a finger into the rectum to feel the gland. The benign gland is enlarged and smooth whereas a cancerous gland feels hard and has irregular areas. A very helpful blood test for detecting malignancy is Prostate Specific Antigen (PSA). A high reading almost certainly means cancer, a low reading almost certainly means benign enlargement. Borderline results or the response to treatment can be monitored by checking the PSA every few months.

TREATMENT

In the case of benign enlargement of the prostate not all men require treatment, especially if the only symptoms are a need to pass urine a couple of times a night and a poor flow of urine. As long as the bladder is not distended and blood tests show that kidney function is normal, it may be several years before treatment is needed, although a slow deterioration in the gland is inevitable.

Benign enlargement

The first choice in medical treatment is using drugs, such as finasteride, that shrink the prostate gland by blocking the action of testosterone on the gland. Other drugs, called alpha-blockers, relax the smooth muscle of the urethra enough to reduce symptoms to acceptable levels, but do not reduce the size of the gland – indoramin is an example.

If these measures fail or if there is complete blockage, a prostatectomy is necessary. This is an operation to trim away the gland. It is usually performed using slim fibreoptic instruments passed into the urethra. The gland is then dissected away by a heated wire or by a laser (see page 365).

There has been interest in implanting metal tubes to prevent the prostate from squeezing the urethra closed but these are not yet fully evaluated. Other possibilities involve heating or freezing the gland and, again, these are relatively experimental but looking promising.

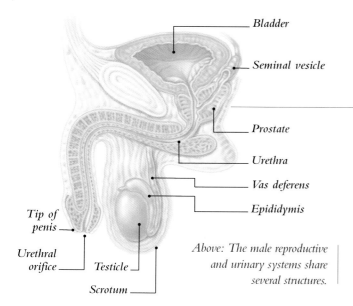

- Bladder
- Seminal vesicle
- Prostate
- Urethra
- Vas deferens
- Epididymis
- Tip of penis
- Urethral orifice
- Testicle
- Scrotum

Above: The male reproductive and urinary systems share several structures.

Cancer of the prostate

It is usual to confirm the diagnosis of prostate cancer by taking multiple biopsies through the rectum, although this is being replaced by high-definition ultrasound images of the gland. It is important to know whether the disease has spread elsewhere, so a bone scan is performed.

If there is just a tiny focus of cancer confined to the gland, the current British approach is to keep it under regular review. In the United States more aggressive treatment is usual, which means removal of the whole gland.

There is a choice either to remove the prostate gland, called a radical prostatectomy, or to irradiate it. Both methods appear to give comparable results. The drawback of surgery is the likelihood of **incontinence** of urine and impotence (see ERECTILE DYSFUNCTION), although improved microsurgical techniques are reducing these risks. Radiotherapy can also cause impotence and there may be radiation damage to the bowel, causing pain and **diarrhoea**. To avoid this, it is now possible to implant radioactive rods into the prostate gland. This novel therapy looks promising for early prostate cancer.

If the disease has spread outside the gland or to bone, then radiotherapy is favoured, together with drugs that reduce testosterone levels. These are cyproterone, taken by mouth, or injectable drugs such as goserelin, which need to be given every three months only. These drugs have thankfully removed the need to perform a castration, which used to be the standard way of reducing testosterone.

Screening for prostate cancer

The discovery of PSA appeared to open the prospect of screening for disease. This is still controversial, however, because not enough is known about the natural history of prostate cancer. As has already been mentioned, up to 80% of men over 80 will have microscopic cancer and may have an abnormal PSA but it is simply not known how many of such deposits may go on to cause problems. Regardless of the lack of scientific evidence to support screening, men over the age of 50 are increasingly asking for screening by way of a yearly rectal examination and PSA.

QUESTIONS

Is surgery/radiotherapy essential?
If cancer is a chance finding, current British practice is to monitor it, because there may be no problems for many years. However, treatment of cancer that is causing symptoms improves survival.

What is the outlook?
Surgery for benign enlargement relieves symptoms for a decade or more and can be repeated. Sixty to eighty per cent of men treated for early cancer are still alive after ten years, which is good considering that these are men already in their 60s and 70s. Unfortunately, once cancer has spread into bone there is a 20% survival to 5 years.

When will screening be recommended?
Currently, screening detects many men with cancer that causes no symptoms and where the rate of progression is unknown. A more specific blood test is under development and should end this still controversial debate, as will safer treatments for early disease.

Complementary Treatment

Cancer: Complementary therapies cannot cure cancer. Herbal and vitamin therapies, however, could be useful for cancer of the prostate, but it is very important to have a conventional medical assessment before embarking on complementary treatment, and to keep conventional practitioners informed of what you are doing. Herbal and vitamin therapies could be provided by a **Western herbalist**, **Chinese herbalist**, **Ayurvedic** practitioner, **naturopath** or **nutritional therapist**. **Reflexology**, **aromatherapy** and **chakra balancing** can all offer support during orthodox treatment for cancer. *Benign enlargement:* Zinc deficiency and/or essential fatty acid deficiency appear to be common factors in the onset of benign enlargement of the prostate. **Nutritional therapists** work to reverse such deficiencies, and might also use herbs, for example clinical trials have shown saw palmetto to be useful. **Homeopathy** can also be of benefit – treatment depends on individual circumstances.

CANCER OF THE TESTICLES AND PENIS

Both of these are unusual, but cancer of the testicles is becoming more common. It is curable, so early detection is important.

CAUSES

In the case of cancer of the testicles, the one agreed cause is undescended testicles. This means that the testicles stayed within the abdomen instead of dropping into the scrotum at or around birth. If untreated, there is about a 5% risk of later malignancy. Other causes of testicular cancer arise from malignant changes in the cells within the testicles that make sperm, although the trigger for this change is not understood. For unknown reasons testicular cancer is more common in men from higher socio-economic groups and is becoming more common.

In the case of cancer of the penis it is thought that poor hygiene contributes to this uncommon tumour. It is extremely rare in circumcised men. The role of environment and heredity is important in other unclear ways. For example, the tumour is up to 20 times more common in parts of South America and Africa than it is in the United States.

SYMPTOMS

In testicular cancer there is a lump in the testicle that may or may not be painful; this testicle often feels heavier than the other. There might be swelling of the scrotum with inflammatory fluid, called a hydrocele. The tumour can spread to bones or lung; if this happens the first symptoms might be pain or breathlessness. Importantly, 10% of tumours cause no symptoms at all but can be detected by self-examination. Most testicular cancers occur in men in their 20s and 30s.

In cancer of the penis there is a persistent sore or ulcer on the penis and often enlarged lymph glands in the groin. The disease is most common in men in their 60s or older.

In both cases the diagnosis has to be confirmed by taking a biopsy, plus scans and chest X-rays to show whether the cancers have spread. This is important in planning treatment and in deciding the prospects for cure.

TREATMENT

Depending on the precise type of the tumour, the treatment for testicular cancer will involve radiotherapy, chemotherapy or both (see pages 370 and 371). Removal of the affected testicle is not always necessary but again it depends on the type of tumour. Treatment is now so good that nearly every man can be cured, although it is important that follow-up for recurrence is continued for many years. Follow-up is aided by the discovery of biochemical substances in blood tests that give early warnings of the recurrence of cancer. These are alpha-fetoprotein and beta-chorionic gonadotrophin, both of which are easily measured.

Many cases of penile cancer can be dealt with by removal of the growth itself, leaving most of the penis intact, depending on the site of the cancer. If it has spread to the glands in the groin these must be removed in a major operation, performed only if the cancer has not spread elsewhere. Chemotherapy or radiotherapy have not proved very effective in the condition. Even so, there is up to a 90% five-year survival, although falling to much less where there is spread to glands or bones.

QUESTIONS

How important is testicular cancer?
Although it ranks far behind lung or bowel cancers, it is the most common tumour in men in their late teens to early 30s (about 1300 cases per annum in the United Kingdom).

Why is early detection of these cancers important?
The prospects for cure of both these conditions is much higher in the case of early disease.

Can these cancers be prevented?
All young men should check their testicles regularly every few weeks. Feel for lumps or ulcers and have anything remotely suspicious checked. Undescended testicles should be surgically corrected at an early age. Any persistent sore on the penis should be reviewed by a doctor. The role of circumcision in preventing cancer of the penis is controversial.

 Complementary Treatment
Complementary therapies cannot cure cancer. However, many of them have a role during treatment. **Chakra balancing** will help with symptom control and energy balance, as well as aiding relaxation during orthodox treatment and offering support during rehabilitation programmes. **Reflexology** can offer support during orthodox treatment. **Aromatherapy**, especially when combined with **massage**, is excellent for reducing stress and tension associated with disease. *Other therapies to try: see STRESS.*

MALE SUBFERTILITY

Subfertility is the failure to conceive despite a year of regular intercourse (once or twice a week). Male causes are a factor for 30–40% of couples having difficulty in conceiving.

CAUSES

First, it is important to distinguish between subfertility in the male as opposed to some problem with sexual technique. There may be impotence (see ERECTILE DYSFUNCTION) or inaccurate ideas about sexual intercourse, so that sperm is being deposited outside the vagina.

Low sperm count

Then it is a matter of whether the man is producing adequate quantities of healthy sperm that can reach their target. Sperm are produced in huge quantities by the testicles, then stored until expelled at orgasm. The life of a sperm is short (90 days) and almost entirely disappointing, bar one brief moment of hope at the time of orgasm. Sperm are little energized cells whose destiny is to race against a hundred million other sperm in order to be the one that fertilizes the egg, thereby passing on genetic material. So what interferes with this?

The testicles need male hormones; any lack of these will affect sperm formation. Many drugs affect the testicles, as do any serious illnesses, especially liver disease, kidney disease and excessive alcohol intake.

A varicocele, a kind of collection of varicose veins behind the testicles, reduces sperm count by increasing the temperature of the epididymis where sperm mature. The sperm themselves may be abnormally formed or lack forward drive. There may be blockages in the pathway from testicle to penis. Antisperm antibodies may be produced by the man against his own sperm or by his partner, which reduce the number of effective sperm despite an otherwise adequate sperm count.

SYMPTOMS

Before focusing on the woman if there is failure to conceive it is essential to look for male causes. Basic investigations are examination of the testicles and penis and a sperm count.

The sperm count should show large quantities of normal sperm. By convention 'normal' is taken to be at least fifty million sperm, of which at least 60% are mobile and most are normally formed. Although it is true that it takes only one sperm to achieve fertilization, the wastage is such that a low sperm count reduces the chances of conception considerably. More sophisticated tests involve measuring sperm antibodies

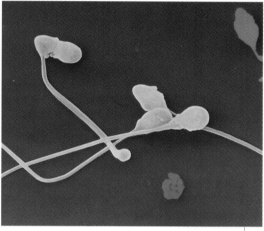

Above: Sperm with abnormal lumps on their heads, which prevent them from successfully penetrating the egg.

and performing a post-coital test – collecting sperm from the vagina after intercourse to establish whether sperm are moving and living within the environment of the vagina.

TREATMENT

Avoiding smoking and alcohol are known to improve the sperm count. The number and quality of sperm improve up to about seven days of abstinence from intercourse, after which they decline. The optimal sperm quality should therefore be timed to coincide with the woman's time of maximum fertility. Treatment is possible in cases of hormone disease such as underactive pituitary gland. Removing a varicocele may improve the sperm count. Attempts to deal with antibodies are not widely successful as yet. The most encouraging work is in artificial insemination (see FEMALE SUBFERTILITY).

Complementary Treatment

Homeopathic remedies include agnus for ineffectual erection, conium for inability to sustain erection and sepia for lack of libido. The effectiveness of these remedies depends on individual circumstances. Diet – low sperm counts may be linked with deficiencies such as vitamin C and zinc; a **nutritional therapist** could advise. **Hypnotherapy** could help if subfertility is linked to subconscious fears about fatherhood. *Other therapies to try: tai chi/chi kung; naturopathy; acupuncture; autogenic training; Ayurveda.*

SEXUALLY TRANSMITTED DISEASES IN MEN

Infections spread by sexual contact, known as STDs. Many are detected through tracing the contacts of those already infected.

CAUSES

These are caused by micro-organisms, most of which prefer living in the genital system and surrounding skin. Some of these are serious, causing gonorrhoea, syphilis and AIDS.

Gonorrhoea is caused by gonococcus, a micro-organism unique to humans and spread only by sexual contact. Syphilis is caused by *Treponema pallidum*, which can also pass from mothers to the unborn foetus, leading to congenital syphilis. In recent years the micro-organism chlamydia has come to be recognized as the most important cause of **urethritis** and, in women, of subfertility. The herpes simplex virus is a common and persistent infection causing much discomfort. The fungus candida is often carried by men, although rarely giving symptoms as annoying as for women, in whom it causes vaginal **thrush**. Then there are viruses that cause warts around the genitalia and those that cause AIDS and hepatitis B and C. Apart from HIV (the virus responsible for AIDS), the above are most common in the West; there are other STDs common in the tropics.

SYMPTOMS

Usually, there is some combination of itching around the genitalia, pain on passing urine and a discharge from the penis. Depending on the cause there may be a rash or warts on the genitalia or the anus, enlarged glands in the groin and possibly a more widespread rash on the body. These symptoms occur any time from a few days after infection to several weeks later.

Urethritis may settle without treatment. Syphilis causes an initial rash and generalized ill health which disappear, only for more serious symptoms to recur years later, for example **ulcers** on the skin, damaged and weakened bones, difficulty with walking, dementia and damage to the heart.

TREATMENT

Genito-urinary clinics deal with diagnosis, treatment and tracing sexual contacts. This is done in the strictest confidence – even your own doctor will not be informed without your permission. Diagnosis is arrived at by taking swabs from the urethra, anus and mouth to try to grow the organism responsible. Blood tests confirm syphilis, HIV and hepatitis B and C.

Treatment may be simply an antifungal or antiviral cream for thrush or herpes. Gonorrhoea is treated by a single short

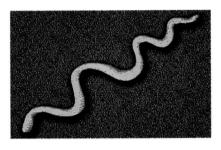

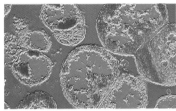

Top left: Spiral-shaped Treponema pallidum *is the micro-organism that causes syphilis.*
Bottom left: Pairs of kidney-shaped gonococci, the bacteria responsible for gonorrhoea.

course of an antibiotic such as amoxycillin or ciprofloxacin. Syphilis requires about 10 days of penicillin injections. Urethritis also responds to antibiotics. There is a very high probability of cure in most cases; even with early syphilis, although the damage done by late syphilis cannot be cured.

Tracing sexual contacts

The importance of this cannot be overstated. Men know when they have a problem but women may not, especially with gonorrhoea and chlamydia, which may silently destroy a woman's fertility. Syphilis and HIV may ruin both partners' lives, and those of future sexual partners. You are encouraged at the clinic to list recent sexual partners. Staff then diplomatically contact them, explain any risks and invite them for investigation. They will not be told who might have infected them.

See also SEXUALLY TRANSMITTED DISEASES IN WOMEN.

Complementary Treatment

There are serious consequences from the inadequate treatment of STDs, so always seek a conventional opinion. Complementary therapies can boost the immune system to help the body resist further attack. **Western herbalism** – echinacea boosts the immune system. In traditional Chinese medicine a combination of **herbs**, **acupuncture** and **tai chi/chi kung** could help. **Ayurveda** would suggest a combination of detoxification, oil massage and yoga. **Aromatherapy** may have some effect on herpes – an experienced practitioner could advise. *Other therapies to try: homeopathy.*

TWISTED TESTICLE

♦

A cause of pain in the groin, with implications for future fertility.

CAUSES

♦

The testicles dangle within the scrotum on the spermatic cord, which is a combination of blood supply, nerves and the vas deferens through which sperm leave the testicles. In theory, this should carry a high risk of the testicle twisting. In fact the testicle is held in place by a surrounding layer of tissue.

It is not known exactly why the testicle sometimes twists but it is thought to follow a vigorous contraction of the muscles that pull up (retract) the testicles. If they contract rapidly enough the testicle twists – called a torsion – cutting off the blood supply, which is a medical emergency. It most often affects boys in their early teens.

SYMPTOMS

♦

There is a sudden severe pain in one testicle, which swells and is extremely tender to even gentle examination. The overlying scrotum becomes reddened, and there may be nausea, vomiting and pain in the lower abdomen. The affected testicle hangs noticeably higher than the other one.

Babies suffering a torsion will cry through pain and draw up their legs. Unless the scrotum is carefully examined it is easy to overlook the diagnosis in a baby.

There are other causes of pain in a testicle: epididymitis gives pain behind the testicle; any injury may cause pain and swelling. Orchitis is inflammation of the testicle and occurs for no obvious reason. These are valid alternative diagnoses to consider in an adult but are unsafe diagnoses in any boy below the age of about 16. This is because it is impossible to tell the difference between these conditions for sure.

In some cases there is little pain, but just a suddenly swollen red scrotum. Within about four hours of torsion there is serious damage to the testicle through blockage of blood flow. Unless torsion is corrected within about 12 hours that testicle will shrink and be permanently less fertile.

It is possible to differentiate these conditions with a radioisotope scan of the testicles but most surgeons prefer to operate to see the situation for themselves.

TREATMENT

♦

It may be possible to manoeuvre the testicle back into position under a local anaesthetic. The more usual treatment is to open up the scrotum, untwist the testicle and stitch it to the

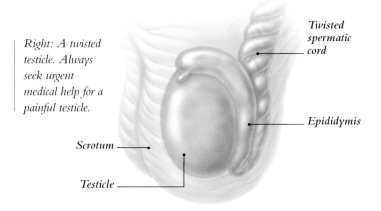

Right: A twisted testicle. Always seek urgent medical help for a painful testicle.

Twisted spermatic cord

Epididymis

Scrotum

Testicle

scrotum to prevent future problems. If one testicle has twisted there is a higher chance of torsion of the other, so it is advisable to stitch both testicles into place.

If the testicle has been irredeemably damaged it may be best to remove it all together.

QUESTIONS

How common is torsion?
Complete torsion is uncommon; minor episodes of pain in the testicle are common and may be the result of twists that correct themselves. Any prolonged discomfort should be taken seriously.

How important is early treatment?
After 12 hours of torsion the testicle will probably be permanently damaged. Therefore pain in a testicle in a young boy should be medically assessed as an emergency.

By how much is fertility affected?
Although a single testicle makes adequate amounts of sperm, losing one will reduce the total sperm count and just tip the odds towards reduced fertility. Of course, it increases the risk of total infertility should an accident happen to the surviving testicle.

Complementary Treatment
Never ignore pain in your testicles. This should always be reported to a conventional practitioner because there are serious long-term consequences from inadequate treatment. Postoperatively, **acupuncture** can be used to control pain. **Chakra balancing** and **healing** can help speed recovery.

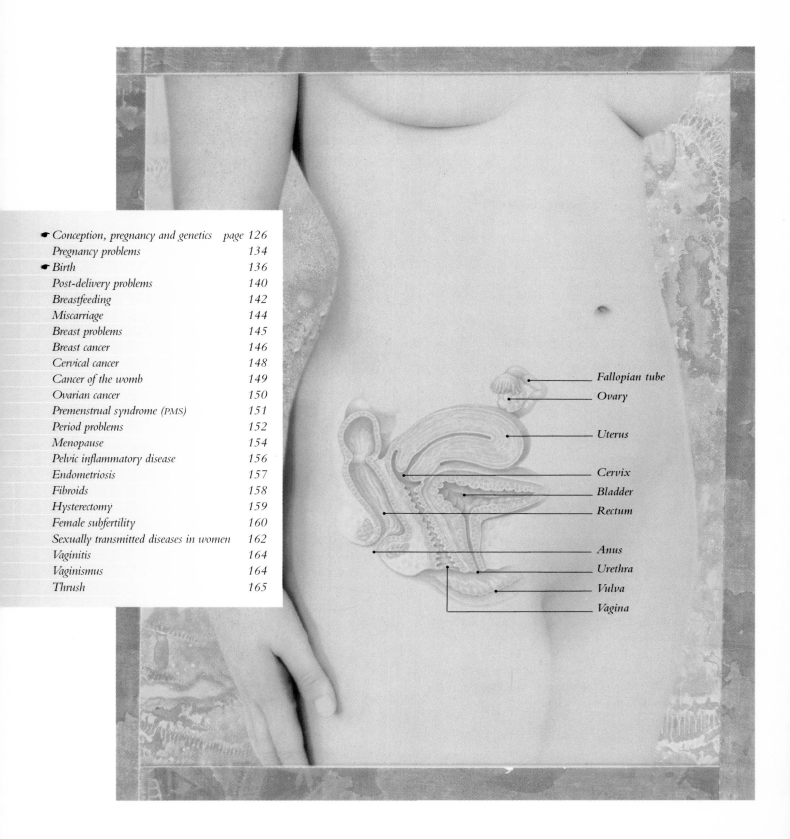

Fallopian tube

Ovary

Uterus

Cervix

Bladder

Rectum

Anus

Urethra

Vulva

Vagina

Most societies regard with awe the menstrual cycle and pregnancy,
an awe enhanced as scientific research reveals the intricate interplay
of hormones and specialized tissues involved.

FEMALE REPRODUCTIVE SYSTEM

THE MAIN COMPONENTS of this system are the womb (uterus), Fallopian tubes and ovaries. The ovaries contain all the eggs a woman will ever have. By just six weeks' gestation the baby girl already has all the genetic material that will be used during her reproductive lifetime. At birth the ovaries contain some two million cells that could turn into eggs; this falls to a few hundred thousand by puberty. During a reproductive life of say 35 years, only about 400 eggs are released. The rest degenerate.

The onset of puberty

Puberty begins when something as yet unknown triggers the hypothalamus in the brain to stimulate the ovaries to produce oestrogen, the female hormone. With this stimulation the girl starts to develop secondary sexual characteristics, such as growth of breasts, pubic hair and, eventually, the commencement of menstruation. Puberty may begin anywhere from nine to sixteen years and is probably triggered in part by the amount of body fat.

The reproductive process

In the mature woman the ovaries work under the influence of hormones from the hypothalamus and pituitary glands, undergoing the cyclical changes of menstruation (see PERIOD PROBLEMS). Most months an egg is released from the ovary and caught by frond-like outgrowths at the end of the Fallopian tubes, which guide it into the tube. Over the next few days the egg travels to the womb; when it occurs, fertilization takes place during this journey.

The womb is where the fertilized egg embeds itself; the womb's walls provide a rich blood supply to the developing embryo via the placenta. The bulk of the womb is made up of muscle which expels the baby at term. The outlet of the womb is the cervix, which projects into the vagina.

The vagina is a muscular tube, guarded at the outside by the labia. The vagina distends during intercourse and, of course, during childbirth to allow the baby to exit. The labia have no particular function, although they do distend during sexual arousal. Tucked just before the entrance to the vagina is the clitoris, which is the female equivalent of the penis and like the penis responds to stimulation, leading to orgasm.

The female reproductive system includes the breasts, which are designed to supply milk to the baby but respond to sexual stimulation as well.

Hormonal control

The whole system is under the control of hormones secreted by the hypothalamus and pituitary glands in the base of the brain, with input from several other sources. Such influences include the adrenal glands, the fat layers, the thyroid gland, growth hormone and the ovaries themselves.

Many women's problems are hormone related, through aberrations in the delicate hormone balance from day to day and from cycle to cycle. The breasts, womb and ovaries are all environments with great cell activity and are subject to tremendous hormonal changes, which is why they are common sites for cancer. Quite unlike in men, infections can gain access to the interior of the body via the vagina and Fallopian tubes; thus pelvic and vaginal infections are common and potentially extremely serious.

At the **menopause** hormonal changes cause women to experience widespread effects throughout the body.

Left: Within the mostly hidden female
system are the structures which produce
eggs and nurture the foetus.

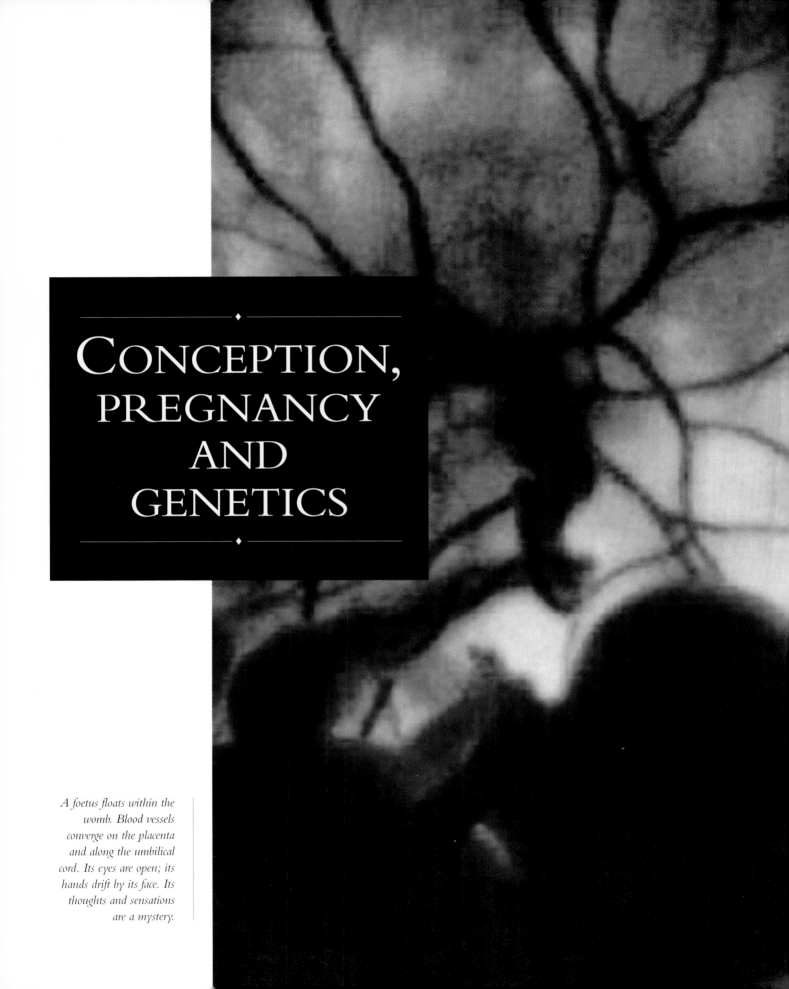

CONCEPTION, PREGNANCY AND GENETICS

A foetus floats within the womb. Blood vessels converge on the placenta and along the umbilical cord. Its eyes are open; its hands drift by its face. Its thoughts and sensations are a mystery.

THE CREATION OF A NEW LIFE begins with the fusion of a sperm and an egg. These two microscopic elements contain between them the blueprint to create over the next 40 weeks that amazing organism called a human being.

At ejaculation, the man deposits 100–500 million sperm into the woman's vagina. The freshly ejaculated sperm must then penetrate the cervical mucus, which is possible only when the vaginal secretions are of a certain acidity and the mucus is of a certain viscosity.

Fertilization

The sperm are capable of living for three days within the genital tract; they swim through the cervix, through the womb and into the Fallopian tube to meet the newly released ripe egg. It is not yet known exactly what drives sperm, but it is thought they are probably responding to a biochemical pull towards the egg.

Of the hundreds of millions of sperm, a mere hundred or so actually reach the egg. One single sperm penetrates the egg by digesting its way through the surface. At that instant of penetration, a biochemical change occurs in the coating of the egg which prevents any other sperm from penetrating it.

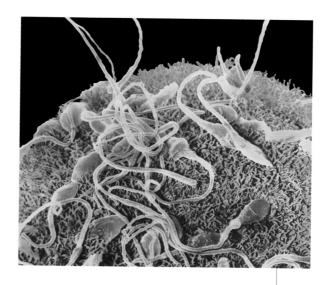

Above: A few successful sperm (green, with tails) on the egg (orange). Of the millions that strove to reach this egg, just one will fertilize it.

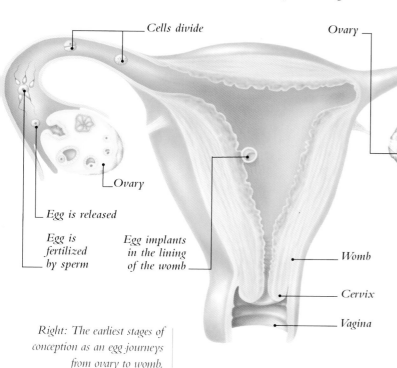

Cells divide

Ovary

Ovary

Egg is released

Egg is fertilized by sperm

Egg implants in the lining of the womb

Womb

Cervix

Vagina

Right: The earliest stages of conception as an egg journeys from ovary to womb.

Egg and sperm then merge, their genetic contents intermingling. Thirty hours later the egg divides in the first critical division into two cells, then into four, then into eight which, within a few weeks, will have formed the billions of cells of the embryo.

Implantation and the placenta

The fertilized egg moves along the Fallopian tube until it reaches the womb after five to seven days. Here it implants into the wall of the womb by sending outgrowths into the womb which mature into the placenta. This remarkable structure combines foetal and maternal tissues to form a large disc where the baby's and the mother's blood capillaries come into intimate contact, but remain separate. The placenta is where oxygen, carbon dioxide and waste materials pass between mother and baby. At the same time the placenta excretes a variety of hormones in order to ensure the continuation of the pregnancy.

Preconception
You can take certain health measures to secure the best possible start for you and your baby even before you are pregnant.

Diet Ensure a balanced intake of fruit, vegetables and protein. Vegetarians may need to take iron supplements.

Folic acid Taking this natural vitamin greatly reduces the chances of having a baby with **spina bifida** – a child whose backbone fails to fuse, leaving the spinal cord exposed. Folic acid should be taken prior to conception and during the first 12 weeks of pregnancy. The dose is 0.4 mg a day.

Alcohol Excess alcohol can cause brain damage in the baby as well as affecting its appearance. The risk increases with the more alcohol you drink; some authorities recommend avoiding alcohol completely during pregnancy.

Smoking If you smoke during pregnancy, your baby will be smaller and weigh less than if you did not smoke and may remain smaller throughout its life – an avoidable legacy.

Rubella *(German measles)* Routine vaccination programmes in childhood now offer protection from this illness, which causes multiple abnormalities in the baby if contracted in the first four months of pregnancy (see page 262). A simple blood test will show whether you are immune.

Exercise: Continue your usual routine of exercise. The first three months is the time of greatest risk of miscarriage, but there is no evidence to suggest that an active lifestyle contributes to this risk. On the contrary, regular exercise is good for maternal and foetal health.

An outline of pregnancy
The course of a pregnancy is normally considered in three sections called trimesters. Each trimester is approximately three months.

The first trimester
The baby These months are the most critical time in the baby's development. All its vital organs are formed, including the brain. Having begun as a single microscopic cell, by just four weeks the embryo has the rough outline of a human baby, although it is just 4 mm/³/₁₆ in long.

How does this happen? It is a process like origami: the twisting and folding of a flattish layer of cells into a cylinder,

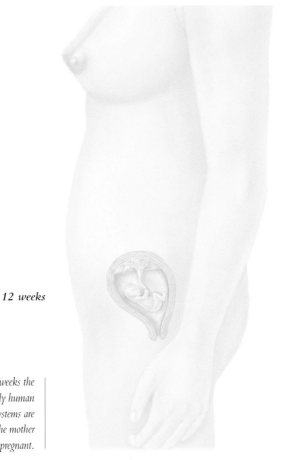

12 weeks

Right: At 12 weeks the foetus is obviously human and most body systems are working, yet the mother hardly appears pregnant.

which further differentiates into the brain, spinal cord and all the internal organs. At eight weeks after conception, the embryo is clearly recognizable as human and is about 2.5 cm/1 in long. Its heart is beating and it can use some muscles. Eyes and ears are present, although primitive. Yet you have only missed one period and may only just suspect that you are pregnant.

By three months' pregnancy the baby will be about 5 cm/2 in long, with well-formed limbs and face. It will be kicking, but too faintly to be felt.

The mother So much is going on yet there is little to show for it except for a few natural, although inconvenient, symptoms caused by hormone changes.

Women vary greatly in how much nausea they experience. Nausea is very rarely serious. Tiredness appears to be a real hormonal effect, although compounded by the need to care for other children or to work.

Bladder irritation is a result of yet more hormonal effects on the neck of the bladder; it is often one of the earliest signs of

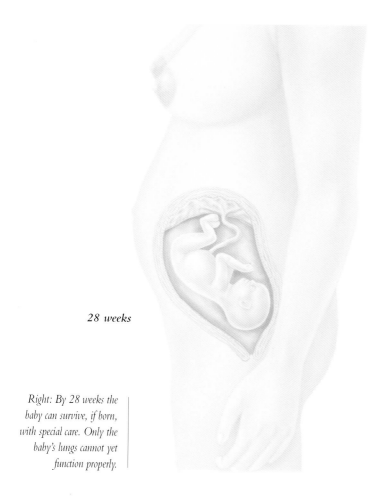

28 weeks

Right: By 28 weeks the baby can survive, if born, with special care. Only the baby's lungs cannot yet function properly.

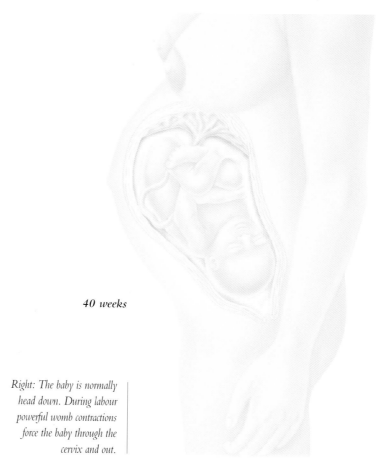

40 weeks

Right: The baby is normally head down. During labour powerful womb contractions force the baby through the cervix and out.

pregnancy. Breast tenderness is from the effect of progesterone causing glands within the breasts to swell up in preparation for producing milk when the baby is born.

The second trimester

The baby All the baby's organs are formed and from now on it is a question of continued growth and maturation. Movements can be felt from about 16 weeks. At 16 weeks' pregnancy the baby has definite limbs, fingers and toes, is 18 cm/7 in long and weighs about 100 g/4 oz; it is recognizably male or female. Its kidneys are secreting urine and it swallows amniotic fluid. At 24 weeks' pregnancy the baby is 24–32 cm/9^1/$_2$–12^1/$_2$ in long and weighs 750–900 g/1^3/$_4$–2 lb. It moves regularly and vigorously, has skin and is covered with fine hair. Its eyes are open, but whether it is able to see or not is not known. Most of its organs are reasonably mature, except for the lungs.

A baby born at 24 weeks has a chance of survival within an incubator but will need artificial respiration because the muscles for breathing are too weak to expand the lungs.

The third trimester

The baby Except for its lungs, the baby is virtually mature and can survive if born at any time during this stage. Over the last three months the main changes are growth and the deposition of fat under the skin. Babies born before 36 weeks may need special care. By 40 weeks the average baby is 50 cm/19^1/$_2$ in long and weighs about 3.4 kg/7^1/$_2$ lb.

The mother You have the increasing anticipation of a happy outcome to your pregnancy which outweighs the discomforts of this last stage. These include backache, feeling ungainly, **constipation**, **piles** or **varicose veins**. Movements are easily felt and often you are aware of contractions of the womb called Braxton Hicks contractions, especially in the last few weeks. In first pregnancies the baby engages at about 36 weeks, which means that its head sinks low into the pelvis, ready for birth. In later pregnancies the baby usually engages only just before labour starts.

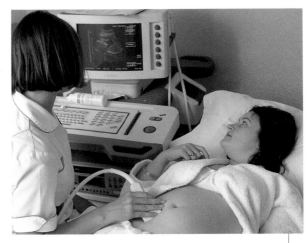

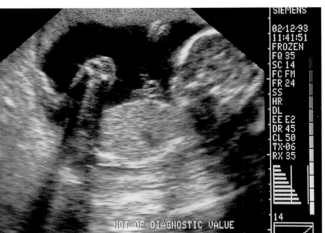

Above: High-definition ultrasound scanning is invaluable for monitoring the health, development and position of the baby. In the lower image the head of a 20-week foetus is visible at the right, knees and feet to the left.

Routine antenatal care

Pregnancy is not an illness, yet there is much that can go wrong: poor growth of the baby, **high blood pressure**, urinary infections, **anaemia**, **diabetes** and many more, quite apart from the hazards of birth itself. Fortunately, serious complications are uncommon but routine antenatal monitoring (see page 356) aims to detect abnormalities as early as possible. In addition to providing time for discussion and reassurance, routine antenatal care includes checks on:

- *Heart*
- *Blood pressure*
- *Urine*
- *Weight gain*
- *Growth of the womb*

Investigations during pregnancy *Pregnancy tests* are done on a urine sample and are highly sensitive and reliable. They detect the presence of HCG (human chorionic gonadotrophin), a hormone released by the fertilized egg and detectable in blood or urine from six days after fertilization, when the fertilized egg is implanting into the womb.

Blood tests are necessary to detect anaemia, blood group, rhesus factor and whether there are unusual antibodies in the blood stream. Later, blood tests can indicate problems with the growth of the baby by measuring a hormone called oestriol, which is an indication of the health of the placenta.

Ultrasound scans allow precise monitoring of the growth of the baby and can detect abnormalities in the heart, back, kidneys and other organs.

Amniocentesis is sampling of the fluid surrounding the baby, performed in cases of suspected abnormality such as **Down's syndrome**.

Chorionic villus sampling can be done from about ten weeks to detect foetal abnormality. A tube is passed through the cervix to take a fragment of the tissue surrounding the foetus as a test for certain genetic disorders such as muscular dystrophy.

IMPORTANT WARNING SIGNS IN PREGNANCY

◆

- *Abdominal pain or bleeding may indicate miscarriage, premature labour or problems with the placenta, depending on the stage of the pregnancy*
- *Rapid weight gain or headaches and blurred vision may indicate pre-eclampsia if there is also a sudden rise in blood pressure*

See also PREGNANCY PROBLEMS *and* MISCARRIAGE.

Right: Pregnancy is a natural sequence of events for which a woman's body is designed. Modern antenatal care makes pregnancy safe while still fulfilling.

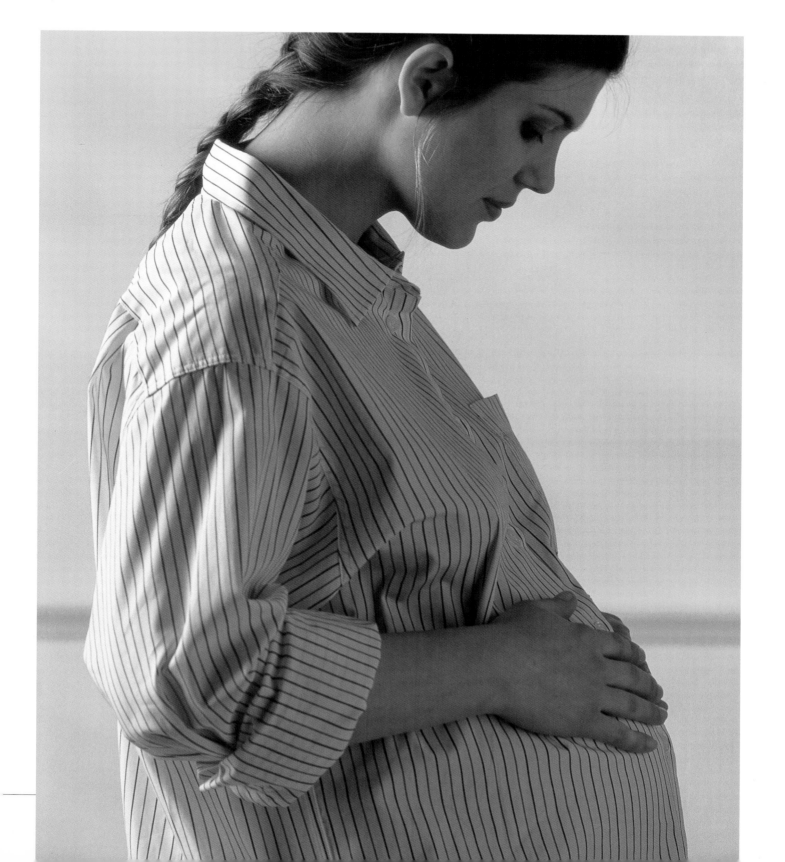

Genetics

There has been an explosion of knowledge about human genetics in the last 20 years. More and more of the genes responsible for human characteristics are being identified and the complete description of DNA has just happened. The following is an introduction to this complex and rapidly changing area of knowledge.

DNA (deoxyribonucleic acid) DNA is made of two molecular strands which spiral around each other in what is called a double helix. It is a record of how to make the proteins that are essential for life. All cells contain DNA because this is the blueprint to which they constantly refer in order to make the myriad proteins required by cells.

DNA is formed using just four simple chemical building blocks called nucleotides. Groups of three nucleotides specify (or code for) particular amino acids (see proteins, below). To translate a section of DNA, RNA (ribonucleic acid) is formed from the DNA in a way that copies the nucleotide sequence. That RNA moves elsewhere within the cell where it is in turn read by other forms of RNA carrying the amino acids specified by the original DNA code. The strand of amino acids lengthens into a protein. A gene is a section of DNA that carries the instructions to build one protein. This is the genetic code.

A strand of DNA contains three to four billion nucleotides, more than enough to code for the one hundred and fifty thousand or so proteins used by life.

Proteins These large molecules are built up from combinations of the 20 different human amino acids. As the amino acids are fitted together, the lengthening chain twists and takes a shape. The shape of a protein is often a vital part of its function, for example four haem proteins join to make haemoglobin, the shape of which allows it to carry iron and oxygen. Other well-known proteins are those in muscles, connective tissue (collagen), blood clotting factors, antibodies and insulin.

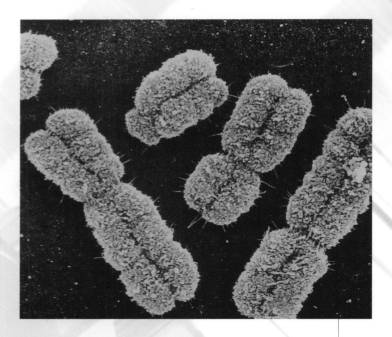

Above: Pairs of chromosomes highly magnified. Each comprises DNA tightly curled in such a way that it can be accessed in order to read the genetic information.

Inheritance

Within most cells the DNA resides in chromosomes, a condensed form of DNA, packaged to make it easier to reproduce itself. Humans have 23 pairs of chromosomes. There is one pair of sex chromosomes, called X- and Y-chromosomes, that determine whether an individual is male or female. A female has two X-chromosomes, while a male has an X- plus a Y-chromosome. The sex chromosomes carry many genes other than those involved in sexual differentiation. These other genes are called 'sex linked' because they are linked with the chromosomes that determine sex. This is why certain genetic conditions are found only in one sex or another. In general, only X-linked recessive genes are of importance in disease, for example haemophilia, which affects males only.

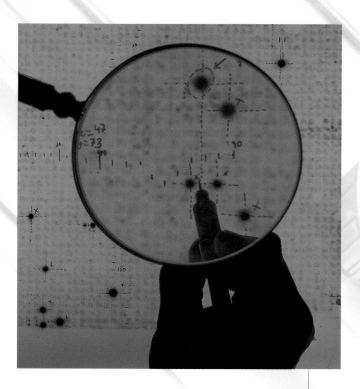

*Above: Close examination of
DNA sequences on a photographic
plate enables scientists to carry out
specialized analysis.*

*A fragment of DNA, enormously enlarged.
Its billions of nucleotides encode the
information needed for life. The elegant
double helix structure was discovered by
Watson and Crick in the 1950s.*

When a cell divides, the double-stranded DNA splits in two, immediately replicating itself from the pool of nucleotides within the cell. Each daughter strand of DNA is a duplicate of the mother DNA, with all its genes.

Eggs and sperm All the eggs a woman will ever have form within the female embryo just a few weeks after fertilization – some seven million in all. Five million of these will have died even before the baby is born; yet more die during childhood. This leaves about 200,000 eggs when puberty begins, just a few hundred of which will ever develop into fully mature eggs during ovulation.

Sperm, on the other hand, are generated continuously from germ cells that activate at puberty.

Eggs and sperm each contain 23 single chromosomes formed by a complex rearrangement of chromosomes and genes and including a sex chromosome. The female egg always carries just an X-chromosome whereas a sperm may carry an X- or a Y-chromosome. It is therefore the father's sperm that determines the sex of a baby – a girl being XX, a boy being XY.

Once fertilized the egg has 23 pairs of chromosomes – a set from the mother and one from the father. Although many of the genes inherited are similar there are subtle differences that will influence how the child will develop – from the shape of his nose, the colour of eyes and overall size to the child's susceptibility to various diseases.

Dominance Certain genes are dominant, that is, they take precedence over the corresponding gene in the other set – for example, the gene for brown hair is dominant over other hair-colour genes, which are non-dominant, or recessive. This means that if the baby gets the gene for brown hair from one parent it will have brown hair whether the hair-colour gene from the other parent is for brown or fair hair. But it may not get that dominant gene because, in the genetic lottery that precedes the formation of eggs or sperm, the gene may not be passed to the particular egg or sperm involved in fertilization.

The genetic diversity from this system is continually altering the human gene bank and is responsible for much of our individuality. However, genetic inheritance is only one strand in human potential, although an immensely important one; environmental factors may help or hinder the expression of natural capabilities. The transmission of culture through the family and society can be regarded as another form of inheritance and is the more important factor in the slow, often painful, evolution of the human race.

PREGNANCY PROBLEMS

◆

There are particular problems associated with each of the three trimesters of pregnancy:

FIRST TRIMESTER

◆

Tiredness, possibly overwhelming, affects most women at this time decreasing by about 12 weeks. It may be due to the hormones of early pregnancy and **anaemia** (see below).

Ectopic pregnancy
Causes: This implantation of the fertilized egg outside the womb occurs in one in three hundred conceptions. The risk is higher if a woman has had an ectopic pregnancy before or conceives with a contraceptive coil in place. The ectopic egg can grow for a few weeks before rupturing surrounding tissue.
Symptoms: There is persistent pain in the lower left or right abdomen (central pain is more suggestive of **miscarriage**). The previous period may have been entirely missed or scanty and brief. There may be other symptoms of early pregnancy – nausea and breast tenderness. Internal examination shows the cervix very sensitive to gentle movement. If the ectopic pregnancy ruptures the Fallopian tube there is sudden severe abdominal pain, vaginal haemorrhage and collapse.
Treatment: An ultrasound scan locates the ectopic pregnancy before emergency surgical removal of the fertilized egg and the Fallopian tube on that side. Sometimes the ectopic egg alone can be removed and the Fallopian tube repaired – preserving future fertility, although it is perfectly possible to conceive with just one Fallopian tube.

WARNING SYMPTOMS IN PREGNANCY, WITH POSSIBLE SIGNIFICANCE
◆

- ◆ *Any bleeding (miscarriage, placenta praevia, premature labour)*
- ◆ *Abdominal pain, especially if one sided (ectopic pregnancy, premature labour)*
- ◆ *Severe nausea (multiple pregnancy)*
- ◆ *Failing to feel baby's movements (problems with foetal growth)*
- ◆ *Fingers or feet that swell rapidly (pre-eclampsia)*
- ◆ *Severe headaches, especially if with flashing lights (pre-eclampsia)*
- ◆ *Breathlessness at rest (anaemia, heart disease, pulmonary embolus)*
- ◆ *A swollen painful leg (deep vein thrombosis)*
- ◆ *A feeling that things are not right (most experienced doctors will respect the mother's instinct about this and arrange tests of the baby's health)*

Nausea
Causes: This is assumed to be due to pregnancy hormones. Severe early nausea may indicate twins or multiple pregnancy.
Symptoms: Nausea is greatest each morning, decreasing during the day. Only occasionally is it so bad that the woman vomits continuously and becomes dehydrated – hyperemesis.
Treatment: It is best to have a snack before getting up in the morning. Antinausea medication is not prescribed unless nausea is severe. Hyperemesis needs intravenous rehydration in hospital, with a scan to detect any multiple pregnancy.

Infection/drug damage
Causes: The baby is insulated from most infections. **Rubella** is the main risk but is virtually eliminated by vaccination. A few drugs can damage the developing foetus; others such as some antibiotics are safe but are best avoided unless essential. Alcohol and smoking to excess affect the baby's growth.
Symptoms: Women who smoke have babies about ten per cent (250 g/8 oz) lighter than predicted. Babies born to heavy drinkers have a recognized abnormal facial appearance.
Treatment: There is such a high risk of foetal damage from rubella (30–40%) that non-immune women exposed to it are offered a termination. If a woman has taken a potentially harmful drug she will be offered a detailed ultrasound scan to try to detect any malformation of the foetus.

SECOND TRIMESTER

◆

Foetal abnormality
Causes: Often, this is pure genetic chance. Drugs, infections and parental age account for just a few foetal abnormalities.
Symptoms: The most serious abnormalities end in miscarriage or failure of the baby to grow normally. Ultrasound scans check the appearance of its organs for **spina bifida**, brain, kidney and heart anomalies or **Down's syndrome**.
Treatment: Some abnormalities can be treated in the womb by foetal surgery. Others give early warning that the baby will need special care, sometimes raising difficult ethical issues.

Placenta praevia
Causes: Placenta praevia means that the placenta is implanted low down in the womb (instead of on the side), covering the cervix and obstructing normal delivery.
Symptoms: Occasionally there is bleeding in late pregnancy. If previously undetected, the first symptom is obstruction at the time of birth. One reason for scanning pregnant women is to check for this condition.

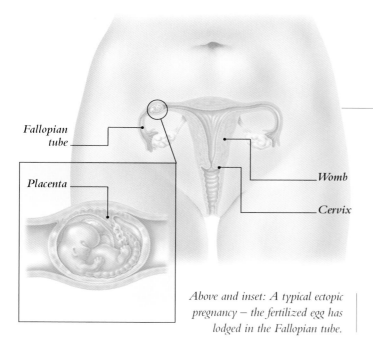

Fallopian tube

Placenta

Womb

Cervix

Above and inset: A typical ectopic pregnancy – the fertilized egg has lodged in the Fallopian tube.

Treatment: Nothing can be done to prevent placenta praevia, but a Caesarean section (see page 139) can be planned in advance and makes safe delivery possible.

THIRD TRIMESTER
◆

Anaemia
Causes: Even in well-nourished women this almost always appears in pregnancy as a result of expansion of blood volume. The risk increases with each pregnancy and in breastfeeding since iron passes into the milk.
Symptoms: There are often none; blood tests show whether it is serious enough to treat.
Treatment: Mild anaemia needs none. Otherwise one or two iron tablets plus folic acid a day are sufficient. It is rare to be so anaemic by delivery that a blood transfusion is needed.

High blood pressure (pre-eclampsia)
Causes: After ectopic pregnancy, this is potentially the most serious complication of pregnancy. The cause is probably an immune reaction against the placenta.
Symptoms: Fingers and feet may swell, appearing and worsening over a few days; there may be severe headaches with flashing lights. Blood pressure is raised, sometimes greatly; there is protein in the urine. This is pre-eclampsia, and may progress to eclampsia with epileptic fits, unconsciousness and a risk of mother and baby dying. Fortunately eclampsia is very rare.
Treatment: Mildly raised blood pressure usually responds to rest as long as there are not the other features above. Severe hypertension is treated with drugs like labetalol. Eclampsia is a medical emergency: the mother has to be deeply sedated and blood pressure controlled by intravenous drugs. The baby must be delivered by Caesarean section immediately.

Premature delivery
Causes: It is not understood why normal labour begins, let alone premature labour. Sometimes the neck of the womb is lax and cannot contain the pregnancy to term.
Symptoms: These are the same as normal labour: a show of mucus, leakage of fluid and blood and rhythmic contractions.
Treatment: The aim is to delay labour until the baby is as old as possible: 32 weeks is desirable, although babies as premature as 24 weeks can survive. A few drugs can delay premature labour which, combined with rest, might gain those vital extra weeks. If the cause is a lax cervix, it is kept closed with a stitch, later removed to allow normal vaginal delivery.

Indigestion, constipation and piles
Causes: The large mass of baby and womb obstructs the gastrointestinal tract. Acid is literally squeezed out of the stomach into the gullet and the bowels are partially obstructed – not helped by taking iron tablets. Piles (see HAEMORRHOIDS) are a direct consequence of the increased abdominal pressure on blood vessels around the anus.
Symptoms: **Heartburn** is common; the bowels may be opened with difficulty, only every few days. Piles are often associated with **varicose veins** at the top of the thighs and in the labia.
Treatment: **Indigestion** lessens once the baby's head engages at about 36 weeks. There are entirely safe antacids available. **Constipation** responds to high fibre or laxatives if necessary. Nothing can be done to reduce piles, which will nearly always disappear after the birth; soothing creams help the itching.

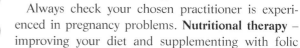

Complementary Treatment
WARNING: In **Western herbalism**, herbs should not usually be taken during pregnancy except under professional guidance. However, ginger tea is a safe and effective remedy for morning sickness.

Always check your chosen practitioner is experienced in pregnancy problems. **Nutritional therapy** – improving your diet and supplementing with folic acid, vitamins B_6 and B_{12} and zinc can help reduce a number of problems, such as nausea and fatigue. **Chiropractic** manipulation can relieve pain in the low and mid-upper back, which is common as a result of enlarging breasts. Specific **yoga** postures can alleviate some symptoms, such as haemorrhoids. **Hypnotherapy** is good at banishing morning sickness. *Other therapies to try: aromatherapy; Chinese herbalism; homeopathy; acupuncture; biodynamics; Bach flower remedies; shiatsu-do; naturopathy; chakra balancing; healing.*

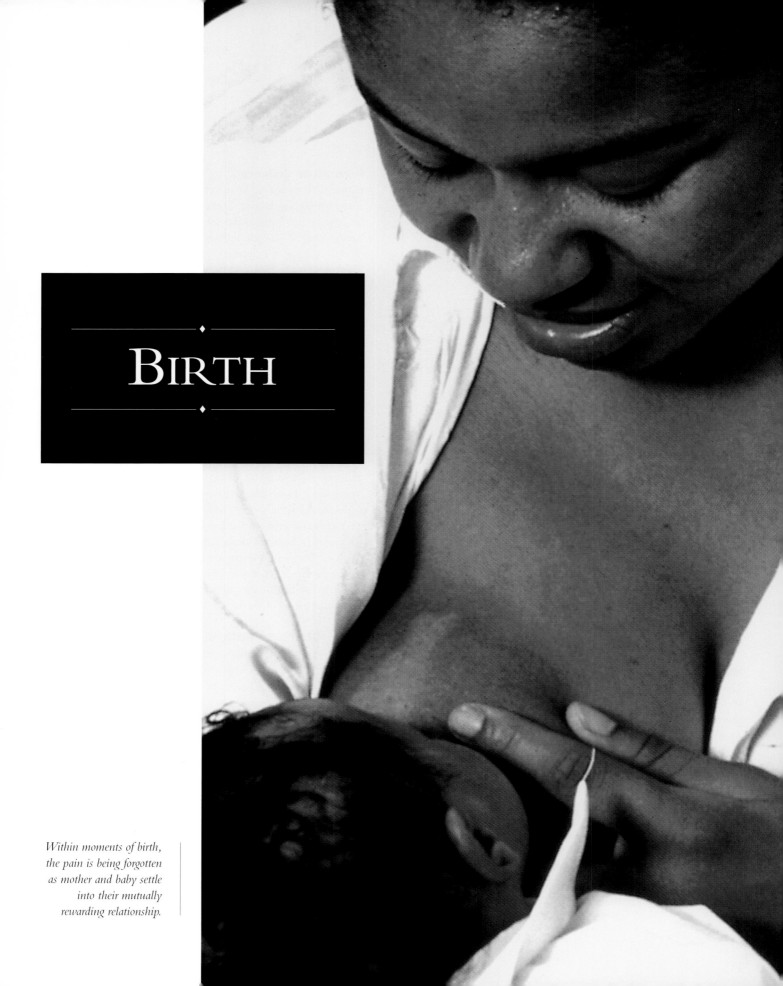

BIRTH

Within moments of birth, the pain is being forgotten as mother and baby settle into their mutually rewarding relationship.

MODERN OBSTETRICS, the care of women in pregnancy, is largely concerned with making birth as rewarding but safe as possible. In most areas of the United Kingdom the expectant mother now has a choice of ways in which to deliver her baby, ranging from the full panoply of medical care in a hospital delivery room to a relatively private event in a birthing pool.

Preparing for labour

By the end of pregnancy the baby is ready to be born; its lungs are the last organs to be mature enough to cope outside the womb. Hopefully, you and your partner are psychologically prepared for the process of birth. Through reading and questioning, try to ensure you know in some detail what to expect – the types of pain and what they mean, who will be dealing with you, the role of the midwife and the obstetrician, the equipment and examinations required. Above all, remember that birth is a natural process and that modern obstetric care aims to assist rather than replace nature.

In most cases the baby lies head down, facing the mother's left or right side. In a first pregnancy the baby should engage at around 36 weeks; the baby's head settles low in the womb in a fixed position. As this relieves pressure at the top of the womb this is also called lightening. In later pregnancies engaging occurs just before birth.

Thanks to the hormone progesterone, the cervix is soft and can dilate easily; the joints between the pelvic bones are relaxed enough to let the baby's head through. Something as yet unknown then triggers the beginning of labour and the mild Braxton Hicks contractions often felt throughout pregnancy become stronger.

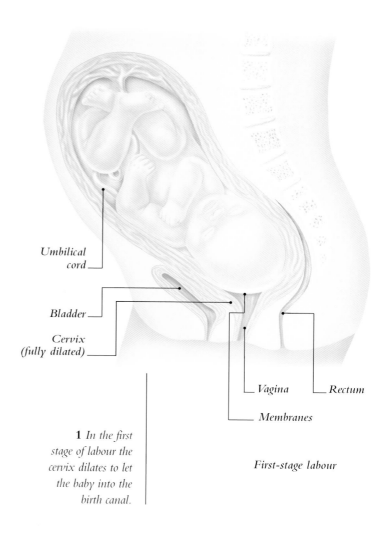

Umbilical cord

Bladder

Cervix (fully dilated)

Vagina   Rectum

Membranes

1 *In the first stage of labour the cervix dilates to let the baby into the birth canal.*

First-stage labour

Monitoring the baby

The use of this technique has waned, but it is still important in higher-risk pregnancies. One element involves monitoring the baby's heart rate during contractions. The other is to take a sample of blood from the baby's scalp. These tests show whether the baby is coping with the stress of birth or whether it is being starved of oxygen and therefore needs to be delivered urgently either by forceps or by Caesarean section (see page 139). During labour your attendants will keep checking to see how the baby is coping. The readings are especially important if there are difficulties such as prolonged labour or exhaustion of the mother.

Early (first stage) labour

With each contraction of the womb the cervix is pulled up towards the womb and then dilates (widens). This process takes between four and eight hours and is not especially painful except towards the end of this time. During this process, the baby drops further into the pelvis, often causing backache and bladder discomfort. In the first stage you may be able to walk and relax in between the increasingly strong contractions. Any urge to push must be resisted until the midwife is satisfied that the cervix is fully dilated to 10 cm/ 4 in, otherwise you would be trying to push the baby through too narrow an opening.

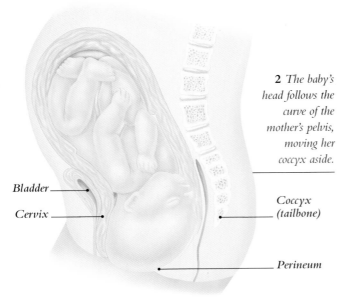

2 The baby's head follows the curve of the mother's pelvis, moving her coccyx aside.

Bladder

Cervix

Coccyx (tailbone)

Perineum

Second-stage labour

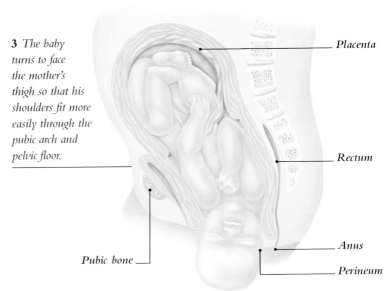

3 The baby turns to face the mother's thigh so that his shoulders fit more easily through the pubic arch and pelvic floor.

Placenta

Rectum

Anus

Perineum

Pubic bone

Third-stage labour

Second-stage labour

Now the active process of birth begins as the womb exerts its maximum effort to expel the baby. It is usually at this stage that the waters break; the amniotic membrane surrounding the baby in the womb ruptures and 500 ml/18 fl oz or so of fluid leaks from the vagina. The urge to push is at a maximum and with each contraction the mother bears down, sending the baby another stage down the birth canal, through the by now fully dilated cervix and into the vagina.

Most babies travel initially looking to one side, a position giving maximum head clearance. Further down the canal, the anatomy alters so that the baby's head should naturally turn to look towards the mother's back, a process called rotation. The midwife may urge you to resist pushing while this takes place.

The head is now visible and the lips of the vagina are fully dilated. This is when the perineum may tear, and a planned cut (episiotomy) may be made. With more efforts the head is pushed out and you will be asked to resist pushing while the baby's body rotates to one side. This allows the shoulders to emerge more easily. With more pushes the whole baby emerges: a moment of exhilaration for the mother, her partner and all her attendants, and one that never loses its magic.

The umbilical cord

Within moments of birth the baby's heart and circulation undergo complicated changes so that the baby no longer relies on the blood coming from the placenta. This process is set off by the baby drawing breath and crying; at that moment the lungs expand and blood begins to flow through them. This is why it is so important for the baby to begin breathing immediately. Once that has happened, blood flow through the umbilical cord ceases, so it can be safely cut and tied.

Third-stage labour

Now all that remains is to expel the placenta, which detaches as a result of the womb's vigorous contractions. It is usually pulled out by gentle tugging on the umbilical cord. There is a risk of bleeding from the raw surface where the placenta was attached. To reduce this risk it is normal to inject a drug called syntometrine to speed up the contraction of the womb.

Afterbirth This is usually a time of rushed activity as the attendants check the baby, examine the mother for tears that need stitching and monitor for excessive blood loss. These initial essential checks finished, the baby is given to the mother

PAIN CONTROL

◆

Women have a choice of using natural methods of pain control such as relaxation techniques or of accepting pain-relieving drugs. Pain control can be given by injection, usually pethidine, or an anaesthetic gas, usually nitrous oxide, under the mother's control. Increasing numbers of women opt for epidural anaesthesia. A tiny tube is introduced by needle into the fluid space around the spinal cord. A continuous infusion of anaesthetic is dripped in, making the mother numb from that point down. An epidural also numbs the desire to push, so the birth has to be more closely monitored and managed by the attendants.

The best preparation for childbirth is to read as much as possible on the subject, to learn some relaxation techniques and to discuss beforehand what pain relief is available.

(ideally with her partner) for a moment of peace in which to gaze at her baby, fondle her then give a first breast feed. Many women are so exhausted physically and emotionally by this stage that they will doze off for a few minutes.

Modern childbirth

Completely natural childbirth can be hazardous. In the under-developed world, the physical damage that most often affects women is tears of the vagina and perineum that do not heal properly and lead to constant urinary **incontinence**.

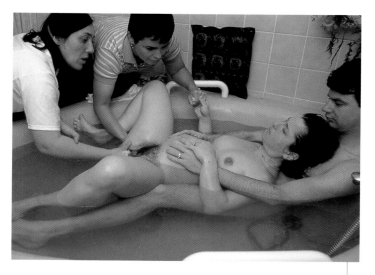

Above: Giving birth in a birthing pool may reduce the mother's pain and allows her partner to be more involved.

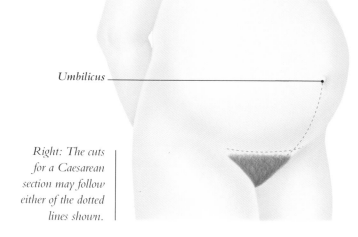

Umbilicus

Right: The cuts for a Caesarean section may follow either of the dotted lines shown.

In the United Kingdom, as recently as the 1930s one in every two hundred women died in childbirth from blood loss, high blood pressure or infection. Now the death rate is less than one in seventeen thousand. Although much of the improvement is due to better general health and more sophisticated anaesthetics, a large measure is as a result of obstetric care. However, many health professionals now accept that managed childbirth went too far in the 1970s and welcome the return to childbirth in an environment with less emphasis on 'high tech' and more on making the experience emotionally rewarding for all involved, while keeping the high-tech equipment available in case it is needed.

Complications in childbirth This vast subject cannot be adequately covered here. It includes multiple pregnancy, poor growth of the baby and maternal ill health, especially **diabetes** and **high blood pressure**; everything that can go wrong during delivery such as the baby getting stuck, the mother getting exhausted or torrential bleeding; and interventions such as forceps and Caesarean section. Fortunately, at least 97 out of every 100 births go normally but the situation during childbirth can change very rapidly. It is with this knowledge that many health professionals are cautious about the current move towards more home births.

CAESAREAN SECTION

◆

This operation removes the baby directly from the womb through a cut just above the bikini line. After the baby and placenta have been removed, the walls of the womb are stitched back together and the abdominal cut is repaired. The wound takes 10–14 days to heal.

Caesarean section is an extremely safe operation, and is done when the risk of vaginal birth, to either mother or baby, appears unacceptable. Some risk factors are clear before labour begins, for example if the mother is carrying triplets or more, or if she has a very small pelvis or high blood pressure. In such a case Caesarean section is a planned procedure for which the mother is prepared.

Often, however, the decision to deliver the baby by Caesarean section is only made once labour has begun, if it is not progressing normally for some reason – for example, the baby may be distressed or stuck, or there may be sudden heavy bleeding. Most obstetricians will recommend Caesarean section at any sign of labour going wrong.

POST-DELIVERY PROBLEMS

Problems for mothers following childbirth — mostly of a minor and easily treatable nature.

CAUSES

There are various kinds of post-delivery problems. To give birth, the vagina has to dilate enough to allow the 10 cm/4 in diameter of the baby's head to pass. During this process tears of the vagina are almost inevitable. An episiotomy, a planned cut at the lower part of the vagina, may be performed to avoid large uncontrolled tears from the vagina to the rectum.

There is always some bleeding at the time of delivery, small amounts of which continue for days if not weeks afterwards.

A Caesarean section (see page 139) involves a cut across the lower abdomen into the womb. Although it heals rapidly, pains are common at the site of incision for several weeks.

Many women who have an epidural anaesthetic to reduce pain during labour suffer headaches and backache for a week or so after. After birth it takes a few days for the hormones that make the breasts secrete milk to build up. For women who are not breastfeeding this engorgement can become intensely painful. Mild infections of the breasts are common, occasionally worsening into a breast abscess. Lastly, whether through hormonal changes or the psychological stress of childbirth, new mothers may have emotional problems.

SYMPTOMS

It is usual to feel tender, especially at the site of an episiotomy. Abdominal tenderness that gets worse and is associated with sweating or shivers suggests infection. Similarly, a bloody vaginal discharge will continue but should gradually lessen as the womb returns to its non-pregnant state over the next eight weeks. An increase in blood flow together with lower abdominal pains and sweats suggests infection of the womb.

If remnants of the afterbirth remain within the womb there will be persistent heavy loss of fresh blood as the womb is unable to contract fully. If the bleeding is severe you may need a curettage, to scrape the walls of the womb clean of any debris. Otherwise minor bleeding can be left for nature to deal with, which is why the first couple of periods after childbirth are often heavy and contain clots.

Breasts

There is often an extra flow of blood from the womb whenever a woman breastfeeds. This is because suckling stimulates the release of the hormone oxytocin, which makes muscles around the milk glands contract and so let down milk. At the same time oxytocin also makes the muscles of the womb contract and so expel blood. This is nature's way of getting the womb back to its usual size as soon as possible.

A breast infection is recognized by increasing pain in the breast, which becomes firm and red over the area of infection. You feel very unwell with shivers and sweats. If you are not breastfeeding the breasts become engorged with milk and very hard and painful for several days.

Psychological symptoms

The elation of birth almost invariably gives way to mild **depression** after a few days. This coincides with going home, getting into the relentless routine of a new baby and coping with all the other domestic responsibilities, too. For the great majority of women this is just a passing phase but about ten per cent of women become more persistently depressed, either immediately after childbirth or within the first three months. They find it difficult to care for the baby, are irritable and cry easily. More extreme, although rare, is puerperal psychosis, which is a very serious depressive illness often accompanied by thoughts of harming the baby.

TREATMENT

The system of postnatal care provided by midwives, health visitors and doctors is intended to pick up problems at an early stage. Many of the above-mentioned problems are dealt

---

SOME WARNING SYMPTOMS AFTER CHILDBIRTH, AND WHAT THEY MAY MEAN

♦ *Pain and swelling in one calf (deep vein thrombosis, see page 51)*
♦ *Heavy, fresh red vaginal bleeding (retained portions of the placenta or infection of the womb)*
♦ *Abdominal or perineal pain, an offensive discharge with or without fever (infection of the womb or perineum)*
♦ *Tender and red breast area with or without fever (breast abscess)*
♦ *Burning sensation on passing urine and a need to go frequently (urinary infection)*
♦ *Sudden breathlessness or sharp chest pain (a blood clot on the lung — a pulmonary embolus, see page 67)*
♦ *Persistent, deepening depression and neglect of the baby (puerperal depression or psychosis)*

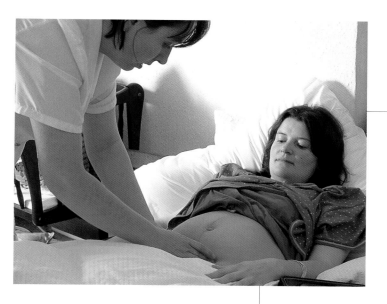

Above: Examining whether the womb has fully contracted, which is one important check after delivery.

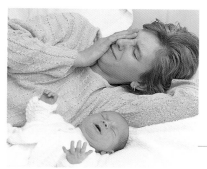

Left: The stresses of a demanding baby can occasionally end in severe depression.

with in this way, perhaps with an antibiotic if appropriate. Hospital intervention is rarely needed unless an episiotomy wound breaks down, there is persistent heavy bleeding that requires curettage or a breast abscess is unresponsive to an antibiotic and needs surgical drainage.

Indigestion, **haemorrhoids** and **constipation** rapidly disappear after birth with the loss of intra-abdominal pressure. Backache is common during pregnancy but should go over a few weeks as the joints and ligaments of the spine and pelvis, which become lax during pregnancy, return to normal.

Psychological treatment

The best and often the only medicine required is the opportunity to discuss worries with the postnatal team. Common queries revolve around feeding schedules, babies who appear demanding and cry all the time, and mild depression. Many women feel inadequate for the heavy demands of motherhood. There is no easy answer to these concerns, which are an inevitable part of the burden of having a new baby.

Women who are isolated from their family, who have unsupportive partners or who live in difficult socio-economic circumstances may especially have problems. Some babies are genuinely difficult and the mother needs help in coping with this. Many mothers find they gain important support from mother-and-baby groups during this demanding time.

Persistent depression that leads the mother to neglect herself and the baby may require treatment with an antidepressant for a few months. Those few women who suffer from puerperal psychosis are best treated in a psychiatric mother-and-baby unit where they can be closely supervised and have intensive medical and psychological therapy.

Sex

It is usually several weeks before sexual relationships are restarted after childbirth, simply because of physical discomfort, tiredness and true lack of sexual desire thanks to the constant demands of a baby. Some men have difficulty seeing their partner in both maternal and sexual roles.

By the routine postnatal check at six to eight weeks the body should be almost back to its non-pregnant state. Contraception and psychosexual queries can be discussed and vaginal pain checked, but there is no need to wait for this to resume sex, which can start as soon as you both feel ready.

In women not breastfeeding periods restart between six and ten weeks after delivery and they are fertile from that time. Breastfeeding suppresses the menstrual cycle so periods do not usually begin in this case for four to six months, but this cannot be relied upon as a method of contraception.

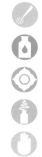

Complementary Treatment

Bach flower remedies – walnut for adjustment to change, star of Bethlehem for shock, Rescue Remedy for general restoration of calm, mustard for 'baby blues', cherry plum for fear of doing the baby harm, elm if you feel overwhelmed with responsibility. **Chinese herbalism** and **acupuncture** are especially good at retuning and rebalancing your hormonal system post-delivery. **Homeopathy** – arnica is good for bruising and soreness, ignatia can help for baby blues. **Chakra balancing** offers energy balancing and relaxation effects. **Aromatherapy** oils can help heal stitches and, in conjunction with **massage**, alleviate the baby blues. **Chiropractic** treatment for backache is common post-delivery, and aims to restore normal joint and muscular function to ease pain and discomfort. **Yoga** can help your body return to normal after pregnancy and delivery. *Other therapies to try: shiatsu-do.*

BREASTFEEDING

This is a natural activity but there may be problems and women will benefit from advice passed on by others.

BACKGROUND

Each breast is made up of 15–25 lobes, each of which is a complete milk-secreting unit. The milk from a lobe drains via tubules, ending in a milk duct in the nipple. Fatty tissue surrounds each lobe, giving the breast its shape. In pregnancy the lobe system enlarges ready to secrete milk. However, milk production only begins in earnest after childbirth, under the influence of the hormone prolactin from the pituitary gland. As long as the baby is regularly suckled, prolactin production is maintained and the breasts continue to secrete milk.

What is breast milk?

Breast milk is a complex mixture of water plus sugar (lactose), protein, fat, sodium, iron, vitamin C, vitamin D and calcium. It has less protein than cow's milk, but 50% of its energy is in the form of fat, a much higher percentage than in cow's milk. Breast milk also contains immunoglobulins – antibodies from the mother – so the breast-fed infant has some protection from infectious illness in the first few months.

In addition, breast milk is on tap at no cost and delivered conveniently at the correct temperature and hygienically.

How does it get out?

Thanks to prolactin, the breasts store milk ready for release whenever the baby suckles. Another hormone, oxytocin, makes muscle surrounding the milk glands contract, so squeezing out the milk. This is called the 'let-down' reflex. The release of oxytocin is controlled by a number of factors. Simply thinking about breastfeeding will stimulate its release, as will hearing the baby cry with hunger and preparing to feed. This is why the breasts start to leak even before feeding begins. Suckling further stimulates the release of oxytocin.

Conversely, **anxiety** and **stress** affect oxytocin and lead to difficulties in let-down, which are easily misinterpreted as an inability to breastfeed. Oxytocin has an additional action in making the womb contract, which is why women may get abdominal cramps and bleeding when breastfeeding.

DIFFICULTIES

Probably the main difficulties that many mothers experience with breastfeeding are getting started, inadequate milk flow, breast infections and pain.

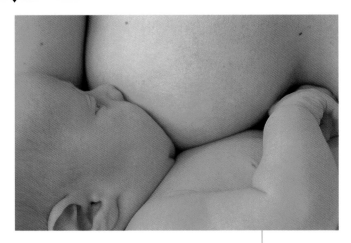

Above: Patience and correct technique should make breastfeeding a pleasure for both mother and baby.

Getting started

It helps to prepare the breasts for feeding before delivery. Some authorities recommend massaging the breasts in the last few weeks of pregnancy, squeezing them towards the nipple. This way you will see some milk expressed. The nipples should be kept soft using moisturizing creams.

After birth it takes two to four days for milk production to get going fully. During this time the breasts secrete a thick yellow type of milk called colostrum, which is adequate for the baby at this time. Thereafter, the more you feed the more you stimulate prolactin and the more milk will be produced.

The technique of breastfeeding is not simply to let the baby latch on to the nipple – by biting on the nipple the baby bites down on to the milk ducts, obstructing them and reducing the flow. The baby needs to suck on the areola, the coloured skin surrounding the nipple, which contains little reservoirs of milk. This way there is no obstruction to the flow of milk through the nipple.

Inadequate milk flow

Rarely a true milk deficiency, this is more likely a result of giving up too soon, which by reflex diminishes the quantity of milk produced; as well, anxiety about feeding inhibits the release of oxytocin. In the first two weeks you can ensure complete emptying of the breasts by manually expressing the milk, which also stimulates maximum secretion of prolactin.

Probably most milk is taken during the first five minutes on each breast; after that the baby continues to get some milk but sucks mainly for pleasure. Time spent on the breast is therefore not an accurate measure of how much milk the baby has actually taken. A better way of judging is whether the baby appears content and comes off the breast without irritation. The most objective measure is obviously whether the baby gains weight at the correct rate of about 175 g/6 oz a week, i.e. doubling its weight in the first three months.

It is tempting to top up breast feeds with bottle feeds 'just in case' but if this is done too much it will have the effect of reducing breast milk production and lead to a vicious circle of diminishing milk production and additional 'topping up'.

Painful breasts and infection

When the milk first comes in the breasts often feel engorged, swollen and tender. This is relieved once the baby suckles. It varies as to how much milk women make and some may have to express some milk initially to relieve discomfort. Those who do not wish to breastfeed will have painful breasts for a few days until prolactin levels diminish. The drug bromocriptine accelerates this process when taken for ten days.

Tender, cracked nipples are common; the cause is not clear. It may be that the technique is at fault, allowing the baby to chew on the nipple rather than the areola. Suckling for too long will lead to sore nipples. Most cases respond to a lanolin cream which is harmless for the baby.

It is easy for infection to enter a lobe of the breast through its duct on the nipple. Once inside, bacteria find the milk an ideal environment in which to grow. The typical breast infection, mastitis, is therefore of one lobe. The symptoms are a red, painful area of one breast and the mother feeling feverish and shivery. Treatment with an antibiotic cures most cases.

A little antibiotic passes across to the baby but it is harmless. It is unusual to require the more extreme measure of draining pus from the breast by a surgical incision. Breastfeeding should continue in mild cases. If severe, stop feeding from that breast but continue to express milk.

Reluctance to breastfeed

Not every woman wishes to breastfeed despite the undoubted benefits for her baby – protection from infection, less chance of **eczema** and fewer episodes of gastroenteritis. Breastfeeding has disadvantages such as tying the mother who wants to work. Other reasons may be lack of success in the past, sheer embarrassment about feeding, the smells and the stains on clothing, and lack of encouragement from family and partner. If it is not for you, do not feel guilty about it but enjoy the warmth and closeness of your baby while you bottle-feed.

QUESTIONS

Does size matter?
Exceptionally small breasts may not produce enough milk; exceptionally large breasts may make it difficult for the baby to grasp the areola without suffocating. These extremes aside there is no evidence to show that size matters.

Do inverted nipples prevent breastfeeding?
Most inverted nipples become sufficiently erect during breastfeeding to be adequate. Massaging or using breast shields to encourage inverted nipples to evert does not work nor is it necessary.

Is breastfeeding a contraceptive?
Breastfeeding suppresses periods for about six months. Although this reduces the chances of conceiving, it is not foolproof. For greater certainty use additional contraception such as the progesterone-only pill or condoms.

How do I know when to stop breastfeeding?
You could breastfeed for a year or more, but most Western women stop sooner, often on return to work. You may need to supplement breast feeds if the baby is not growing satisfactorily. Your breast milk will diminish naturally as you introduce solids.

Complementary Treatment

Chinese herbalism and **acupuncture** both help restore and maintain your hormonal balance; an experienced practitioner could advise. **Western herbalism** can help increase both the quantity and quality of breast milk: try infusions of nettle or raspberry leaves. When you want to stop breastfeeding, red sage tea will help reduce the milk flow. **Homeopathy** – use calendula cream for sore or cracked nipples. In conjunction with orthodox treatment, **aromatherapy** might be able to help alleviate mastitis – consult an experienced practitioner. **Yoga** can help by promoting relaxation and enhancing confidence. **Hypnotherapy** – hypnotic suggestion can help increase milk flow, and alleviate mastitis. Many **Ayurvedic** preparations are available to improve the quality and quantity of breast milk. General self-help – chilled cabbage leaves or grated carrot can be placed on engorged breasts to reduce discomfort. *Other therapies to try: Bach flower remedies; shiatsu-do; chakra balancing.*

MISCARRIAGE

◆

A pregnancy that ends prematurely with the loss of the foetus.

CAUSES

◆

Early miscarriages, up to about 14 weeks' gestation, are usually due to fundamental abnormality with the foetus or placenta. The baby may be seriously malformed; the placenta may be unhealthy or poorly attached to the womb. These factors affect at least one pregnancy in six. The risk of two consecutive miscarriages is about one in thirty-six – uncommon but not rare and may happen through pure and sad chance. Fewer than one in two hundred women have three miscarriages in a row. Although this may still be through chance, such mothers may have Hughes' syndrome (see below).

Late miscarriage means a miscarriage between 14 and 26 weeks. (From 26 weeks the baby may survive, so technically it is premature labour.) Late miscarriage is still usually because of abnormality of the baby or placenta. Additional possibilities are infection such as toxoplasmosis, trauma to the abdomen or serious maternal disease. The cervix may be too lax to retain the contents of the womb, a condition called cervical incompetence.

SYMPTOMS

◆

There is vaginal bleeding, slight initially and often brown (from altered blood) rather than bright red. There is a 50% hope of these symptoms stopping (threatened miscarriage). Later there are abdominal cramps, increased bleeding and backache (signs of inevitable miscarriage). The symptoms of complete miscarriage are passing large clots and jelly-like material. Late miscarriages resemble labour.

Abdominal pains on one side as opposed to mid-line warn of an ectopic pregnancy (see PREGNANCY PROBLEMS).

TREATMENT

◆

It is likely that many very early miscarriages are experienced as a slightly delayed, heavier-than-usual period. No treatment is required in these cases. There is about a 50% hope of a threatened miscarriage settling down. Although no treatment has been shown to influence this, it seems both sensible and kind to rest. An internal examination may show that the neck of the womb is open; this means that miscarriage has occurred or is inevitable. Where there is doubt, an ultrasound scan of the womb shows whether the pregnancy is still there and whether the baby is still alive (see page 349).

After definite miscarriage or where a scan shows the foetus has died, the contents of the womb should be removed by curettage to avoid any possible infection of the womb.

The treatment of cervical incompetence involves a purse string stitch around the cervix, called a Shirodkar suture, which is removed in later pregnancy. In cases of recurrent miscarriage investigations are necessary. These may show an abnormal anatomy of the womb or Fallopian tube that interferes with the implantation of the egg. Research has shown that some women having recurrent miscarriages have antibodies to a protein called cardiolipin (Hughes' syndrome) and can be helped by taking aspirin during early pregnancy.

In the hurried physical treatment of miscarriage it is easy to overlook the psychological consequences. Miscarriage means the loss of a baby and parents may need to mourn as much as after losing a full-term infant. It may help to reflect that miscarriage will usually have been nature acting for the best.

QUESTIONS

Does a threatened miscarriage affect the pregnancy?
Be reassured that the pregnancy will be unaffected and that there is no more risk of abnormality than in any uncomplicated pregnancy.

Is it important to wait before falling pregnant again?
It is reasonable to allow one normal period; this is often heavy as it carries away any remaining debris from the womb. There is no need to wait three months as used to be advised.

Does physical activity lead to miscarriage?
There is no evidence that ordinary sport, sex or stress affect the overall chances of miscarriage at all. Women who have recently had a miscarriage would be sensible to avoid excessive physical activity during the first 12 weeks of their next pregnancy.

Complementary Treatment
Complementary therapies cannot halt a miscarriage once it has begun, but they can help while you are recuperating. **Chakra balancing** and **healing** can help you through both emotional and physical pain and can also help with reactions such as insomnia, tension, guilt and anxiety. **Hypnotherapy** can be used to lessen anxiety in future pregnancies. **Ayurveda** can offer help in preparing your body for the next pregnancy, as can **acupuncture** and **Chinese herbalism**.

BREAST PROBLEMS

Pain, skin changes and discharge from the breasts – problems for which there are many innocent reasons.

CAUSES

The desirability of large or small breasts varies with all the fickleness of fashion. Very large breasts can cause back and neck pain. Many women suffer breast pain during the second half of the menstrual cycle, when the breasts enlarge under the influence of hormones. This is usually just a mild inconvenience, although some women actually suffer severe pain for two to three weeks every month.

Localized pain

The breasts are easily bruised so localized pain often follows an overlooked injury. It is less likely that pain is due to disease but a new or persistent pain should be assessed. There is absolutely no evidence that breast injuries lead to cancer.

Sore skin or discharging nipples

The skin of the nipples is subject to any of the afflictions of skin suffered elsewhere, for example **eczema** or infection. A sweat rash under the breasts is extremely common, especially if they are full. It is sensible to have these diagnoses confirmed by a doctor the first time they happen.

An abnormal secretion of prolactin (the hormone that stimulates the breasts to produce milk) from a (benign) growth in the pituitary gland may result in a milky discharge. A green or yellow discharge is usually harmless and comes from glands within the breast.

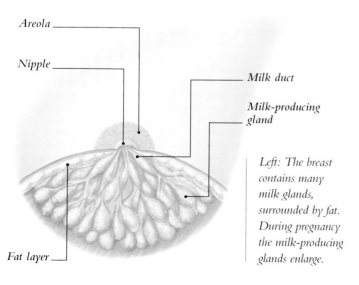

Areola

Nipple

Milk duct

Milk-producing gland

Fat layer

Left: The breast contains many milk glands, surrounded by fat. During pregnancy the milk-producing glands enlarge.

SYMPTOMS

Pain that is definitely cyclical is usually benign, especially if associated with firm glandular tissue within the breast. Pain localized to one portion of the breast is potentially more serious and should be brought to medical attention. The common sweat rash under the breasts is sore, red and itchy.

Any persistent discharges call for a careful medical assessment, possibly including measurement of prolactin in the blood. Bleeding from a nipple is a very important symptom that should always be investigated as it may be the first symptom of cancer within a duct of the nipple. The general rule is to seek medical advice if you notice any unusual change in your breasts, be it a lump, discharge, tenderness of the breast or of the nipples, or an altered appearance such as dimpling.

TREATMENT

A well-fitting and supportive bra helps mild cyclical pain and reduces discomfort caused by very large breasts. Breast reduction surgery might be a sensible option for extreme cases.

Oil of evening primrose is a therapy for cyclical breast pain; it has to be taken continuously for three months for full effect. Of course if there is anything unusual to feel in the breast you may require mammography or biopsy of a suspicious area (see page 353). Danazol and bromocriptine are drugs for severe breast pain, but have many side effects (see PMS).

Many skin problems respond to a mild steroid cream such as hydrocortisone, often combined with an antibiotic cream and antifungal agent.

Persistent pain and especially a bloody discharge need full assessment by a breast specialist. The treatment for abnormal prolactin depends on the cause.

See also BREAST CANCER.

Complementary Treatment

Chinese herbalism and **acupuncture** have much to offer – consult a reputable practitioner in Chinese medicine. **Homeopathy** – arnica cream is useful if breasts are bruised following an injury, calendula cream is useful for general soreness. **Nutritional therapy** – coffee, tea and chocolate have all been linked with increased risk of breast lumps and cysts. **Yoga** promotes relaxation and enhances confidence. **Ayurveda** offers detoxification and *marma* therapy. *Other therapies to try: naturopathy; chakra balancing.*

BREAST CANCER

The most common cancer among women, affecting about one in fourteen women. With treatment, about 50% of patients survive 10 years or more.

CAUSES

Cancer happens when cells grow independently of the body's control. A breast remains a breast because all the millions of cells that make it – skin, blood vessels, muscles – continue to do their jobs as skin cells, muscle cells and so on, maturing and dying as determined by their position in the breast. Cancer begins when a cell breaks free of that control and duplicates itself endlessly. What the trigger for this escape may be is the main concern in cancer studies. In breast cancer a number of factors increase the risk of that happening.

Heredity

Women with a mother or sister with breast cancer are two or three times more likely to get it themselves, having a one-in-five risk. However, there is no single gene that causes cancer. Rather it appears that inheriting a number of genes that control cell growth determines the risk in any one individual. These genes are called either oncogenes or tumour suppressor genes. A woman may inherit such defective genes or they may be mutated by radiation. Women with a family history of breast cancer should be medically examined annually.

Hormones

Being born female is the greatest risk for breast cancer. Men do get it but very rarely. Female hormones are involved in most, though not all, cases and the longer women are exposed to their female hormones, the greater their risk. Thus breast cancer is rare below the age of 30 and becomes more common upward of 40. Women are at greater risk the earlier their periods began, or if they have few or no children, or if they have a late **menopause**. These factors all increase the length of time their breasts are exposed to oestrogen.

Hormone replacement therapy (HRT) slightly increases the risk of breast cancer. This has to be weighed against the protective effects of HRT on heart disease and **osteoporosis**. The risks from the pill are debatable: it possibly increases the risk slightly in women who start it in their teens.

Environment

The incidence varies greatly from country to country. The United Kingdom and United States have some of the highest rates whereas, for unknown reasons, it is uncommon in Japan.

SYMPTOMS

Most cancers are diagnosed after finding a lump in the breast. It is a good idea to examine your breasts regularly – the best time is midway between periods. There is no set time interval; just be aware of your breasts in order to detect early changes.

Bear in mind that breast lumps are common and only about one in ten proves to be cancerous, even fewer in women under thirty. The normal glandular tissues of the breast feel firm and slightly irregular but in a continuous sheet through the breast, whereas a lump feels firm but separate from the rest of the breast tissue. Most breast lumps are benign overgrowths of the normal milk-secreting glandular tissue of the breast. Cysts, fluid-filled lumps, are also common. Breast pain is usually innocuous, but it is suspicious to have pain over a breast lump.

FEATURES OF A POSSIBLY CANCEROUS LUMP

- *Hard and irregular as opposed to smooth*
- *Feeling tethered to one place as opposed to mobile*
- *Associated with inversion of a previously normal nipple*
- *With puckered skin over it*
- *Associated with bleeding from the nipple*

Discharge from the nipple

This always needs to be medically examined. Bleeding from a nipple has to be regarded as coming from breast cancer until proven otherwise, and is not to be ignored. Green or yellow discharges, however, are usually benign.

Further investigation

Mammography is a specialized X-ray of the breast which distinguishes between benign and cancerous lumps. In the United Kingdom this is offered every three years to women between the ages of 50 and 65, which is the time of greatest risk. The benefit from breast screening is controversial and not all authorities agree that it makes a difference to survival rates as opposed to early detection rates.

A biopsy can be taken through a special needle as an outpatient procedure (see page 353) and allows the direct microscopic analysis of a suspicious area of tissue. Sometimes the only way of being sure is to remove the lump under anaesthetic for full analysis.

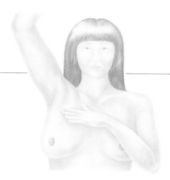

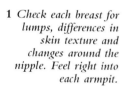

1 *Check each breast for lumps, differences in skin texture and changes around the nipple. Feel right into each armpit.*

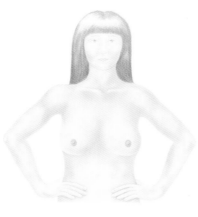

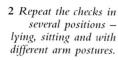

2 *Repeat the checks in several positions – lying, sitting and with different arm postures.*

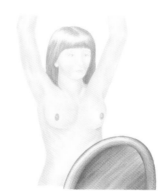

3 *Standing in front of a mirror helps you to become familiar with the usual appearance of your breasts.*

Above: It is important to learn how to examine your breasts yourself.

TREATMENT
◆

The aims are to remove the cancer itself and to detect and treat any spread (metastases or secondaries) to bones, liver and the brain. In planning treatment it is essential to know if and where there are metastases. Examination of the liver and armpits is the first step but only detects large secondaries. To detect small secondaries without symptoms it requires a bone scan and a CT scan of the liver, lungs and brain.

In the case of localized disease, the cancerous lump plus any glands within the armpit that may be involved are removed. After the wound has healed a course of radiotherapy (see page 370) is given to the armpit and breast in order to kill any remaining cancerous cells.

Hormone therapy
Hormone therapy is used if the disease has spread. Commonly used is tamoxifen, which is an anti-oestrogen, the use of which is believed to be responsible for the large increase in survival in the last 10 years. A similar effect is achieved by removing the ovaries, which immediately decreases the amount of oestrogen in the body. There are additional drugs if the woman is post-menopausal, for example anastrazole. Tumours vary in their responsiveness to oestrogen; this is discovered by analysing the tumour and helps predict how likely it is to respond to hormone treatment. Tamoxifen is widely used even for localized disease and may be taken for several years.

Chemotherapy
Formerly reserved for women whose disease recurred after surgery, evidence now points to the value of giving chemotherapy (see page 371) at the same time as initial surgery. American results suggest this improves survival by 25%. The drugs are given every week or two, commonly methotrexate, cyclophosphamide and 5-fluorouracil. In addition, steroid drugs shrink secondaries and reduce the effects in, for example, the brain.

Prevention
There are a few women whose family history of breast cancer is so poor that their chances of getting cancer are extremely high. After suitable counselling these women may opt to have both breasts removed. Although this sounds extreme, the logic behind it is scientifically sound and understandable.

Complementary Treatment
No woman should spurn conventional assessment or approaches of her condition. However, many complementary therapies have a role during treatment. Check that your chosen practitioner is experienced in treating breast cancer. **Chakra balancing** helps with symptom control and energy balance, aids relaxation during orthodox treatment and offers support during rehabilitation programmes. **Massage** can help promote self-esteem and a positive body image, especially after surgery. **Aromatherapy** massage with scented oils can reduce stress and tension associated with this disease. **Reflexology** can offer support during orthodox treatment. Diet is extremely important and a **nutritional therapist** or **naturopath** would tailor a diet to suit your particular needs and circumstances – any diet is likely to feature plenty of wholefoods and fresh fruit and vegetables. *Other therapies to try: see* STRESS.

CERVICAL CANCER

Cancer of the neck of the womb, which is treatable and often curable if detected early enough.

CAUSES

Since the cervix projects into the vagina, the cells of the cervix are exposed to any infection within the vagina and to sperm; both may be involved in causing cervical cancer. The cancer is slow growing and alters the microscopic appearance of the cells of the cervix in its early stages. This is why the cervical smear screening programme is valuable. Untreated cancer spreads through the cervix and eventually invades the surrounding tissues. The disease is more common in smokers, although it is not known why.

Viruses and sexual activity

The human papilloma virus can be detected in the cervix in many cases of cancer. The same virus causes genital warts and can therefore be sexually transmitted. Cervical cancer is less common in women whose partners use condoms, supporting the notion of a viral cause. However the virus is also commonly found in women (and men) who are perfectly well.

Evidence suggests that the women at greater risk of cervical cancer are those who began sexual activity early and who have had many partners. This further supports the theory that a sexually transmitted agent contributes to the condition.

SYMPTOMS

Early cervical cancer does not cause any symptoms at all. Symptoms only appear once the cancer is fairly well established, causing a raw area on the cervix. Possible symptoms then include a heavier-than-usual vaginal discharge, intermenstrual bleeding and bleeding after intercourse (from rubbing of the cervix). Pain is not a feature of the condition unless the cancer has spread into surrounding tissue. There are, however, many innocent causes of these same symptoms.

Cervical smears

Scraping the cervix with a spatula painlessly gathers cells for microscopic examination, so as to detect any early changes. The spatula is usually a wooden stick specially shaped to allow it to pass into the cervix; the scrapings are transferred on to a glass slide. Smears are graded on the appearance of the cells from normal, through possible early malignancy to frank cancer. Sexually active women should have regular smears, normally every three years, until the age of 65.

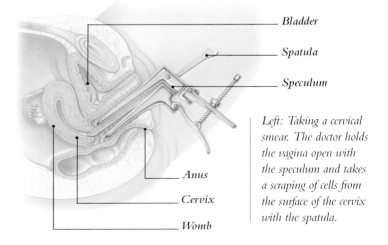

Bladder

Spatula

Speculum

Left: Taking a cervical smear. The doctor holds the vagina open with the speculum and takes a scraping of cells from the surface of the cervix with the spatula.

Anus

Cervix

Womb

TREATMENT

Suspicion that areas of the cervix contain pre-cancerous cells can be confirmed using a colposcope, an instrument that gives a magnified view of the cervix. The surgeon looks through this while applying acetic acid to the cervix; abnormal areas turn white and biopsies are taken for more detailed analysis. Pre-malignant or early cancer cells are destroyed by laser beam or by cauterizing or by freezing (cryotherapy). These modern techniques can be used to perform a cone biopsy, whereby if problem areas are numerous, a whole cylinder of abnormal cells can be cut out, without causing any significant damage or affecting future fertility. More advanced disease is treated by removal of the cervix in a **hysterectomy**, followed by radiotherapy (see page 370) to the pelvis.

In theory, regular cervical screening should make cancer of the cervix an avoidable disease. Treatment of early disease virtually guarantees cure. Of the women who have advanced disease (i.e. invasive) at least 80% will survive 5 years.

Complementary Treatment

   Keep up regular screening. If cancer is diagnosed, do not spurn conventional approaches – complementary therapies cannot cure cancer. However, many therapies have a role during treatment. **Chakra balancing** can help with symptom control and energy balance, and aid relaxation during orthodox treatment. **Reflexology** can offer support during orthodox treatment. **Aromatherapy** reduces stress and tension associated with this disease, especially when linked with **massage**. *Other therapies to try: see STRESS.*

CANCER OF THE WOMB

Uterine cancer accounts for about 3000 deaths per annum in the United Kingdom, making it the second most common cancer in women after breast cancer.

CAUSES

The cancer arises in the cells in the lining of the womb, the endometrium. These are influenced by the hormones oestrogen and progestogen, which regulate the menstrual cycle. It appears to be this regular pattern of hormonal stimulation that predisposes to malignancy. Growing slowly, the cancer eventually spreads through the womb (uterus) to surrounding pelvic tissues and finally to the lungs, liver and bones.

Some women are at greater risk of cancer of the womb than others by virtue of an increased lifetime exposure to oestrogen. This means women who began their periods at an early age, who have a late **menopause** or who have no children. The risk is also higher in those women who are overweight because fat tissues produce oestrogen.

Early types of hormone replacement therapy (HRT), when it was given as oestrogen alone, caused an increased risk. Now, in the United Kingdom, women with a womb have HRT containing progesterone for ten to twelve days each month which is sufficient protection.

SYMPTOMS

The alerting symptom of womb cancer is unusual vaginal bleeding, especially after the menopause. In fact any vaginal bleeding after the menopause is suspicious, even if the bleeding is occasional or just enough to cause a blood-tinged vaginal discharge. This does not mean that all post-menopausal bleeding is from cancer. Far from it; mostly it is caused by innocent post-menopausal thinning of the walls of the vagina or by benign changes within the womb.

Cancer of the womb is less common before the menopause (25% of cases) and less likely to be suspected. This is because the symptoms – irregular bleeding or heavier-than-usual bleeding – are common from the late 30s onward anyway. The best advice is to take account of any uncharacteristic and persistent change in your menstrual pattern.

Pain is not a feature of this cancer unless it is advanced.

Diagnosis

The diagnosis is established by ultrasound scan of the womb (see page 349) to detect areas of unusual thickness in the walls. An essential further investigation is endometrial biopsy, which means sampling cells from the lining of the womb. This can be done as an outpatient procedure in the gynaecology clinic in contrast with the older dilation and curettage (D&C) (see PERIOD PROBLEMS), which required a general anaesthetic.

TREATMENT

In almost all cases the womb must be removed (a **hysterectomy**), together with the ovaries, because these produce oestrogen, which would encourage the spread of the cancer elsewhere. It is usual to have a course of radiotherapy to the pelvis (see page 370) to destroy any cells remaining within the pelvis and the lymph nodes. Because of its side effects, chemotherapy (see page 371) is reserved for those with advanced disease that has spread widely within the pelvis or elsewhere.

The chances of cure are excellent if the cancer of the womb is diagnosed early. At least 85 of every 100 women treated will survive 5 years or more.

QUESTIONS

Can womb cancer be screened for?
There are no blood tests currently available. Women taking HRT should have a regular pelvic examination to detect any enlargement of the womb. This can be combined with having a smear (see CERVICAL CANCER).

Is every change in menstrual pattern significant?
All women experience variations, especially as they get older, the vast majority of which are innocent in nature. Therefore minor month-to-month changes are not likely to be important. You should take notice of any persistent change that involves periods getting heavier or irregular. In the case of post-menopausal bleeding, you should report even the tiniest episode to your doctor.

Complementary Treatment

You should not spurn conventional approaches – complementary treatments cannot cure cancer. However, many therapies have a role during treatment. **Chakra balancing** will help with symptom control and energy balance, and aid relaxation during orthodox treatment. **Reflexology** can offer support during orthodox treatment. **Aromatherapy** is excellent at reducing the stress and tension associated with disease. *Other therapies to try: see STRESS.*

OVARIAN CANCER

Malignant growths of the ovary are among the most common cancers in women.

CAUSES

Cancer of the ovary is a particularly complex subject, because there are many different types of growth, each with its own natural history, progression, response to therapy and outlook.

The ovary produces a number of cysts every month, each containing an egg. It is therefore not surprising that many cancers begin as cysts: fluid-filled growths that can reach a large size before causing any problems. The diagnosis is complicated because ovarian cysts are common and what appears to be a benign cyst may become malignant over time.

As with **breast cancer** and **cancer of the womb**, ovarian cancer seems stimulated by the female hormone oestrogen and so the women at higher risk are those who have been longest exposed to oestrogen: those who began to have periods early, experience a late **menopause** and have few or no children. Having a close relative with the condition increases the risk several times over.

Taking the contraceptive pill reduces the incidence of ovarian cancer by about 40% – a much under-publicized benefit of this contraceptive. Ovarian cancer is mainly a disease of women who are in their 50s upwards, but cases of the cancer in younger women or even children are not rare.

SYMPTOMS

Unfortunately, ovarian growths may reach a considerable size without causing any suspicious symptoms. Even with a growth several centimetres in diameter there may be no features. In cases where symptoms are present they manifest as lower abdominal swelling, discomfort and urinary frequency, caused by pressure on the bladder. Periods may or may not be affected. Advanced tumours lead to swelling of the legs and gross abdominal swelling.

It is possible to feel the ovary on a vaginal examination, but it is not possible to tell by examination alone whether or not an enlarged ovary is malignant or caused by an innocent cyst.

TREATMENT

An ultrasound scan of the ovaries (see page 349) is a useful aid for confirming an ovarian swelling but this diagnostic tool alone cannot tell if the swelling is malignant or benign. For this, laparoscopic surgery is required (see page 372) so that the swelling can be inspected by the gynaecologist. Once diagnosis is certain, treatment is always removal of the affected ovary and often of the womb as well, if it looks as if the tumour has spread. After this, it is usual to direct radiotherapy at the pelvis. Chemotherapy is used to try to eradicate any remaining cells and any that may have spread (metastasized) elsewhere in the body. (See pages 370 and 371.)

Taxone, a drug from the bark of the Western Yew, is now available for treating advanced ovarian cancer.

Some ovarian cancers produce a biochemical marker in the blood stream called Ca 125, which can be used to measure response to treatment and is an early indication of recurrence.

QUESTIONS

How curable is the condition?
This depends very much on the exact type of tumour, varying from a 95% five-year survival to just 10%. In general ovarian cancer carries a poor prognosis because it tends not to be diagnosed until the cancer is well established.

Is there any screening test?
The only recognized test is to have a pelvic examination of your ovaries every year. This should also be done whenever you have a cervical smear test. With the discovery of Ca 125 it was thought that this could be extended to general screening of the population and a screening programme is now being planned.

How serious are ovarian cysts?
Small cysts are more common than once thought. However, in younger women they are nearly always benign. A gynaecologist will perform a laparoscopy if in doubt or if cysts are detected in older women.

Complementary Treatment

No complementary therapy can cure ovarian cancer. However, many have a role during conventional treatment. **Chakra balancing** will help with symptom control and energy balance, and aid relaxation during orthodox treatment. **Reflexology** offers support during orthodox treatment. **Aromatherapy** is excellent for reducing stress and tension, especially when combined with **massage**. There are **homeopathic** treatments for benign ovarian cysts, if the diagnosis is certain. *Other therapies to try: see STRESS.*

PREMENSTRUAL SYNDROME (PMS)

Various symptoms as a consequence of the effects of hormone changes during the menstrual cycle.

CAUSES

While it seems self-evident that it is the cycle of hormones that causes PMS, it has proved difficult to pinpoint just what is responsible for what. Most women experience tension and irritability during the second half of their menstrual cycle, which coincides with rising levels of oestrogen and progesterone. If fertilization does not happen the levels of these hormones fall until menstruation occurs. Numerous studies have tried to relate concentrations of hormones to symptoms but without reaching generally accepted conclusions. Such evidence as is agreed increasingly suggests that the level of oestrogen is more important than those of other hormones.

In addition, women vary as to how well they tolerate these changes; it may be that swings in mood that would normally be coped with become intolerable for women who have other stresses in their life such as children, marital or money problems. Surveys show that women aged in their 30s and 40s are most affected by PMS.

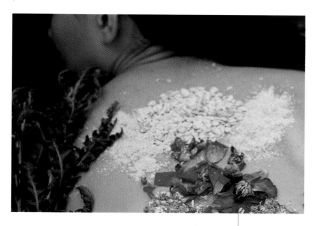

Above: Many women with PMS find that herbal remedies are helpful. It may be worth trying them for yourself.

SYMPTOMS

To make the diagnosis it is essential to show that symptoms fluctuate in a regular cycle. Certain symptoms are especially frequent: feeling bloated, depressed, irritable and anxious and getting headaches. Cravings for sweet things is common.

These symptoms should begin from mid-cycle onward, reach a maximum just before menstruation and disappear within a couple of days of the onset of menstruation. The severity of symptoms often varies from cycle to cycle.

Despite PMS being a probably universal experience for women, most cope well. An estimated 10% suffer more severely; for perhaps 1–3% of women PMS is a major problem each month, disrupting relationships and family and work responsibilities.

TREATMENT

The treatment for PMS is as controversial as the explanations offered. Women must be prepared to try a variety of treatments to find one that works well for them.

One scientifically validated treatment is vitamin B_6, essential for enzymes that form the neurotransmitters serotonin and dopamine, important in depression. There is no agreed reason why women should become cyclically deficient in B_6 but many women do benefit from taking a small dose.

Diuretics reduce fluid retention, relieving bloating and breast tenderness, but should be taken for only a few days each time. Danazol is a drug that suppresses oestrogen and progestogens. It is an effective treatment for some women but its side effects such as nausea and weight gain make it unacceptable for many. The same goes for bromocriptine, which is good for breast tenderness but causes nausea.

Oil of evening primrose is a rich source of gamma linoleic acid. This theoretically reduces prolactin levels, which some researchers believe are a cause of the breast tenderness and mood changes. Oestrogen taken in the form of tablets helps some women.

Fluoxetine (prozac) has recently been licenced for treatment of PMS for women who are not helped by non-drug therapy.

Complementary Treatment

Western herbalism can encourage hormone regulation before periods and help with specific symptoms. In **Chinese herbalism** a useful remedy is *Xiao Yao Wan* (free-and-easy wonder formula). **Bach flower remedies** – mustard for depression for no reason, cherry plum for loss of control, beech for intolerance, impatiens for impatience and irritability, and willow for self-pity. Useful **aromatherapy** oils include chamomile, geranium, rose, bergamot and clary sage. *Other therapies to try: most therapies have something to offer.*

PERIOD PROBLEMS

◆

Upset of the delicately balanced menstrual cycle – caused by emotion, dieting, medication or hormonal fluctuations.

BACKGROUND

During the menstrual cycle changing levels of hormones prepare the ovaries and womb for pregnancy. This cycle reaches a peak about 14 days after the first day of the previous period. Up to this stage the ovaries are stimulated by follicle-stimulating hormone (FSH), a hormone which comes from the hypothalamus, and which makes a few eggs mature. A pituitary hormone, luteinizing hormone (LH), then induces the release of one egg.

Meanwhile, the maturing eggs themselves release oestrogen, which makes blood vessels grow within the lining of the womb, ready to supply nutrients to a fertilized egg. The ovary also begins secreting progesterone, the hormone of pregnancy, which further prepares the womb to receive an egg.

By mid-cycle the body is in an optimal state for fertilization. If this fails to occur levels of progesterone and oestrogen fall; the rich blood supply of the womb lining degenerates to a point where the lining dies and is shed as the menstrual flow. This, as it were, wipes the lining clean ready for the next cycle.

It is only by convention that 28 days is considered the 'normal' length of a cycle. It is perfectly normal to have a cycle of 21 days or of 35 or more days.

TYPES OF PROBLEMS

◆

Periods may be absent or infrequent, or prolonged. They may be scanty or heavy, painless or painful. Many period problems are the result of fluctuations of the interplay of hormones, so hormones play a useful role in dealing with them.

Absent or infrequent periods

Causes: When periods first begin and towards the **menopause**, the ovaries often fail to produce an egg. The resulting lack of oestrogen and progesterone makes for menstrual irregularities – and often for heavy periods, too.

Absent or scanty periods are also common for several months after stopping the contraceptive pill. Alternatively, periods may be made irregular by emotional problems, dieting (in anorexia nervosa they stop altogether) or heavy athletic training. Much less likely is the failure of hormone production by the pituitary gland. Another possibility, and more common than once thought, are polycystic ovaries – causing an excess secretion of male hormones, suggested by a combination of absent periods, hairiness, acne and obesity.

Pregnancy always has to be borne in mind, too. In women past the age of 30 with previously regular periods, the abrupt cessation of periods could be due to an early menopause.

Symptoms: These can range from total lack of periods to infrequent scanty periods, which may or may not be painful.

Treatment: A girl who has reached 16 and not begun menstruation should have a full gynaecological assessment, looking for hypothalamic failure, hormone disorders and abnormal anatomical or genetic make-up. Otherwise, if infrequent periods are not a source of worry treatment is not essential.

Infrequent periods can leave a niggling doubt about pregnancy, allayed only by pregnancy tests. If treatment is desired, the contraceptive pill will give a regular cycle.

Older women with a previously regular cycle should have a full hormonal assessment looking especially for premature menopause and hyperprolactinaemia, the abnormal secretion of prolactin from the pituitary gland. During pregnancy prolactin stimulates the breasts to make milk but can be secreted at other times by disease of the pituitary gland. Treatment is with bromocriptine, which blocks production, or removal of a pituitary tumour by surgery or radiotherapy.

Treatment for polycystic ovaries includes the pill, steroids or clomiphene to stimulate egg production and improve fertility.

Heavy or painful periods

Causes: Painful periods are common in the first few years of menstruation. If occurring later the combination suggests **fibroids**, **pelvic inflammatory disease** or **endometriosis**. The contraceptive coil causes heavier periods, too. A rarer reason is **cancer of the womb**, a possibility in women over 40 with significant changes in their menstrual pattern.

Symptoms: What is a heavy period for one woman is considered normal by another. The average blood loss of the whole period is 30–80 ml. Symptoms that are suggestive of truly heavy periods are becoming anaemic, flooding or clots, or high use of tampons or sanitary towels. Pain on intercourse plus heavy, painful periods suggests disease of the womb as opposed to benign hormone disorders.

Treatment: Assuming other disease is excluded, the treatment is with hormones. The contraceptive pill gives a regular moderate period. Progestogen tablets, such as norethisterone or dydrogesterone, are helpful taken for several days each month. Effective non-hormone treatments include mefenamic acid and tranexamic acid, both of which reduce bleeding and pain if they are taken in the first few days of the period. Most promising is a coil containing the hormone levonorgestrel which reduces heavy periods while providing contraception.

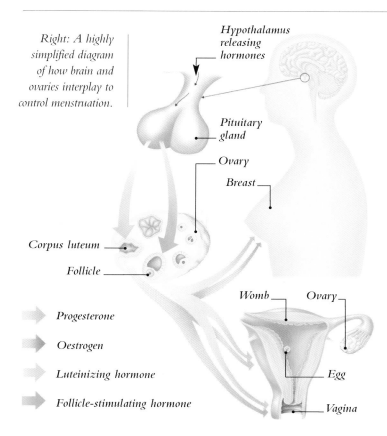

Right: A highly simplified diagram of how brain and ovaries interplay to control menstruation.

Hypothalamus releasing hormones

Pituitary gland

Ovary

Breast

Corpus luteum

Follicle

Womb — Ovary

Egg

Vagina

Progesterone

Oestrogen

Luteinizing hormone

Follicle-stimulating hormone

At one time a D&C was both routine investigation and treatment in older women; this is a scraping (curettage) of the womb via the widened (dilated) cervix and was used to exclude cancer of the womb. The operation is becoming obsolete thanks to smaller sampling syringes, which give just as reliable results but do not require a general anaesthetic.

If these strategies fail, one option is ablation (destruction) of the lining of the womb using a laser or similar heat source (see page 365). Although this is a safe and effective treatment, symptoms tend to recur after a year or so.

Finally, there is **hysterectomy** – removal of the womb. Many doctors favour it as it removes a possible site for cancer. In young women the ovaries are kept to avoid an abrupt, early menopause. The levonorgestrel coil may avoid hysterectomy in future.

Irregular periods

This refers to bleeding without any regular pattern.
Causes: Most cases are due to fluctuations of hormones. This is common in women who are approaching the menopause or who are in the first few years after starting to menstruate, and it is unlikely to be serious.

It is important to distinguish irregular, which means unpredictable, from intermenstrual bleeding. The latter means bleeding in between an otherwise normal menstrual cycle; it may be spotting mid-cycle or bleeding after intercourse. Intermenstrual bleeding is important since it may be caused by erosion on the cervix, **cervical cancer**, polyps in the womb or cancer of the womb.

Bleeding after the menopause is never ever 'normal' and it is essential to have investigation for even the slightest blood loss, to exclude cancer of the womb.
Symptoms: The menstrual cycle may be completely irregular, or there may be a relatively regular cycle with additional episodes of blood loss mid-cycle, i.e. intermenstrual bleeding.
Treatment: In younger women, as long as health and a physical examination are normal, it is not necessary to treat irregular periods other than to provide the convenience of having a predictable cycle. This is achieved with the contraceptive pill.

Innocent hormonal fluctuations are still the likeliest explanation for irregular periods in older women but it is advisable to have further investigation because disease of the cervix or the womb is more common than in younger women. This is all the more important if the bleeding is intermenstrual. The treatment for a cervical erosion, as for polyps, is cauterization (burning it away). A sample of the lining of the womb should be taken either by a D&C or by an outpatient procedure, to exclude cancer.

Complementary Treatment

Ayurveda and **Western** and **Chinese herbalism** all offer preparations to reduce pain and spasm and regulate both the menstrual cycle and the severity of bleeding. In **acupuncture** an important point is Spleen 6, above the ankle, at the meeting point of three energy channels that all connect to the womb. In **auricular therapy** needling points on the ear is thought to influence the hormonal system, so this is of great value in treating period problems. **Chiropractic** treatment can provide relief, back pain being frequently associated with period problems. **Yoga** can cure period problems if practised regularly. **Healing** helps regulate the menstrual cycle and restore a balanced hormonal picture. **Hypnotherapy** visualization and suggestion therapy can help if the problems are linked to negative conditioning about periods. *Other therapies to try: homeopathy; tai chi/chi kung; shiatsu-do; nutritional therapy; naturopathy; chakra balancing.*

MENOPAUSE

♦

The cessation of menstrual periods, which affects all women by the time they are in their mid-50s.

CAUSES

♦

Most women menstruate from the menarche (the time of first menstruation) for the next 35–45 years. This is controlled by an elegant system of hormones in the hypothalamus and pituitary glands, which act on the ovaries and womb (see PERIOD PROBLEMS), becoming erratic as the 'biological clock' ticks on.

By the mid-40s, the number of immature eggs within the ovaries has diminished and those remaining are relatively unresponsive to the hormones that should bring them to maturity. As a consequence oestrogen levels fall, while levels of other hormones rise. Eventually menstruation ceases, which occurs on average when women are in the early 50s.

From this point the ovaries no longer produce eggs but they continue to secrete some oestrogen. Oestrogen is also formed within fatty tissue and the skin so that it does not completely disappear after the menopause but, except in the obese, it decreases to pre-pubertal levels.

It is not known why the menopause happens when it does, nor why some women experience an early menopause and others a late one. A fair guide to when to expect the menopause is the age your mother or sisters reached it. Menopause occurring in women in their 30s is premature. There is rarely any serious reason for this, although it may be distressing, meaning as it does the end of the woman's childbearing days.

Any woman who has to have her ovaries removed will experience an abnormally abrupt menopause with correspondingly severe symptoms. This might be required as treatment for **cancer of the womb**, **ovarian cancer**, **breast cancer**, **endometriosis** or **pelvic inflammatory disease**.

SYMPTOMS

♦

By convention the menopause is taken to be definite when periods have finished for a year. Before then periods might occur just every couple of months until ceasing. Some women experience clear menopausal symptoms such as hot flushes while continuing to menstruate, presumably because of falling levels of oestrogen. Where there is doubt, blood tests can confirm that you are entering the menopause by measuring the levels of stimulating hormones which rise at the menopause.

The following symptoms last for two to five years. Although all women experience some symptoms, for only about one-third of women are they a serious inconvenience.

Hot flushes

There is a feeling of heat that sweeps across the body within seconds and is accompanied by sweating, especially at night. They are the result of instability of the circulatory system, which usually controls the dilation of blood vessels in response to emotions, changes of temperature and tension.

Physical changes

With the fall in oestrogen, the parts of the body sensitive to oestrogen return to a pre-pubertal state. The breasts diminish in size with reabsorption of fatty tissue, becoming thinner and shapeless. The walls of the vagina depend on oestrogen to remain thick and supple; after the menopause these become thin and drier. This leads to discomfort during intercourse and, not uncommonly, slight bleeding from the vagina's walls, which look dry and shiny, and also to recurrent cystitis.

Heart disease

Women are relatively protected from this before the menopause, perhaps because of a positive protective effect from oestrogen. It may also be that oestrogen shields against the harmful effects of women's natural male hormones (androgens) until the menopause, after which falling oestrogen levels remove this buffer. After the menopause the risk of heart disease for women rises rapidly to equal that of men.

Osteoporosis

After the menopause women lose bone mass, which becomes thin and lighter (see OSTEOPOROSIS). This process continues for decades after the menopause but the loss is especially rapid at the time of the menopause and for a couple of years afterwards. Accompanying the bone thinning it is common for post-menopausal women to notice a general stiffening of their joints and aches all over. This is partly the effect of ageing, but some of it is due to oestrogen deficiency.

Mood changes and psychological adjustment

Symptoms often recounted are irritability, emotional instability, worsening memory, **depression** and tiredness. It is hard to decide which of these are from hormonal changes as opposed to being coincidental effects from psychological adjustments.

TREATMENT

♦

It is vital to bear in mind that the menopause is a natural and inevitable event. However inconvenient its symptoms and however distressing the psychological effects, it is not a med-

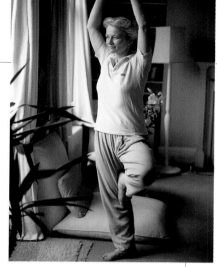

Below: HRT *is popular as pills or patches, as well as implants or gels.*

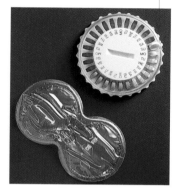

Above: Exercise, relaxation and a good diet are all important strategies for post-menopausal health.

ical abnormality. Indeed, many women welcome the end of menstruation. What is important is to reduce the impact of the most upsetting symptoms and to deal with those aspects of the menopause that may have long-term health implications – essentially osteoporosis and cardiovascular disease.

Hormone replacement therapy (HRT)

HRT reliably alleviates many of the most distressing symptoms of the menopause. The hormone being replaced is oestrogen and it can be supplied as a tablet, a pellet implanted into the lower abdomen, a patch worn on the hip or a gel rubbed into the arm. A woman who has had a **hysterectomy** can take just oestrogen daily (known as unopposed oestrogen). A woman who still has her womb has to take additional tablets containing progestogen for ten to twelve days each month; this is to counteract the effect of pure oestrogen on the womb, which otherwise increases the risk of womb cancer. The effect of the additional tablet is to cause a light menstrual bleed each month; there are now several formulations that reduce the bleeding to just once every three months or not at all.

Advantages: It gives a sense of wellbeing, improves skin texture and reduces aches in the joints. Hot flushes are virtually abolished, it reduces vaginal dryness or soreness and often relieves **cystitis** due to drying of the urethra. It prevents osteoporosis and, combined with an appropriate diet, may actually reverse it. While on HRT women continue to enjoy the relative protection from heart disease they had before the menopause.

Drawbacks: Weight gain, breast tenderness and nausea are all common side effects in the first few months but usually disappear. HRT carries a slightly increased risk of thrombosis

(see DEEP VEIN THROMBOSIS and PULMONARY EMBOLISM). Evidence suggests that HRT slightly increases the risk of breast cancer which may be significant after about eight years.

Conclusion: On balance, if HRT is taken for two to five years its benefits outweigh its disadvantages. Thereafter the balance is still overall in favour of HRT because its continuing protection against heart disease and osteoporosis outweigh the risks of breast cancer. However, the individual woman must consider the pros and cons herself. It is a personal decision that needs thorough discussion with her medical advisor, and the picture will change as more research is done.

Other treatments

Vaginal dryness can be treated with an oestrogen cream but this should not be used for more than a few years. Many women find a non-hormone lubricating gel is sufficient. (Regular sex after the menopause reduces dryness without the need for hormones. As many women find their sexual interest is the same or greater after the menopause as those who lose interest.)

Hot flushes can be reduced by taking blood pressure medication (clonidine). Osteoporosis is delayed by giving up smoking, maintaining a high calcium and vitamin D intake and regular weight-bearing exercise. Oestrogen-rich bread is interesting, although its long-term benefits are unproven.

See also WOMEN: THE MENOPAUSE AND AFTER, page 20.

Complementary Treatment

Chinese and **Western herbalism** both offer herbs to reduce the severity of a range of problems such as hot flushes and fatigue. **Chakra balancing** – often psychological balancing is needed here and this can definitely help. **Auricular therapy** – needling points on the ear is thought to influence the hormonal system, so it is of great value during menopause. For severe symptoms such as hot flushes, treatment should be daily initially, but the severity should lessen within days. **Aromatherapy** can help adjustment to change by balancing nerves and hormones; oils to try include chamomile, cypress, rose, geranium, fennel and juniper. **Nutritional therapy** – supplements of vitamins B, D and E often alleviate menopausal symptoms. Cut out coffee. **Yoga** can be useful. **Hypnotherapy** can help, especially cell regeneration therapy. **Ayurveda** offers detoxification, oral treatments, and yoga meditation. *Other treatments to try: tai chi/chi kung; acupuncture; homeopathy; healing; shiatsu-do; Bach flower remedies.*

PELVIC INFLAMMATORY DISEASE

Infection of the womb and ovaries, which can start and progress with minimal symptoms. Abbreviated to PID.

CAUSES

The female genital tract is especially liable to infection, because germs easily gain access from the outside. They ascend through the vagina into the womb, then to the Fallopian tubes and ovaries. They can then gain entry to the interior of the abdomen. Infections lead to scar tissue and bands of fibres which tether the womb or block the Fallopian tubes or ovaries, reducing their normal function and leading to chronic pain and **female subfertility**.

Sources of infection
Sexually transmitted diseases are the most important causes of infection and include gonorrhoea and chlamydia.

Following a **miscarriage** or a termination of pregnancy, not uncommonly fragments of the placenta remain in the womb. In the majority of cases these will be expelled with the next menstrual cycle, otherwise the dead tissue is a fertile breeding ground for bacteria. This is why it is recommended to have a D&C (see PERIOD PROBLEMS) after a miscarriage to clear the womb thoroughly.

The contraceptive coil carries a risk of pelvic inflammatory disease in women who have had PID before.

As with any part of the body with a rich blood supply, the womb and tubes can be subject to infection purely by chance, although this is a relatively uncommon cause of PID.

SYMPTOMS

The diagnosis of pelvic inflammatory disease is suggested by a combination of aching over the lower abdomen and an offensive yellow or green vaginal discharge. The woman may feel ill with fever and shivering. The diagnosis is straightforward with such symptoms but PID can follow a much less obvious course with just a transiently abnormal vaginal discharge and other symptoms emerging over several months. These are increasingly heavy and painful periods and pain on intercourse, felt deep inside.

One possible consequence of pelvic inflammatory disease is subfertility, because the ovaries cannot release their eggs properly or sperm cannot reach the egg because the Fallopian tubes are blocked. The disease may be first detected on investigation for subfertility, when special X-ray studies of the womb and Fallopian tubes reveal the blockages.

TREATMENT

The first step in treatment is to identify the infection responsible by taking a swab of vaginal secretions. This gives guidance as to the most appropriate antibiotics to use. These are then given in high dosages for at least ten days. Tests will also identify any sexually transmitted infection. Sometimes the infection is so severe that the woman needs intravenous antibiotic therapy in hospital.

The same approach is used if the disease is chronic. In addition, it may be possible to release the ovaries surgically from any fibrous bands or to reopen the Fallopian tubes in order to restore the woman's fertility. Where pain and discomfort on intercourse is persistent, **hysterectomy** may be the woman's only option.

QUESTIONS

Is the diagnosis of PID straightforward?
Given classic acute symptoms it should be easy. The diagnosis is more difficult if there is just slight abdominal discomfort and a mildly abnormal discharge. In such cases the diagnosis should be confirmed by a laparoscopy, which means looking inside the pelvis to see if the internal organs are inflamed.

Is PID invariably due to sexually transmitted disease?
There is a great deal of overlap between pelvic inflammatory disease and sexually transmitted disease (see page 162) but it would be wrong to regard them as identical since PID can arise simply through chance.

What are the risks of subfertility?
There should be no problem with promptly and vigorously treated acute pelvic inflammatory disease. The risks increase with more chronic or repeated episodes of PID.

Complementary Treatment
If PID is diagnosed, antibiotics should not be shunned. **Chinese** and **Western herbalism** can both offer herbs to help fight infection – experienced practitioners will be able to advise. **Chakra balancing** can help ease pain and aid relaxation and should reduce discomfort during intercourse. **Shiatsu-do** techniques can help. **Naturopathy** has much to offer. *Other treatments to try: homeopathy; aromatherapy; Bach flower remedies.*

ENDOMETRIOSIS

Deposits of cells from the womb that seed within the pelvic organs and elsewhere, causing pain and subfertility.

CAUSES

Endometriosis is being increasingly recognized. The lining of the womb, the endometrium, consists of cells sensitive to oestrogen and progesterone, which regulate the menstrual cycle. Towards the end of the cycle these cells degenerate and bleed, forming the menstrual flow. For unknown reasons, these same endometrial cells can lodge elsewhere in the body and still go through a menstrual cycle, including bleeding.

There are many theories to account for this. One theory is that some cells escape during menstruation and, instead of leaving in the menstrual flow, ascend the Fallopian tubes into the pelvis. They lodge on the ovaries, the outside of the womb or the intestine. The groups of cells are often small, but endometriosis can spread across the pelvic organs, forming large cysts.

SYMPTOMS

Minor endometriosis is quite common and asymptomatic. If the deposits are large they give rise to pain at the time of menstruation, because the blood they produce accumulates as a painful cyst. In more extensive disease, there is the formation of scar tissue which binds the womb and ovaries in a way similar to **pelvic inflammatory disease**. There is pain felt deep inside on intercourse, and periods become painful and heavier. There is a risk of **female subfertility** through blockage of the Fallopian tubes by scar tissue.

Deposits can be felt on internal examination but more often the diagnosis is established by laparoscopy, which gives a full idea of the extent of the condition.

Although most cysts lodge within the pelvis, endometrial deposits can turn up anywhere in the body; they have been known to cause such bizarre symptoms as a belly button that bleeds in exact sequence with the menstrual cycle.

TREATMENT

Until recently, there was no treatment to reverse the condition and only **hysterectomy** and removal of the Fallopian tubes could be offered to relieve pain. Now hormone treatment is available with drugs that block oestrogen. The first was danazol, taken by mouth but with many side effects. There are now injectable drugs with fewer side effects, such as goserelin, which shrink the deposits so they no longer cause symptoms.

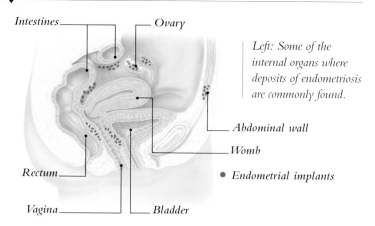

Left: Some of the internal organs where deposits of endometriosis are commonly found.

Intestines — Ovary — Abdominal wall — Womb — Rectum — Vagina — Bladder — Endometrial implants

In addition, large deposits can be destroyed by laser under laparoscopy. It may be possible to reopen blocked Fallopian tubes, with improvement in fertility. The contraceptive pill is effective for women whose only symptom is painful periods.

QUESTIONS

How common is endometriosis?
Up to 20% of women who need a laparoscopy because of gynaecological symptoms prove to have endometriosis. It is the cause of subfertility in about 10–15% of subfertile women.

How serious is it?
Often an unexpected, incidental finding, it is not dangerous in itself but is important because of the pain and subfertility it may cause. Treatment is not necessary if it is not causing symptoms.

Is endometriosis becoming more common?
Endometriosis used to be diagnosed by the combination of symptoms plus feeling cysts on internal examination. The increased use of laparoscopy is revealing how common endometrial cysts are that are too small to be felt on internal examination alone.

Complementary Treatment

Traditional Chinese medicine (**herbs**, **acupuncture** and **tai chi/chi kung**) can have a good effect, especially in lessening pain. **Homeopathy** can help but treatment depends on what brings on the pain, how it presents, what makes it better or worse, and so on. **Chakra balancing** helps ease pain, aids relaxation and reduces discomfort during intercourse. **Hypnotherapy** can be used in pain control, and to lessen anxiety.

FIBROIDS

Benign overgrowth of muscle in the womb that can reach an enormous size.

CAUSES

The walls of the womb are mostly composed of tough muscle, which enlarges during pregnancy. It is this muscle that gives rise to minor contractions during pregnancy and eventually expels the baby during labour. A fibroid begins when a number of muscle cells start to expand and grow into a tumour within surrounding healthy muscle. This is not a cancerous process; the tumour is entirely benign. Fibroids grow very slowly and can reach the size of a small melon before causing any symptoms. Untreated they can continue to grow up to 20 kg/44 lb in weight. It is common to have several fibroids in the womb of varying sizes; the larger they are the more they distort the shape of the womb and the more they project into the cavity of the womb, giving rise to symptoms.

Just what sets off the process is unknown, but fibroids are more common in women who have had no children or who have delayed having children until after 30 (which remarkably now includes the majority of women in the United Kingdom). This suggests that prolonged exposure to oestrogen has something to do with it, in support of which is the fact that fibroids tend to shrink after the **menopause**, when oestrogen levels diminish. Nor are they that rare: about 20% of women will have them.

SYMPTOMS

Small fibroids do not cause any symptoms and are a chance finding on gynaecological examination or on a scan of the womb. If larger, the most common symptoms are heavy and irregular periods (see PERIOD PROBLEMS). Pain is not a feature of fibroids except in the uncommon instances of the fibroid degenerating through outgrowing its blood supply. The largest fibroids will cause abdominal swelling and put pressure on the bladder leading to a constant desire to pass urine.

There is no agreement as to whether fibroids can affect fertility. A large fibroid might prevent implantation, affect the growth of the baby or prevent normal delivery.

TREATMENT

Treatment is only needed if fibroids are causing symptoms or if they might interfere with a future pregnancy. It is difficult but possible to cut out each individual fibroid in an operation

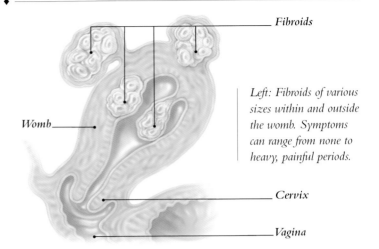

Left: Fibroids of various sizes within and outside the womb. Symptoms can range from none to heavy, painful periods.

Fibroids — Womb — Cervix — Vagina

called myomectomy. Many fibroids can be removed at the one operation. Myomectomy is suitable for women who contemplate a future pregnancy or who do not want a **hysterectomy**.

Many women do opt for a hysterectomy, to avoid the 10–15% chance of fibroids regrowing.

It may be possible in the future to make fibroids shrink using the same drugs used in **endometriosis**, for example goserelin, which reduce oestrogen levels.

QUESTIONS

Can the diagnosis be made on examination only?
There is a typical feel to most fibroids that allows gynaecologists to be confident about the diagnosis simply on internal examination. If in doubt they can order an ultrasound scan of the womb or, if there is pain, perform a laparoscopy.

Do fibroids cause pain on intercourse?
This is not a recognized symptom of fibroids; if you are experiencing this, other diagnoses such as endometriosis or pelvic inflammatory disease must be considered.

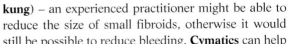

Complementary Treatment
Chinese medicine (**herbs**, **acupuncture** and **tai chi/chi kung**) – an experienced practitioner might be able to reduce the size of small fibroids, otherwise it would still be possible to reduce bleeding. **Cymatics** can help by focusing corrective sound waves at your womb. **Hypnotherapy**, especially visualization techniques, can be effective – consult an experienced therapist.

HYSTERECTOMY

An operation to remove the womb – necessary for various reasons and one of the most commonly performed operations on women.

CAUSES

Hysterectomy is almost always a planned operation; there are few situations that call for an emergency hysterectomy. The operation is performed when there is a problem within the womb which cannot be isolated. Probably the most frequent reason is persistent heavy periods, but the levonorgestrel-releasing coil is already making this much less common (see PERIOD PROBLEMS). The next most common reason is probably large **fibroids**, where again the periods are heavy.

Women tend to be prone to urinary **incontinence** due to anatomical drooping of the outlet from the bladder. Although operations to correct this do not necessarily require a hysterectomy, it often makes technical sense to do this at the same time.

Cancer of the womb of course requires hysterectomy, as does **cervical cancer** if it is invading tissues outside the cervix itself. **Endometriosis** and **pelvic inflammatory disease** are conditions in which the womb becomes chronically inflamed or tethered and it is sometimes best to remove it.

A pre-menopausal woman considering hysterectomy must be convinced that it is the necessary treatment for her, in the understanding that it brings her childbearing days to an end.

SYMPTOMS

The conditions described above usually produce heavy, painful or irregular periods or else the symptoms of cancer of the womb or cervix.

TREATMENT

The womb can be removed either by abdominal surgery or via the vagina. The abdominal approach is technically easier, because the field of view is greater. It involves an incision just above the bikini line. The Fallopian tubes are cut where they join the womb and the vault of the vagina is stitched closed where it meets the womb. Vaginal hysterectomy is technically more complicated but is a preferred method if the woman is also having the walls of the vagina tightened for prolapse. Also, there is no external scar.

In both cases recovery takes a couple of weeks. Hysterectomy can be a debilitating operation and it may take eight to twelve weeks to recover completely from the operation.

The ovaries

Usually the ovaries are left in pre-menopausal women so as to allow them to continue to produce oestrogen. To do otherwise would start an abrupt menopause. If removal is unavoidable, for example if they are caught up with endometriosis or pelvic inflammatory disease, hormone replacement therapy (HRT) would be given at or about the time of surgery.

Complications

Serious complications after hysterectomy are uncommon. Possible minor complications include urinary infections, wound infections and loss of belly muscle tone. Several important structures, for example the bladder, lie near the womb and could be damaged by surgery. However, such problems are exceptionally rare.

QUESTIONS

Does hysterectomy affect sex?
Many women fear it will, imagining that they are in some way less female or more delicate. This is not at all the case and a normal sex life can resume within a month or so.

Is hysterectomy done for trivial reasons?
Removal of the womb takes with it all future problems of menstruation and cancer of the womb or cervix; many women find that an unalloyed blessing. However, you must feel comfortable that the gynaecologist has covered all non-surgical options.

Will I still have a menopause?
When your ovaries fail, you will get symptoms such as hot flushes. Because you no longer have periods, it can only be confirmed with blood tests to detect levels of relevant hormones.

Complementary Treatment

Many therapies can help postoperatively. **Chakra balancing** can help with pain control and aid healing of wounds. **Homeopathy** uses arnica to reduce bleeding and bruising, staphisagria if healing is slow. In **aromatherapy** bergamot and sandalwood are both useful for alleviating postoperative fatigue. **Bach flower remedies** – for emotional aftercare, star of Bethlehem for shock and grief, willow for weepy introspection. After recovery, **yoga** can be beneficial – tell your teacher you have had a hysterectomy.

FEMALE SUBFERTILITY

This means difficulty in becoming pregnant. In cases of couples who appear subfertile about 40% are the result of problems within the woman.

BACKGROUND

A successful pregnancy is the end result of a process of extraordinary complexity. The ovaries have to bring a normal egg to maturation under the influence of hormones from the brain and from the ovaries themselves. This egg has to be picked up by the Fallopian tubes and swept along towards the womb. At some point in this journey a sperm, one of a hundred million that began the journey, will meet the egg and enter it, merging the genetic material from both parents.

The fertilized egg has to implant in the womb, and will gain its nutrition and blood supply from the placenta, whose growth and efficiency has to keep pace with the baby's development for the next nine months. Problems can arise at every step of the way.

Before embarking on the uncomfortable and often disappointing trail of subfertility investigations, it is important to make sure about the fundamentals: that intercourse is taking place regularly and with a correct technique and at mid-cycle, when the egg has been released. **Male subfertility** is a factor in about 30–40% of all couples experiencing problems with conception. Not all subfertility is understood – in at least 20% of cases no convincing reason can be found to explain subfertility yet the couple fail to conceive.

Subfertility must be distinguished from repeated early **miscarriage**, which has its own investigations and treatment.

REASONS FOR SUBFERTILITY

Failure to release eggs (ovulate)

Causes: Failure to ovulate is quite common and means that the woman has all the right hormones but that an egg is not reaching maturity. The problem is recognized by measuring the hormone progesterone in the second half of the menstrual cycle. Any serious generalized illness, for example **diabetes**, **stress** or abnormal dieting, might cause ovulation to fail.

The ovaries might be malformed or might even be absent, as a result of the chromosome abnormality of Turner's syndrome. More common are polycystic ovaries, where the ovaries are covered in small cysts containing immature eggs which do not progress to full maturity. Women with polycystic ovaries have an excess of male hormone, leading to acne and hairiness as well as irregular periods and subfertility.

Symptoms: Congenital problems are suspected if a woman fails to begin menstruating and has poor breast development. The diagnosis is confirmed by blood tests showing low levels of female hormones and by making a chromosome analysis, using cells scraped from the inside of the cheek. Abnormalities of the ovary might be to blame if menstruation is irregular or absent and can be confirmed by ultrasound imaging of the ovaries or by examining them via a laparoscope.

Treatment: Ovulation can be improved by using drugs such as clomiphene which stimulate the release of more eggs. This has to be done very carefully, however, to avoid stimulating too many eggs at once, leading to multiple pregnancy. The treatment of polycystic ovaries also uses clomiphene plus steroids to enhance egg production.

If the problem is a congenital absence or malformation of ovaries, unfortunately nothing can be done.

Barriers to eggs implanting

Causes: Essentially this means a physical barrier within the Fallopian tube or the ovary so that the egg cannot reach the womb. The likeliest reasons for this are chronic **pelvic inflammatory disease** or **endometriosis**, both of which tether the Fallopian tubes with fibrous material that blocks them. Much less commonly, the barrier to implantation lies within the womb, which might be misshapen, for example with an abnormal division up the middle – a bicornuate womb.

Symptoms: The woman fails to become pregnant despite having a normal menstrual cycle. There is a history of pelvic infection, periods are heavy and painful and she suffers internal pain during intercourse.

A malformed womb is undetectable without a specialized dye test to show the outline, called a hystero-salpingogram. A dye that shows on X-ray is injected into the womb and outlines the shape of the womb. The dye should emerge from each Fallopian tube. This test is sometimes combined with laparoscopy to inspect the Fallopian tubes carefully.

Treatment: It is sometimes possible to release the tethered tubes or to enlarge the channels through them. A malformed womb might also be surgically correctable. Otherwise such cases are best handled by artificial fertilization techniques (see below).

Other factors

Some women appear to develop antibodies to their partner's sperm, which are destroyed. This is diagnosed by a post-coital test, which samples semen from the vagina several hours after intercourse and analyses how many sperm are still alive and

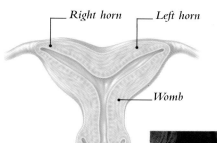

Right horn — Left horn

Womb

Vagina

Left: A bicornuate womb. The abnormal shape makes it difficult for an egg to implant.

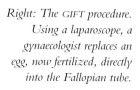

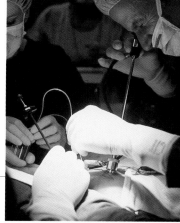

Right: The GIFT procedure. Using a laparoscope, a gynaecologist replaces an egg, now fertilized, directly into the Fallopian tube.

active. At present there are no treatments to improve this situation other than some experimental techniques.

If a woman has irregular or prolonged menstrual cycles it can be difficult to judge the most fertile time for intercourse. Urine-based tests are now available that indicate ovulation and therefore the best time to have intercourse.

Age affects fertility: there is a marked decline in a woman's natural fertility from the age of 35 onward. Whatever the economic and personal reasons for wishing to postpone conceiving, it is important to bear in mind that the older you get the more likely it is you will have difficulty conceiving.

IN VITRO FERTILIZATION
♦

Artificial fertilization techniques go by a variety of names, for example GIFT. The process involves harvesting an egg via laparoscopy. This egg is fertilized by the man's sperm within a test tube, hence *in vitro* fertilization. The fertilized egg is returned to the woman and reimplanted within her womb or within the Fallopian tubes.

The development of *in vitro* fertilization and other similar techniques has been a tremendous advance in dealing with subfertility and, despite the ethical problems, they offer new

hope to many couples. The technology is still new and, like all new technologies, is imperfect but continually improving. The success rate is still quite low – a 20–25% success rate is considered good. The procedure is expensive and the whole process can seem mechanical. This makes it particularly important that couples embarking on this route should ensure they are attending properly accredited clinics where their treatment is supervised by doctors who, as well as being technically proficient, offer the combination of optimism and realism required by subfertility treatment.

QUESTIONS

How common is subfertility?
After one year 90% of all couples will have achieved a pregnancy. Of the remaining 10% just under half will eventually conceive, either through chance or through treatment. One in thirteen couples will remain infertile.

For how long is it worth trying treatment?
After five years, whatever the treatment, the chances of success are very low. Moreover, most couples find that the emotional and financial stresses of subfertility treatment are too much to bear after that length of time. Unexpected pregnancies have been known to happen years after all hope and treatment have been abandoned.

Complementary Treatment

You may feel that it is worth trying gentle complementary approaches, which can be very effective, before resorting to disruptive, and possibly expensive, conventional interventions. A qualified practitioner of traditional Chinese medicine (**herbs**, **acupuncture**, **tai chi/chi kung**) may be able to help. **Chakra balancing** may make you more likely to conceive by relaxing you, and could help by balancing energy from your hormones and enzymes. **Healing** – an experienced practitioner may be able to help you come to terms with the emotional implications. Diet – nutritional deficiencies such as zinc and vitamin A may be implicated in subfertility and a **nutritional therapist** would be able to advise on supplementation. **Hypnotherapy** – hypnotic regression and suggestion can help if the subfertility is caused by subconscious fears of birth or motherhood. *Other therapies to try: homeopathy; naturopathy; Ayurveda; see also* STRESS.

SEXUALLY TRANSMITTED DISEASES IN WOMEN

Diseases spread by sexual contact, known as STDs.

BACKGROUND

Although many sexually transmitted diseases in women are more inconvenient than serious, a significant number do pose an important threat to health. Unfortunately those with long-term health consequences are the ones that usually produce the least symptoms, for example gonorrhoea and chlamydia. Therefore there is an onus on men with STDs to alert their partners to the possibility that they too may be infected. This is also why genito-urinary clinics put so much emphasis on tracing the contacts of men or women with STDs. (See SEXUALLY TRANSMITTED DISEASES IN MEN.)

DIFFERENT TYPES OF STD

Trichomonas

Causes: This is a single-celled organism that is usually, but not always, spread venereally.
Symptoms: The symptoms are **vaginitis** – pain and inflammation of the vagina – plus a green or yellow and often frothy vaginal discharge.
Treatment: Treatment is with the antibiotic metronidazole.

Herpes simplex

Causes: The herpes virus responsible is a type of herpes virus that causes cold sores on the lips. The virus is spread by sexual contact with someone with active genital herpes or by oral sex with someone with cold sores. As with other herpes viruses, it is able to live for many years within the nervous system and can be reactivated from time to time, meaning that symptoms can recur several times a year for several years.
Symptoms: After a few days of burning discomfort, a very tender group of blisters appears on the genitalia. The blisters take seven to ten days to dry and disappear; they are infectious during this time and for a few days after disappearing. The blisters recur at times of stress or simply at random, each time being preceded by a few days of warning painful irritation that sufferers come to recognize with foreboding.
Treatment: Antiviral drugs, if taken early enough, reduce the severity of each appearance. The best-known drug is acyclovir, used as a cream applied to the skin or as tablets. Fortunately, with time attacks become less frequent and less severe. If a pregnant woman has active herpes at the time of delivery the baby must be delivered by Caesarean section to avoid the serious consequences of infecting him with herpes.

Thrush

Causes: This is one of the most common causes of vaginal symptoms (see THRUSH). By no means all cases are via sexual contact because the fungus responsible is a natural inhabitant of the body. In cases of recurrent infection, sexual transmission may be to blame.
Symptoms: The symptoms are vaginal itch and a vaginal discharge containing white curd-like deposits.
Treatment: Treatment is with antifungal agents in the form of creams or pessaries, for example clotrimazole, and, for resistant cases, tablets such as fluconazole.

Gonorrhoea

Causes: Whereas gonorrhoea in men produces discharge from the penis and burning on passing urine, in women infection can persist in a low-key manner. The gonococcus lives within the female genital tract, so that the first the woman may know of infection is when she develops **pelvic inflammatory disease** (PID) or is found to be subfertile.
Symptoms: There may be an infected vaginal discharge plus **urethritis**. If there is PID there will be pelvic pain and a high fever. Unfortunately in about 70% of women infected with gonorrhoea there are no specific symptoms.
Treatment: This is with a single dose of amoxycillin with probenecid as tablets. The cure rate is very high. If the disease becomes chronic with PID it is difficult to eradicate. The effects on fertility are irreversible, although all the treatments given for subfertility are available (see FEMALE SUBFERTILITY).

Syphilis

Causes: The initial infection is even less likely to produce symptoms than gonorrhoea. The organism responsible, *Treponema pallidum*, causes long-term damage to the nervous system and will infect the baby of any future pregnancy.
Symptoms: There is a small sore on the lips of the vagina, which occurs one to three months after infection. There may be a sparse generalized skin rash, which lasts for several weeks, then warts appear around the genitalia and there is enlargement of lymph nodes in the armpits and the groin. There are often no further problems for many years but eventually there may be difficulty with walking, generalized body pains and, ultimately, dementia. This is called tertiary syphilis. The diagnosis is made by blood tests.
Treatment: Treatment of early syphilis requires injections of penicillin for two weeks. Even the established disease can be cured by the same treatment but the effects on the nervous system are irreversible.

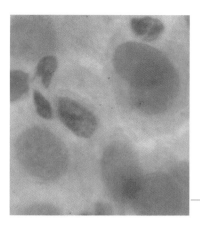

Left: Abnormal cells that have been affected by chlamydia, an organism responsible for pelvic inflammatory disease and subfertility.

Chlamydia

Causes: This micro-organism is being increasingly recognized as one of the most common causes of PID and sterility. Estimates suggest that up to 30% of sexually active women have had it, especially younger women, while 1–5% are at risk of active chlamydial infection and its consequences.

Symptoms: The organism can cause urethritis, with burning on passing water and a discharge, but only in a minority of cases. Otherwise it causes inflammation of the cervix, then inflammation of the womb and Fallopian tubes. In 70% of cases, all this takes place silently, with no symptoms. There may eventually be chronic pelvic pain and irregular bleeding.

Chlamydial infection appears to increase the risks of ectopic pregnancy (see PREGNANCY PROBLEMS). There is an estimated 10% chance of subfertility, the risk rising rapidly with each infection. The diagnosis is difficult even using specialized swabs. Blood tests are becoming available to assist in diagnosis.

Treatment: Chlamydia responds well to antibiotics such as tetracycline and erythromycin, taken for 7–21 days. The disease is so widespread that there will soon be screening for it on the basis that it is common, carries a high risk of causing ill health and is readily treatable.

Genital warts

Causes: These extremely common STDs are caused by the wart virus and arise spontaneously. (Syphilis can cause multiple genital wart-like lesions.)

Symptoms: There are collections of flat warts around the genitalia. Warts cluster around the anus in those who practise ano-genital intercourse. The warts vary from just a few in number to enormous quantities.

Treatment: You must be screened for other STDs. Although most warts can be distinguished from those of syphilis by appearance alone, blood tests should be done. Treatment is

with paints containing the drug podophyllin; if there are large numbers they may have to be cauterized (burnt off). The wart virus can invade the cervix and predispose to **cervical cancer**, so it is important to have regular cervical smears.

See also AIDS.

QUESTIONS

How can I avoid sexually transmitted disease?

Know the sexual habits of your partners. Anyone who has several sexual partners in a short period of time is at significant risk of getting an STD. Use condoms unless you are in a stable long-term relationship. Report any unusual vaginal discharge or bleeding.

What if I have an STD?

You should seek help as soon as possible from a genito-urinary diseases clinic. Such clinics are completely confidential, will check for any coincidental STDs and, crucially, will trace contacts.

Can STDS affect pregnancy?

Apart from reducing fertility some may have serious consequences for the foetus. It is important to inform your doctor if you have genital herpes and if there is any risk of syphilis or HIV/AIDS.

Complementary Treatment

There are serious consequences from the inadequate treatment of STDs, so always seek a conventional opinion. Complementary therapies can both boost the immune system to help the body resist further attack and alter the acidity of the vaginal secretions so they become hostile to harmful organisms. **Western herbalism** – echinacea boosts the immune system, and herbal douches can change the environment of the vagina. Traditional Chinese medicine (a combination of **herbs**, **acupuncture** and **tai chi/chi kung**) could help. **Ayurvedic** treatment might involve a combination of detoxification, oil massage and yoga. Various **aromatherapy** douches are available, and this therapy may have some effect on herpes – an experienced practitioner could advise. In some instances, **homeopathy** can be helpful, especially for genital warts, where useful remedies include thuja, medorrhinum, nitric ac and sabina. *Other therapies to try: nutritional therapy; naturopathy; Alexander Technique.*

VAGINITIS

Inflammation of the vagina, most often caused by infection of the walls of the vagina.

CAUSES

Trichomonas is a micro-organism that causes vaginitis; bacterial vaginosis is the term for infection by one of several other non-specific bacteria that cause inflammation. Another common infectious cause is **thrush**. Many irritants can inflame the vagina, such as vaginal deodorants, bubble baths or even condoms.

SYMPTOMS

There is itchy discomfort, often with a vaginal discharge. There may be internal discomfort from inflammation of the cervix, called cervicitis. The colour of the discharge provides a clue: a frothy yellow-green discharge suggests trichomonas; a grey smelly discharge bacterial vaginosis and a thick white discharge thrush. The diagnosis is confirmed by a swab.

TREATMENT

The antibiotic metronidazole is effective against both trichomonas and bacterial vaginosis; clindamycin vaginal cream is a more specific treatment for bacterial vaginosis. Treatment is continued for a few days and recurrences are common. Obviously any irritants such as bubble baths and vaginal deodorants should be avoided.

Treatment is essential. Even asymptomatic trichomonas should be treated or it will eventually provoke symptoms. Bacterial vaginosis may affect the unborn baby and complicate gynaecological surgery so should be treated in those circumstances, but otherwise not unless it is causing symptoms.

Complementary Treatment
Chakra balancing can help ease pain and aid relaxation, and should reduce discomfort during intercourse. **Naturopathy** – dietary changes might be recommended, along with fasting, **yoga** and hydrotherapy. **Hypnotherapy** can help.

VAGINISMUS

Spasm of the vagina, associated with psychosexual problems.

CAUSES

Apprehension about having sexual intercourse normally underlies this fairly common problem. There may be logical reasons: a woman may be rejecting intercourse with a man she has mixed feelings about or worrying about pregnancy. There is spasm of the muscles around the vagina, preventing entry or making entry very uncomfortable. This should be distinguished from normal entry followed by pain felt deep inside during intercourse, which suggests a pelvic problem such as **endometriosis** or **pelvic inflammatory disease**.

SYMPTOMS

Nothing appears out of the ordinary until intercourse is attempted and entry has to be abandoned. The muscles around the vagina are seen to be in spasm. This is sometimes noticed during routine gynaecological examination, for example taking a smear, when the vagina goes into spasm when the doctor tries to examine internally or to pass an instrument.

TREATMENT

It is important to exclude causes of localized pain such as unhealed tears from childbirth, herpes or **vaginitis**. Otherwise it is a matter of discussing the psychological factors that might contribute to the condition. These could be ignorance and therefore apprehension about sex, previous pain or rape, or lack of foreplay leading to inadequate lubrication.

Treatment involves the woman getting used to feeling her own anatomy, using vaginal dilators of graduated size, plus explanation of sexual technique for both partners.

Psychological therapy helps by diverting attention away from intercourse, substituting other sexual activity such as manual stimulation or cunnilingus. The couple return to sexual intercourse once they have mutual trust.

Complementary Treatment
Acupuncture relaxes your muscles and calms your mind. **Chakra balancing** eases pain, aids relaxation and reduces discomfort during intercourse. **Hypnotherapy** – suggestion and regression techniques can find the cause, and deal with the symptoms.

THRUSH

◆

A widely found fungal organism that commonly affects women.

CAUSES
◆

Thrush is caused by a member of the yeast family of fungi, called *Candida albicans*. Candida thrives in warm, moist conditions with the food supply those areas provide and grows by putting out filaments on which new bodies bud.

Candida is a normal inhabitant of the intestinal tract and of the mouth. It is not an infection 'picked up' from somewhere, nor is it a typical sexually transmitted disease (STD), although it often goes to and fro between sexual partners.

Candida is but one of hordes of micro-organisms found on the body and which compete for available food sources. Its moment of glory comes if other organisms are reduced in number, for example following antibiotic treatment. Antibiotics destroy susceptible organisms all over the body and not just in the infection targeted. This is why vaginal (and oral) thrush is so common after an antibiotic, although women vary greatly in how liable they are to this side effect.

Thrush will overgrow if there is a superabundant food supply, as when someone has excess sugar in the body – **diabetes**.

Finally, the damper and warmer the body's climate the more thrush thrives. This applies particularly to the areas under the breasts, in skin folds of the upper thigh and in the vagina.

SYMPTOMS
◆

There is an itchy red rash under the breasts or on the inner thighs. Vaginal thrush causes an itchy discharge, with white curd-like deposits. The diagnosis is confirmed by taking a swab of the vaginal discharge. Thrush can actually live within the vagina without causing symptoms, and only be discovered if a smear or swab is taken for some other reason.

TREATMENT
◆

Thrush on the skin is treated with drugs called imidazoles, which kill the fungus. Drug names are clotrimazole and imidazole and are often combined with stronger antiseptic agents and with hydrocortisone to reduce itching.

Vaginal thrush is treated with pessaries containing an imidazole. Pessaries are inserted at night for one to six nights. Often an antifungal cream needs to be applied to the vagina, too. Thrush resistant to these methods can be eradicated with an antifungal agent taken by mouth, such as fluconazole. This may be taken as a single large dose or spread over several

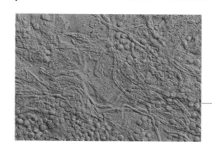

Left: The fungus causing thrush, showing the filaments on which new buds eventually form.

days. Sexual partners should use an antifungal cream on the penis. Anyone, female or male, who keeps getting thrush should be tested for diabetes.

Wearing loose-fitting clothing helps reduce heat and sweating in skin folds. Since candida lives in the intestinal tract, after opening the bowels a woman should wipe from front to back, otherwise she may self-infect the vagina.

QUESTIONS

Do antithrush treatments lose effect?
In general they do not; the organism does not develop resistance in most cases. Recurrent problems are more likely a result of reinfection rather than of resistance.

Why don't antibiotics kill thrush too?
Antibiotics are very specific in their targets and those that kill bacteria do not have antifungal effects. The same is not quite true in reverse: antifungal drugs often have a weak antibacterial activity.

Is self-treatment a good idea?
Certainly for women who get occasional, typical thrush. Anyone getting frequent or apparently resistant thrush should see a doctor to consider diabetes or other rarer causes of recurrent thrush.

Complementary Treatment
Chinese and **Western herbalism** both offer remedies with antifungal effects. Western herbalism offers a range of teas to be used as effective washes: try lavender, marigold, rosemary or thyme. **Aromatherapy** – try tea tree oil in pessary form, or one of the following in a daily sitz bath (six drops): frankincense, myrrh, lavender, tea tree. **Nutritional therapy** might suggest cutting out sugar, fermented foods and yeast. Garlic and live yogurt have antifungal properties. *Other therapies to try: naturopathy; homeopathy; hypnotherapy.*

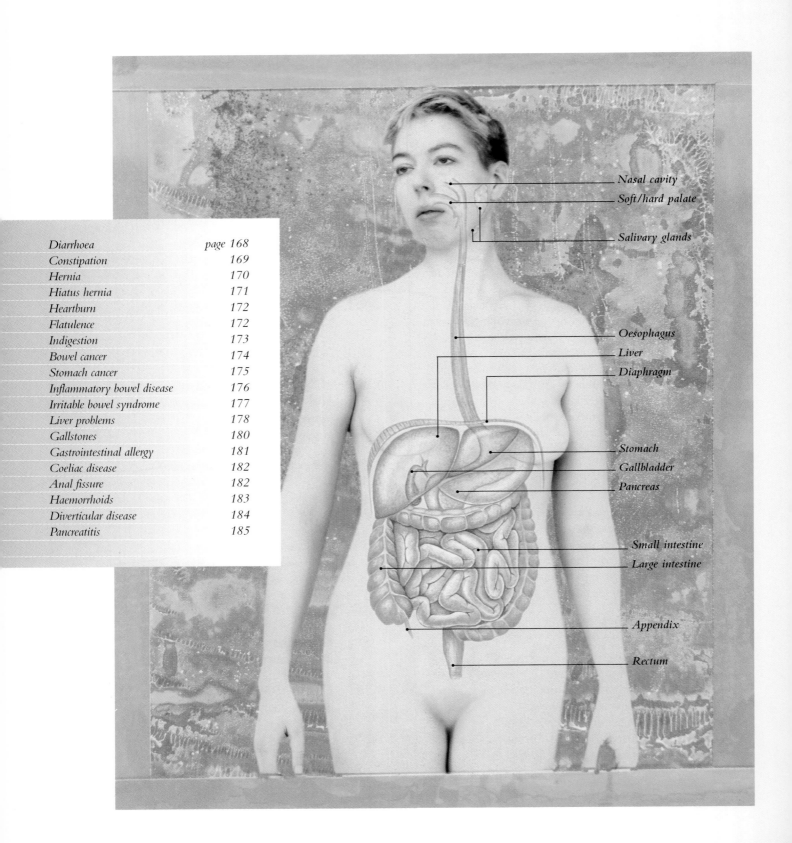

Nasal cavity

Soft/hard palate

Salivary glands

Oesophagus

Liver

Diaphragm

Stomach

Gallbladder

Pancreas

Small intestine

Large intestine

Appendix

Rectum

All the ingenuity of food presentation and the inventiveness of cooks is reduced by the digestive processes to certain fundamental materials. These are carbohydrates, fats, proteins, minerals and vitamins.

DIGESTIVE SYSTEM

THE BASIC MATERIALS we need to function are carbohydrates, fats, proteins, minerals and vitamins. *Carbohydrates* (starchy foods) are large molecules that can be turned into sugar (glucose) to provide the main energy source of the body. Glucose can also be transformed into fat and protein.

Fat is a very high energy source used throughout the body.

Proteins are found in, for example, meat, pulses and grains. They are complex molecules formed from amino acids. Amino acids are like building bricks that, once digested, become available to make all the other body structures, such as muscles, nerves, organs, blood and skin.

Minerals include calcium, potassium, sodium, iron and many more. Each mineral has an important role to play in the body's metabolism, so there are specialized digestive processes that harvest them from food.

Vitamins are biochemicals of a particular type which the body cannot, on the whole, make for itself, but which are essential to cell metabolism. Even though tiny amounts are required, they are vital for making blood, bones, skin, the nervous system, energy production and much more.

The digestive process

Enzymes break the raw food molecules into smaller fragments, which are absorbed and transported all around the body. This begins in the mouth, where saliva starts the breakdown of starch. Digestion begins in earnest in the stomach, where food plunges into a warm highly acidic bath of hydrochloric acid mixed with enzymes.

The liquid mass now passes into the small intestine, the site of the bulk of both digestion and absorption. Yet more enzymes from the pancreas attack the food, breaking down protein. Bile from the liver dissolves fat molecules.

The lining of the small intestine is composed of billions of frond-like outgrowths, which vastly increase the surface area. The outer layer of each frond contains specialized cells that actively transport molecules from the food slurry into the blood stream. Within the blood stream yet more specialized proteins pick up the newly digested food and carry it mainly to the liver for further processing.

The digestive process is by and large complete by the time that material reaches the large intestine – called the colon. Huge quantities of bacteria live in the large intestine and complete the digestion of tough carbohydrate fibres. Water and minerals are also reabsorbed there.

Control

The process of digestion is under an array of biochemical and nerve controls, which are far from fully understood. These cause the right enzymes to appear at the right times and regulate acid and bile production. They influence the complicated muscle layers in the walls of the bowels, which sweep food through the system and which expel it at the end.

Digestive disorders

Many bowel problems revolve around the production of excess acid (ulcers, **indigestion** and **heartburn**), the upward escape of acid (**hiatus hernia**) and disordered movements of the intestine (**constipation**, **diarrhoea** and **irritable bowel syndrome**). The rapid turnover of cells within the digestive tract predisposes to cancer, especially of the stomach and large intestine.

Left: The chemical resources of the digestive system break food down within hours into usable components.

DIARRHOEA

Liquid motions that occur if the bowel fails to reabsorb fluid.

CAUSES

For much of its passage through the intestinal tract food moves as a liquid slurry, totalling about 8 litres/1¾ gallons a day. Water is reabsorbed in the large intestine until the motions are solid or semi-solid. This process is affected by infection, inflammation or growths in the bowel. The over-whelming majority of cases of diarrhoea are caused by minor and self-limiting infection.

Infection and inflammation

Many germs can cause a temporary inflammation of the bowel, which interferes with fluid absorption. Even the common cold viruses do this, especially in children. More serious infections such as cholera or typhoid are unusual in the developed world. These lead to dangerously high fluid loss in a very short period of time.

Food poisoning may be caused by a definite germ or by poisons (toxins) within the food that do not infect the bowel but cause it to be overactive. The terms gastroenteritis and food poisoning largely overlap. Chronic diarrhoea is a feature of **inflammatory bowel disease**.

Growths

Growths, benign or cancerous, in the bowel cause diarrhoea by interfering with its normal function. Much less common than gastroenteritis, these bear consideration if an older person has diarrhoea lasting more than a couple of weeks.

Miscellaneous causes

Less common reasons include worry ('my bowels turned to water'), malabsorption (as in **coeliac disease**) or an overactive thyroid gland (see THYROID PROBLEMS). In the elderly diarrhoea often coexists with **constipation**.

SYMPTOMS

The motions are semi-formed if not pure liquid. Abdominal cramps are relieved by opening the bowels urgently many times a day. Blood is not uncommon with gastroenteritis; recurrent blood loss or mucus in the motions suggests inflammatory bowel disease or a growth, as does persistent diarrhoea, diarrhoea at night, abdominal pains and weight loss. Thirst and tiredness with prolonged diarrhoea suggest serious fluid and mineral loss and require medical attention.

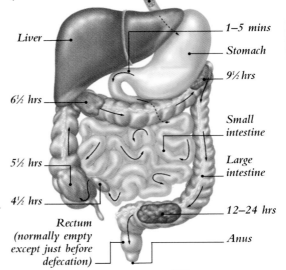

Oesophagus (gullet)
Delay of 3 secs
Liver
1–5 mins
Stomach
9½ hrs
6½ hrs
Small intestine
5½ hrs
Large intestine
4½ hrs
12–24 hrs
Rectum (normally empty except just before defecation)
Anus

Left: Timed progress of the first part of a meal through the digestive system, after leaving the mouth. (The latter part of the meal takes 3–5 hours to leave the stomach.) Food reaches the large intestine as liquid. If water is not properly absorbed there, diarrhoea results.

TREATMENT

The vast majority of cases of diarrhoea settle without any medication over a few days. The individual should simply drink 2–3 litres/3½–5 pints a day of bland drinks such as water, tea, or fizzy drinks gone flat. It is best to avoid milk and sweet drinks, which can make diarrhoea worse. It is especially important for both the elderly and children to take extra fluids containing the minerals lost in diarrhoea, such as potassium.

Various antidiarrhoea remedies work on the nervous system, which controls the bowels, slowing it down. They are useful for short-term control but see a doctor for diarrhoea lasting more than a few days. Drugs include loperamide and codeine. Analysing a stool sample may reveal infection treatable by an antibiotic. Antibiotics such as ciprofloxacin are helpful if diarrhoea acquired abroad is persistent and severe.

See also page 334 for diarrhoea in children and babies.

Complementary Treatment

Most complementary therapists will offer dietary advice along with treatment: **nutritional therapists** and **naturopaths** can be especially helpful. Commonly used **acupuncture** points are Stomach 25, on the abdomen, and Stomach 36, below the knee. **Chinese herbalism** remedies to strengthen a weak digestive system include *Dang Shen* and *Bai Zhu*, both part of the formula called *Si Jun Zi Tang* (four noble formulae). *Other therapies to try: homeopathy; Western herbalism; shiatsu-do; cymatics; hypnotherapy; auricular therapy; Ayurveda; chakra balancing.*

CONSTIPATION

Bowels that open infrequently with hard, uncomfortable motions.

CAUSES

Whereas **diarrhoea** results from excess fluid in the large intestine, constipation is quite the opposite. The contents of the bowel stay so long that excess fluid is absorbed, leaving the motions so hard that they are difficult to pass. Constipation also occurs if something obstructs the passage of motions or reduces the normal rhythmic contractions of the intestines.

Delayed transit time

This extremely common cause affects everyone at some time and the elderly more than most. There is a reduction in the bowel's rhythmic contractions that normally push food through the system. Faeces accumulate within the large intestine; the longer they stay the more water is extracted and the harder they become. Eventually the bowels open through sheer weight of material, although it can be painful and leaves the individual feeling that the bowel is incompletely emptied.

Children often deliberately withhold opening their bowels for reasons clear to Sigmund Freud but unclear to everyone else. The resulting pain on defecation leads to a vicious circle of further retaining of motions.

Obstruction and other factors

In an older person, persistent change of bowel habit to constipation (or diarrhoea) could indicate a growth in the large bowel, especially if the change in bowel habit is accompanied by pain or bleeding. Rarely, children are born with congenital malformations of the bowel which interfere with defecation.

Constipation is a feature of both severe **depression** and an underactive thyroid gland (see THYROID PROBLEMS). Most powerful painkillers also cause constipation, for example codeine, morphine and co-proxamol. This can be a problem for those individuals who need to take such painkillers for chronic pain. Constipation is a feature of **irritable bowel syndrome** and is common during pregnancy (see PREGNANCY PROBLEMS). Constipation can also be an indicator of inadequate dietary fibre.

SYMPTOMS

There is no definition of constipation in the sense of how much, how often. People vary from having a bowel action twice a day to having one once a week. Therefore constipation is defined by reference to your usual bowel habit and not by reference to any rules. If the bowels are opened only infrequently but without straining there is no reason for concern, whereas a daily struggle may indicate a problem.

Constipation plus blood in older people needs full investigation. Sudden constipation plus abdominal pain and distension is typical of a bowel obstruction needing emergency care.

TREATMENT

Temporary constipation responds to increased fluid or a laxative. Some laxatives, for example senna, stimulate the muscle of the bowel to move faeces faster and can lead to uncomfortable cramps. Others, such as lactulose or fibre drinks, draw water back into the motions. If necessary a suppository will stimulate the bowel quickly; an enema literally washes out the bowel. Sometimes children with constipation resistant to mild laxatives may have emotional problems that need unravelling. All cases benefit by increasing the amount of fibre in the diet.

Techniques for investigating possible **bowel cancer** include sigmoidoscopy, colonoscopy to look at the lining of the bowels (see page 355) or a barium enema (see page 348).

QUESTIONS

Are regular laxatives harmful?
Stimulant laxatives such as senna lead to reduced muscular activity of the bowel and are not advisable. Those that retain fluid and fibre drinks are safe for long-term use.

Why is constipation so common in the elderly?
Older people eat less and often take less bulky foods. They exercise less (immobility is constipating) and may be on painkillers that have constipation as a side effect.

Complementary Treatment

Consult a **nutritional therapist** or **naturopath**; boost your fibre intake. **Acupuncture** and **Chinese herbalism** – see DIARRHOEA. **Chakra balancing** reduces pain and relaxes the abdominal wall, stimulating defecation. **Aromatherapy** oils to stimulate digestion are black pepper, marjoram and rosemary. **Hypnotherapy** can get the bowel moving regularly. **Ayurveda** offers bowel cleansing with various enemas and laxatives. *Other therapies to try: homeopathy; tai chi/chi kung; auricular therapy; cymatics; shiatsu-do; yoga.*

HERNIA

◆

Protrusion of an internal organ through muscle wall covering it.

Inguinal hernia ———

Right: A soft swelling in the groin is typical of an inguinal hernia.

CAUSES

◆

The common types of hernia occur in the groin, where there is always a weakness of the muscle wall. A hernia here is called an inguinal hernia. In men the testicles descend from the abdomen into the scrotum a few weeks before birth or shortly afterward. They descend along a path called the inguinal canal, which always remains a little weak. Anything that increases abdominal pressure pushes away at that potential weakness, for example **chronic bronchitis** with its persistent cough, or constant heavy lifting. Eventually the muscle weakens so much that a loop of intestine gets inside and appears as a bulge. Women do get inguinal hernias but much less often.

For similar reasons the other common sites for hernias are the umbilicus (belly button), which passes through the muscles of the abdominal wall, and at the site of surgery over a muscle – an incisional hernia.

SYMPTOMS

◆

An inguinal hernia begins as a small uncomfortable bulge in the groin, which steadily increases in size. It aches when the person is standing, becoming particularly uncomfortable if he is straining, but disappears when he is lying flat and relaxing.

A hernia is termed incarcerated if a loop of intestine becomes stuck, unable to retract back inside the abdomen: the lump is firm and feels tender. More serious again is a strangulated hernia, when the loop of intestine is not only stuck but its blood supply has become obstructed; the lump is then extremely painful and hard. This is a surgical emergency, marked by severe pain then vomiting from bowel obstruction. In theory hernias elsewhere can become incarcerated or obstructed, but this is much less common.

Inguinal hernias are quite common in baby boys and often grow smaller without treatment or even disappear.

TREATMENT

◆

Once an inguinal hernia has appeared in an adult it is only a matter of time before it gets bigger and needs repairing. Although trusses were once the vogue treatment, most doctors now regard them as obsolete and recommend surgery. In surgery the weakness in the muscle layer is repaired either by stitching it together or using an artificial plastic or metal mesh. Laparascopic (key hole) surgery (see page 372) now

allows this with just a tiny incision and internal stitching.

An incarcerated hernia can be treated by a whiff of general anaesthetic which makes the surrounding muscles relax. A strangulated hernia has to be dealt with as an emergency before the bowel dies through lack of blood flow. There is a chance of a hernia recurring in people who are constantly coughing or who are overweight, although improved surgical techniques are making this less likely.

Hernias elsewhere are in general less likely to run into problems of pain or obstruction so surgical repair is not essential.

QUESTIONS

What are the advantages of key-hole surgery?
It is as strong as conventional repair, less painful and recovery is much quicker – a matter of days if not hours. Technically it is more complicated than open surgery, so choose an experienced surgeon.

Must hernias be repaired?
Other than in cases of incarceration or strangulation, there is no medical need for repair except for the knowledge that you may eventually have too much discomfort to bear. This is bound to happen at the most inconvenient time for you.

Complementary Treatment

Alexander Technique – hernias can be helped by improved postural balance and a decrease in contractions along the spinal column. **Reflexology** treatment is aimed at reflex points associated with the adrenal glands and the affected area. **Homeopathy** – depending on circumstances, suggested remedies might include nux or aesculus. **Hypnotherapy** can lessen anxiety and hence help reduce problems. **General self-help** – avoid lifting heavy objects.

HIATUS HERNIA

◆

A weakness in the diaphragm that allows stomach contents to wash upward into the gullet.

CAUSES

◆

This extremely common condition follows from the inevitable weakening of the diaphragm as people get older.

The diaphragm stretches across the upper abdomen, roughly in line with the lower ribs. It is a sheet of tough muscular fibres, which marks the boundary between the chest and the abdominal contents. One important function of the diaphragm is in breathing: as the diaphragm moves up and down it draws air into the lungs.

Certain structures have to pass from the chest into the abdomen, notably major blood vessels, nerves and the gullet. The junction between the gullet and the stomach is especially important since without a tight seal, the contents of the stomach will wash up into the gullet, the walls of which are not designed to withstand the powerful stomach acid.

A hiatus hernia alone does not necessarily lead to symptoms unless other factors increase the chances of acid washing back up, known as reflux. These include **obesity**, smoking and high alcohol intake (see ALCOHOL AND ALCOHOLISM).

SYMPTOMS

◆

Acid in the lower gullet produces **heartburn** with belching and pain localized behind the breastbone. It is typical that the symptoms are worse when you are lying flat or bending over, circumstances in which the stomach contents can more easily reflux. Having a hiatus hernia does not inevitably mean that you will get symptoms; nor is it necessary to have a hiatus hernia to get symptoms from reflux, although having one does make reflux for any other reason worse.

A hiatus hernia is diagnosed on a barium swallow, which shows a characteristic appearance. The constant irritation of the gullet can lead to inflammation and oozing of blood which can, in turn, lead to **anaemia**. Endoscopy (see page 355) is necessary to establish how inflamed the lower gullet is and to look for complications such as ulceration or constriction.

TREATMENT

◆

This can be as straightforward as avoiding wearing tight clothes around the waist, reducing smoking and raising the head of the bed slightly, all of which reduce the chances of acid refluxing through the hiatus hernia. Otherwise treatment is similar to that for **indigestion** or heartburn. Initially there are antacids, especially those containing alginate, which form an insulating layer on the acid, reducing the chances of reflux. Next steps include acid-reducing drugs such as H2 blockers (cimetidine and ranitidine) and proton pump inhibitors (lansoprazole and omeprazole). Other drugs increase the rate at which food passes through the stomach, again reducing the chances of reflux; these include cisapride and metoclopramide.

Surgery

It is possible to repair the weakness of the diaphragm and restore the normal anatomy. This is not surgery to be lightly undertaken without tests to make quite sure that the hiatus hernia is the cause of the symptoms and that all medical avenues have been explored. The repair can now be done laparoscopically (key-hole surgery) (see page 372), avoiding the previous extensive surgery that required opening both the chest and the abdomen.

QUESTIONS

How important is reflux?
Symptomatically reflux is greatly annoying by interfering with the enjoyment of food. Constant irritation can lead to narrowing of the gullet and difficulty in swallowing. This has been shown to be more common than once thought, stimulating research into improving diagnosis and treatment.

Are there other risks?
Constant irritation of the gullet by acid may predispose the cells to become cancerous. A great deal of research is currently addressing the problem as to which people should have endoscopy to detect these changes and how often.

Complementary Treatment

In **cymatics** corrective soundwaves will be focused on your abdomen, thus rebalancing its energy to promote healing. **Alexander Technique** – hernias can be helped by improved postural balance and a decrease in contractions along the spinal column. **Reflexology** treatment is aimed at reflex points associated with the adrenal glands and the affected area. You will find that a **nutritional therapist** or a **naturopath** could tailor a diet to help you reduce acidity. *Other therapies to try: homeopathy; Chinese herbalism.*

Heartburn

Raw feeling behind the breastbone from an inflamed gullet.

Causes

Swallowed food progresses down the gullet to the stomach. There is a muscular system that should prevent stomach contents from escaping back into the gullet, but this mechanism frequently fails. Strong stomach acid then irritates the walls of the gullet and is felt as heartburn. It can happen that the gullet becomes inflamed spontaneously, called oesophagitis, when the mere act of swallowing causes discomfort.

Symptoms

Soon after eating a burning sensation spreads across the front of the chest. Belching often accompanies the pain; acid may rise into the mouth. It is important to distinguish it from chest pain arising from exertion, which may come from the heart.

Treatment

Often it is enough simply to avoid the foods you find cause your heartburn, for example acidic foods and alcohol. Simple antacids are the next step in treatment. These work by neutralizing the stomach acid and providing the walls of the gullet with a protective coating. Acid-blocking drugs such as ranitidine may be needed for the most severe symptoms.

See also INDIGESTION and HIATUS HERNIA.

QUESTION

How easy is the diagnosis?
The close relationship to eating normally clinches the diagnosis. Heartburn in older people for the first time can be indistinguishable from angina (see page 41) and doctors may order heart checks.
If you vomit blood or have difficulty in swallowing your doctor will arrange for endoscopy of the gullet in case the symptoms are caused by a growth in the gullet.

 Complementary Treatment
Western herbalism – the following herbs improve digestion and reduce acid production and inflammation: meadowsweet; caraway; dill; aniseed; ginger; chamomile and peppermint. *Other therapies to try: most have something to offer.*

Flatulence

A common problem of excess intestinal gas and its consequences.

Causes

Gas is formed during the digestion of food: within the large intestine bacteria complete the digestive process with gas as a byproduct. The gas is methane, with a little hydrogen sulphide, nitrogen and carbon dioxide. Eating a high-fibre diet predisposes to excess gas and abdominal distension. Another source of wind, said to be important, is from swallowed air that accumulates within the intestines.

Symptoms

The abdomen feels swollen; relief is obtained by belching and by passing wind through the rectum. People become aware of what appears to be excessive amounts of both – as judged by the reaction of others. General health is normal.

Treatment

Reducing the amount of vegetable fibre in the diet helps to relieve the problem of flatus, although reducing too much may lead to **constipation**. It is really a matter of trial and error, eliminating high-fibre foods.

Try to eat without talking, since you may be swallowing large amounts of air unconsciously. In terms of medication, peppermint is a natural deflatulent and aid to digestion; charcoal tablets are used on the basis that charcoal absorbs gases.

Antacids containing alginates reduce stomach wind, limiting the quantity of wind entering the intestines.

 Complementary Treatment
Nutritional therapy – steer clear of pulses, onions and cabbage. Helpful **aromatherapy** oils include peppermint, fennel, chamomile, cardamom and basil. *Other therapies to try: most have something to offer.*

INDIGESTION

Problems from excess acid production, including peptic ulcers.

CAUSES

Indigestion is very common and progresses in only a fraction of cases to ulceration and on to stomach and duodenal ulcers.

The stomach secretes highly concentrated hydrochloric acid, which begins the process of digestion and sterilizes the food. Thick mucus coats the walls of the stomach, protecting it from this acid. Good as this protection is, it commonly breaks down where there are persistently high levels of acid production. Anything that further irritates the lining of the stomach, like alcohol and acidic foods, adds to this. The gullet has less protection against acid, so any acid there causes **heartburn**. Similarly, acid in the duodenum irritates its walls.

For many years the organism *Helicobacter pylori* was thought to be an innocent inhabitant of the stomach and duodenum but it is now recognized as a potent source of gastric irritation, peptic ulcers and possibly even of **stomach cancer**.

Certain drugs irritate the stomach – most commonly anti-inflammatories such as aspirin and ibuprofen – and vary in how irritant they are. Stress, alcohol and smoking all greatly increase the risks of indigestion and peptic ulcers.

SYMPTOMS

At its mildest there is a burning, gnawing sensation in the pit of the stomach. There may be heartburn. The sensation may be provoked or relieved by eating.

Symptoms suggesting a peptic ulcer are more persistent pain, especially one that wakes you at night and seems to gnaw into the back. However, it is now known that the symptoms bear a poor relationship to the severity of the condition. The diagnosis requires endoscopy, a breath test to detect *H. pylori*, which gives off a characteristic gas, or biopsy of an ulcer, which is to exclude malignancy and is one reason why endoscopy has replaced barium studies. Duodenal ulcers are almost certainly benign; a stomach ulcer may be malignant.

If an ulcer erodes through a blood vessel in the lining of the stomach or duodenum, there may be vomiting of blood or the passage of blood in the stools, colouring them jet black. If the bleeding is seen at endoscopy to be slight, treatment with tablets alone will be sufficient. If it is more severe, urgent surgery will be required. Potentially, a peptic ulcer can erode through the stomach or duodenal wall, to become a perforated peptic ulcer. This surgical emergency causes sudden severe upper abdominal pain and peritonitis.

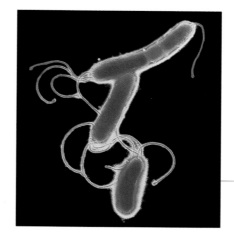

Left: Helicobacter pylori. These common micro-organisms probably cause chronic indigestion, peptic ulcers and possibly some stomach cancers.

It is easy to dismiss the importance of indigestion. The symptoms of stomach cancer exactly mimic it. Anyone over 40 with unusual or persistent indigestion should see a doctor.

TREATMENT

Remedies for mild indigestion neutralize the acidity of the acid, reducing burning. Often they are sufficient. It is essential to reduce smoking, alcohol and **stress**, which is also a factor.

A more efficient way to reduce acid is to block its production with drugs called H2 blockers, such as ranitidine or cimetidine. More potent are the rapidly acting proton pump inhibitors like omeprazole and lansoprazole.

There is much research at present looking into the best way of destroying *H. pylori*. Current regimes combine antibiotics (amoxycillin or metronidazole) with a powerful antacid such as omeprazole. Eradicating *H. pylori* cures peptic ulcers in about 90% of cases for at least a year. Surgery is now a rarity for peptic ulcers. It involves severing the vagal nerve, which controls the secretion of acid by the stomach. Surgery is essential for the emergency of a perforated peptic ulcer.

Complementary Treatment

Western herbalism – try peppermint or psyllium. See a **nutritional therapist** or a **naturopath** for dietary advice. **Chiropractic** – mid-upper back pain can come with indigestion; treating the spinal irritation and muscle spasm in the mid-thoracic area with manipulation helps ease pain and settle the indigestion. *Other therapies to try: homeopathy; tai chi/chi kung; chakra balancing; cymatics; hypnotherapy; Ayurveda; acupuncture; Chinese herbalism; auricular therapy.*

BOWEL CANCER

Malignant growths within the intestines are common in the West and are curable if detected early.

CAUSES

The small intestine is where the bulk of digestion takes place; despite its great activity it is unusual to develop cancer here. Cancer is far more common in the large bowel, even though it is a less energetic environment. Most growths arise in the final part of the large bowel, called the descending colon, the rectum and just inside the anus itself.

Bowel cancer, the second most common cancer in the United Kingdom, is rare in Africa and Asia, which suggests that environmental factors are involved. Possibly the Western low-fibre diet means that faeces remain in the large intestine for longer so that any cancer-producing agents in the diet have longer to influence the cells of the bowel wall.

There is a genetic tendency to bowel cancer: people with a close relative who has it have a two to four times increased risk themselves. People with ulcerative colitis (see INFLAMMATORY BOWEL DISEASE) have as much as a 40 times increased chance of bowel cancer once they have had colitis for more than 15 years.

SYMPTOMS

The disease is most common after the age of 60, and is rare below 40 except in the high-risk groups above.

Change of bowel habit is the prime symptom to be aware of, whether it is towards **diarrhoea** or towards **constipation**. Temporary changes of this sort are extremely common; changes lasting more than a couple of weeks need investigating. Bleeding from the bowel is another 'must investigate' symptom, even though there are plenty of benign causes.

Anaemia in an otherwise healthy adult with a good diet is a possible indication of internal bleeding from a silent growth and investigation would be recommended. Other symptoms may include weight loss and abdominal pains, although these are features of more advanced disease.

A rectal examination picks up about one-third of all bowel tumours. Other bowel investigations include checking the stools for traces of blood, sigmoidoscopy, colonoscopy (see page 355) and barium enema (see page 348).

TREATMENT

If caught early, when the cancer is confined to the surface layer of the bowel, bowel cancer is virtually curable – there is a better than 95% five-year survival. Treatment involves an abdominal operation to cut out the tumour with part of the bowel and to rejoin the healthy bowel. Modern surgical techniques mean that it is now uncommon to need a colostomy, other than as a temporary measure, except for tumours that are sited very close to the anus.

Once the cancer has spread deeper inside the wall of the bowel or into the surrounding tissue, the chances of a cure are less, there being a 30–65% five-year survival. Radiotherapy and chemotherapy (see pages 370 and 371) are slowly improving these figures, however.

QUESTIONS

Is screening worthwhile?
Trials are now testing the value of regular screening of people after the age of 50, for example by testing a stool sample for blood or by using sigmoidoscopy every five to ten years. People at high risk of bowel cancer should have regular colonoscopy of their bowel in order to detect early disease – every three years at least.

What happens with untreated cancer?
It erodes into surrounding tissue, causing pain and bleeding, and may obstruct the bowel. It eventually spreads to the liver, causing liver failure.

Complementary Treatment
See STOMACH CANCER

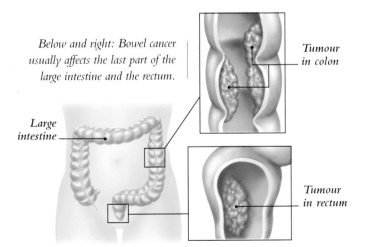

Below and right: Bowel cancer usually affects the last part of the large intestine and the rectum.

Tumour in colon

Large intestine

Tumour in rectum

STOMACH CANCER

A common cancer, although becoming less common worldwide.

CAUSES

Wide international variations in how common stomach cancer is have led to a search for triggers. Diet has been closely studied and factors under suspicion include preservatives in food and alcohol intake. The evidence for these, however, is currently slim and controversial.

There is a hereditary tendency but not as much as with **bowel cancer**. People with type A blood group have a slightly increased risk, as do people with pernicious **anaemia**.

The trigger that has been receiving most attention in recent years is the *Helicobacter pylori* infection. This organism is found in people with gastric irritation; indeed it has become recognized as a major cause of peptic ulcer (see INDIGESTION). Researchers believe that inflammation induced by *H. pylori* increases the risk of malignant change in cells.

SYMPTOMS

Early cancers are silent but eventually there is indigestion and later actual stomach pain. Stomach cancers tend to ooze blood, so that anaemia may be the first symptom of disease. Later in the illness there is persistent pain over the stomach, and loss of appetite and weight.

Indigestion is such a common symptom that it is understandably difficult for a doctor to decide whether or not to investigate. As a rule, an individual over 40 who develops indigestion for the first time or whose indigestion is unusually persistent or intense should have further investigation. The preferred investigation is endoscopy (see page 355) for a thorough inspection of the gullet, stomach and duodenum; samples can be taken from any suspicious areas. Endoscopy is replacing barium meal as the investigation of choice.

TREATMENT

In early disease it is possible to remove the part of the stomach containing the cancer, preserving the function of the rest of the stomach reasonably well. In more advanced disease it is possible to remove the whole stomach (a gastrectomy). This serious and risky operation offers a chance of cure, providing the cancer has not spread outside the stomach, for example to the liver. If cancer has spread it will recur despite gastrectomy, making it hard to justify exposing a patient to risk and discomfort for no gain. Sometimes this decision can only be

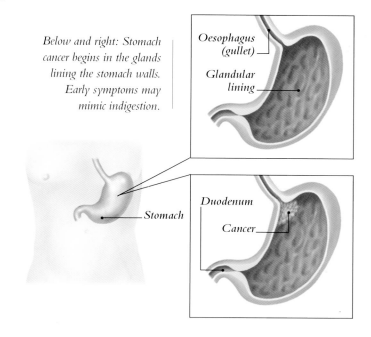

Below and right: Stomach cancer begins in the glands lining the stomach walls. Early symptoms may mimic indigestion.

Oesophagus (gullet)

Glandular lining

Stomach

Duodenum

Cancer

made after opening the abdomen to explore the cancer.

Even if the cancer is inoperable, surgery can divert the flow of food past the diseased part of the stomach. This gives relief from vomiting and obstruction, which are otherwise such distressing symptoms of advanced disease. Chemotherapy (see page 371) has been found to improve the survival by a few months but at the cost of severe side effects.

The outlook for early stomach cancer is about 90% five-year survival; this falls to about 30% in people who have more advanced disease but where surgery still appears justified. Overall, there is a 10% five-year survival, which is a grim outlook. For this reason many surgeons advocate aggressive investigation of older people who have symptoms that are suggestive of early stomach cancer.

Complementary Treatment

No complementary therapy can cure cancer, but many have a role during orthodox treatment. **Chakra balancing** will help with symptom control, energy balance and relaxation, and offer support during rehabilitation programmes. **Reflexology** can offer support during orthodox treatment. **Aromatherapy**, especially when linked with **massage**, can be excellent at lessening the stress and tension associated with disease. Diet – a **naturopath** or **nutritional therapist** should be consulted. *Other therapies to try: see STRESS.*

INFLAMMATORY BOWEL DISEASE

Illnesses that are characterized by pain, diarrhoea and bleeding from the lining of the intestines.

CAUSES

The two recognized forms of inflammatory bowel disease are Crohn's disease and ulcerative colitis. Crohn's disease can affect any part of the digestive tract from the mouth to the anus; ulcerative colitis affects only the large intestine. Some specialists believe that these are related diseases differing in severity. It is possible that both are caused by an auto-immune condition. Many sufferers lead mainly normal lives in between flare-ups, although severe flare-ups are potentially dangerous. Life expectancy is little affected by ulcerative colitis, whereas people with Crohn's disease are twice as likely as the general population to die prematurely.

Crohn's disease

Crohn's disease became more common during the 20th century, leading to a search for a causative factor such as a virus. Currently the measles virus is suspected but there is no definite proof. There is a strong family tendency in white racial groups, less so in black groups. It is four to six times more common in smokers, whereas smoking appears to have a protective effect against ulcerative colitis. The peak incidence is between 20 and 40 years of age.

Ulcerative colitis

Ulcerative colitis is also more common in families and certain racial groups, for example Jews. Smokers are half as likely to get the condition. (See LUNG CANCER, however, for the great dangers of smoking.)

SYMPTOMS

Abdominal pains and **diarrhoea** are prominent features of both conditions, although these tend to be worse in ulcerative colitis. Bleeding and the passage of mucus with diarrhoea are particular symptoms of ulcerative colitis. In both diseases there are periods of ill health, weight loss and **anaemia** interspersed with remissions when you feel quite normal. People may also have inflammation of their joints and eyes.

The diagnosis is confirmed by blood tests, which show inflammation, and by colonoscopy whereby the bowel can be inspected and biopsies taken. As Crohn's disease can extend outside the large intestine, barium studies are useful to show the extent of the condition (see page 348).

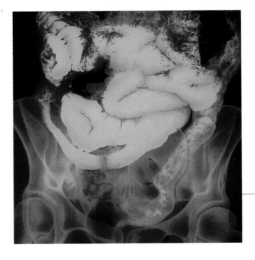

Left: A barium enema of the intestines. The narrow intestine on the left is typical of Crohn's disease.

TREATMENT

In acute attacks antidiarrhoea compounds such as loperamide or codeine are needed, plus steroids to reduce inflammation and drugs like mesalazine or salazopyrin to reduce overall bowel inflammation. Disease confined to the rectum can be treated with enemas containing steroids. People can become very ill very quickly through dehydration, bleeding and the bowel rupturing, so hospital treatment is often needed. Many people find that taking mesalazine or similar daily reduces the frequency and severity of the condition. Such drugs are more effective for ulcerative colitis than for Crohn's disease.

Surgery is avoided if possible because the bowel does not heal well, but it may be a last resort for severe persistent ulcerative colitis. The whole large bowel and rectum are removed, leaving an ileostomy – a bag worn on the abdomen into which the small intestine empties. For Crohn's disease it may suffice to cut out areas of localized disease.

Ulcerative colitis has a greatly increased risk of **bowel cancer** after 15–20 years, so that regular screening is advisable.

Complementary Treatment

Useful **acupuncture** points are Stomach 25, on the abdomen, and Stomach 36, below the knee. In **Chinese herbalism** helpful herbs include *Dang Shen* and *Bai Zhu*, both part of the formula called *Si Jun Zi Tang* (four noble formulae.) **Chakra balancing** can help reduce inflammation of the gut and aid healing of the gut wall surface. Diet – consult a **naturopath** or **nutritional therapist**. *Other therapies you could try: homeopathy; healing; shiatsu-do; chiropractic.*

IRRITABLE BOWEL SYNDROME

◆

A blanket term for many abdominal disturbances for which no other cause can be found.

CAUSES

◆

There are no agreed causes for the condition of irritable bowel. The general medical thinking is that it is a disorder of the system that controls mobility of the bowel – the nerve layer within the walls of the bowel that makes the muscle of the bowel contract.

Many sufferers appear to be under **stress**, if not definitely suffering **depression**. Since irritable bowel syndrome is what is wrong with the majority of patients seen by gastroenterologists worldwide, it is unlikely that some simple cause such as candida has been overlooked. More likely it is a non-specific, humble part of the human condition.

SYMPTOMS

◆

Most people with irritable bowel are young women. The core symptoms are recurrent abdominal pains, often with minor changes in bowel habit from **constipation** to **diarrhoea**. A consistent finding is that pain is relieved by defecation and made worse by stress. There is a feeling of abdominal distension and bloating. The motions may be pellet-like and individuals need to keep opening their bowels.

The symptoms are experienced for months, if not years, despite which the individual looks well, does not lose weight and there are no abnormalities to be found on examination apart from non-specific abdominal tenderness.

TREATMENT

◆

It is important to have some basic investigations, not only to exclude other disease, but to reassure individuals that their symptoms are being taken seriously, since no one doubts that they do experience pain.

The main differential diagnosis is **inflammatory bowel disease**; in such cases the individual usually feels ill and loses weight. Investigations involve blood tests, which show inflammation, and sigmoidoscopy to inspect the lower bowel and perhaps take biopsies from the bowel wall.

The older the individual the more extensive the testing, as the risk of cancer grows, but with average individuals in their teens or twenties the diagnosis can be made with reasonable confidence and minimal investigations.

Treating the condition can be difficult. For many people simple reassurance is enough. Others might try more or less fibre in their diet. Numerous drugs, for example mebeverine, are said to relax the muscles of the bowel; some people derive benefit from such drugs, others do not. Recently, specialists have been subdividing irritable bowel into separate syndromes, which may lead to more focused treatment. If there are symptoms of depression or stress a course of anti-depressants can be helpful.

One of the pitfalls with the condition, of which surgeons are well aware, is to indulge in ever more extensive investigations. Their reluctance to do more should not be interpreted as being uncaring; operations carry hazards and can lead to abdominal pains themselves. With reassurance many people find the condition decreases over a few years.

SYMPTOMS TO BE TAKEN SERIOUSLY

◆

The following symptoms should be taken seriously, even if a diagnosis of irritable bowel syndrome has previously been given. (Possible diagnoses are given in brackets – these are not fully comprehensive.)

◆ *Abdominal pain unrelieved for more than about six hours, especially if accompanied by fever, loss of appetite and vomiting (peritonitis)*
◆ *Abdominal pain with the passage of blood or mucus from the rectum (inflammatory bowel disease below the age of 40, cancer of the bowel above 40)*
◆ *Lower abdominal pain after missing a period or having an unusual period (ectopic pregnancy)*
◆ *Pain with fever, vaginal discharge (pelvic inflammatory disease)*
◆ *Abdominal pain accompanied by weight loss (inflammatory bowel disease, cancer)*

Complementary Treatment

Diet – consult a **nutritional therapist** or **naturopath**. **Auricular therapy** relieves anxiety and regulates digestion, in conjunction with dietary changes following traditional Chinese principles. **Chiropractic** can help if the condition is accompanied by low back pain. **Ayurveda** offers oral preparations, *panchakarma* detoxification, yoga meditation and *marma* therapy. *Other therapies to try: homeopathy; tai chi/chi kung; cymatics; hypnotherapy; acupuncture; Chinese and Western herbalism; autogenic training; chakra balancing.*

LIVER PROBLEMS

Disease of the liver caused mostly by infection, alcohol and cancers.

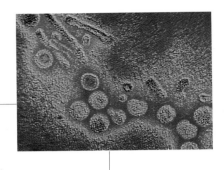

CAUSES

The largest internal organ of the body, the liver is a power-house of activity. It is a storage site for glucose, the fuel of the body, and can synthesize it rapidly if stores are insufficient. It makes bile, later kept in the gall bladder. Bile is necessary for the absorption of fat from food. The liver also makes the fats needed for cell metabolism, including triglycerides and cholesterol. The bulk of protein synthesis takes place in the liver and, crucially, it makes the proteins needed for blood clotting such as fibrinogen.

Also, the liver contains cells that catch and destroy bacteria and viruses from the intestine and so prevent them gaining access to the rest of the body. Lastly, the liver inactivates many hormones once they have done their jobs and this caretaking function extends to the destruction of drugs, alcohol and old blood cells. These are the main source of the pigment bilirubin, which is responsible for the jaundice of liver disease and which eventually makes the motions and urine brown.

With its huge blood supply and never-ending activity, it is to be expected that the liver is prone to disease. Many infections and drugs cause temporary effects on the liver, which may be felt simply as a vague discomfort over the liver or detected on monitoring of liver function blood tests.

Infections

Many infections, including the common **glandular fever** virus, cause a mild hepatitis – inflammation of the liver. Some specific viruses cause a more severe hepatitis. New hepatitis viruses are occasionally discovered and now range from A to G. Some are acquired through pure chance; others such as B and C are transmitted by sexual contact (especially male homosexual activity) in semen or saliva or through blood products and intravenous drug abuse. Internationally, hepatitis B is a huge cause of chronic hepatitis, cirrhosis and liver cancer, affecting hundreds of millions of people mainly in the Far East and Africa. It carries a 1% risk of death from liver failure and a permanent risk of future cirrhosis (up to 50%) and liver cancer. Mothers positive for hepatitis B almost always pass on the virus to their unborn baby.

Alcohol, drugs and immune conditions

These can all lead to cirrhosis of the liver. Cirrhosis is a degeneration of the active cells of the liver, being replaced by fibrous tissue, which is of course non-functioning. Although

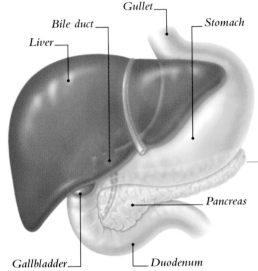

Above: A cluster of the viruses that cause hepatitis B. After invading cells, they reproduce in enormous numbers.

Gullet — Bile duct — Liver — Stomach — Pancreas — Gallbladder — Duodenum

Left: The liver occupies the right upper abdomen. It is vital for digestion, blood formation and handling toxins.

early cirrhosis may be reversible, established cirrhosis is permanent. In the case of paracetamol poisoning the effects may be fatal rapidly. Chronic cirrhosis is a risk for people regularly drinking more than about 30 units of alcohol per week, i.e. 15 pints of beer or 5 bottles of wine.

Tumours

In the West the majority of tumours within the liver have spread there via the rich blood supply from cancers elsewhere, especially bowel tumours. This so-called secondary liver cancer is often the way in which people with cancer finally die. Worldwide, primary cancer of the liver is common and often follows previous infection with the hepatitis B virus.

SYMPTOMS

Viral infections produce hepatitis of rapid onset. There is an incubation period from the time of infection with the virus. In the case of the common hepatitis A this is two to three weeks; in the cases of hepatitis B, four to twenty weeks. There is a week or so of nausea, vague ill health, **fever** and upper abdominal discomfort, after which the individual becomes jaundiced (yellow) from the deposit of pigments that the liver would ordinarily handle. In most cases the illness settles over another week or so. It is rare for people suffering from hepatitis A to have other problems.

Alcohol, drugs, immune conditions and tumours

The immediate effects on the liver of a serious drug or alcohol overdose are nausea, jaundice and itching, followed by bleeding because blood-clotting factors are no longer being made. As toxins build up in the blood stream there may be confusion and a slide into unconsciousness.

Chronic poisoning has more subtle and widespread effects. Itching is common and there may be a hint of jaundice. Men notice breast development and may suffer from impotence (see ERECTILE DYSFUNCTION) because female hormones normally broken down by the liver are at higher than usual levels. The palms become red – also related to female hormones.

Tiny dilated veins appear on the hands, face and chest, called spider naevi. As the cirrhosis worsens, there is accumulation of fluid in the abdomen called ascites and in the ankles. There is a risk of bleeding, leading to widespread bruising and possibly bleeding into the gullet. Eventually the liver fails, with increasing jaundice, confusion, then unconsciousness.

Means used to confirm and measure liver disease are blood tests of the chemicals produced by the liver and markers of any viruses responsible. An ultrasound scan (see page 349) can show typical features of cirrhosis. A liver biopsy (see page 353) is the best way of establishing the exact diagnosis.

TREATMENT

◆

Acute liver damage is usually due to viral infection or drug damage, especially overdose of paracetamol. The drug itself is neutralized by biochemical means in a drip. Patients then have to be nursed in intensive care, receiving correction of the widespread biochemical changes in the blood stream that accompany acute liver failure. They need infusion of clotting factors to prevent internal bleeding and measures to reduce swelling of the brain, which is the main reason for death. Liver transplantation may be the final hope (see below).

Acute liver failure is a very serious condition, with a high mortality rate even in the best centres. If the liver disease is caused by spread of a cancer, there is little that can be done other than general supportive care.

Chronic damage (cirrhosis)

You must stop any behaviour contributing to the cirrhosis, i.e. give up alcohol. This will not reverse the changes in the liver, but will reduce the load it has to bear. Outlook is poor: a 50% five-year survival. A major risk from chronic cirrhosis is bleeding from dilated veins in the gullet called oesophageal varices, which may bleed torrentially and need emergency repair.

Liver transplantation

This now offers hope to those facing inevitable liver failure, from many causes. It is not suitable in cases of liver failure caused by spread of cancer, which will invariably spread into the new liver, but it can be done in cases of people with primary liver cancer.

The risk from the surgery is low; the major risk is from rejection of the liver. The results now offer a remarkable 90% survival to 1 year and better than 70% five-year survival, figures that are improving all the time. (See also page 363.)

(See also page 363.)

QUESTIONS

What is a dangerous dose of paracetamol?
As little as 10 g (20 standard tablets) can be enough to cause serious liver damage. Just 15 g (30 tablets) can be a fatal dose. Urgent treatment is needed within hours of a suspected overdose.

What vaccination is there against hepatitis?
Hepatitis A vaccination is for travellers who might eat shellfish and poorly washed salads, and protects for up to ten years. Vaccination against hepatitis B is for healthcare workers who face exposure to contaminated blood, needles and body fluids.

Are women's livers weaker?
They have to handle the breakdown of the female hormone oestrogen, and therefore have less capacity to cope with alcohol or drugs.

Complementary Treatment

No complementary therapies can prevent or cure hepatitis in its various forms. **Chinese herbalism** can be very helpful, but note a reputable practitioner will insist on regular blood tests to monitor liver function. **Shiatsu-do** strengthens the blood quality through improved organ functioning and toxin discharge. In **nutritional therapy** the liver is considered to be stressed by an excess of saturated fat in the diet; a number of foods and herbs could be used to help drain these fats, for example beetroot and dandelion. **Hypnotherapy** – anxiety interrupts the free flow of enzymes; hypnotherapy can lessen anxiety, and hence help reduce problems. **Ayurveda** – liver tonics and special preparations for inflammatory liver disease are available; detoxification is an essential part of healing. *Other therapies to try: acupuncture; tai chi/chi kung.*

GALLSTONES

◆

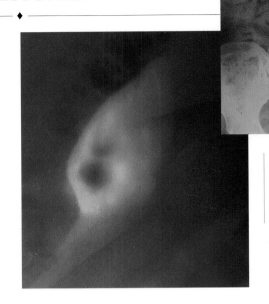

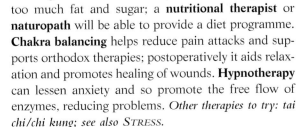

Gallstones are seen as dark shadows under the ribs (above) and in X-ray (left).

Greasy stones within the gall bladder, sometimes causing pain.

CAUSES

◆

Gallstones form within the gall bladder as a result of precipitation of cholesterol and bile salts from the bile. Women are twice as likely as men to get them, but in later life there is a roughly equal chance of gallstones.

Most bile is formed by the liver from cholesterol. It mixes with yellow and green pigments derived from the breakdown within the liver of old blood cells. Bile makes fat soluble, which is an important step in the absorption of fat from the intestinal tract. The liver secretes a remarkable 1 litre/1¼ pints a day of bile, half of which is stored temporarily in the gall bladder, the rest going directly into the duodenum via a network of ducts from the liver.

There are a few rare conditions where an excessive load of bile pigments increases the risk of gallstones, for example certain types of **anaemia**. Gallstones are extremely common: 10–20% of the adult population have them, and only a fraction cause symptoms.

SYMPTOMS

◆

Many gallstones are silent. They lie within the gall bladder and are simply a chance finding on investigation for other abdominal symptoms.

A stone obstructing the gall bladder causes severe upper right-sided abdominal pain, which comes and goes in waves as strong muscular contractions try to overcome the obstruction. Other classic symptoms are mild intermittent pain under the right ribs, which is worse after eating – especially after fatty foods because fat in the diet provokes a reflex contraction of the gall bladder. The pain is from partial obstruction of the flow of bile from the gall bladder into the duodenum.

If there is complete obstruction, infection of the gall bladder invariably results after 24 hours, causing **fever** and jaundice (see LIVER PROBLEMS).

TREATMENT

◆

Fewer than 20% of silent gallstones will cause problems, even over 15 years, and treatment is unnecessary. By contrast if you are getting pains, most surgeons recommend removal because there is a much higher chance of eventual obstruction.

During an acute attack, you will need powerful analgesics to deaden the pain until the gallstone falls away from the bile duct. This usually takes a few hours. If there is infection an antibiotic is given. Mild episodes of pain can be left to settle themselves. Meanwhile the diagnosis is confirmed by an ultrasound scan (see page 349) of the gall bladder, showing stones.

Surgical opinion differs as to whether to remove the gall bladder immediately the acute attack has settled or to defer surgery for a few months. Both attitudes are widespread.

Dissolving gallstones was popular when drugs for this were first found. It takes up to two years of continuous treatment with a 50% chance of recurrence once treatment is stopped, so they are rarely used now that surgery is so safe.

Surgery for gallstones

The usual procedure is laparoscopic removal of the gall bladder (see page 372). Occasionally the older-type operation has to be performed, which involves a long incision under the ribs and from which it takes several weeks to recover.

Gallstones lodged in the duct between the gall bladder and duodenum can be removed by endoscopy (see page 355).

Complementary Treatment

Diet – gallstones are linked with the consumption of too much fat and sugar; a **nutritional therapist** or **naturopath** will be able to provide a diet programme. **Chakra balancing** helps reduce pain attacks and supports orthodox therapies; postoperatively it aids relaxation and promotes healing of wounds. **Hypnotherapy** can lessen anxiety and so promote the free flow of enzymes, reducing problems. *Other therapies to try: tai chi/chi kung; see also STRESS.*

GASTROINTESTINAL ALLERGY

Adverse reaction to certain foods, although the conventional view is that true gastrointestinal allergy is rare.

CAUSES

It is a matter of common experience that certain foods make other conditions worse, for example **eczema**, **asthma** and migraine (see HEADACHES AND MIGRAINE). Beyond that, the subject is bedevilled by lack of agreement as to what else constitutes a reaction and the possible mechanisms whereby the food alleged to be responsible has that effect.

Certain people clearly experience a true allergic reaction; others have more of an intolerance of certain foods. Acute gastroenteritis with **diarrhoea** leaves the lining of the intestine unable to handle the absorption of milk for a few days and the resulting persistent diarrhoea can be misinterpreted as allergy.

Coeliac disease is a true allergic reaction to gluten in the diet. Allergy to peanuts has for unknown reasons become more common in recent years. Other substances identified as possible causes of gastrointestinal allergy are tyramine in cheese, tartrazine (a food additive), egg protein and histamine in strawberries. The widespread concern about E numbers has not been scientifically substantiated.

SYMPTOMS

There may be a true allergic reaction: within minutes there is a blotchy skin rash, tingling in the mouth, swelling of the lips and throat and wheezing. At its most severe there may be collapse through a fall in blood pressure, called anaphylaxis.

Food intolerance would be suspected by the appearance within hours or days of diarrhoea, bloating, or a worsening of asthma or of eczema. The diagnosis is supported by showing regular and repeated reactions to the foods in question. Individuals can be tested by exposure to dilute samples of the foods to which they might be intolerant.

A child who is suspected of cow's milk or lactose intolerance with accompanying poor growth and diarrhoea should show catch-up growth and loss of bowel symptoms when a substitute is given. Lactose intolerance can also happen in adults, causing diarrhoea and **flatulence**.

There is no scientifically proven link between the many other symptoms, such as headaches and behavioural disturbances, that people complain of and true sensitivity to certain foods. For example, in double-blind trials individuals have unknowingly had foods they say they are allergic to, yet they have not shown the expected reaction.

TREATMENT

Where there is a definite association with a particular food, avoid the offending substance. The more severe the reaction the more scrupulously this must be done, for example people with an acute anaphylactic reaction to eggs or nuts must be obsessive about avoiding them. Such people should wear a bracelet with medical details. There are self-injection devices containing adrenaline for immediate treatment. Lesser degrees of allergy are treated with antihistamine tablets or steroids for stronger reactions.

There is little orthodox medical support for diets that exclude a wide range of common foods on the basis that they cause arthritis, malaise, tiredness, hyperactivity and so on.

QUESTIONS

What is an exclusion diet?
It is a very simple diet with just a few foods. The idea is to see whether symptoms disappear, then to introduce a single food from fortnight to fortnight until one provokes the symptoms.

What is wrong with this?
Few people manage to do it properly for the many weeks that are necessary. The interpretation is difficult as the symptoms are often vague and not easily objectively assessed. Extreme exclusion diets may not be nutritionally complete if followed for long periods.

Are other tests available?
Blood tests may show abnormal reactions, but their interpretation is controversial. Scientific studies of hair analysis and many other complementary and alternative procedures do not support the faith some therapists have in them.

Complementary Treatment

A registered **homeopath** could greatly reduce, or even eradicate, your food sensitivity. **Nutritional therapy** can help you identify food intolerance; if you have multiple allergies they could be linked to toxic overload and you will need to undertake work to improve your bowel, liver and digestive system. **Hypnotherapy** can be used in conjunction with a desensitizing programme. **Ayurveda** treats gastrointestinal allergy through detoxification, and oral preparations and *marma* therapy are also important.

COELIAC DISEASE

A hypersensitivity to gluten leading to destruction of the food-absorbing surface of the small intestine.

CAUSES

Coeliac disease is an allergy to gluten, a protein found in most cereals, principally wheat and rye. The disease was confirmed in The Netherlands during the Second World War. The health of certain children improved because bread was scarce and they were therefore no longer exposed to gluten.

The surface of the lining of the small intestine is made of innumerable finger-like outgrowths called villi, which greatly increase the surface area for absorption of food. Gluten makes these villi disappear, leading to malabsorption of food.

SYMPTOMS

In children there is failure to grow, which coincides with the introduction of cereals. Adults, usually women, become tired, and have abdominal pains and **diarrhoea** but it is likely that many sufferers are just anaemic. On investigation there is **anaemia** and often **mouth ulcers**. Diagnosis follows a biopsy of the small intestine (see pages 353 and 355). A blood test showing antibodies to parts of the bowel is a useful screening test.

TREATMENT

Gluten is excluded from the diet and replaced by any of the wide range of gluten-free foods now available. Within three to four months the surface of the small intestine will have recovered. This gluten-free diet has to be lifelong.

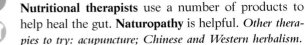

QUESTION

How common is coeliac disease?
Rare in non-Caucasians, the disease affects at least one in 1500–2000 of a Caucasian population. In some areas it is far more common, for example affecting one in three hundred Irish people. There is a strong family association, suggesting a genetic tendency. However, the exact mechanism whereby gluten affects the villi is not known.

Complementary Treatment
Nutritional therapists use a number of products to help heal the gut. **Naturopathy** is helpful. *Other therapies to try: acupuncture; Chinese and Western herbalism.*

ANAL FISSURE

A tear of the back passage, usually through straining.

CAUSES

The anus is held closed by muscular tissue, which distends to allow motions out of the rectum. Passing a large hard motion may be too much, with the result that the canal tears. Recurrent or multiple tears may be caused through bowel disease, in particular Crohn's disease (see INFLAMMATORY BOWEL DISEASE).

SYMPTOMS

There is pain after passing a large motion and bleeding is visible on cleaning. The pain recurs each time the bowels are opened. The tear can be seen as a raw area in the anus and it is extremely tender if the doctor examining it attempts to pass a finger inside the rectum.

TREATMENT

Small tears are common and heal spontaneously, maybe with an anaesthetic gel to reduce pain. Glycerine trinitrate gel has recently been shown to be more effective. It is important to keep the motions soft with a bulk-forming laxative.

Large tears that won't heal are dealt with by dilating the anus under anaesthetic. This reduces the extent to which the fissure stretches on defecation, and so allows it to heal over a couple of weeks. It is unusual to need more than this, but it may be necessary to stitch up a chronic fissure. Never ignore rectal bleeding, although benign causes are common.

Complementary Treatment
Nutritional therapy would reccomend boosting fibre intake and adding natural laxatives to your diet for a while until regular bowel habits are established. These include linseed products and blackstrap molasses.

HAEMORRHOIDS

Swollen veins, popularly known as piles, are the most common cause of bleeding from the back passage.

CAUSES

There are two types, internal and external piles. The causes are the same. External piles are visible as swellings around the back passage and can be felt. They are veins that have become dilated and varicose, similar to varicose veins on the legs. Internal piles are a little more complicated. They are pillars of cushioning tissue supporting the rectum and cannot usually be felt unless they prolapse (drop) through the anus.

Anything that increases the pressure of blood within the abdomen increases the chances of piles, for example spending much time standing, pregnancy (see PREGNANCY PROBLEMS) and chronic **constipation** with accompanying straining.

Piles are more often a nuisance than anything else, unless they prolapse. When this happens to internal piles the piles become trapped by the muscles of the anus and remain as large painful swellings that cannot be pushed back inside. External piles can thrombose – meaning that the blood inside them clots.

SYMPTOMS

Often there is slight discomfort around the back passage, itching and occasional bleeding after defecation. Prolapsed piles are felt and seen as large tender swellings at the anus.

TREATMENT

Mild piles are common and cause little by way of symptoms. Even though they occasionally prolapse they are easily pushed back inside. No treatment is needed apart from avoiding constipation and straining, by increasing fibre and fluid intake. It may be possible to spend less time standing. Piles appearing during pregnancy will go after birth.

If the pile has prolapsed and is tender, treatment is with painkillers and creams containing a local anaesthetic rubbed into the pile. It will shrink over a few days. Occasionally, a pile causes so much pain that a surgeon will need to cut it open to let out the blood, but this does prolong the healing process.

Various treatments for piles that give recurrent problems all cause the blood to clot inside the pile, which will then shrink away. Piles can be burnt, gripped with tough rubber bands, frozen or injected. Whatever is done, piles tend to recur after a few years and haemorrhoidectomy, offering a good chance

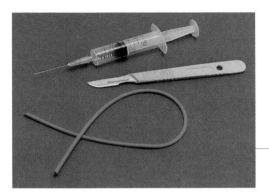

Left: Injections, scalpel and rubber band – all are treatments for haemorrhoids.

of permanent cure, may be necessary. This involves cutting a portion of the rectal lining, taking the pile with it. The operation has a reputation for being painful, as has the first opening of the bowels afterwards. Good anaesthetic technique avoids this by blocking the pain nerves at the time of surgery.

QUESTIONS

Should I worry that I often get bleeding from piles?
It is tempting to ascribe rectal bleeding to piles. While this is safe in young people with obvious piles, older people should have further checks to exclude other causes of bleeding.

Are piles dangerous?
Theoretically there is a risk of anaemia through constant blood loss but this is very unusual unless significant bleeding is neglected.

Is there any harm in self-treatment?
If you know you have piles and if the symptoms are familiar, there is little harm. The older you are the more seriously you should take any change in the amount or pattern of bleeding or discomfort.

       Complementary Treatment
Homeopathy – paeonia ointment for external piles, or paeonia suppositories for internal piles. **Chakra balancing** aids pain control and healing; the relaxation effect eases defecation. **Aromatherapy** – try a daily sitz bath with one of the following oils (six drops): cypress, chamomile, lavender. A **nutritional therapist** would suggest boosting your fibre intake. **Ayurveda** – oral preparations are given, plus dietary advice. **Yoga** is especially helpful, together with pelvic floor exercises. *Other therapies to try: shiatsu-do.*

DIVERTICULAR DISEASE

Weakening of muscle of the walls of the large intestine, allowing the formation of small stagnant pockets.

CAUSES

This appears to be a disease of the West, almost certainly caused by a lack of fibre in the diet. The theory is that high fibre leads to bulky, soft stools, which are expelled by the colon with little effort, whereas the small hard stools of a low-fibre diet require strong muscular effort for the same result.

The walls of the large intestine contain muscle which does the propelling and churning of the faecal material, prior to defecation. Under pressure, the wall weakens and a pouch may form. It is more common in older people because the walls of the colon naturally weaken with age.

Most people over the age of 50 have a few of these pouches of just 1 cm/½ in diameter. In diverticulitis there are dozens if not hundreds. For much of the time these diverticulae are asymptomatic. They are a potentially stagnant area – if faeces lodge in them it is only a matter of time before infection occurs, when symptoms and possible complications arise.

SYMPTOMS

Few with diverticular disease have symptoms. Mild effects may be pains in the left lower abdomen of a colicky nature that come and go over a few hours, and there may be rectal bleeding. These symptoms are from mild irritation of diverticulae. If there is a serious infection, then there is much more pain plus **fever**. The lower left side of the abdomen is tender.

Considering how common the condition is complications are rare. One is peritonitis with very severe stomach pains and collapse. This only happens if one of the diverticulae has burst (perforated), allowing faeces to spill into the abdomen, and is

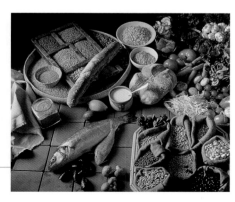

Right: High-fibre foods protect against constipation and therefore diverticular disease.

a surgical emergency. The other complication is obstruction with colicky pains, vomiting and loss of bowel action.

A barium enema shows up the diverticulae (see page 348); symptoms should also be investigated by sigmoidoscopy and colonoscopy (see page 355) as this is the same age group risk as for **bowel cancer** and the symptoms can be very similar.

TREATMENT

Mild attacks need only painkillers and an antibiotic. Once the diagnosis is established, doctors recommend a high-fibre diet and an antispasmodic such as mebeverine to relieve any occasional colicky pains. Usually nothing more is necessary. Only in patients with severe and persistent problems is it necessary to remove the diseased portion of colon – a colectomy.

In cases of sudden severe pain hospital admission may be necessary for intravenous antibiotics and to exclude obstruction or the dangerous complication of perforation and peritonitis, needing emergency surgery.

QUESTIONS

Diverticulitis/diverticular disease – what are they?
Diverticular disease means simply having multiple diverticulae, but without experiencing symptoms, the condition being discovered while investigating other abdominal symptoms such as rectal bleeding. Diverticulitis is inflammation of one of those diverticulae, giving rise to symptoms as above.

What are the risks?
It is estimated that of the 50% of over 50s who have it, only 10% will get any symptoms at all and only 1% will run into serious complications requiring surgery or intensive treatment. Asymptomatic disease is best left alone.

  Complementary Treatment
 Diet – consult a **nutritional therapist** or **naturopath**. Useful **acupuncture** points are Stomach 25, on the abdomen, and Stomach 36, below the knee. **Chinese** **herbalism** remedies include *Dang Shen* and *Bai Zhu*. If the condition is accompanied by low back pain, **chiropractic** can help. **Ayurveda** – *panchakarma* detoxification, oil laxatives and enemas are used, often with oral medicines. *Other therapies to try: chakra balancing; Western herbalism; homeopathy.*

PANCREATITIS

◆

Inflammation of the pancreatic gland, which is always serious.

CAUSES
◆

The pancreas lies behind the stomach at the back of the abdomen. It secretes insulin, which is of fundamental importance in the handling of glucose. It also secretes pancreatic enzymes into the small intestine which are important in digesting protein and fat. These are powerful juices; the seriousness of pancreatitis lies in the fact that the release of these juices leads to auto-digestion of whatever they come into contact with, for example the lining of the abdomen, the liver, the intestines and other internal organs. Pancreatitis is divided into acute and chronic.

Acute pancreatitis
Sudden inflammation of the pancreas is thought to be related to liver or gall bladder problems. This may be because the ducts through which pancreatic juices flow lie close to these structures and become blocked or irritated by bile. A few drugs can cause pancreatitis and it can be a rare consequence of viral infections including **mumps**.

Chronic pancreatitis
This is nearly always associated with alcoholic liver disease (see LIVER PROBLEMS), when the pancreatic gland becomes converted to fibrous tissue.

SYMPTOMS
◆

In the case of acute pancreatitis the illness begins with upper abdominal pain, which appears to radiate into the back. It is impossible at this stage to distinguish it from the condition of severe **indigestion** without investigations. The pain may be mild but persistent or it may be excruciating, accompanied by collapse of blood pressure and nausea, and so severe that peritonitis is suspected.

The diagnosis is very difficult to make without measuring enzymes released by the inflamed pancreas into the blood stream. The most useful one is amylase, which should be measured in all cases of severe upper abdominal pain.

Chronic pancreatitis is characterized by recurrent upper abdominal pain in a heavy drinker (see ALCOHOL AND ALCOHOLISM). As the gland deteriorates there is weight loss because the juices are no longer available to digest food. **Diabetes** develops through lack of insulin. The diagnosis is difficult to make without a CT scan (see page 350).

TREATMENT
◆

Acute pancreatitis is a very dangerous condition, with mortality at best 1%, and in severe cases 50% or higher. Treatment is with drip feeding to maintain blood pressure and energetic treatment of any internal infections, which are common. Sometimes fluid-filled cysts within the abdomen need be surgically drained. Recovery takes weeks or months.

To treat chronic pancreatitis, it is essential that the individual stops drinking alcohol to avoid further progression of the disease, although this will not reverse the damage done. Diabetes is treated with insulin, drugs or diet depending on how bad it is. Capsules are available containing the digestive enzymes no longer being produced by the pancreas. Painkillers are needed for persistent pain, which can also be helped by surgically removing diseased parts of the pancreas. The pain of chronic pancreatitis can be intense – a painkiller as strong as morphine may be required at times. The outlook is quite good as long as the individual gives up alcohol.

QUESTIONS

Is pancreatitis related to cancer of the pancreas?
There is no evidence for this; cancer of the pancreas is steadily increasing in frequency for unknown reasons, but there has been no such increase in the incidence of pancreatitis.

How risky are gallstones?
Considering how common gallstones are (see page 180) – affecting 20% of an adult population – very few actually cause pancreatitis. However, anyone with gallstones who has even mild pancreatitis would be well advised to have the gall bladder removed as soon as possible. Investigations for gallstones are routine in anyone presenting with pancreatitis.

Complementary Treatment
Acute pancreatitis is a medical emergency, and should be treated by a conventional practitioner. **Chakra balancing** helps reduce pain attacks and supports orthodox treatment; postoperatively it aids relaxation and promotes healing of wounds. **Cymatics** could help for chronic, long-term pancreatitis. You should use all means of support to give up alcohol, and **hypnotherapy** can have a role here, too. *Other therapies to try: see ALCOHOL AND ALCOHOLISM.*

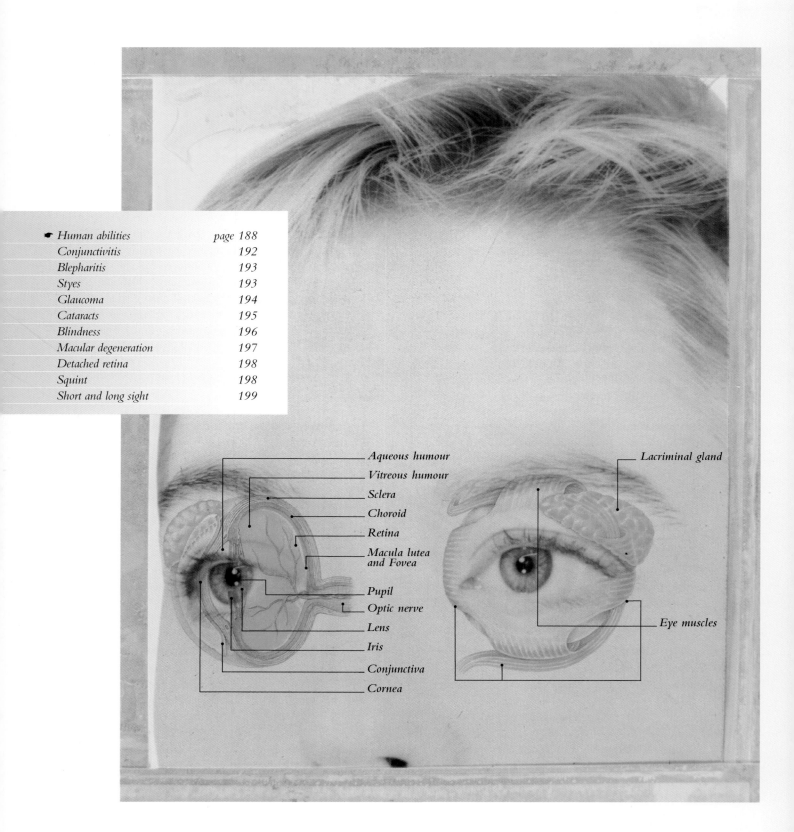

Aqueous humour

Vitreous humour

Sclera

Choroid

Retina

Macula lutea and Fovea

Pupil

Optic nerve

Lens

Iris

Conjunctiva

Cornea

Lacriminal gland

Eye muscles

The visual system is rightly seen as one of the wonders of the human body. As more is known about it, our sense of astonishment grows at its complexity. But eyes are fragile organs, subject to disorders and injuries that can cause the loss or curtailment of vision. This makes their care vital.

EYES

THE EYES ORIGINATE as outgrowths from the brain, and are specialized to detect light. Each is a fluid-filled globe of intricate design. Light enters through the transparent cornea; it strikes the lens, which focuses light on to the retina, the light-sensitive surface at the back of the eye. From there electrical signals leave via the optic nerve which goes to the brain.

The retina
Within the retina there are two types of receptor called rods and cones – this refers to their shape. Each receptor is a single cell that contains a pigment that reacts to light by firing an electrical impulse. The pigment in the rods is called rhodopsin and is derived from vitamin A.

Rods give black and white vision. Bright light reduces the amount of rhodopsin in the rods: when you go into the dark it takes 20 minutes for quantities of rhodopsin to rise to a maximum. This explains why it takes time for eyes to adapt to the dark. The fully dark-adapted eye is about 100,000 times more sensitive to light than the light-adapted eye.

Cones are responsible for colour vision and for detailed vision. It is believed that there are three types of cone, each one containing pigments that respond best to a particular colour. Colour vision is the result of the integration of the output of all three types of cone.

Each eye contains about 120 million rods and 6 million cones. The electrical output flows through nerve cells within the retina, which begin the process of analysing vision by sharpening up the output from the receptors. However, the great bulk of analysis of information takes place in the brain by processes that are still far from well understood. There are specialized collections of cells that deal with visual output all the way from where the optic nerves enter the brain to the visual cortex, which is at the back of the brain. Some centres appear to coordinate eye movements, while others seem to deal with the interpretation of images.

Other parts of the eye
The eye contains many structures other than the retina, although all structures are designed to maintain efficient vision. The cornea is crystal clear; there are no blood vessels in it. Its cells are unique because they gain their nutrition and oxygen from the fluid beneath them. The lens is a semi-liquid structure surrounded by muscles that change its shape and so alter the focus of light. The amount of light entering the eye is varied by the iris, which is another sheet of muscle; the pupils are the aperture through the iris. The surface of the eyes is bathed constantly by tears, which are antiseptic. Six muscles control the movements of each eyeball.

Eye problems
Most eye problems result from degeneration with age of the structures of the eye, especially the lens – causing **cataracts**, and the retina – causing **macular degeneration**. The increased pressure of fluid within the eye causes **glaucoma**. The eyes and eyelids are prone to infections and allergies.

Left: No computers can yet remotely match how eyes and brain interpret patterns of light.

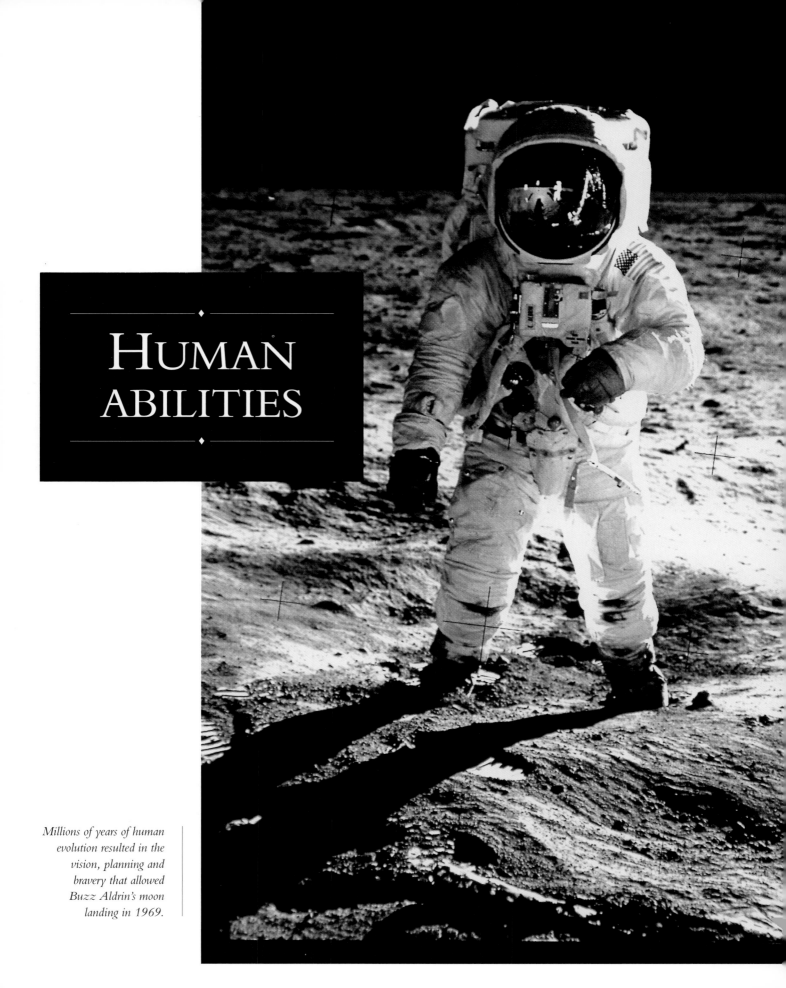

HUMAN ABILITIES

Millions of years of human evolution resulted in the vision, planning and bravery that allowed Buzz Aldrin's moon landing in 1969.

W E HUMANS ARE NOT the most distinguished when it comes to physical abilities. A rabbit can outrun us, a flea (proportional to size) can outjump us, and a monkey can out-shriek us. What we do have in our favour is exceptional brain capacity and powers of understanding. As a result we can use our intellectual abilities to outwit our would-be predators and to dominate our environment.

The senses

Vision The eye detects light with extraordinary efficiency, all the more remarkable since only 10% reaches the light-sensitive retina. The rest is lost in passage through the eye. More remarkable again, the light receptors face away from the incoming light as a quirk of the evolutionary development of the eye. In its most sensitive parts there are 150,000 colour-detecting cones per mm² of retina and 160,000 rods.

Night vision is 100,000 times more sensitive than day vision, although it lacks the capability of discerning colour and fine detail. It takes 20 minutes for the eyes to adapt fully to the dark, by which time they can detect just a few photons of light energy as a flash. The fully dilated pupil lets 32 times more light into the eye than when constricted.

The eyes can detect shifts of position with impressive accuracy – an object moving a few centimetres/inches can be seen from a distance of 1.6 km/1 mile.

The brain analyses the signals from the eyes and this is how we learn to recognize things under different conditions of light and position. So important is this that 10% of the brain is devoted to processing information from the eyes.

Our eyes produce a binocular, stereoscopic image of what we see, because when we look at something the image falls on approximately the same part of each eye. However, this reduces our field of vision. Many animals and insects have eyes that each see a different scene, giving the impression of having eyes at the back of the head – and some almost do.

The skin The skin contains nerve receptors that detect temperatures up to 45°C/113°F and down to 10°C/50°F. Pain is recorded by nerve endings scattered through the skin and internal organs, although there are none in the brain itself. Touch varies greatly over the body. On sensitive regions such as the fingertips you can distinguish between objects just 2 mm/¹/₁₆ in apart, whereas on the back of the hand they must be 50 mm/2 in apart before they are identifiable as more than one object. The fingertips can detect vibration of as little as one ten-millionth of a metre.

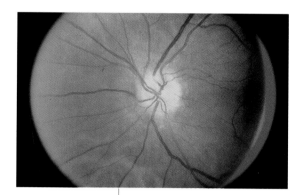

Above: The retina of the eye. Blood vessels and the optic nerve emerge from the yellowish optic cup.

Right: Optical illusions make the brain misinterpret visual information. Here, flat wavy lines give the illusion of three-dimensional depth.

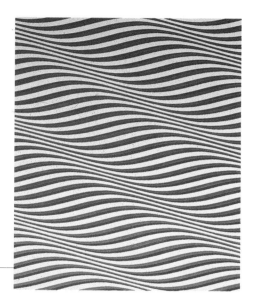

Smell and taste Specialized cells in the nose transmit straight to the brain, into a system also involved with emotions. Humans can detect up to ten thousand different smells, sometimes recognizing just one single molecule of an odour. One of the smelliest substances is mercaptan, a sulphurous compound smelling of sewage and rotting fish, which is detectable at just one part in over four hundred million parts of air.

Taste alone detects only sweet, bitter, salt and sour, relying on smell for all the subtleties. This is why you lose your sense of taste when you have a cold.

Hearing The human ear detects sounds in the range of 20–20,000 waves per second, sometimes higher. The quietest detectable sound moves the eardrum by just one-millionth of a millimetre. The trained ear can tell the difference in sounds that differ by just 0.3% in frequency (pitch) and can detect the loudness of sounds from barely audible to sounds billions of times louder. We can tell where sound comes from: by analysing the difference in the way a sound strikes both ears, we can tell the direction of sounds to within a few degrees.

Thought

A Japanese man has memorized Pi to forty thousand places, which he can recite. Others can calculate multi-digit numbers in seconds. These feats seem extraordinary, but remember that we nearly all pick up language with its complex rules and tens of thousands of words and most of us can recognize thousands of different objects instantly.

Structure Neurones are nerve cells that run from the spinal cord and brain around the body. They transmit impulses along an axon, which is like an electrical wire, to other cells. The shortest axons are under 1 mm/^{3}/$_{64}$ in, the longest over 1 m/39 in. Electrical current flows at between 1 m/3^1/$_4$ ft per second, for example in the fibres which make the pupil contract, to 100 m/328 ft per second in the knee-jerk reflex. The electrical flow depends on chemical pumps in the cell wall, which exchange electrically charged atoms – ions – of sodium and potassium. A typical neurone has a million of these pumps; nerves may fire up to 300 electrical impulses per second, the pumps exchanging 200 million ions per second.

Jumping gaps Nerves meet at junctions called synapses, or on muscles at end plates. How does electricity jump that gap? Nearly always it is by chemical transmission with minute globules of a transmitter. Some ten thousand are released with each signal down the nerve; they cross the gap in about ^{1}/$_{2000}$ of a second, setting off the electrical wave in the next fibre. Many drugs work by affecting transmitters.

The average brain weighs 1.3–1.6 kg/3–3^1/$_2$ lb. This is about 2% of total body weight, but it gets 20% of the heart's output of blood. The brain contains a hundred thousand million neurones with billions of additional supporting cells. You are born with all the neurones you will ever have. From the time of birth ten thousand a day die – two hundred and fifty million over a seventy-year lifetime. It sounds enormous, yet that still leaves you with over 99.9% of all those you began with.

The number of interconnections is beyond comprehension – about a hundred million million. It is within these interconnections that we experience emotion, thought and memory, expressed as electrical brain waves at a frequency of 4–25 cycles per second.

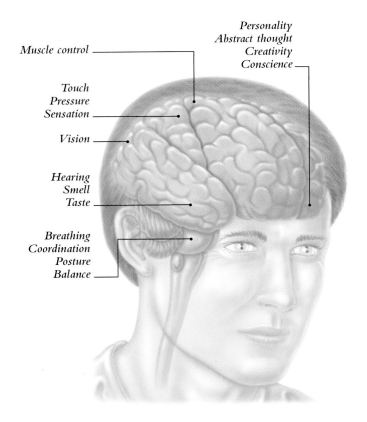

Muscle control

Touch
Pressure
Sensation

Vision

Hearing
Smell
Taste

Breathing
Coordination
Posture
Balance

Personality
Abstract thought
Creativity
Conscience

Above: A very general map of the brain showing where it handles various senses, activities and abilities.

Circulation

At rest, the heart pumps 5 litres/8 pints of blood every minute through an estimated 96,500 km/60,000 miles of blood vessels, comprising arteries, veins and capillaries. The total surface area for exchange of blood and fluid in an adult is 2600 km^2/1000 sq miles.

In each cubic millimetre of blood there are over 5 million red blood cells, thousands of white cells and 250,000–450,000 platelets for blood clotting, quite apart from a horde of biochemicals, hormones, proteins, cholesterol, fats and glucose. Every second 2.5 million new red blood cells are released from the bone marrow, replacing a similar number that are destroyed or damaged.

Per day the heart pumps 7000–8000 litres/12,300–14,000 pints, which increases greatly on exertion. Normally 20% of blood flow goes to the brain, 25% to the intestines and liver, 20% through the muscles and 4% through the heart itself. The rate of blood flow to the heart increases fivefold during exercise.

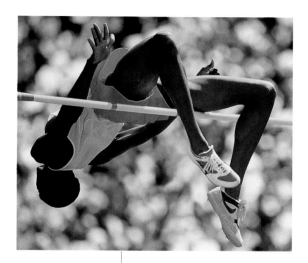

Above: A purely human feat – a demanding, unnatural target, elegantly achieved through sheer determination. Right: The competitive urge spurs us on.

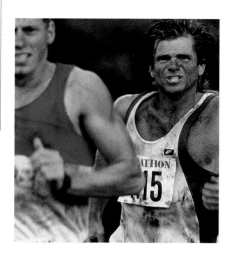

What goes in to the body and what comes out

What goes in . . .

♦ *Adults need 1200–5000 calories of energy a day, depending on the physical work they do. An average is 2000–2800 calories*

♦ *At rest you need 250 ml per minute of oxygen, obtained by breathing 6 litres per minute of air. On exertion this increases to 100–200 litres of air per minute, absorbed through 40–80 m^2/430–860 sq ft of lung surface*

♦ *Your kidneys filter the whole blood volume every 40 minutes, equivalent to filtering 180 litres/315 pints of blood a day*

♦ *You digest food with 7–9 litres/12–16 pints a day of saliva and digestive juices, passing through 4 m/13 ft of short intestine and 1.5 m/5 ft of large intestine, totalling 200 m^2/2150 sq ft of absorptive surface*

♦ *You need about 150 g/5 oz a day of carbohydrate, 80 g/3 oz of fat, 40–50 g/1½–1¾ oz of protein and minute amounts of vitamins and minerals*

♦ *You have over seven billion billion defensive cells ready to act against invading germs*

What comes out . . .

♦ *You use energy at the rate of 2–10 calories a minute. A brisk walk uses 5 calories a minute, gardening 6, aerobic dancing 6.5, jogging 10 and competitive football 15*

♦ *You expend this energy via some 600 muscles acting on some 206 bones*

♦ *You produce 1.5 litres/2¾ pints of urine a day on average but this can be varied from 23 litres/40 pints a day to just 400 ml/14 fl oz a day depending on fluid intake and loss through sweating. Your bladder can hold 700–800 ml/1¼–1½ pints of fluid. You produce 200 ml/7 fl oz of fluid a day in motions*

♦ *Other fluid is lost through the lungs and the 19,350 cm^2/ 3000 sq in of skin*

♦ *Your eye muscles move 100,000 times a day*

♦ *You have more thoughts, plans and dreams than we can possibly measure*

Exercise and muscles

During heavy exertion the heart beats harder and faster, increasing the flow of blood to 25 litres/44 pints per minute. The heart gets a fivefold increase, but blood flow to the main muscles increases by 20 times. Most of the increased output is through the heart beating faster but there is a limit to this, which decreases with age. Regular exercise increases the volume the heart can pump with each beat, which is why trained athletes can pump high volumes of blood without having very high heart rates.

Muscles Muscles comprise thousands of muscle fibres, organized into bundles that are controlled by nerve fibres.

How do muscles move? The process is very complex and not entirely certain but seems to involve the ultra-rapid formation of chemical bridges between proteins within muscle fibres that pull one strand of protein along another, so shortening the muscle fibre. This movement is triggered by the electrical activity of the nerves.

CONJUNCTIVITIS

Inflammation of the eyes as a result of an infection or allergy.

CAUSES

An inflammation of the outer surface of the eye, conjunctivitis may be bacterial, viral or allergic, or caused by a foreign body. Bacterial infections are common in children and often spread rapidly in schools and nurseries. They also occur after a foreign body – even a speck of dust – gets into the eyes. Babies often have sticky eyes after birth, having been infected via the birth canal. Viral conjunctivitis often arises in local outbreaks. It is resistant to standard antibiotics but is often self-limiting.

An allergy and an infection produce a similar appearance in the eye – the clue is the seasonal nature of the redness and its persistence. Sources of allergy are pollens, fumes and dust (see HAY FEVER).

SYMPTOMS

The eyes feel prickly and uncomfortable. Redness then spreads over the whites of the eyes as a result of the dilation of normally invisible blood vessels. The greatest redness is at the eye's margins – this pattern is important in confirming diagnosis. Redness concentrated around the iris of the eye (the coloured portion) may be due to different diseases – iritis or an ulcer on the cornea. A yellow or green discharge sticks the eyelids together, which have to be gently bathed open.

Viral conjunctivitis causes similar symptoms but lasts for weeks rather than the few days of bacterial infection. Allergic conjunctivitis leads to persistent irritation as well as redness. The eyes stream tears and the person keeps sneezing or has a persistent runny nose. In all types of conjunctivitis the under surface of the eyelids, seen by flicking down the eyelid, is red and inflamed. In allergic conjunctivitis the under surface has many small cysts that give a 'cobblestoned' appearance.

TREATMENT

Tears contain a natural antiseptic that cures most minor infections within a day or two. Where there is a lot of discharge and redness, an antibiotic is used in the form of drops or an ointment. Drops need to be used four to six times a day, ointments two to four times a day – the choice is a matter of personal preference and convenience. Drops are easier for treating children, because they are simply dripped on to the eyelids and allowed to soak through on to the eyeball. Viral conjunctivitis will not respond to antibiotic drops and will

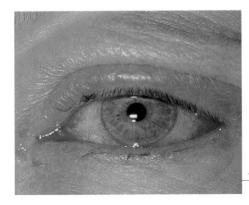

Left: In conjunctivitis, the redness gets worse further away from the iris.

take several weeks to settle down. Treatment for allergic conjunctivitis depends on its severity and the associated symptoms. Use antiallergic eye drops or ointments such as cromoglycate three to five times a day. Try an antihistamine first; it is often enough to relieve itching and redness as well as any other symptoms of hay fever. The sticky eyes in newborn babies respond to bathing with salt water or antibiotic drops; a swab should be taken first to confirm diagnosis.

WARNING SIGNS ABOUT RED EYES

Seek medical opinion if, as well as redness, the following occurs:
- *Only one eye is red*
- *The redness is concentrated around the coloured part of the eye*
- *There is blurred vision*
- *The eye feels painful, rather than itchy*
- *The redness follows any injury to the eye*
- *There is profuse watering of the eye and light irritates intensely*

Such features could indicate iritis, an ulcer of the cornea, injury of the cornea or glaucoma.

Complementary Treatment

WARNING: Never use aromatherapy oils near the eyes. **Western** and **Chinese herbalism** – anti-inflammatory herbs can supplement, not replace, orthodox treatments. **Homeopathy** – make an eyewash using a level teaspoon of salt and ten drops of euphrasia mother tincture in 300 ml/½ pint boiled, cooled water. **Nutritional therapy** – zinc supplements may help; seek advice. **Ayurveda** – try herbal eyewashes and drops. *Other therapies to try: acupuncture; chakra balancing.*

BLEPHARITIS

Inflammation at the roots of the eyelashes that spreads into the eyelids.

CAUSES

Blepharitis is caused by infections that enter the eyelids through the base of the eyelashes. It can occur at all ages and the condition can become chronic.

People who have **eczema** and dandruff may get blepharitis, because of their general skin sensitivity. Any cosmetic preparations that reach the eyelids, for example moisturizing creams, perfumes and nail varnish may cause eczematous blepharitis, but people with eczema may get blepharitis without any obvious irritant. Similarly, blepharitis can be caused by an allergic reaction to eye make-up or skin preparations. However, often the cause is obscure.

SYMPTOMS

The edges of the eyelids are swollen, red, scaly and itchy. There may be crusting of the eyelids but, unlike **conjunctivitis**, this crusting tends to spare the eyes themselves. They are rarely affected and are therefore neither red nor sticky. There may be eczema elsewhere – dry, irritant flaking skin and scalp, or dandruff. In severe cases small ulcers may develop at the root of the eyelashes and the lashes may fall out.

TREATMENT

Work antibiotic eye drops or ointments into the eyelashes. For severe infection an antibiotic is given by mouth. If the cause is eczema, it can be very hard to treat. Consider irritants that have transferred to the lids; mild steroid creams on the lids should cure the condition. If there is dandruff, the blepharitis may be helped by using an antidandruff shampoo on the scalp.

Good eyelid hygiene is important. Clean the eyelids twice daily with a cotton-wool bud and warm water to remove all crusts, especially before applying any ointment. Removing the crusts reduces the risk of reinfection.

 Complementary Treatment

WARNING: Never use aromatherapy oils near the eyes. **Homeopathy** – bathe your eyes with saline solution and lightly apply calendula ointment. *Other therapies to try: Western and Chinese herbalism; nutritional therapy; naturopathy; chakra balancing; Ayurveda.*

STYES

Infections of eyelash roots, similar to skin infections elsewhere.

CAUSES

Eyelash roots are a convenient entrance site for bacteria, as are any hair-bearing parts of the body. The bacteria proliferate into a small abscess called a stye, which people often get as a result of rubbing at their irritated eyelids.

SYMPTOMS

The base of one eyelash feels uncomfortable. In a few hours it swells into a visible abscess with a yellow head on it; the lid is often a little swollen, too.

TREATMENT

Pull out the eyelash to allow the pus to drain. Antibiotic eye drops or eye ointment help deal with the infection, as does irrigating the eye with salty water. The great majority of styes settle with this treatment within three to five days. Only very occasionally does the infection spread deeper within the eyelid, causing greater swelling. In these cases an antibiotic by mouth is required.

QUESTION

Are styes infectious?
They are only mildly infectious and much less so than conjunctivitis. Thorough and regular handwashing greatly reduces the risk of spreading the infection.

 Complementary Treatment

WARNING: Never use aromatherapy oils near the eyes. **Bach flower remedies** – try a dilution of crab apple and Rescue Remedy in water, or apply Rescue Remedy to the affected area as a cream. *Other therapies to try: homeopathy; chakra balancing; naturopathy.*

GLAUCOMA

Raised pressure of fluid within the eye that affects vision and can end in blindness. It occurs in 1% of the population.

CAUSES

There is a circulation of fluid, called aqueous humour, within the eyes, between the cornea and the lens. This fluid is continually being produced and normally drains through channels at the edge of the iris – the coloured portion of the eye. In many people this drainage system deteriorates with age, ultimately resulting in increased pressure of fluid. This is chronic glaucoma. Acute glaucoma is a type of glaucoma where the drainage is abruptly obstructed, causing sudden symptoms; fortunately acute glaucoma is rare.

Glaucoma affects vision by damaging the optic nerve where it leaves the back of the eyeball. This causes a loss of the outer (peripheral) field of vision. Unless it is treated, deterioration continues until blindness occurs.

People who use steroid eye drops for long periods of time may develop glaucoma. Some drugs, for example antidepressants and certain drugs prescribed for **Parkinson's disease,** worsen pre-existing glaucoma by widening the iris, thereby reducing drainage of fluid. There is also a strong family tendency to glaucoma.

SYMPTOMS

Early glaucoma does not produce any noticeable symptoms. Even though peripheral vision is being lost, the brain compensates as long as central vision remains good. However, at night, when pupils are dilated to a maximum, fluid drainage is reduced. People may notice haloes around lights and there may be slight discomfort in the eye.

Acute glaucoma causes dramatic symptoms – sudden blindness or extremely hazy vision, the eyeball is intensely painful and red and the normally clear cornea becomes cloudy. Increased pressure within the eyeball makes it feel very hard.

Screening

The best way to detect early glaucoma is with regular tests of the field of vision using special charts. There is a screening test where air is directed at the eyeball, depressing it briefly; pressure within the eye is calculated from the degree of depression. A more accurate measure is by applying a pressure gauge to the eyeball under local anaesthetic. Glaucoma causes characteristic appearances at the back of the eye as seen through an ophthalmoscope.

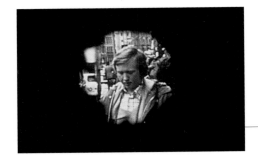

Left: Tunnel vision in advanced glaucoma. Outer vision has been lost.

TREATMENT

Chronic glaucoma is controlled with eye drops that reduce the pressure within the eye. Some drugs reduce the rate of production of the aqueous humour fluid, thereby keeping pressure low. Other drugs keep the pupil constricted and drainage at a maximum. Similar treatment is used for acute glaucoma, with higher doses and sometimes using drugs taken by mouth. When surgery is required, it involves cutting the edge of the iris with a small scalpel or laser to improve drainage.

QUESTIONS

When should people be screened?
If you have a close relative (for instance a parent or a sibling) with glaucoma you should be screened every three years from the age of forty onwards – the condition runs in families. Everyone else should see their optician for an eye check specifically for glaucoma when they reach sixty.

Can glaucoma be cured?
There is no permanent cure for glaucoma, but drugs can help to control the condition. Even after surgery you will need to see an ophthalmologist regularly.

 ### Complementary Treatment

WARNING: Never use aromatherapy oils near the eyes. Acute glaucoma is a medical emergency – see your doctor immediately. Complementary therapies provide options for long-term glaucoma. A **nutritional therapist** might recommend cutting down on protein and/or supplementing vitamins A, B_1 and C, and the minerals chromium and zinc. *Other therapies to try: homeopathy; reflexology; naturopathy; yoga.*

CATARACTS

The normally clear lens of the eye becomes opaque, causing hazy and indistinct vision. It affects 20% of people by the age of 60.

CAUSES

Light passes through the cornea, lens and fluid in the eyes with great efficiency, but eventually the clarity of the lens deteriorates. Exposure to daylight over many decades may be the main cause of the condition, probably because ultraviolet light changes the protein within the lens.

Diabetics are at greater risk of cataracts, developing them ten to fifteen years earlier than otherwise expected (see DIABETES). Those who take steroids by mouth, for example for **rheumatoid arthritis**, run a significant risk – perhaps up to 75% – of developing cataracts. They should be checked regularly by a doctor to detect cataracts early.

Injury that has penetrated to the lens will leave scarring. There are a few rare congenital or biochemical causes of cataracts that might be suspected if cataracts appear at an unusually early age.

SYMPTOMS

The effect of a cataract is similar to looking through frosted glass. Light is scattered so that the edges of objects look blurred. Bright light causes a glare and objects are indistinct unless brought very close to the eyes, and even then may be fuzzy. As well as loss of clarity there is deterioration of colour vision, which again can be reproduced by looking through frosted glass. Lesser degrees of cataract can be indicated by a non-specific change in vision and difficulties with close work. Changing the prescription of glasses makes no difference.

Cataracts seen through an ophthalmoscope appear as a white opacity to the bright light. The usual tests of visual acuity will show how much vision has been affected in order to judge how urgently surgery might be required.

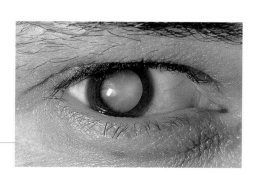

Right: An advanced cataract. The lens is hazy and white, vision is greatly reduced.

TREATMENT

Cataract surgery is a highly developed and delicate branch of ophthalmology that can, in most cases, restore good vision. Surgery involves removing the opaque lens, usually by very fine dissection, from its attachments. Increasingly, surgeons do this by a technique that liquefies the lens so it can be sucked out, causing less disruption to surrounding structures. An artificial lens is replaced within the capsule that contained the natural lens (a lens implant).

Unlike the natural lens, which can of course vary focus, the replacement lens is a fixed focus. Therefore you may need glasses in order to deal with distant or close vision, but you will notice that your overall vision will be restored to its normal clarity and normal colour.

Cataract surgery is a relatively safe procedure that is usually done under local anaesthetic. Any surgery carries a risk of infection or bleeding. For this reason, if you have cataracts in both eyes, surgeons will normally defer dealing with the second eye until after full recovery from the first operation.

QUESTIONS

What are 'ripe cataracts'?
This was a term that meant cataracts bad enough to justify surgery and the heavy cataract glasses that were inevitably necessary following surgery.

Will I need thick-lensed glasses?
These date from when cataract surgery removed the lens and did not replace it. Therefore the only way to achieve focusing was by using very thick lenses. Thanks to lens implants, these type of glasses are now rarely required.

Complementary Treatment

WARNING: Never use aromatherapy oils near the eyes. Eye surgery is the only effective treatment for cataracts, although complementary therapies do play a supportive role. **Chakra balancing** – there is evidence that cataracts may become less opaque for a few days following treatment but this is not yet proven. **Nutritional therapy** – boosting the intake of antioxidant vitamins (A, C and E) can aid prevention. **Yoga** and **massage** are both therapies that are beneficial postoperatively. *Other therapies to try: see STRESS.*

BLINDNESS

While some loss of vision is fairly common, complete loss of vision is relatively unusual.

CAUSES

Blindness can result from disease anywhere along the visual pathways from the eyes to the brain. Causes therefore include not only diseases of the eyes but brain disorders as well.

Retinal damage

Most blindness in the developed world results from damage to the retina, which is the light-receiving surface at the back of the eye. This is a densely packed structure where specialized light receptors – the rods and cones – react to light. Much of the initial processing of information takes place in complex nerve interconnections within the retina that begin the recognition of shape, movement and position. The retina needs a good blood supply to function, and interference with it underlies much acquired blindness.

The major causes of blindness are **glaucoma**, diabetic eye disease (see DIABETES) and **macular degeneration**. These all affect blood supply to the critical receptors through disease of the blood vessels.

Trauma

Direct injury to the eye will cause blindness if it damages the lens or destroys the eyeball. This includes **detached retina**.

Brain disease

The information from the eyes reaches the brain through the optic nerve and is finally analysed in specialized regions of the brain. A **stroke** may damage some of those fibres. This is unlikely to produce total blindness but it can destroy part of the field of vision. A tumour of the pituitary gland also causes gradual loss of part of the field of vision.

Other causes

Other important causes are parasite infection of the eye and deficiency of vitamin A, required to make the visual receptors.

SYMPTOMS

Abrupt blindness is immediately recognized but a slower onset blindness can be easily overlooked. This is especially true if only one eye is affected because the brain compensates. This happens with glaucoma, diabetic eye disease and also a slow-growing **brain tumour**.

Blindness after a stroke typically affects only part of the field of vision – one-half or one-quarter – and this too can be overlooked unless specifically tested for. This is done by measuring the whole field of vision with special charts.

The reflexes of the pupils of the eye and the appearance of the back of the eye viewed through an ophthalmoscope give some clue as to the likely cause of blindness.

TREATMENT

Emergency treatment may help when the cause is a detached retina or blockage of blood flow to the retina. Blindness as a result of strokes in the brain cannot be treated but there is a high probability of improvement with time and as the brain compensates. The treatment of trauma, brain tumours and parasitic infections varies from case to case. Early treatment is essential for glaucoma and diabetic eye changes to reduce the risk of deteriorating vision.

QUESTIONS

How common is blindness?
In the United Kingdom about 140,000 people are registered totally blind; many more are registered as severely visually impaired. Such individuals can often cope well if they are given input from specialized advisers. Similar percentages of blindness apply elsewhere in the developed world.

When can temporary blindness occur?
Migraine can cause loss of vision, usually in one eye, accompanied by headache and nausea. Vision returns after an hour or two. Sudden painless loss of vision that recovers within hours is almost certainly due to a stroke. Since this may herald a larger stroke, it is important to have an urgent medical assessment.

Complementary Treatment

WARNING: Never use aromatherapy oils near the eyes. No specific therapy is recommended as treatment, but some can ease the stress associated with increasing blindness and help you come to terms with your deteriorating vision – **aromatherapy massage** to the body can be beneficial in promoting positive acceptance; **arts therapies**, **chakra balancing**, **healing** and **hypnotherapy** also have a role here. *Other therapies to try: see STRESS.*

MACULAR DEGENERATION

Progressively poor vision due to disease of the fovea, the most light-sensitive part of the retina.

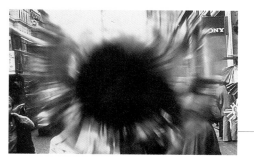

Left: Macular degeneration affects central vision but peripheral vision remains normal.

CAUSES

The whole of the retina is a light-sensing surface, the most sensitive part of which is the fovea. This is a tiny pit in the retina, which is surrounded by a reddish area called the macula. Macular degeneration is caused by disease of the fovea and the surrounding macula.

Within each fovea there are only about 4,000 cones, but each one is individually wired into the optic nerve. This makes the fovea the area of the most precise vision and with the highest visual acuity. Paradoxically, this part of the eye is the least sensitive to light and needs bright light to work properly.

So important is the fovea that it has its own dedicated blood supply. Age is the usual reason for the blood supply to degenerate, through leakages or blockages. This leads to the death of a number of cones which are irreplaceable. Age-related macular degeneration may run in families.

Conditions that weaken blood vessels increase the risk of macular degeneration. The most common one is **diabetes**, the other is **high blood pressure**.

SYMPTOMS

There is usually a gradual loss of visual acuity – the sharpness and clarity of vision. This cannot be corrected by new prescription glasses, because the problem is not one of focusing light but rather of the light receptor itself.

Vision outside the macula is unaffected so you can still walk along a crowded street or take in a whole visual scene. Awareness of movement at the corner of the eye also remains efficient because this does not rely on the macula. However, as soon as you try to focus on something there is difficulty, because you are focusing light on to the macula.

A way of demonstrating retinal changes is with fluorescein angiography, where fluorescent dye is injected into a vein and photographed passing through the retina. Blood vessels show up as bright strands and the circulation around the macula is visible. (Leaking vessels can be treated by laser – see below.)

TREATMENT

There has been recent progress in transplanting blood vessels to improve blood flow to the macula; this is still experimental. Efforts still have to be directed instead at preventing poor

blood flow in the first place. As there are no warning signs with macular degeneration, it is vital for diabetics to have annual eye checks to see whether diseased blood vessels are encroaching on the macula. If this is so, it can be arrested with laser treatment. This entails placing a precise burn directly on to the diseased blood vessel that is threatening the macula. People with macular degeneration should have treatment for any high blood pressure and also stop smoking, since both of these increase the risks of progression of the condition.

QUESTIONS

I have been diagnosed with macular degeneration; will it make me blind?
Rest assured that this will not happen, because you will still retain all the rest of the retina outside the fovea. However, you will find that you will have problems in fine work and in reading.

How can I best cope with this condition?
It is important to have good light for reading and also magnifying devices. Over time you will learn how to look at things slightly off centre so that the image is focused off the macula and on to a part of the retina which still has efficient vision.

Complementary Treatment

WARNING: Never use aromatherapy oils near the eyes, although **aromatherapy massage** to the body can be beneficial. You must follow the advice and treatment programme put forward by your orthodox practitioners. Complementary therapies have a supportive role. **Hellerwork** relaxes the facial muscles and helps to reduce eyestrain. **Chakra balancing** has a deep relaxation effect and rebalances energy. *Other therapies to try: see* STRESS.

DETACHED RETINA

Occurs when the retina loses its adherence to the back of the eye.

CAUSES

The retina – the light-sensitive inner layer – rests on the back of the eye and is mainly held in place by the pressure of fluid in the eye. The usual reason for detachment is a hole in the retina through which the fluid of the eye enters and forces the retina off the back of the eye. Short-sighted people are at greater risk of holes, because their retina is thinner.

A sudden blow to the head could also detach the retina and it is a recognized hazard of bungee jumping and boxing.

SYMPTOMS

When the retina becomes detached, you see flashing lights as it tears away from the eyeball. People talk of a curtain falling across part of their field of vision; the remaining vision is distorted because of ripples in the retina. Detachment is often preceded by an increased numbers of 'floaters', those otherwise innocent objects that drift across the field of vision and are in fact cells shed into the fluid of the eye.

TREATMENT

A detached retina is a surgical emergency: the retina will need to be repositioned on the back of the eye by an operation. Early treatment has a high chance of success.

QUESTION

How quickly should a detached retina be dealt with?
Unless reattached within hours, the detached part of the retina will suffer irreversible damage from lack of blood supply. Therefore seek an urgent opinion if you experience flashing lights or sudden distortion of vision. The unaffected eye will need careful assessment, as there is an increased risk of detachment on this side as well.

Complementary Treatment

Seek immediate orthodox treatment. Complementary treatment is not appropriate for a detached retina but post-operatively any stress-reducing therapy could help you to overcome the trauma.

SQUINT

Imbalance of the muscles that move the eyeballs, leading to misalignment. The condition runs in families.

CAUSES

Each eye is moved by six muscles that swivel it in all directions. Squint happens if, through an imbalance of muscles, one eye fails to move precisely in line with the other. The other main cause of squint is poor vision in one eye as the brain will tend to favour the better focused eye.

Temporary squints are normal in newborn babies but after three months they should be taken seriously, as should a newly appearing squint which may signal brain or eye disease.

SYMPTOMS

One eye turns in or out more than the other and does not move in coordination with the other. Double vision is rare.

Gross squints are obvious, but minor squints are difficult to quantify without specialist assessment.

TREATMENT

Children do not grow out of a squint, and if the condition is left untreated, the vision will be permanently affected.

If the cause is poor vision, the good eye is patched (covered over) and glasses are worn to correct the weaker eye. Patching forces the brain to accept signals from the poorer eye and to learn to control its muscles better. If the cause of squint is muscle imbalance, this can be corrected by surgically shortening or lengthening the muscles responsible.

Squints occurring in adults will need to be investigated for a brain disorder. Any double vision will require special glasses or surgery.

Complementary Treatment

WARNING: Never use aromatherapy oils near the eyes. **Hellerwork** will help to relax the facial muscles and reduce eyestrain. There is some evidence of the power of traditional Chinese medicine but more research needs to be done in this area.

SHORT AND LONG SIGHT

Variations in the shape of the eyeball are the cause of these extremely common problems.

CAUSES

The eyeball is a slightly elongated globe, the size of which should match the focusing power of the lens. Ideally the lens of the eye will focus light precisely on the retina, regardless of the distance of the object being looked at. It does this by using muscles that alter the thickness of the lens and therefore its focusing power.

In the case of long sight the eyeball is slightly too short. Despite maximum power the lens cannot focus objects on the retina; the point of focus actually lies behind the eyeball.

Short sight, or myopia, is where the eyeball is too long, so that light is focused in front of the retina except when objects are held very close to the eye. In both cases the lens mechanism of the eye tries to compensate as best as possible.

The focusing ability of the eye changes over time, as the lens becomes less elastic. This is illustrated by measuring the near point of vision: the closest position on which the eye can focus. At age eight this is about 8 cm/3 in, by age twenty this is 10 cm/4 in, and by age sixty, 83 cm/33 in. This is why children can read with the book pressed up to their face while their parents, anxious to know if this is normal, have to consult their book of child development at arm's length!

SYMPTOMS

The vision is blurred looking either at distant or close objects (myopia or long sight respectively). There may be discomfort in the eyes as well as headaches, through overwork of the muscles in the eye that are trying to pull the lens into the best shape for focusing.

In children, a **squint** may be the first clue to poor vision, whether through long or short sight.

Eye charts will define the precise degree of the problem.

TREATMENT

Glasses and contact lenses are still the most widely used and tested methods for dealing with poor vision. The artificial lens is shaped to bend light enough to compensate for the visual problem, bringing the image to focus precisely on the retina. Treatment is especially important in children in order to avoid the brain disregarding the information from a poorly focusing eye. Rapid changes in vision also need investigation.

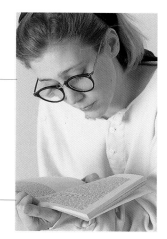

Right: Glasses can effectively compensate for changes in the focusing ability of the eyes.

Photo-refractive keratectomy

This is a new surgical technique to correct short sight. It works almost immediately and is increasing in popularity. A laser is used to shave a wafer-thin disk off the cornea and effectively shorten the eye and improve its focussing ability. It is a novel and promising technique that offers an alternative to wearing glasses or contact lenses.

QUESTIONS

Does a lot of studying weaken the eyes?
This is a controversial question. In surveys, children who are of above-average intelligence tend to be short sighted more often than others. This observation has not been explained. It is thought unlikely that their eyes have become weakened by studying.

How safe is photo-refractive keratectomy?
In skilled hands the technique has a good success rate for mild short sight. The risks are infection, subsequently finding bright light dazzling and failure to provide sufficient correction and in any case it will not obviate the need for reading glasses as people grow older. The technique will probably become more widely used as the laser technology improves and its long-term safety is well established.

Complementary Treatment

WARNING: Never use aromatherapy oils near the eyes. The **Alexander Technique** teaches you to unlearn habits of overstraining, which can have a beneficial effect on the neck and facial muscles, helping reduce problems associated with eyestrain. With **autogenic training** improved short sight has been reported, but more research is needed. **Hellerwork** relaxes the facial muscles and reduces eyestrain. *Other therapies to try: rolfing; naturopathy; nutritional therapy.*

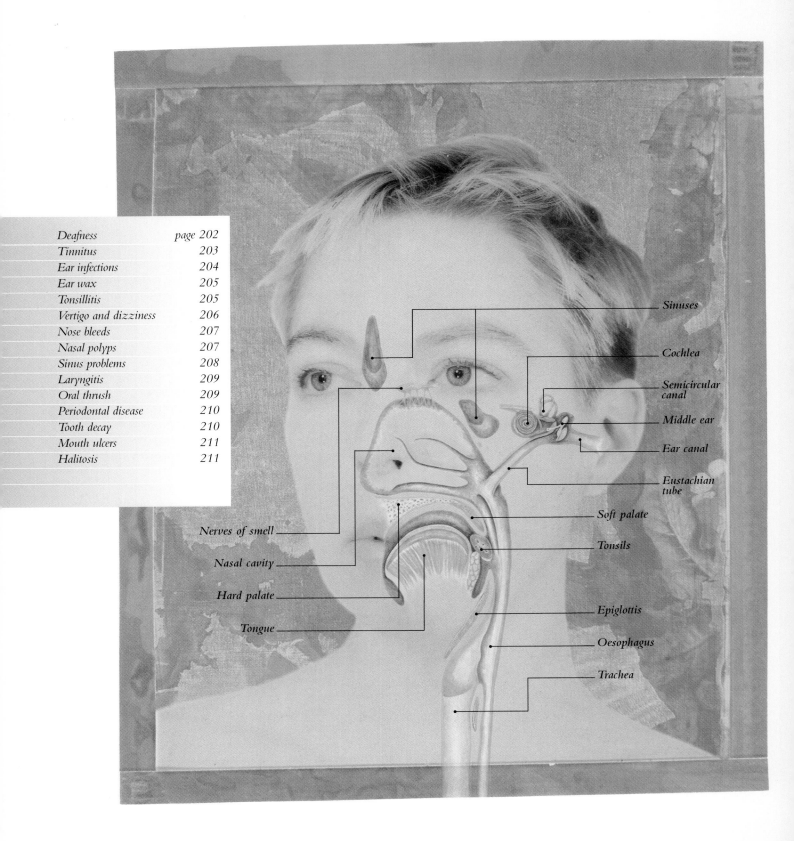

Sinuses

Cochlea

Semicircular canal

Middle ear

Ear canal

Eustachian tube

Soft palate

Tonsils

Epiglottis

Oesophagus

Trachea

Nerves of smell

Nasal cavity

Hard palate

Tongue

Shared embryonic development and shared connections mean that problems in one of these structures frequently affect the others. Hence ENT (ear, nose and throat) specialists deal with all three areas.

EAR, NOSE AND THROAT

THESE STRUCTURES ARE GROUPED together because they are so closely interconnected that diseases in one part often influence other parts – for example, nasal congestion leading to ear infection. The most common ENT problems are those to which all hollow organs are liable – namely infections and blockage. The following pages concentrate on infections of these structures, rather than malformations or cancers.

The ears

These miracles of micro-engineering turn sound waves into nerve impulses for interpretation by the brain. Sound waves make the eardrum vibrate. A tiny bone, the stapes, lies against the eardrum and moves as the drum vibrates. Through a series of joints with two other bones those vibrations are amplified and finally applied to the inner ear, the cochlea, a bony organ that looks like a snail shell.

The cochlea is filled with fluid that picks up the amplified vibrations. What happens next is complicated and still not completely understood. The cochlea has a lining of specialized nerve tissue covered in hairs, called the organ of Corti. Sounds of different frequency set up waves in the fluid which bend the hairs at different sites of the organ of Corti; the site stimulated is interpreted by the brain as pitch. The degree of bending of the hairs is interpreted as loudness. The electrical output goes to the brain for this sophisticated analysis.

Close to the cochlea are the semi-circular canals, three more fluid-filled structures and, oddly, a number of tiny crystals.

Head movements cause movements of the fluid and crystals to be sensed by yet more specialized cells and turned into nerve impulses. These are interpreted to give us our sense of position and direction of movement.

The nose

Inhaled air passes over the blood-rich lining of the nose, which warms it and extracts odours for the sense of smell. Tiny hairs in the nose trap larger dust particles, while other particles are absorbed on to the moist surface of the back of the nose and throat. The sense of smell is provided by cells in the roof of the nose which respond to just a few molecules in the air. The resulting nerve impulses go straight to a part of the brain also involved with mood and emotion for analysis, which explains why smells can have such an evocative or disturbing effect.

The throat

Here channels from the mouth, nose and sinuses meet before dividing up into the trachea leading to the lungs, and the gullet going to the stomach. Some slick muscular coordination takes place during swallowing to keep airways and food intake separate: food in the lungs is dangerous. Being a first port of call for bacteria and viruses, the throat is not surprisingly the place where many infections begin.

Speech is produced as exhaled air makes the vocal cords vibrate and is given power and resonance by the shape of the nose, throat, mouth and sinuses.

Left: These related structures handle hearing, balance, breathing, speech and swallowing, via amazingly clever muscle and brain control.

DEAFNESS

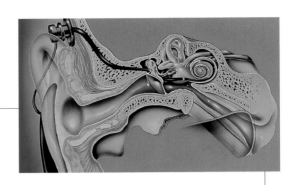

Above: A cochlear implant, showing the microphone and wiring going to the cochlea.

Loss of hearing through natural decline or disease.

CAUSES

Hearing, like other systems, is subject to deterioration with age. Hearing relies on the conversion of sound into electrical impulses. Sound waves cause minute movements of the eardrum, amplified by a chain of bones (the ossicles) which transmit movements to the cochlea. Deafness from problems with the ossicles or eardrum is called conductive. The cochlea turns sounds into nerve impulses; diseases from this region onward cause sensori-neural deafness.

Conductive deafness
In otosclerosis, joints between the ossicles stiffen with age. The eardrum and bones may be damaged by severe infection or trauma. Accumulated **ear wax**, middle ear infections and glue ear (see EAR INFECTIONS) decrease hearing temporarily.

Sensori-neural deafness
The most common cause is presbyacusis, the hearing loss from ageing, due to the degeneration of nerves within the cochlea. An accelerated form of this is from acoustic trauma – constant exposure to loud noises. Ménières disease is a disorder of blood flow to the ear associated with **tinnitus**. Several drugs affect the nerves of hearing, for example gentamicin. Tumours of the auditory nerve are uncommon. Some children are born deaf as a result of malformation of the inner ear. **Rubella** is one cause, although unusual. At any age infection can destroy the nerve pathways, for example **mumps**, **shingles** and meningitis (see BACTERIAL and VIRAL MENINGITIS).

SYMPTOMS

Within a few weeks of birth a child should be startled by sudden loud noises and by three to four months he should turn to interesting sounds. Children should be babbling by about nine months and saying a few words by one year. If these milestones are not met or if the child's speech starts to deteriorate, immediate investigation is needed. Modern techniques can confirm hearing problems in babies as young as three to six months, especially if their hearing might be at risk from premature birth. Immediate investigation is needed so that the child can begin a programme to acquire skills. Older children can say if their hearing is indistinct. Certain children are at high risk of hearing difficulties and should be screened, for example following an illness such as meningitis.

In adults sudden hearing loss is obvious. A more gradual loss, for example presbyacusis, is easily overlooked and is as likely to be picked up by others as by yourself. Presbyacusis reduces sensitivity for high tones, the ones important in conversation and telephone listening. Deafness that is associated with pain or discharge should never be ignored.

TREATMENT

Conductive deafness is more likely to be treatable than sensori-neural deafness. With the former there are operations to replace diseased ossicles, repair the eardrum and remove fluid from within the ear caused by infections.

Sensori-neural deafness is treated with hearing aids (both behind-the-ear and within-the-ear devices) that amplify sound. However, these are limited by the efficiency of the remaining nerve pathways, which cannot be repaired. Cochlear implants (see page 362) may help to overcome this.

QUESTIONS

When should a deaf child be treated?
The sooner the child gets into a deafness programme, the better it is for language acquisition, performance and social skills.

What is a cochlear implant?
A microphone leading to electrodes implanted in the cochlea, stimulates the nerves directly. These ever-more sophisticated devices are becoming standard treatment for the totally deaf.

 Complementary Treatment
Always seek orthodox medical advice for any kind of deafness. **Hellerwork** can help improve hearing although results, as with other therapies, depend on the level of deafness; it cannot restore hearing to someone who is profoundly deaf. *Other therapies to try: auricular therapy; reflexology; osteopathy.*

TINNITUS

◆

Ringing in the ears — a common problem and difficult to treat.

CAUSES

◆

Tinnitus appears to be somewhat similar to the feedback noises of other types of amplification system. It can accompany any other ear disorders, such as presbyacusis – the deterioration of hearing with age. Other common associations are with otosclerosis, where the chain of bones transmitting sounds gets stiff. Tinnitus after noise trauma is common – think of the ringing in your ears after some loud noise such as an explosion or a pop concert, which may take a day to disappear. Ringing in the ears can become permanent in people constantly exposed to noise, for example gunnery officers.

Ménières disease

This poorly understood disease, thought to come from deterioration of blood flow to the ear, causes **deafness** together with tinnitus and vertigo (see VERTIGO AND DIZZINESS).

Other causes

Drugs can cause tinnitus, the most common being aspirin and alcohol. Even **ear wax** and **ear infections** may also provoke it.

SYMPTOMS

◆

Ringing affects both ears, one usually more than another. It is frequently a high-pitched ringing noise that varies in intensity but rarely disappears. People with severe tinnitus often get depressed for understandable reasons. Tinnitus plus deafness and vertigo suggest Ménières disease. Tinnitus affecting only one ear is uncommon and may be a feature of disease of the nerve in that ear, especially if accompanied by deafness.

There are no objective ways to measure tinnitus; doctors must rely on what the patient reports.

TREATMENT

◆

It is worthwhile removing ear wax and any other source of irritation within the ear. Hearing tests can be done and will determine whether the tinnitus is a consequence of conductive deafness or of sensori-neural deafness. Treating deafness with a hearing aid may relieve the tinnitus.

One-sided tinnitus should be investigated for the rare cases caused by a tumour on the nerve of hearing, called an acoustic neuroma. This search, once extremely difficult, is now straightforward with a brain scan.

After investigation there will remain many people for whom no definite cause can be found and for whom treatment is unlikely to be curative. Nevertheless, there are a number of ways in which people with tinnitus can be helped.

In people who suffer **high blood pressure** this should be treated. It is worth trying a number of drugs that reduce pressure within the ear, such as betahistine and cinnarizine; however, these drugs do not work for everyone.

If a hearing aid has not helped, then a masking device might be able to. This looks like a hearing aid and is worn behind the ear. It generates white noise, which is noise that has neither pattern nor content. The idea behind this is to find a pitch and loudness that will cancel out the tinnitus. It may seem odd to attack one noise with another, but it is a form of treatment that does work.

Finally, a few very unfortunate people, usually with Ménières disease, have so much upset from tinnitus and vertigo that they are willing to have the hearing nerve destroyed on that side; this is a drastic, very carefully considered last resort that is rarely needed.

QUESTIONS

What should I do if I hear other constant noises?
Various sounds bear medical consideration if the noise heard is unusual. For example, a rushing noise may be transmitted from the carotid arteries in the neck or from a heart murmur.

Are antidepressants helpful if you have tinnitus?
Depression often accompanies severe tinnitus, for obvious reasons. Treatment helps reduce the mental burden of the constant noise, but people should also consider self-help organizations.

Complementary Treatment

Auricular therapy treatment can be effective at weekly intervals, but once it stops the symptoms may return. **Nutritional therapy** might suggest supplementing B vitamins, magnesium, manganese and potassium, and essential fatty acids. **Chiropractic** – treating the neck using manipulation and soft tissue massage cannot clear tinnitus, but it can help to make your life more bearable. **Hypnotherapy** has worked when all other methods have failed: you learn to turn down, and turn off, the ringing. *Other therapies to try: tai chi/chi kung; healing; acupuncture; chakra balancing.*

EAR INFECTIONS

These comprise internal infections and external skin complaints.

CAUSES

Although ear infections are a common childhood problem, treatment is still controversial. Adults are less frequently subject to infection, but commonly suffer **eczema** of the outer ear.

Middle ear infections (otitis media)

The inner ear communicates to the outside world via the Eustachian tube, a channel that ends at the back of the throat. Each time you swallow this tube opens, allowing air to enter or leave the inner ear. A child's narrow tube predisposes to the stagnation of secretion and infections of the eardrum.

Outer ear infections (otitis externa)

The outer ear skin can suffer from eczema, boils (see BOILS, SPOTS AND ABCESSES) and **fungal infections**. Over-vigorous cleaning of the ear with cotton-wool buds increases the chances of infection by scratching the skin of the canal.

SYMPTOMS

With middle ear infection, pain is the prime symptom, typically in a child who has a cold. It begins abruptly and is very distressing, and is due to the pressure of fluid within the middle ear. A severe infection may lead to rupture of the eardrum, with discharge of pus and blood but also relief of pain.

With outer ear infections there is itching and a watery discharge; scaling may spread from the ear canal on to the ear. A boil in the canal is painful out of all proportion to its tiny size.

TREATMENT

Treatment for middle ear infections ranges from painkillers and time to an appropriate antibiotic. If the eardrum has burst, letting out pus, a follow-up check-up is necessary to ensure that the eardrum perforation has healed up. This should take a few weeks. In the rare cases of failure to heal an operation may be needed to put a graft in place.

Many children experience infections every few weeks during childhood. As long as each infection resolves entirely it is best to wait for the child to outgrow these naturally as the air passages of the ears and nose enlarge. However, some children are so much affected that they merit having their adenoids (glands at the back of the nose that can obstruct the air passages of the ears) removed and grommets inserted in their

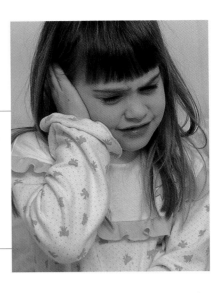

Right: Children with distressing earache should have painkillers sooner than antibiotics.

eardrums. Some children have persistent mucus within the ears, termed a glue ear, which reduces hearing. If it persists for several months, involves both ears and causes significant hearing loss then most ENT surgeons would once again perform an adenoidectomy and insert grommets.

With outer ear infections it can be difficult getting the medication to where it is needed. Medicated drops containing an antibiotic and an antifungal settle most minor infections or eczema. Any but the most minor infections need an antibiotic by mouth, especially boils in the canal. Chronic infections or eczema need specialized ENT treatment to remove debris from the ear canal and to pack it with antiseptic gauze.

QUESTIONS

Can acute ear infections be avoided?

These are more common where the parents smoke, although the precise relationship is uncertain. While courses of antibiotics or decongestants are often prescribed, they may have little value.

What are grommets?

These are tiny tubes placed in the eardrum to let air into the middle ear and to let secretions out. Although ENT surgeons tend to disagree on the use of grommets, there is agreement on their value in selected cases of chronic ear disease.

Complementary Treatment

Chinese and **Western herbalism** can be very effective in helping the body fight infections: seek professional advice for specific remedies. **Homeopathy** can be extremely effective but treatment depends on what brings the problem on, how it presents, what makes it better or worse and so on. **Chakra balancing** can help with pain control and healing. *Other therapies to try: naturopathy; acupuncture.*

EAR WAX

Discharge of wax is normal, but sometimes causes difficulties.

CAUSES

Glands within the ear canal continuously secrete wax, which keeps the eardrum supple. Wax is swept towards the ear opening where its bitter taste repels insects and traps any that get into the ear. Some people produce more wax than others. In dusty or dry conditions it may become hard and accumulate.

SYMPTOMS

Wax may be to blame if hearing becomes muffled or if, after a shower or swimming, the ear feels blocked, due to water trapped behind wax. Nearby wax melted by the warmth of **ear infections** can be mistaken for an infected discharge.

TREATMENT

Wax should only be treated if it is causing a problem, for example muffled hearing. Avoid removing wax with cotton-wool buds, which can push wax into a firm plug over the eardrum and make hearing worse. Buds often scratch the ear canal and introduce infection, leading to chronic irritation or **eczema**. Wax softens in warm water; letting water into the ears when washing may keep levels down. There are many eardrops that dissolve it. Syringing should be a last resort.

QUESTION

Does wax cause pain?
This is unlikely; more often pain signifies an infection of the eardrum or in the ear canal. Doctors avoid syringing a painful ear, even if there is a clear plug of wax, until antibiotics have settled any infection. Similarly they will not syringe a discharging ear.

 Complementary Treatment
Auricular therapy – needling the ear to treat any condition will often produce sensations of warmth and increase local blood circulation; treatment focused specifically on the ear can lead to improvements. *Other therapies to try: reflexology.*

TONSILLITIS

An infection of the tonsils, which can be very painful.

CAUSES

The tonsils and adenoids are part of a ring of specialized tissues surrounding the throat and nasal passages, that trap infection before it gets further into the lungs or gullet. The frequent sore throats of childhood are this system mopping up germs. Sometimes this leads to severe inflammation of the tonsils. In teenagers, **glandular fever** is a common cause of tonsillitis; generally, sore throats are caused by viruses, but full-blown tonsillitis may be the result of bacterial infection.

SYMPTOMS

A mild sore throat rapidly becomes severely painful, with the feeling of a lump in the throat and difficulty swallowing. Often pain is felt in the ears and breath smells bad (see HALITOSIS). White spots or a white slough are all over the tonsils, but appearances do not always correlate with the severity.

TREATMENT

If the cause is a bacterial infection treatment is with penicillin. Painkillers and throat sweets give relief. For a run of bad throats or an unusually inflamed one a blood test could exclude glandular fever or a blood disorder.

QUESTION

When is removal of tonsils advisable?
If you have more than six attacks of tonsillitis a year with severe symptoms and are losing time from school or work.

 Complementary Treatment
Aromatherapy – try a gargle of sage, myrrh or thyme (two drops in half a glass of water). *Other therapies to try: naturopathy; nutritional therapy; Western and Chinese herbalism; acupuncture; homeopathy; healing.*

VERTIGO AND DIZZINESS

Sensations most commonly experienced by older people.

CAUSES

True vertigo means a sensation of spinning. Dizziness is a much vaguer term, which includes light-headedness and feeling faint. There are many possible causes but experience shows that the great majority result from a few conditions which, although inconvenient, are not dangerous.

A viral infection, labyrinthitis, causes abrupt vertigo with nausea. Similarly, vertigo may accompany an ear infection or congestion of the ear. Deterioration of blood flow to the ears is believed to account for many cases of vertigo. An acute **stroke** may cause vertigo and unsteadiness, along with other symptoms. The long list of less likely causes of vertigo includes drugs affecting the ear, tumours on the auditory nerve and neurological disease.

Osteoarthritis of the neck, universal in older people, can squeeze the major arteries to the brain in certain neck positions and the resulting fall in blood flow causes dizziness. In many older people postural hypotension (see below) results in light-headedness. Vague dizziness is a frequent complaint of people under **stress** or with **depression**.

SYMPTOMS

The pattern of symptoms is the best clue to the likely cause. Most diagnoses can be made after assessing the patient's ears, blood pressure, heart sounds, neck and limb movements and psychological status. Brain scan and specialized tests of the organs of balance within the ear are available for puzzling disabling vertigo or dizziness but are of little help in diagnosing most acute cases. Acute vertigo with nausea and no ear inflammation is probably viral in origin. Acute vertigo with slurred speech or limb weakness may be a result of stroke or brain disease. Osteoarthritis of the neck can cause dizziness when looking up, which goes on looking level again. Light-headedness on standing, with a measurable drop in blood pressure, suggests postural hypotension or anaemia. Vertigo plus **tinnitus** and **deafness** is the triad of Ménières disease.

TREATMENT

Medication to relieve the giddiness and nausea of an acute attack of vertigo includes prochlorperazine and domperidone. These drugs are available as tablet, injection or by pellet that dissolves in the mouth. Treatment continues for as long as

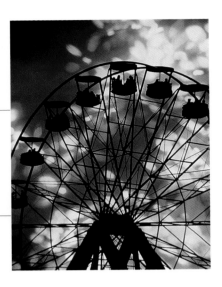

Right: Providing the thrill of vertigo is the basis of a section of the leisure industry.

necessary, but most acute vertigo passes after a week or two.

The problems associated with postural hypotension and osteoarthritis of the neck are difficult to treat effectively. Strategies include learning to stand up slowly and to wait a few seconds for blood pressure to adjust, wearing support stockings to keep blood pressure up when standing and having adjusted any medication for **high blood pressure**, which may be contributing to the problem. People with osteoarthritis of the neck need to learn to avoid sudden neck movements.

Psychological causes may respond to counselling or anti-depressants.

QUESTIONS

Why is it so important to differentiate between the terms 'vertigo' and 'light-headedness'?
It is necessary for the doctor to first work out what a patient mean by these terms in order to avoid diagnostic blind alleys for what may simply be a problem of stress or tension.

Is low blood pressure bad?
British and American doctors consider it a good thing unless it causes dizziness. European doctors blame it for widespread ill health and treat it. There is no common ground on this intriguing cultural difference.

Complementary Treatment
See your doctor if you have recurrent vertigo. **Chiropractic** may help since vertigo can be aggravated by neck stiffness and muscle spasm. Vertigo responds particularly well to **hypnotherapy** regression and suggestion therapy. **Western herbalism** – ginkgo may help dizziness caused by poor blood flow to the brain. *Other therapies to try: tai chi/chi kung; acupuncture; homeopathy; cymatics.*

Nose bleeds

A common occurrence, which only rarely has a serious cause.

CAUSES

Several arteries run very close to the surface near the front of the nose and bleed readily if irritated through inflammation or trauma – typically when having a cold or picking at the nose.

Nose bleeds are more common in children, and in the elderly. Every adult with a nose bleed without an obvious cause should have their blood pressure checked, although in fact most people with **high blood pressure** do not get nose bleeds. People who have profuse or recurrent nose bleeds should be tested to ensure their blood is clotting normally.

SYMPTOMS

Blood drips painlessly for several minutes and there may be a blood-tinged ooze which lasts for a day or two.

TREATMENT

The first aid treatment (see page 400) is to pinch the soft part of the nose, just below the bridge, hard enough to close the blood vessel for about ten minutes. Most bleeding will stop provided that probing fingers are kept away from the scab.

A profuse nose bleed will require the nose to be packed tightly with a long ribbon of gauze to put pressure on the blood vessels. It is removed after 48 hours. The curative treatment for nose bleeds is to burn the offending blood vessel with silver nitrate or an electric cautery.

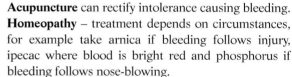

QUESTION

Is a nose bleed dangerous?
Bleeding for more than a few hours causes significant blood loss – it may be due to the rare cases of poor blood clotting and must be dealt with appropriately. High blood pressure (probably coincidental) should be handled in the standard way. The majority of nose bleeds are otherwise merely inconvenient rather than dangerous.

Complementary Treatment

Acupuncture can rectify intolerance causing bleeding.
Homeopathy – treatment depends on circumstances, for example take arnica if bleeding follows injury, ipecac where blood is bright red and phosphorus if bleeding follows nose-blowing.

Nasal polyps

Fleshy benign growths in the nose that cause obstruction.

CAUSES

The surface lining of the nose reacts naturally to dust or fumes by secreting mucus. Often the surface overgrows into a polyp in people who are continuously exposed to irritant atmospheres, or in those with **hay fever** who have a perpetually overactive mucus surface. Each polyp has a 0.5–1 cm/¼–½ in diameter, is pinkish-grey, hangs on a stalk and blocks the nasal passage. Where there is one there are often several.

SYMPTOMS

Someone whose nose keeps running or who is forever sneezing eventually finds that their nose constantly feels blocked. Often one side is worse affected than the other. An ENT specialist can see how many polyps there are and plan treatment.

TREATMENT

If the nasal polyps are small, there is a fair chance that a steroid nasal spray such as fluticasone or beclomethasone will make them shrink. Some people have so many polyps that sprays are unlikely to work sufficiently. If medical treatment with steroid sprays fails or you are simply fed up with having to use the spray daily surgery is possible. The polyps can be removed under a local anaesthetic. Each one is snared and cut off. If necessary, this can be repeated every few years.

The mucus surface of the nose can also be removed for a permanent cure, although this quite extensive operation is less commonly performed.

Complementary Treatment

Aromatherapy inhalations could help ease symptoms: try eucalyptus, thyme or myrrh (two to four drops in a bowl of hot water or on a handkerchief).

SINUS PROBLEMS

Disorders of these cavities in the skull, mostly caused by infection.

CAUSES

There are three main sinuses: the maxillary in the cheekbones, the frontal sinus above the eyes and the ethmoidal behind the bridge of the nose. The linings of the sinuses produce a mucus secretion, which carries away any infection and dust that have penetrated the sinuses. The secretions drain through ducts into the posterior part of the nose.

Sinusitis often follows a cold which has obstructed the drainage ducts. The roots of the upper molar and premolar teeth end very close to the floor of the maxillary sinus and inflammation may spread into it from the teeth. In addition, jumping or diving into water can force water up the nose and into the sinuses.

The function of the sinuses is unclear. It may be to make the skull lighter or to add resonance to the voice. During sinusitis a person may sound like Donald Duck.

Chronic sinusitis

Chronic sinusitis may be congenital, for example unusually narrow ducts, or it may be provoked by allergies such as **hay fever**, which thicken the mucus surface around the drainage channel, or by **nasal polyps**, which block the channel.

SYMPTOMS

In the case of acute sinusitis, a few days after a cold, pain increases over one of the sinuses, most often the maxillary sinus. Pressure is felt in the skull, and there are aching teeth and pain behind the eyes. On bending forward you feel a rush of fluid within the sinus and increased pain. The nasal discharge becomes particularly offensive and yellow and drips down the back of the nose to the throat, creating a foul taste.

Pain that occurs at the top of the nose or deep behind the eyes suggests an infection of one of the deeper sinuses. If there is pain and swelling of the eye, then this will point to a very serious internal infection.

In chronic sinusitis there is persistent nasal obstruction and discharge of infected mucus, plus the pressure symptoms mentioned above. Often the individual is a smoker, has allergies or is under some degree of tension (see STRESS).

The diagnosis of sinusitis on clinical grounds alone is not terribly accurate. The definitive test is a CT scan (see page 350) to demonstrate fluid; these show that many presumed diagnoses of sinusitis are wrong.

TREATMENT

For acute sinusitis an antibiotic is used to penetrate the pus in the sinus. This requires a high dosage over ten days of, for example, amoxycillin or doxycycline. Decongestant nose drops and tablets are helpful, as are steam and menthol inhalations to improve the effectiveness of medication.

Infection of the frontal sinuses or ethmoidal sinuses is treated similarly but with higher doses of antibiotic and with drainage of the sinus if infection worsens.

Chronic sinusitis

Scans first prove the diagnosis and exclude an underlying cause such as allergy or **tooth decay**. The treatment is as for acute sinusitis but given for longer. If this fails, you will need a wash out of the sinus with a hollow needle under local or general anaesthetic. Failing this, a more permanent drainage channel can be made through the nose or via the upper gum.

Endoscopic instruments allow the surgeon to inspect the interior of the sinus, remove polyps or to enlarge the drainage channels. Similar techniques can be used to drain the frontal or ethmoidal sinuses in cases resistant to antibiotics.

QUESTIONS

Do children get sinusitis?
The sinuses do not begin to form until about five years of age and are not fully formed until about twelve. Thus sinusitis is impossible below the age of five and unusual before the age of twelve.

Is sinusitis dangerous?
Prompt treatment with antibiotics makes complications unusual, but in theory infection could spread into surrounding bone or into the brain. A bloody discharge should not be attributed to sinusitis without investigation for a possible tumour.

Complementary Treatment

Aromatherapy – try inhaling cajeput or eucalyptus oil (two to four drops in a bowl of hot water, or on a handkerchief). **Nutritional therapy** – food allergy might be the underlying cause: seek advice. **Chiropractic** helps alleviate pain and tension as part of the overall treatment plan. **Ayurveda** offers herbal steam inhalations, oral preparations and dietary advice. *Other therapies to try: most have something to offer.*

LARYNGITIS

Inflammation of the larynx, the part of the tube through which air passes to the lungs, which contains the voice box.

CAUSES

The upper airways bear the brunt of what the atmosphere can throw at them – smoke from cigarettes, fumes from pollution, pollen in the air, bacteria or viruses such as the common cold. Some people find that dry or air-conditioned atmospheres give them persistent discomfort in the larynx. Using the voice a lot will also lead to inflammation of the airways. Laryngitis can be acute or chronic and is more common in smokers.

SYMPTOMS

There may be pain of a burning nature that is felt all the way from the back of the throat down behind the breastbone. The voice of someone with laryngitis varies from hoarse through every type of squeak to even complete loss.

Children, whose airways are narrower than adults, may cough more and feel more unwell.

Hoarseness lasting more than three weeks may be caused by cancer of the larynx and you should see your doctor.

TREATMENT

Stop smoking. Most cases are due to viral infections, so antibiotics are of little use. It is better to rest your voice, keep the throat moist with drinks or lozenges and avoid smoky or dry atmospheres. Children benefit from being in a steamy room. The rare cases of airways obstruction need hospital treatment.

QUESTION

Is whispering a good idea when you have laryngitis?
Whispering actually puts a similar strain on the voice as talking normally and arguably more if you have to keep repeating yourself! Reconcile yourself to pointing, gesturing or holding up signs during the three to five days that it takes for the condition to improve.

Complementary Treatment
Western herbalism – helpful astringent and antiseptic herbs include myrrh and thyme. **Aromatherapy** – see SINUS PROBLEMS. *Other therapies to try: naturopathy; acupuncture; homeopathy; Chinese herbalism.*

ORAL THRUSH

A common fungal infection affecting all age groups.

CAUSES

The organism that causes oral thrush, candida, also causes vaginal **thrush** and **nappy rash**. Some cross-infection may occur in these cases. Babies are especially prone to oral thrush by transfer from their mother's skin. It is common after taking an antibiotic, which kills germs that compete for the food supply, and affects asthmatics using steroid inhalers. Persistent or recurrent oral thrush may be a warning of **diabetes** or, less commonly, a deficiency in the immune system.

SYMPTOMS

The inside of the mouth is coated with small white deposits, which are the thrush organisms. If they are scraped off, the underlying surface bleeds. The mouth feels sore; babies may be reluctant to feed because of this.

TREATMENT

Babies are treated with mouth drops and adults with lozenges; resistant cases require antithrush tablets. Thrush elsewhere is treated to avoid reinfection. Severe cases need investigation.

QUESTION

How contagious is oral thrush?
There is no risk of spread as long as cups and glasses are kept clean and not shared. Babies' teats should be sterilized.

Complementary Treatment
Homeopathy – try an aloe vera mouthwash. **Aromatherapy** – gargle myrrh or tea tree (two drops in half a glass of water). *Other therapies to try: naturopathy; Western and Chinese herbalism; acupuncture.*

PERIODONTAL DISEASE

Disease of the gums around the teeth, leading to teeth loosening.

CAUSES

Teeth make a special joint with the bone of the jaw called a gomphosis, meaning a nail or bolt. Fibres grow from the bone into the tooth, securing it in place. Periodontal disease begins when food debris accumulates around the tooth, allowing in chronic bacterial infection, which works its way down the root and loosens the tooth fastening. Eventually it involves the tooth, the gum and the bone of the jaw, resulting in ever looser teeth and increased risk of infection.

SYMPTOMS

The gums feel tender through an inflammation called gingivitis. They bleed easily, even on brushing, and the teeth feel loose. Persistent infection causes **halitosis**. There may be pus around the teeth, but only in totally neglected conditions.

TREATMENT

Unfortunately, the damage from chronic infection cannot be repaired. Teeth loosened by infection cannot be tightened up and the same goes for loose gums around the teeth or erosion of the jaw bone. Dental hygiene can, however, help to prevent progression of the process, which would otherwise end in loss of teeth or chronic gingivitis.

Since periodontal disease cannot be reversed, prevention is the best step. Remove food residue every day, using a toothbrush and floss to remove debris from between teeth. Tartar (accumulated food debris) should be regularly removed by a dental hygienist. Antiseptic mouthwashes may help.

Complementary Treatment

A **nutritional therapist** might recommend boosting your intake of vitamin C. **Bach flower remedies** – try Rescue Remedy. *Other therapies to try: Western herbalism; homeopathy.*

TOOTH DECAY

Destruction of the teeth caused by enamel erosion and infection.

CAUSES

The basic cause of tooth decay (dental caries) is acid that dissolves the hard enamel coating teeth. Acid comes from bacteria growing in plaque around the teeth, which feed on sugar. Once enamel erosion has occurred, bacteria invade deeper into the tooth, eventually reaching the pulp. The resulting inflammation destroys the pulp, leaving the tooth fragile.

SYMPTOMS

Decay does not cause pain until it inflames the nerve-rich pulp. Throbbing pain may worsen into the excruciating pain of an abscess and swelling of that part of the face. The diagnosis is confirmed by examination and X-ray.

TREATMENT

Antibiotics can reduce the degree of infection, but almost certainly the tooth will need drilling in order to let out the pus. In less severe cases, filling the tooth should stop further decay.

With more serious decay, the tooth can be capped. In very severe cases, prompt root canal work can save the tooth even though the pulp has died; extraction is the only sensible option for a badly decayed tooth.

QUESTION

How can decay be prevented?
You should avoid sweets, sugar, starch and sugary drinks on which bacteria thrive. Daily careful brushing with a fluoridated paste is very worthwhile in preventing tooth decay. Plaque should be removed regularly by a dental hygienist. Fluoridated water is a highly effective public health measure and worries about its safety have little scientific support.

Complementary Treatment

There are no alternatives to conventional dentistry. Aim for prevention by cutting out sugary foods and drinks, and maintaining good dental hygiene with regular flossing and cleaning of teeth. A variety of herbal toothpastes is available.

MOUTH ULCERS

Open sores, most of which, though irritating, are benign.

CAUSES

The majority of mouth ulcers are caused by viral infections or by scratches, whether from a toothbrush, hard food or sharp teeth. Common viral causes include herpes and Coxsackie. Rarely, the mouth may ulcerate because of disease elsewhere in the gastrointestinal system, for example Crohn's disease (see INFLAMMATORY BOWEL DISEASE), Behçet's disease, **coeliac disease** or **systemic lupus erythematosus**.

SYMPTOMS

Crops of tiny painful ulcers appear over the walls of the mouth and tongue. Ulcers clustered over the soft palate and back of the mouth are probably caused by a herpes virus. Mouth ulcers with itchy spots on the palms and feet are typical of the alarming sounding but benign **hand, foot and mouth disease**, caused by the Coxsackie virus. Mouth ulcers can last for up to seven to fourteen days. Recurrent or large ulcers associated with ill health or abdominal pains need investigating for an unusual bowel or immune cause.

TREATMENT

Mouth ulcers are treated with a steroid gel or pellet held in contact with the ulcer. Children badly hurt by mouth ulcers may stop eating until the pain subsides, after about three days.

QUESTION

When should you see a doctor about changes in the mouth?
Any ulceration of the mouth, white patch or area of irritation that lasts more than about a fortnight should be seen by a doctor or dentist. This is to pick up the rare serious ulcers caused by cancer or to consider the unusual bowel or immune diagnoses.

 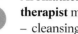

Complementary Treatment

Aromatherapy – see ORAL THRUSH. A **nutritional therapist** may suggest avoiding citrus fruits. **Ayurveda** – cleansing medications would be prescribed, along with dietary advice. *Other therapies to try: homeopathy; chakra balancing; naturopathy; hypnotherapy.*

HALITOSIS

Bad-smelling breath with many causes – several preventable.

CAUSES

The mouth has an effective self-cleansing mechanism in the antiseptic properties of saliva. If it breaks down then poor dental hygiene is the number one cause (see PERIODONTAL DISEASE) – the smell comes from bacteria around the teeth. Bacterial colonization is also the reason for halitosis in people with chronic nasal discharges, **tonsillitis**, sinusitis (see SINUS PROBLEMS) and chronic lung infections. Less likely is halitosis from stomach disease or peptic ulcers. Diet, alcohol and smoking may also contribute.

SYMPTOMS

These may be those of periodontitis, gingivitis, sinusitis or indigestion. You might be aware of your own halitosis. Some people imagine they have halitosis when others say this is not the case; this may be a self-image problem. However, people are mostly unaware of their own halitosis because the nose rapidly becomes accustomed to ever-present odours, including the smell of one's own breath, which is why it takes an outsider to point out the problem.

TREATMENT

Good oral hygiene is the key, plus treatment for any focus of infection whether in the teeth, sinuses or lungs. It may take reassurance or other psychological treatment to help someone who imagines they have halitosis; they may need the reassurance of mouthwashes and oral deodorants to allay their fears.

Complementary Treatment

Homeopathy – treatment will depend on the specific details of your case; useful remedies include nux, mercurius, pulsatilla, quercus and arnica. *Other therapies to try: hypnotherapy; nutritional therapy; naturopathy.*

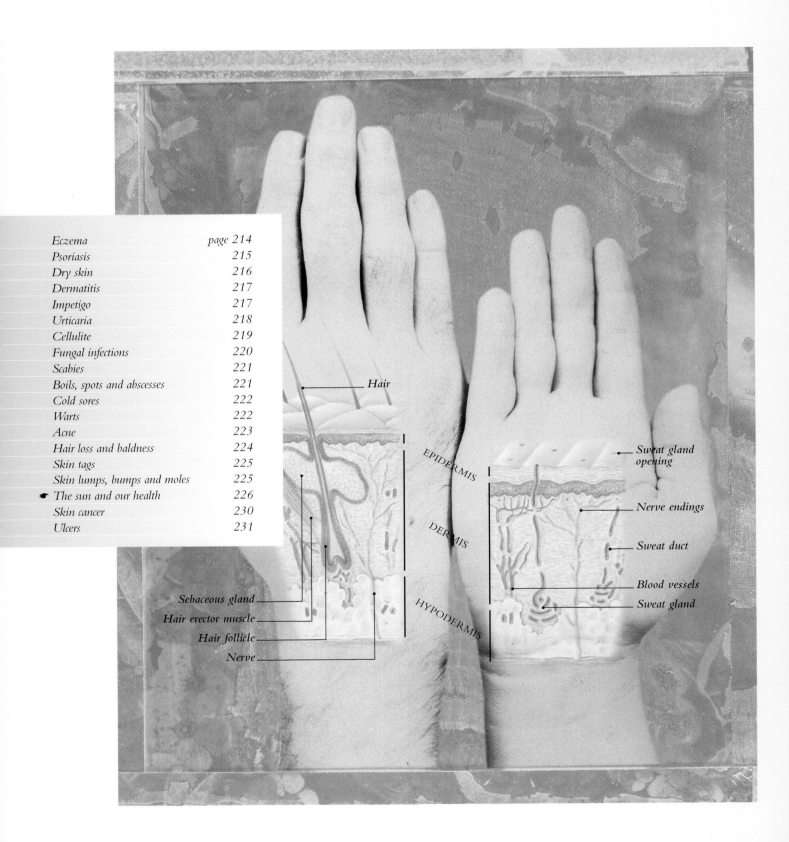

Hair

Sweat gland opening

EPIDERMIS

Nerve endings

DERMIS

Sweat duct

Blood vessels

Sweat gland

HYPODERMIS

Sebaceous gland

Hair erector muscle

Hair follicle

Nerve

*While the other organs of the body enjoy a high profile, the
skin is relatively undervalued, despite it being the largest organ
of the body in terms of weight. It performs many vital roles
that we rarely think about — from keeping our bodies cool to
protecting against infection.*

SKIN AND HAIR

SKIN NOT ONLY ACTS as a covering for the body's
organs, it also maintains a vital interface between the
ever-changing external environment and the relatively more stable internal environment.

The skin is a three-layered and multi-function structure.
The outer epidermis comprises cells rich in keratin, which
render it waterproof. They migrate from a deeper level, die at
the surface and are shed continuously, the process taking
about 30 days. In this layer are cells that pigment the skin and
cells that mount immune responses to infection.

Below the epidermis is the dermis, a complex layer combin-
ing elasticity and flexibility with many other functions as follows. Hair grows from hair follicles in cycles up to three years
long (see HAIR LOSS AND BALDNESS). Nails, which are modified
keratin, are generated from specialized cells below the nail
folds. A greasy secretion called sebum keeps the skin supple;
this is derived from the sebaceous glands within the dermis
and excreted into hair follicles.

The sweat glands, which are found all over the skin, regulate body temperature and salt balance. A particular variety of
sweat gland is found around the armpits, genitalia and breasts
and may have a sexual function producing pheromones, the
animal equivalent of nectar to a bee.

The deepest layer of skin, the subcutaneous tissues, is made
of fat, blood vessels and yet more sweat glands.

In addition, skin also plays an important role in calcium
balance (and therefore bone formation), by synthesizing
vitamin D using ultraviolet light. Pigmented skin acts as a protection against harsh sun.

Scattered throughout the skin are multitudes of sensory
receptors for touch, pressure, movement and pain. The dense
blood supply rushes clotting factors and protective cells to
any breach in the surface of the skin.

Skin problems

The most common skin diseases arise from the rate of cell formation (which greatly increases in **psoriasis**), immune reactions causing **dermatitis** and **eczema**, and infections leading
to boils (see BOILS, SPOTS AND ABSCESSES). Overactivity of certain cells leads to excessive sweating and to the many **skin
lumps, bumps and moles** to which skin is prone.

The skin is one organ, even though the delicate skin of the
eyelid looks very different from the callused skin of the soles
of the feet. This is why an irritation in one part of the skin
often causes reactions elsewhere, for example a flare-up of
eczema from a skin irritation will bring out a sympathetic
eczematous response in more distant parts.

The state of the skin's health is something we notice immediately: its greasiness, dryness, flaking, blushing and weeping.
Although few skin diseases are actually infectious, we experience an almost instinctive reaction to both poor and excellent
skin health, influencing social isolation or acceptance.

*Left: Skin and hair protect, insulate and
cool the body, enhance its appearance and
give much of our individuality.*

ECZEMA

Inflammation of the skin through an inherent hypersensitivity.

CAUSES

In eczema the skin reacts unusually vigorously to external irritation, or it may even react without any external irritation at all. This differentiates eczema from **dermatitis**, where the cause is clearly an external irritant.

People who are most liable to eczema are atopic, meaning they have a heightened immune system, and often also suffer from **hay fever** and **asthma**. Blood tests confirm high levels of proteins involved in immune responses, called IgE, which release inflammation-provoking substances called cytokines and interleukins that cause the skin changes.

There is a large genetic component: if both parents have eczema there is up to a 60% chance of their children having it.

SYMPTOMS

Infant eczema can begin within weeks of birth, with the baby having red and scaly rashes over her cheeks, scalp, chest, groin and eyebrows. The baby appears unsettled and irritable, not surprisingly given the tenderness of the skin. As the baby grows into a child, the skin looks less greasy and more red and dry. The parts of the body that are then most affected are the skin creases of the elbows and knees, with rashes scattered elsewhere. In areas where there is particular irritation the skin becomes thickened and cracked, called lichenification. The eczema will have greatly improved in at least 50% of children by the age of 5 and in 80–95% by adolescence.

Adults who have suffered lifelong eczema will have areas of lichenified skin. There will be the same red, dry patches anywhere on the body or face. These will vary in severity with external influences, such as dry or cold weather and irritant clothing. Adult eczema may involve the palms of the hands and soles of the feet, causing tiny itchy fluid-filled lesions. Eczema can accompany **varicose veins**. Individuals will often have associated asthma and hay fever.

TREATMENT

The aim at all ages is to keep the skin moisturized and to avoid obvious irritants. It is usual to start with moisturizing creams, for example aqueous creams combined with bath lotions, that go all over the body. There are many proprietary brands of varying degrees of greasiness. These help keep the condition under control, but require meticulous application.

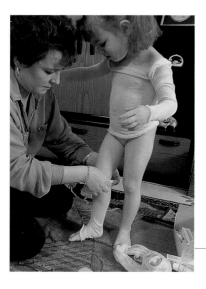

Left: Children with severe eczema need careful daily treatment. Fortunately, eczema often improves with time.

It is also very important to wear materials, such as cotton, that are non-irritating and absorbent.

Since the 1960s steroid preparations, in the form of creams and ointments, have revolutionized the treatment of eczema. However the use of these strong steroids is kept to a minimum because, on the face for example, they will thin the skin and cause pimples. As treatment for acute flare-ups, however, steroids are unsurpassed.

For more regular treatment, mild hydrocortisone preparations are safe for all ages, can be used for months and can be applied to the face. However, preparations of ever-increasing potency may be required – even, rarely, on the face. The strongest of these preparations, for example betamethasone or clobetasol, are reserved for the most resistant cases, especially eczema of the hands. Anti-itch drugs may be needed at all ages, for example chlorpheniramine or terfenadine.

In recent years the role of infection has been recognized in causing flare-ups of eczema, so there is renewed interest in steroid/antibiotic preparations.

Complementary Treatment

Chinese herbalism – see DERMATITIS. **Western herbalism** – your medical herbalist is likely to ask you to drink teas or infusions, as well as applying ointments or pastes to the affected area. **Homeopathy** – use calendula cream as a moisturizer and rub evening primrose oil on to unaffected areas of skin as a preventive measure. **Ayurveda** – see SCABIES. *Other therapies to try: healing; shiatsu-do; naturopathy.*

PSORIASIS

A problem characterized by skin scaling and red patches, affecting about 2% of the population.

CAUSES

As a result of an increased rate of cell growth in the outer layers of the skin, cells pile up in characteristic plaques. Many people with psoriasis have a genetic tendency to the condition, which makes them up to seven times more likely than average to suffer from it. In susceptible people a streptococcal throat infection can trigger it, as can constant pressure on or rubbing of the skin. Psoriasis may prove to be an auto-immune condition, that is, one where the body reacts against its own tissues. Many people find that emotional upsets will cause a deterioration. Others find that the cold makes it worse by drying out the skin. Certain drugs can bring on psoriasis, notably lithium and beta-blockers. But however bad psoriasis looks, it is not catching and there is no risk to others.

SYMPTOMS

Psoriasis does not begin until late teens or adult life. Silvery plaques of skin accumulate over the elbows, knees and pressure areas such as the base of the spine. Similar plaques form around the hair margins on the scalp. Plaques can affect skin anywhere, from the chest to the palms, soles, groin and the genitalia. People may get joint pains and their nails often have tiny pits in them. In severe psoriasis, where there is chronic scaling and disfigurement, significant loss of protein through the shed skin and disabling joint stiffness, people may become reclusive through psychological and physical distress.

TREATMENT

Unfortunately, psoriasis is not curable. It is difficult to treat well and the treatment has to be tailored to the individual. This calls for trust and patience on the part of patient and doctor.

Steroid creams

These are used where there are just a few small plaques giving little trouble. They are unsuitable on the face or for long use.

Coal tar preparations

A mainstay of treatment, these are applied as pastes, creams, lotions and bath additives to reduce inflammation and the amount of scaling. Pure coal tar is messy and cosmetically unacceptable, so preparations have been made that both smell

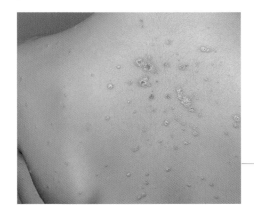

Left: Plaques of psoriasis, showing the typical scaling and redness.

better and do not stain skin or clothing, for example alphosyl and dithrocream. Cosmetically acceptable scalp preparations are now available.

Calcipotriol

This is a form of vitamin D applied as a cream. It is pleasant to use and effective for small plaques or on the scalp, but it is impractical for widespread psoriasis.

Psoralens with ultraviolet A (PUVA)

This is treatment with ultraviolet light in a special booth; tablets containing psoralens, which increase skin sensitivity, are taken a couple of hours beforehand. Ultraviolet A refers to the wavelength of the light. PUVA, which has excellent results, takes about three months for full effect; thereafter treatment every few weeks should keep the condition under control.

Other forms of treatment

Acitretin is a hospital-only treatment for severe psoriasis but with many side effects, for example dry skin and liver damage. Because it damages the foetus, acitretin must not be taken during pregnancy; this risk persists for two years after treatment. Cytotoxic drugs, as used in certain cancers, are increasingly used for otherwise unresponsive severe psoriasis.

Complementary Treatment

Chinese herbalism – see DERMATITIS. **Shiatsu-do** – skin disorders worsened by stress, including psoriasis, are responsive. **Chakra balancing** can help with skin healing and pain control. **Auricular therapy** could help, especially in conjunction with **acupuncture**. A **nutritional therapist** could recommend a diet to enhance liver function. **Cymatics** could help. **Ayurveda** – see SCABIES. *Other therapies to try: see STRESS.*

DRY SKIN

❖

The natural self-lubricating glands of the skin tend to become inefficient with age.

CAUSES

❖

The skin is kept oiled by slightly greasy secretions of the sebaceous glands. With age, these glands become less efficient and, combined with loss of the skin's natural elasticity and water content, this results in dry skin that cracks easily. Exposure to strong sunlight and harsh weather also accelerates drying of the skin. The skin of smokers ages more rapidly and looks drier and more wrinkled at an earlier age. Many women find that their skin becomes drier after the menopause.

Dry skin is rarely due to disease, with the exception of **eczema**, where there is dryness combined with redness and inflammation. A severely underactive thyroid gland leads to dry skin (see THYROID PROBLEMS).

Anything that degreases the skin inevitably leads to dryness; common degreasants are detergents, washing-up liquids and industrial solvents.

Very occasionally people have congenitally abnormally dry, cracked skin structure, the condition of ichthyosis.

SYMPTOMS

❖

Dry skin feels irritable and cracks easily. It looks flaky and cells may be shed on to clothing. Itch can be a big problem, especially in the elderly, but severe itch and dry skin should trigger a search for an underlying problem such as an underactive thyroid gland, **anaemia** or kidney problems (see KIDNEY DISEASE). Secondary infections can get into large cracks.

TREATMENT

❖

Emollients are preparations to lubricate the skin. Some are medical formulations, others have been developed by cosmetic companies; use whatever you find most effective.

Broadly speaking, there are creams where lubricants are dissolved in water, or ointments where lubricants are dissolved in oil. Creams rub into the skin, leaving no residue, whereas ointments leave a greasy layer that may be inconvenient for people employed in certain occupations, for example those handling paper or film.

These preparations are fine for small areas but difficult for widespread dryness. This is where liquid emollients are helpful, as they are put on immediately after showering or are dissolved in the bath water. These tend to be oil based. You

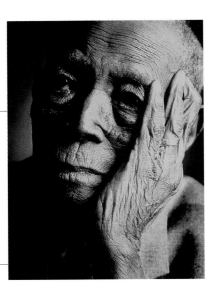

Right: Sun-damaged skin. With care, even aged skin can remain supple and self-repairing.

may find you need a combination of preparations: a liquid for all-over lubrication, a cream for your hands and an ointment for your arms or your face.

If you get itch or inflammation after using an emollient, you might be allergic to something in the skin preparation that is causing **dermatitis**. The substances most often responsible are lanolin and perfumed preparations. If you have become allergic to one of these you should avoid other skin preparations containing it by checking the detailed ingredient list. This is easy in the case of medical preparations but it may be more difficult with patented preparations.

QUESTIONS

Should children routinely use emollients?
These are necessary only for children with eczema whose skin is dry and inflamed.

What is the secret of delaying the ageing of skin?
Moisturizing the skin is a fundamental strategy; avoid excessive exposure to sunlight, wind and cigarettes. If you work with detergents or industrial cleaners, apply emollients liberally; remember that too much washing with soap or bath detergents is degreasing.

Complementary Treatment

Chinese herbalism – see DERMATITIS. **Homeopathy** – use calendula cream as a moisturizer and rub evening primrose oil on to unaffected areas of skin, as a preventive measure. **Aromatherapy** – try a massage oil made up with one of the following: sandalwood, rose or neroli (three drops to 10 ml carrier oil). **Ayurveda** – see SCABIES. Skin disorders that are worsened by stress, including dry skin, are responsive to **shiatsu-do**. *Other therapies to try: Western herbalism; cymatics.*

DERMATITIS

Irritation of the skin through environmental stimuli.

CAUSES

Dermatitis is the general term for an inflammation of the skin caused by some external factor. The most common irritants are oils, greases, soaps and perfumes, metal, plants and ultraviolet radiation. These are all potent sensitizers in some people and once the skin has been sensitized in one area it is likely to show signs of dermatitis elsewhere. It is also the case that people with skin that is sensitive to one agent often prove to be sensitive to several others.

Dermatitis can be cured once the irritant has been identified, unlike **eczema** where there is a congenital tendency to inflamed skin and which is often a permanent problem.

SYMPTOMS

The skin is red and itchy and may flake or ooze tissue fluid. Through repeated scratching the surface of the skin breaks down so that secondary bacterial infection is common, with increased redness and pain.

TREATMENT

Often the offending agent is easily identifiable, for example if hands are raw where gloves end, or the skin is red just underneath a metal watch or the skin improves on holiday and deteriorates on return to work. Skin testing helps identify otherwise obscure agents. Avoidance of the agent is obviously necessary. The symptoms respond to moisturizing creams or steroid creams plus antihistamine tablets to reduce itching.

Complementary Treatment

WARNING: Chinese herbalism – herbs can be extremely effective, but a few people have an adverse reaction that affects the liver. Reputable practitioners insist on regular blood tests to monitor liver function. Formulas are person specific, depending on the skin condition and underlying intolerance, and often change during treatment. **Homeopathy** – use calendula cream as a moisturizer and rub evening primrose oil on to unaffected areas of skin as a preventive measure. *Other therapies to try: naturopathy; healing; chakra balancing; Ayurveda; auricular therapy; shiatsu-do.*

IMPETIGO

A highly contagious infection of the skin.

CAUSES

Impetigo is especially common in children, through the acquisition of skin infections with streptococcus or staphylococcus bacteria. Once these have invaded the skin they cause it to blister and burst, leaving a raw surface that is open to secondary infection. Most cases of impetigo are caught by cross infection from others; hence it spreads fairly easily around schools and homes.

SYMPTOMS

The face is the site that is most commonly affected. What begins as a small spot grows into a cluster of angry-looking lesions within hours. These have a red raw base with a crusted yellow coating and they leak tissue fluid. The infection then spreads easily by direct contact to the hands and arms – in fact anywhere that infected fingers may roam.

TREATMENT

Use an antibiotic cream for a single spot and oral antibiotics for more extensive infection. Do not share a towel and avoid skin-to-skin contact with others. Most cases are cured by a week's worth of antibiotic treatment.

QUESTION

Is impetigo dangerous?
The spots just look unpleasant, and only children with low resistance to infection might become ill. Treatment should be vigorous, however, because it can quickly spread through a community.

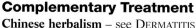

Complementary Treatment

Chinese herbalism – see DERMATITIS. **Naturopathy** or **nutritional therapy** can help. **Ayurveda** – see SCABIES. *Other therapies to try: homeopathy; Western herbalism.*

URTICARIA

Skin rashes that result from an allergic reaction.

CAUSES

Also known as nettle rash or hives, urticaria is the response of the skin to something that triggers an allergic reaction. During the reaction, the skin throws defending cells against a supposed invader and supplements these with chemicals that further affect the skin, for example histamine, prostaglandins and others. This accounts for the skin reactions of swelling and fluid retention.

Often urticaria is an obvious response to a definite substance, either directly on the skin or that has been eaten, for example strawberries or shellfish, irritant plants or aspirin-type drugs. More likely, however, the cause is obscure and remains so even after allergy testing.

Emotion and exercise can cause a particular type of urticaria, called cholinergic urticaria after the nerves involved. Other forms are in reaction to cold, to sunlight and even to water. There are a few uncommon inherited reasons that are important to identify because of the lifelong implications.

Urticaria is most common in children and young adults but occurs at all ages.

SYMPTOMS

The skin reaction usually occurs within minutes of exposure but may take hours, making it harder to identify the cause.

The skin feels itchy and rapidly swells into a weal that is pale in the middle and red around the margins. A sufferer may have a few large weals or multiple small ones of all shapes – more usually called hives. Weals wax and wane within minutes; the whole experience can last minutes, hours or even days.

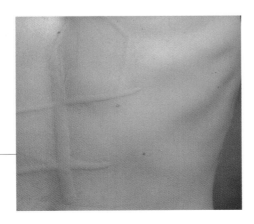

Right: Severe urticaria, showing how even minimum contact with an irritant causes weals.

Soft tissues

It is not unusual for the lips and eyelids to swell. This is called angioedema and is a sign of a widespread allergic response. More severe again, although relatively uncommon, is swelling that may extend to the soft tissues of the throat and trachea, causing difficulty in breathing.

Anaphylaxis

This is the most severe reaction: a collapse of blood pressure through whole-body release of histamine-type substances. Although rare, it most often occurs as a result of insect stings and, more recently recognized, from eating nuts.

TREATMENT

This depends on the severity of the condition. Mild to moderate urticaria is treated with antihistamines by tablet or injection. The older antihistamines such as chlorpheniramine are sedating, which is helpful at night; the modern non-sedating antihistamines are better in the day, for example astemizole. Soothing lotions like calamine are helpful for children.

In the more severe case of angioedema a short course of steroids will rapidly dampen the reaction. The slightest hint of difficulty in breathing or swallowing must be taken seriously and hospital care arranged.

Anaphylaxis

This most serious association with urticaria is a medical emergency. The immediate treatment is to inject adrenaline, which restores blood pressure, after which steroids and antihistamines can be given. People who know they are at risk should wear medical bracelets that alert to the fact and carry an adrenaline self-injection kit.

Many people react to aspirin-type drugs, widely used for arthritis, and it is important to consider whether these might be causing severe urticaria in an adult.

Complementary Treatment

Chinese herbalism – see DERMATITIS. **Homeopathy** – a registered homeopath should be able to help, and will try to find out what triggers your condition, what makes it better or worse, and so on. As a **self-help** measure, urtica ointment relieves itchiness. You can also try applying an ice-pack to the affected area. **Chakra balancing** can help with relaxation and healing. **Ayurveda** – see SCABIES. *Other therapies to try: auricular therapy.*

CELLULITE

A non-medical term for the unwelcome aspect of fat in the body.

CAUSES

At a biochemical level, fat is a highly concentrated means of storing energy (1 g of fat supplies over twice as much energy as 1 g of protein or carbohydrate). It also provides heat, insulation and protection, as well as buffering organs from movement by being distributed under the skin and around many organs. Finally, it forms the external shape of the body and contributes to the texture, as with the hips and the breasts.

But in spite of fat's beneficial roles, people are more concerned about its negative aspect – cellulite. Cellulite is not a medical term but we all know what it means. Medically it refers to the adipose tissue, wherein fat cells hang within a loose connective tissue framework. Each fat cell is a great globule of fat, squeezing the cell nucleus to one side. As we get older the connective tissue framework becomes laxer, while fat tends to accumulate. The result is cellulite.

SYMPTOMS

Cellulite causes a characteristic dimpled appearance over fat-bearing areas, typically the thighs and hips. It is more visible on standing, when the weight of the fat pulls on the connective tissue framework, and from certain angles when light picks out the dimpling. Paradoxically, dieting may actually worsen the appearance, because connective tissue has less fat to support, so the dimpling tends to become deeper.

Cellulite is not the same as **obesity**; even slim people will have plumper parts where cellulite may lurk.

Cellulite is a particularly female phenomenon, because of the way in which the female body is shaped by strategically placed layers of fat.

TREATMENT

It is claimed by some manufacturers that certain creams, when rubbed into the skin, make cellulite disappear. This claim appears improbable: even if you apply something that succeeds in bursting the fat cells, this fat will only be reabsorbed by the surrounding cells. It will *not* slosh around in a liquid form that drips out if you cut yourself!

Dieting to remove cellulite is not an option, as it can actually make it appear more obvious, as mentioned above.

Liposuction is still a controversial surgical technique to remove cellulite or indeed fat in general. Under anaesthetic a

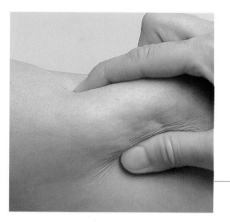

Left: If pinching fat causes dimples like the ones here you may have cellulite.

tube is inserted into the fat-bearing area – the hips, abdomen or thighs – and the fat is literally vacuumed out under suction. The technique carries the risks of bleeding, infection and uneven tissue removal. However, it has become a popular treatment of choice for some and the results in the hands of the very skilled are very impressive.

QUESTIONS

Can early action reduce cellulite?
Evidence suggests that the number of fat cells is determined during foetal development. Possibly, therefore, children born to mothers with a fat-rich diet have more fat cells, which will predispose them to obesity and cellulite in later life.

Why is it relatively difficult to lose fat by dieting?
If you eat less the body turns to using carbohydrate for the energy it needs. The body only begins using fat significantly when these carbohydrate stores are exhausted. This means that you need to follow a very low-calorie diet for this to occur.

Complementary Treatment
Chinese herbalism – see DERMATITIS. **Aromatherapy** – try making up a massage oil with one of the following – cypress, fennel, juniper (three drops to 10 ml base oil). Alternatively, many proprietary creams contain essential oils for their detoxifying and fluid-reducing properties, and their ability to balance hormones. Diet – a **nutritional therapist** or **naturopath** could help. **Healing** promotes elimination of wastes, which helps keep the skin clear. *Other therapies to try: cymatics.*

FUNGAL INFECTIONS

Infections from fungi that can be mild or severe.

CAUSES

Fungal infections can occur in the skin, nails or scalp.

The most common skin infection is caused by candida, a natural skin inhabitant (see THRUSH and ORAL THRUSH). It thrives in warm, moist conditions and where other food competitors are reduced, for example after antibiotic treatment. It grows around the genitalia and groin and under the armpits and breasts. The other common skin fungus is ringworm, which is usually transmitted by close contact with infected animals. Athlete's foot is an infection between the toes caused by yet another family of fungi.

Several different fungi grow in the nails. They are unlikely to spread and are usually caused by self-infection.

Ringworm of the scalp used to be common but it is now found only in cases of gross personal neglect.

Skin and scalp infections are spread by close skin contact. People with unusually widespread or persistent fungal infections should have medical advice, as they may have **diabetes** or an underlying immunity problem.

SYMPTOMS

Fungal skin infections cause an itchy red rash with a definite margin; the margin is the actively growing part of the fungus. Athlete's foot causes intense itching between the toes and flaking of the skin. Fungal infections of the soles or palms can look like **eczema**. The diagnosis of fungal rashes is usually straightforward and confirmed by examining skin scrapings.

With nail infections, the nails thicken, the ends break in a ragged margin and the nail may detach itself slightly from the nail bed. The toenails are more often affected than the fingers. The diagnosis is confirmed by examining nail clippings.

In infections of the scalp, the infected area is itchy and scaly and the hairs break off at the roots. In more severe infection the skin is crusted. Under ultraviolet light the affected scalp fluoresces blue-green, which is a useful confirmatory test.

TREATMENT

Many antifungal creams are available for these skin infections, often combined with a mild antiseptic and a mild steroid to reduce itching. These are very effective for fungal infections of the groin and under the breasts and for athlete's foot. Continuing treatment for at least a week after the rash

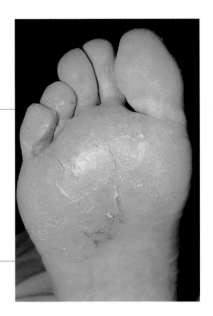

Right: Athlete's foot – the fungus makes skin cracked, itchy and inflamed.

has gone ensures complete eradication of the fungus. In really resistant cases, it may be worth taking an antifungal by mouth, such as fluconazole; this treatment is more widely used for vaginal thrush.

Nails are the most difficult to treat, because they are slow growing. If only a few nails are affected, treatment is with an antifungal lacquer containing, for example, tioconazole or amorolfine. This has to be used for at least three months. Otherwise there are oral antifungals such as terbinafine, also taken for at least three months. Recurrence is common and the nails may remain thickened, yellow and unsightly.

Treatment for scalp infections is with an antifungal taken by mouth, such as itraconazole.

QUESTION

How safe is antifungal medication?
Creams and nail lacquers are very unlikely to cause any side effects apart from stinging caused by skin sensitivity. Antifungal tablets are effective but may have significant side effects, especially inflammation of the liver.

 Complementary Treatment
Complementary therapies generally attempt to boost the immune system, so treatment is constitutional. **Chinese herbalism** – see DERMATITIS. **Western herbalism** – echinacea boosts the immune system. Unless you are already immune suppressed, **chakra balancing** can promote healing by strengthening the immune system. Diet – either a **naturopath** or a **nutritional therapist** could help. **Ayurveda** –see SCABIES. *Other therapies to try: see* THRUSH *and* ORAL THRUSH.

SCABIES

A not uncommon insect infestation of the skin, which is highly contagious.

CAUSES

The bug responsible is the scabies mite which, however nasty it looks at a distance, is a thousand times worse in close-up. The female of the species burrows within the skin, laying eggs; the itch of scabies is actually caused by the eggs.

Scabies is spread by close contact and the infection involves just a few mites. A more severe form of scabies involving infection by thousands of mites is associated with a deficient immune system. Scabies is most common in children and young adults, and those who live in an institutional setting where it can spread more easily.

SYMPTOMS

There is intense itching over the skin creases of the wrists and ankles, between the fingers and around the genitalia. The burrows are visible as tiny tracks a few millimetres in length. If you wish you can extract the mite with a needle. Often a generalized sensitivity occurs, leading to widespread itching.

TREATMENT

Treatment is with an antiscabies lotion such as malathion. This is applied all over the body from the neck down and kept on for 24 hours. The standard advice used to be to wash all potentially infected bedding or clothing, but the exact value of this is debatable.

QUESTION

When does the itching stop?
This can take weeks, because it is not just from the eggs but from a hypersensitivity reaction of the body. Similarly, itching only starts a few weeks after infection. Persistent itching should be re-treated.

 Complementary Treatment
Ayurveda treats skin conditions by considering the right diet, right lifestyle and right process for the individual person. Ointments and oral preparations are used. Full *panchakarma* detoxification is effective, especially with yoga meditation and *marma* therapy.

BOILS, SPOTS AND ABSCESSES

All of these are types of skin infection.

CAUSES

Considering how many contaminants occupy the skin, infection is relatively unusual thanks to various protective mechanisms. Fat on the skin surface is a natural antibacterial; 'friendly' germs produce substances which hinder the growth of germs muscling in on the neighbourhood. The dry outer layer of the skin inhibits penetration by bacteria. Yet nicks, cuts and abrasions forever breach these security features while hair shafts offer a direct route into the inner skin. Staphylococci and streptococci are the common invaders.

SYMPTOMS

Infection begins as a small tender swelling. Then a yellow head appears; this is pus, which is a mixture of dead defending cells and bacteria. The more extensive the infection, the larger the collection of pus and surrounding inflamed tissues, forming a boil or abscess. There may also be discomfort or pain at the affected site.

TREATMENT

Small spots and boils respond well to antibiotic creams rubbed over them. Spots and boils that are larger than 1 cm/ ½ in merit treatment with an antibiotic by mouth such as flucloxacillin. An abscess has a large collection of pus that cannot be penetrated by antibiotics. It should be incised and allowed to drain to relieve pain and speed recovery.

 Complementary Treatment
Chinese herbalism – see DERMATITIS. **Western herbalism** – try pastes of either slippery elm powder or marshmallow root powder. **Aromatherapy** – tea tree oil is effective. *Other therapies to try: homeopathy; auricular therapy; naturopathy; Ayurveda.*

COLD SORES

Skin blisters usually affecting the area around the mouth.

CAUSES

The herpes simplex type 1 virus is the cause of cold sores. After a first infection it continues to live in the nerves in a dormant state until it is reactivated by some external irritant. This may be sunlight or another infection. Cold sores can appear premenstrually. The virus regrows rapidly, leading to the appearance of new sores.

SYMPTOMS

For the first few days you are aware of a tingling sensation typically on one lip, then a rash of small but painful spots appears. Crusts form on these spots and secondary infections may lead to swelling of the lip. It takes ten to fourteen days for the rash to disappear.

TREATMENT

Treatment is typically with aciclovir, a modern antiviral drug that reduces the pain and duration of an attack. It is available as an ointment or as tablets for severe cases. It should be used when the tingling begins, because this is when the viruses are reproducing. A separate antibiotic cream may be necessary if there is a secondary infection. In time the severity of the attacks will diminish until they eventually stop altogether.

QUESTION

Can cold sores lead to genital herpes?
They are both caused by the herpes virus, but genital herpes is more often from a different strain – herpes simplex type 2. It is possible to transmit cold sores to the genitalia although it is not as easy as the transmission of genital herpes to someone else. The treatment of genital herpes is the same as for cold sores.

Complementary Treatment
Chinese herbalism – see DERMATITIS. A **nutritional therapist** might suggest supplementing lysine, an amino acid, vitamin C, zinc and bioflavinoids. Avoid peanuts, chocolate, seeds and cereals. **Aromatherapy** – apply neat lavender oil to the sore with a cotton-wool bud. *Other therapies to try: shiatsu-do; homeopathy; acupuncture; Ayurveda.*

WARTS

Fleshy skin outgrowths of viral origin.

CAUSES

Warts are caused by the many strains of the papilloma virus. The infected skin generates the dense tissue that forms the wart. Warts around the anus and genitalia may be caused by **sexually transmitted diseases** and should be seen by a doctor, although many will prove as innocent as warts elsewhere.

SYMPTOMS

The typical wart is a few millimetres in diameter and height. The surface is rough; the tiny black dots visible in the centre are capillary blood vessels in which blood has clotted. Warts on the face tend to be longer and slimmer, for example the filiform wart, which can grow up to 1 cm/½ in long. A verruca is a wart on the sole that has been flattened by pressure.

TREATMENT

The majority of warts disappear once the body has developed an immunity to the virus responsible. For this reason the treatment should not be worse than the condition itself. Over-the-counter wart preparations destroy the thick skin; they do work but it may take months.

It is possible to freeze warts, including verrucas, with liquid nitrogen, but this is a painful process that is only worth it for particularly unsightly or persistent warts.

Warts on the face may need to be carefully excised in order to avoid scarring.

Complementary Treatment
Homeopathy – apply thuja mother tincture twice daily to the wart and cover with a plaster. **Aromatherapy** – apply neat tea tree oil to the wart with a cotton-wool bud. **Ayurveda** – see SCABIES.

ACNE

There is still uncertainty as to the fundamental cause of these pimples that haunt the teenage years.

CAUSES

Acne results from bacterial colonization of the sebum-producing glands of the skin. The bacteria are emphatically not there through lack of personal hygiene, but rather because increased male hormones (androgens) at puberty stimulate sebum (grease) production, which favours bacterial invasion. This applies to youngsters of both sexes.

Acne may persist into adult life as a result of a continuing excess of androgens. Polycystic ovaries in women cause a combination of acne, hirsutism and absent periods (see PERIOD PROBLEMS). The role of food is debatable: it is really an individual matter as to which foods worsen one person's acne.

SYMPTOMS

The first sign is a blackhead, a dot in the base of a skin pore. This is caused by a colour change in a blocked sebaceous gland. The surrounding area becomes inflamed and swells into the familiar acne pimple: red with a yellow tip. Small spots come and go within days; larger ones may pit and scar the skin. Acne mainly affects the greasier parts of the face, forehead, back and chest. It is not infectious, but infectious secondary bacteria may invade large cysts.

TREATMENT

Although lack of cleanliness is not the cause, the skin should be kept clean with a degreasing agent, and lotions to dissolve the blackheads. Avoid greasy make-up which blocks the pores. Washes containing, for example, benzoyl peroxide induce peeling of a surface layer of skin, taking blackheads with it. Another directly applied preparation is retinoic acid, which reduces the formation of blackheads; this must not, however, be used during pregnancy.

Antibiotics are invaluable for more extensive or resistant acne. That they do work is undeniable, but it cannot be proved they reduce colonization by acne-producing bacteria. For mild to moderate acne antibiotics are applied as a roll-on lotion, for example erythromycin. Otherwise they are taken as tablets. The antibiotics most used are tetracyclines, which are well tolerated and have few side effects. A drawback is that some common foods, for example milk, reduce absorption. Minocycline overcomes this problem, but is more expensive

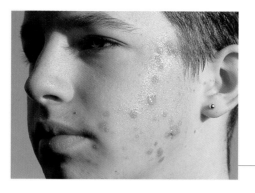

Left: Severe acne should be treated so as to avoid permanent scarring.

and carries a slight risk of arthritis. An antibiotic may lose its effect after a few years, requiring a switch to an alternative.

For women, acne can be greatly reduced with a contraceptive pill that contains an antiandrogen, called cyproterone. Different types of contraceptive pill also vary in their natural antiandrogen activity, so changing brands can help.

Retinoic acid tablets are now the best treatment for severe acne, especially if causing scarring. A few months' treatment can clear acne for over two years but it has significant side effects of dry skin and liver upsets. It also harms the foetus, so if you are planning to conceive, you should wait a month after finishing treatment with retinoic acid; again it must not be taken during pregnancy.

Acne usually improves in the summer with ultraviolet light, which can also be given as therapy in special light cabinets.

QUESTION

Does chocolate or greasy food make acne worse?
There is no scientific evidence for this but individual experience may suggest otherwise. If you have bad acne and eat a lot of chocolate and/or greasy food, try eating less of it and see what happens.

Complementary Treatment

Chinese herbalism – see DERMATITIS. **Western herbalism** – see ECZEMA. **Auricular therapy** works well in combination with **acupuncture**, especially if some points are bled. **Ayurveda** – see SCABIES. A **nutritional therapist** might suggest supplementation with zinc; other nutritional elements might control excess sebum production. Many therapists offer a cleansing diet, or a course of treatment aimed at expelling toxins from the skin. *Other therapies to try: homeopathy; healing.*

HAIR LOSS AND BALDNESS

While partial hair loss is common, complete hair loss is rare.

CAUSES

While a healthy head of hair may appear very stable, hair growth is in fact constantly changing. Each hair follicle goes through phases of growing, shedding and resting. During the growing phase the hair lengthens by about 1 cm/½ in a month; this phase, and therefore the life of an individual hair, is up to three years. Then growth stops, the hair goes into a state of limbo and is soon shed. The follicle rests for three to four months before hair growth recommences. Fortunately these phases are randomly distributed among the 300,000 scalp hair follicles so that only 50–300 hairs are shed each day.

The most common reason for hair loss is the influence of male hormones, which shorten the growing phase and lengthen the resting phase. It is this, plus family tendencies, that accounts for the severity and age of onset of male hair loss.

From the menopause onward, women experience hair loss for similar reasons, as the male hormones become more predominant in their system. Women can also lose a lot of hair after pregnancy, because abnormally large numbers of follicles enter the shedding phase.

Any serious generalized illness may cause hair loss. Other possible causes of a diffuse hair loss are an underactive thyroid gland (see THYROID PROBLEMS), iron deficiency, **eczema** of the scalp, ringworm, **systemic lupus erythematosus** and the side effects of chemotherapy (see page 371).

Hair loss can occur as a result of different types of trauma. This can include chemical damage from perms and hair colouring, heat treatments, brushes that snag the hair, pulling the hair tightly and extreme stress and shock.

Localized hair loss (alopecia areata) is thought to have an auto-immune origin, with a strong family association. Occasionally alopecia extends to complete loss of all body hair.

SYMPTOMS

Male pattern baldness starts at the temples, spreading to involve the rest of the scalp margins and then the crown. It follows a similar pattern in women, although at an older age, and can cause much distress. Alopecia areata is characterized by areas of complete hair loss within otherwise normal hairs. A moth-eaten appearance suggests infection of the scalp.

Except in cases of classic male hair loss or localized alopecia, you should have tests performed in order to exclude thyroid disease, auto-immune conditions and **anaemia**.

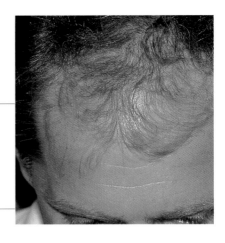

Right: Male pattern baldness: hair recedes from the temples, leaving a fine down.

TREATMENT

Not all hair loss needs treating. If it follows severe illness or pregnancy, regrowth can be expected after the follicles have had their three to four months' rest. Small areas of hair loss may respond to steroid lotions or steroid injections.

Treatment of larger areas is a triumph of hope over evidence although, of course, hormone or iron deficiencies must be dealt with. Steroid lotions may help. Minoxidil, a drug originally used for high blood pressure, stimulates regrowth in about one-third of cases, but has to be used continuously.

Other alternatives include hair transplants, which take hair from the back of the scalp and replant it in the frontal area, as well as wigs and hair pieces.

QUESTIONS

Can hair regrow after alopecia?
It often does after several months or a year. The new hair is initially unpigmented, growing as a white patch. Pigmentation comes in after some months.

Why does shock cause hair loss?
It stimulates loss at one go of all those hairs that have stopped growing but are yet to be shed. This leads to an alarming thinning, but hair can be expected to recover after a few months.

 Complementary Treatment
Complementary therapies will not be able to restore lost hair. **Chinese herbalism** – see DERMATITIS. **Aromatherapy** can help if baldness is stress induced. Make up a massage oil for the scalp using the following, alone or in combination: wheatgerm, juniper berry, jojoba, lavender, rosemary or chamomile (three drops in 10 ml carrier oil). **Western herbalism** – herbal shampoos made from catnip, nettle or thyme can stimulate growth.

SKIN TAGS

♦

Tiny growths on the skin that are of cosmetic rather than medical importance.

CAUSES

♦

Constantly irritated skin often responds by forming small growths. These are most common in areas of greatest friction, typically around the collar. By middle age most people have several of these. They are also found in other less obvious sites of friction, such as the armpits, groin and the back.

Babies are sometimes born with small tags on their ears that have been left from the developmental process. These can be removed for cosmetic reasons if parents wish.

SYMPTOMS

♦

Skin tags are more of a cosmetic nuisance than one that causes symptoms. Sometimes they itch. Bleeding may occur if a lesion is torn off, but should stop quickly. Persistent bleeding in a lesion that does not disappear is suspicious and requires further investigation.

TREATMENT

♦

This is only necessary if you are bothered by the lesion or if it is in an awkward place where it keeps getting rubbed. It can be frozen off or surgically excised under local anaesthetic.

QUESTION

Does it hurt to pick off skin tags?
A better remedy is to cut off the blood supply by tying fine thread around the tag – they drop off within days. Be sure that the tag has none of the suspicious features shown by skin cancer and is not where scarring would be unacceptable, for example on the face.

 Complementary Treatment
Ayurveda is an excellent therapy for skin problems; even someone with healthy skin should have full detoxification four times a year, with seasonal changes. See SCABIES for further details.

SKIN LUMPS, BUMPS AND MOLES

♦

Most skin lumps and moles are completely harmless and do not need treatment.

CAUSES

♦

Any of the cells of the skin may multiply in benign growths. In general the larger the lump the less likely it is to be malignant. The most common growths are from fat cells, called lipomas, and sebaceous glands, called sebaceous cysts. Many other types of firm lumps can be seen in the skin or felt inside it, for example at sites of previous injury.

Some people have an inherited tendency to lumps, for example neurofibromas from nerve fibres, or lipomas.

SYMPTOMS

♦

There is a smooth nodule in or on the skin. The skin is unbroken and does not bleed or crust. The lesion may be colourless or red from blood vessels in it. If it grows at all it is very slowly. The term mole refers to any coloured skin lump that is not a wart.

TREATMENT

♦

Lumps can be removed, but the size of scar might not make it worthwhile. An exception is for lipomas, which can grow large and unsightly, or sebaceous cysts, which often get infected.

QUESTION

When should a lump be biopsied?
If it grows steadily, itches, is crusted, bleeds or changes colour. Size is no guide – often smaller lesions are more suspicious than larger ones. Biopsy may be warranted for lesions that are unusually hard or have irregular pigmentation.

 Complementary Treatment
WARNING: Do not massage directly over the lump or bump. Diet – a **nutritional therapist** or a **naturopath** could advise you if food intolerance is a contributing factor for skin lumps and bumps.

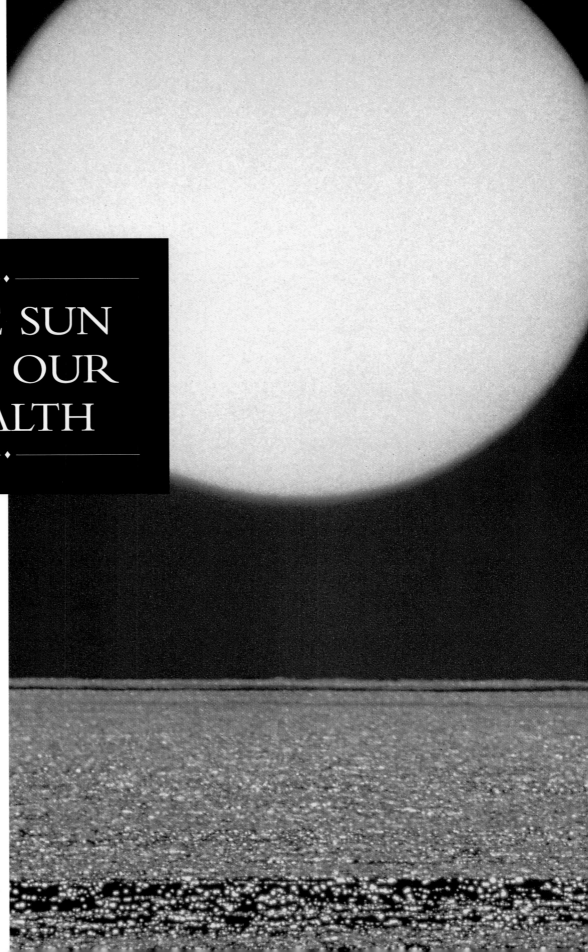

THE SUN AND OUR HEALTH

We need the light provided by the sun but in terms of health there can be too much of a good thing.

M UCH OF THE SUN'S ENERGY hits the earth as heat: part is visible light, part is ultraviolet light. Ultraviolet light causes sunburn on brief intense exposure. Long-term modest exposure ages the skin and predisposes to **skin cancer** in white people. Cloud and humidity are partially protective, otherwise we would risk burning even during the winter.

The fashionable tan

In response to sunlight – or artificial ultraviolet light – the skin tans. Cells called melanocytes produce increased amounts of a pigment known as melanin. Melanin protects against burning from the sun's rays, but does not abolish the risks of long-term damage from sunlight.

Until the 20th century it was actually unfashionable to have a tan. The classic hero or heroine was pale and wan. Even in naturally sunny countries, being pale carried a social cachet by implying that you were wealthy enough not to have to work in the sun.

Now a tan says the complete opposite: not that you have to labour from dawn to dusk but quite the contrary – that you can lounge in the sun at any time of year. And, as a result of foreign travel, we are exposed to sun of an intensity for which many of us are unprepared. The last few decades have also seen a gradual increase in average temperatures, with warmer summers. Because of these factors white skins are exposed to more sun than they can handle (black and brown-skinned people being protected by their natural melanin).

The benefits of sunshine

Humans need light and those who lack daylight suffer. The recently described seasonal affective disorder appears to be a real depression caused by lack of sunshine during the winter months which responds to artificial daylight from light boxes. This treatment works possibly by stimulating the pineal gland in the brain, and/or by increasing serotonin levels.

Sunshine and vitamin D Vitamin D, which is necessary for calcium balance, is formed by the action of sunshine on the skin. Not much exposure is needed – just a few minutes a day to the forearms is sufficient. Without this people are at risk of rickets, especially dark-skinned people having a poor intake of calcium and vitamin D from milk and dairy products.

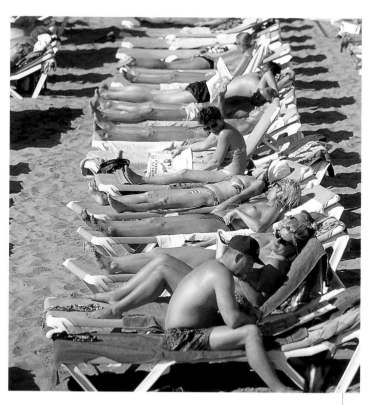

Above: Sunbathing is a fairly recent but enthusiastically followed pastime, which carries a major health risk.

Skin disease Sunlight helps several diseases, especially **psoriasis** and **acne**; some sufferers from **eczema** derive similar benefit. So useful is this that one treatment for psoriasis is to use an ultraviolet light box.

The drawbacks

Sunburn is a true burn, with tissue destruction, and it happens a few hours after exposure to sun. Severe and repeated sunburn in childhood increases the risk of malignant melanoma (see SKIN CANCER).

Sensitivity rashes Many individuals have a sensitivity to ultraviolet light and react with redness, rashes and itch. Unlike sunburn, this reaction occurs after just brief exposure to strong sunshine. Many substances and drugs increase the sensitivity of the skin and worsen this type of reaction, for example perfumes, certain plants (wild parsley being one), drugs such as oxytetracycline and thiazide water tablets. A few rare illnesses are notable for light sensitivity, for example **systemic lupus erythematosus** and porphyria.

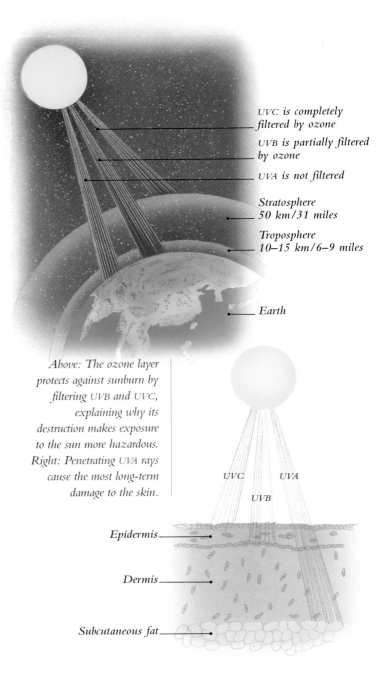

UVC is completely filtered by ozone

UVB is partially filtered by ozone

UVA is not filtered

Stratosphere 50 km/31 miles

Troposphere 10–15 km/6–9 miles

Earth

Above: The ozone layer protects against sunburn by filtering UVB and UVC, explaining why its destruction makes exposure to the sun more hazardous. Right: Penetrating UVA rays cause the most long-term damage to the skin.

UVC   UVA

UVB

Epidermis

Dermis

Subcutaneous fat

Ageing skin Relentless exposure to radiation damages collagen and permanently alters the cells of the skin. Eventually the skin is prematurely aged – dry, wrinkled, tough-looking and with colour variations.

Skin cancers The risk of skin cancer is very high for white people living in high-sunshine areas. Fortunately, the majority of cases are relatively benign cancers (squamous or basal cell) and comparatively few are aggressive (malignant melanoma).

The risk of squamous or basal cell cancers reflects the total lifetime exposure to ultraviolet light. They are common in outdoor workers such as farmers and fishermen, appearing on the face and back of the hand as small persistent areas of

rough skin or small ulcers. Although common – skin cancer has reached epidemic proportions in Australia, South Africa and parts of the United States – they are nearly always curable by freezing or surgical removal and serious spread is rare.

Malignant melanoma is a different problem altogether. These dark skin patches are aggressive and infiltrate the skin. Worse, they spread to other parts of the body, especially the liver, and the risk of death is high. Melanomas have become more common due, most specialists believe, to our increased tendency to expose ourselves to sunshine. Another factor may be that raised public awareness sends people to seek help sooner for early suspicious skin change.

Certain people are at a higher risk of melanoma: the fair-skinned and blue-eyed, and those who were severely sunburnt in childhood. People who sunbathe occasionally but inten-

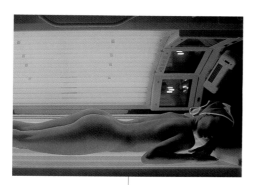

Above: Regular use of sunbeds can pose risks as strong as exposure to tropical sunshine.

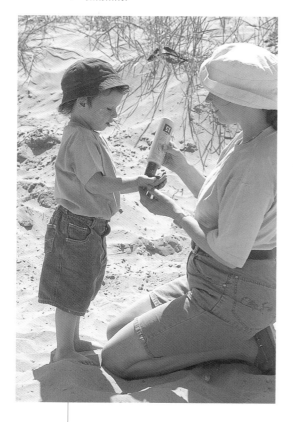

Above: Sensible precautions allow children to play outdoors while reducing later risks of skin cancer.

sively are probably at higher risk than people who are exposed to the sun more regularly. Anyone with more than a hundred moles runs a higher risk, but freckles are not a risk factor.

Sun creams

Sun creams containing titanium reflect or completely block ultraviolet light and do not allow tanning. For tanning as well as protection you need a cream or lotion that only partially absorbs ultraviolet light. The degree of protection is expressed as a factor number. For example, Factor 6 means you could stay exposed for six times longer than the length of time at which unprotected skin would burn. Factor 6 or higher gives reasonable protection but in extreme sunlight you need Factor 25 or higher.

Ordinary sun screens protect against medium-wavelength ultraviolet light (ultraviolet B), which causes sunburn. They do not protect against longer-wavelength ultraviolet light (ultraviolet A) which, while not causing sunburn, does cause long-term skin ageing and cancer. For complete protection either cover up or use sun screens that protect against both UVB and UVA.

SUN PROTECTION – DO'S AND DON'TS

Do . . .

♦ *Encourage your children to enjoy being outdoors, but to wear protective clothing, sun hats and sun screen; the greater their exposure to sun, the greater their risk of skin cancer 20 or more years later*
♦ *Wear cotton or silk; it is a better barrier than looser weaves*
♦ *Cover your limbs or use sun screen*
♦ *Watch your skin and report unusual changes to a doctor*

Don't . . .

♦ *Swim at midday, thinking water protects your back; it does not*
♦ *Have short intensive sunbathing holidays, especially if you are fair-skinned or have more than a hundred moles*
♦ *Forget to renew your sun screen after swimming and after every few hours*
♦ *Use ultraviolet sunbeds all year long. Excessive use is more damaging to the skin than lying under the African sun*

SKIN CANCER

One of the most common forms of cancer, and on the increase.

CAUSES

The main types of skin cancer are squamous cell, malignant melanoma and basal cell. The first two cancers are stimulated by sunlight or weather beating on the skin; environmental factors are less important with basal cell cancers.

Squamous cell cancer begins in the surface layer of skin in areas of chronic irritation, such as the face, parts of the body previously irradiated for cancer or skin exposed to chemicals. They may arise in skin irritated by **varicose veins** or leg **ulcers**.

A malignant melanoma arises from pigment cells deeper in the skin. Skin that has been severely sunburnt at some time may carry the increased risk of malignancy years later. Certain individuals inherit a tendency to pigmented patches on their body, which carry a small risk of turning malignant.

Basal cell cancer arises from cells in the epidermis for reasons similar to squamous cell cancer. Another type of skin cancer is Kaposi's sarcoma. This is a malignant nodule that was once very rare but is now common in people with **AIDS**.

SYMPTOMS

Basal and squamous cell cancers occur most often by the eyes and on the ears. They are persistently crusted patches a few millimetres in diameter and may stand slightly proud of the skin. They are painless and do not normally bleed.

A malignant melanoma is a deeply pigmented patch in or just proud of the skin. It often itches and may bleed. A malignant melanoma can occur anywhere on the body, including the neck and the soles of the feet. Individuals may have many pigmented spots, but a subtle change in colour or itch may single one out in particular.

Kaposi's sarcoma looks like a bruise that becomes darker and raised; it may occur in several sites at once.

TREATMENT

Basal and squamous cell cancers are treated by surgical removal, irradiation or, most recently, by chemotherapy creams, with very high cure rates. If neglected, they damage local tissues extensively, requiring skin grafting. It is unusual for them to spread distantly (metastasize), but if this happens the metastases are removed or treated with radiotherapy.

A melanoma always has to be cut out for analysis in order to see how deeply it has invaded the skin, because this

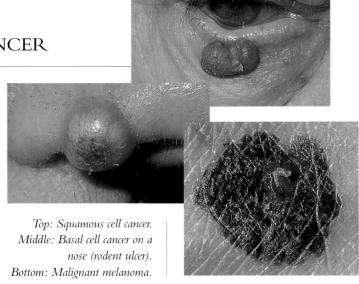

Top: Squamous cell cancer.
Middle: Basal cell cancer on a nose (rodent ulcer).
Bottom: Malignant melanoma.

WARNING SIGNS OF MALIGNANT SKIN CHANGE

- *Itching, bleeding or colour change in a pre-existing spot*
- *A persistently crusted lesion, especially on the face or the back of the hands*
- *A mole that turns dark and starts to itch*
- *A mole in a position where it keeps getting irritated*
- *A dark, newly appeared spot on the soles of the feet*
- *A patch of dry skin on the face that never goes away*
- *Having multiple moles (more than 100)*

determines the outlook. If it is less than 1 mm/³⁄₆₄ in deep, the cure rate is greater than 90%. The deeper the melanoma invades, the wider the margin around the lesion must be cut out. In more advanced disease chemotherapy is given to the affected limb. Unfortunately generalized radiotherapy or chemotherapy does not appear to be very effective.

Treatment of Kaposi's sarcoma is by radiotherapy or chemotherapy, despite which recurrence is common.

Complementary Treatment

Any changes in the skin must be seen by an orthodox practitioner. Complementary therapies cannot cure cancer, but can have a supportive role during orthodox treatment. **Chakra balancing** helps with symptom control and energy balance, promotes relaxation during orthodox treatment and offers support during rehabilitation programmes. It is especially good at helping the healing of skin grafts. **Massage** can be very supportive, especially when it is combined with **aromatherapy**. *Other therapies to try: see* STRESS.

ULCERS

The outermost surface of an area of skin which has broken down and does not heal within a few days.

CAUSES

There are two broad reasons for this breakdown: problems with venous blood flow or problems with arterial blood flow.

Venous ulcers

The blood returning to the heart through the venous system is depleted of oxygen and carries other waste products from the tissues. Anything interfering with this return of blood predisposes to stagnation, lack of oxygen and tissue breakdown. Common causes are **varicose veins** and previous **deep vein thrombosis** in a limb.

Arterial ulcers

Here the cause is poor flow of fresh arterial blood because of disease of the arterial blood vessels, for example **high blood pressure**, **atherosclerosis** or **diabetes**.

Pressure sores (bed sores)

Constant unrelieved pressure closes the capillary circulation and leads to very rapid breakdown of skin.

Other causes

Several rare auto-immune illnesses cause ulcers and might be suspected because of the unusual appearance of the ulcer or characteristic symptoms elsewhere.

SYMPTOMS

Venous ulcers are found mainly on the lower leg and around the ankle. A central raw core, which can be quite large, is surrounded by an irregular margin; the skin is mottled with white and brown stains from abnormal blood leakage.

Arterial ulcers are also usually found on the legs and feet, although these tend not to be on the ankles. These ulcers are smaller, with more sharply defined edges. The limb has other features of poor blood flow such as absent pulses and thin, hairless skin. If there is doubt, blood flow can be assessed by sound scanning devices called Dopplers.

Pressure sores are found directly over the bony parts of the hips, back and ankles. They can be very deep, even extending into muscles and bone.

The smell of infected ulcers comes from particular bacteria that inhabit the oxygen-starved environment.

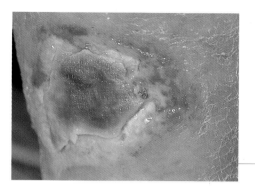

Left: A chronic leg ulcer will take many months to heal.

TREATMENT

Treat a small ulcer with antiseptic cream, but if it persists, see a doctor to exclude other diseases and to have it dressed by a nurse who has particular expertise in ulcer treatment.

An ulcer must be kept clean with antiseptic solutions and treated with an antibiotic if there is resistant infection, suggested by surrounding redness and pus and confirmed with swabs. A dressing should be worn both to allow air to get to the ulcer and to provide a protective cover that soaks up discharge without sticking to the ulcer. This encourages new skin to grow, which is not pulled off when the dressing is changed.

For venous ulcers it is important to improve blood flow by keeping the legs raised and by wearing stockings or bandages which compress the leg. These may have to be worn permanently. Such treatment is inappropriate for arterial ulcers, as compression would reduce blood flow. Where necessary, arterial flow is improved by arterial grafts or varicose veins are surgically removed. It is possible to put skin grafts on to otherwise resistant ulcers. The individual should keep as active as possible and be on a good diet to encourage healing.

Once a bed sore has developed, the pressure must be relieved to help it heal. Change the individual's position every two to three hours, and strategically place cushions and sheepskin on, between or under affected areas.

     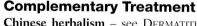

Complementary Treatment

Chinese herbalism – see DERMATITIS. **Reflexology** is an especially good therapy for leg ulcers. **Naturopathy** treatment would be based on nutrition and dietetics, especially cleansing programmes with fasting. Exercise – after recovery, **yoga** and **tai chi/chi kung** are both gentle forms of exercise which can be beneficial. **Ayurveda** – see SCABIES. *Other therapies to try: Western herbalism; homeopathy.*

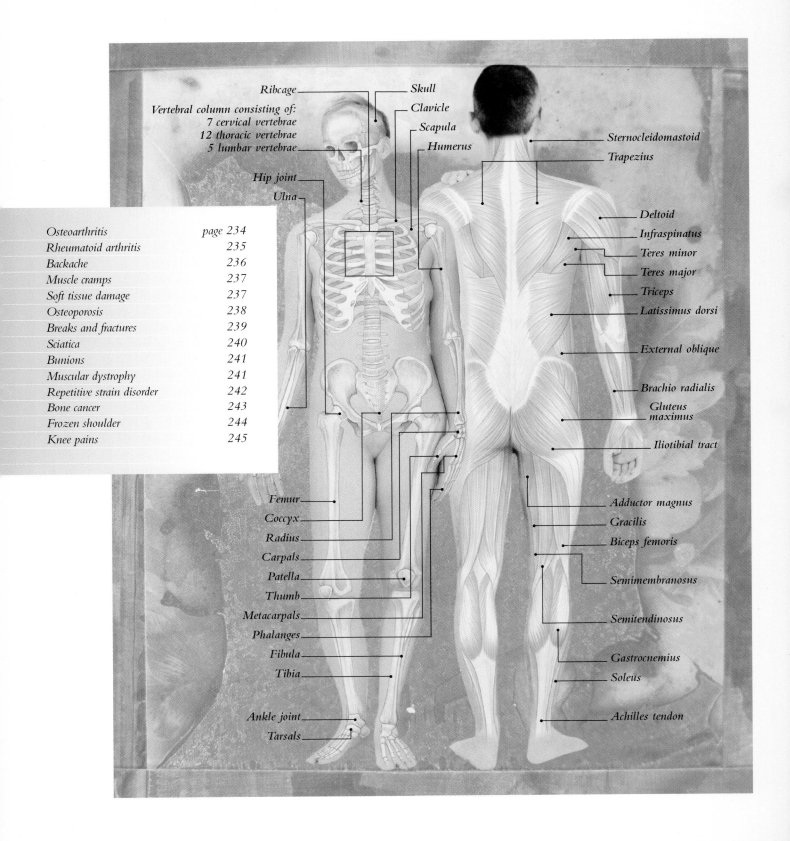

If our sophisticated internal organs, blood vessels, nerves and pipework are not to collapse, something has to keep them supported. This something is the bony skeleton, which is like a building's girders providing support for the walls and floors.

MUSCULO-SKELETAL SYSTEM

A LTHOUGH THE SKELETON can be likened to structural girders, buildings are not noted for walking. Such activity in humans requires another system – that of muscles, tendons and ligaments to convey movement to bones. The nervous system is the interface between brain and body, transmitting the brain's demands for movement to the muscles and thence to bone.

Bone

Bones consist of a tough outer cortex a few millimetres thick and a more sponge-like interior. Most bones end in cartilage, a plastic-like material that lets bone move against bone without grating. Bones seen after death give the impression of being completely inert structures, but this is misleading. Most parts of the bone are actively replacing and remodelling. Bones heal from fractures thanks to cells which throw out fresh material to knit the fracture together, followed by specialized cells which remodel the bone to its correct shape.

Within the hollow interior is the bone marrow, a tremendously active environment where much of the blood is made – the red and white blood cells and the platelets so important in blood clotting. It is this dynamic activity which makes the bone marrow susceptible to disease and poisons. It is where **leukaemia** begins and where drugs that affect bone marrow have their devastating effect.

The two main problems that affect bones and joints (apart from **breaks and fractures**) are **osteoarthritis** and **osteoporosis**. Bone infections are relatively uncommon. **Bone cancer** is also uncommon but secondary cancer frequently spreads from cancer elsewhere. Bone diseases are intimately connected with the metabolism of calcium and phosphate and are affected by several hormones – parathyroid hormone, calcitonin, thyroid, growth hormone and vitamin D, which is necessary for the absorption and deposition of calcium.

Muscle

Muscle is tissue that is specialized for the process of turning energy into movement. There are three types: skeletal muscle, which is considered here, heart muscle and lastly smooth muscle, which is the type of muscle surrounding hollow structures like the intestines and bladder.

Seen under magnification skeletal muscle is made of array after array of fibres, each composed of innumerable microfibres. These in turn are composed of the special proteins actin and myosin, which have the property of contracting when stimulated to do so by an electrical signal. Movement is transmitted from the muscle to bone through tendons, which are fibrous bands that grow from muscle into bone.

Muscle is everywhere in the body, from the minute muscles in the ear to the great back muscles, all of which are under electrical nerve control. The degree of nervous control varies so that, for example, the fine muscles of the eye can be moved more precisely than the thigh muscles. In the case of the latter, power is more important than delicacy of movement. Muscle is a reliable structure and disease of muscle is comparatively uncommon, compared to diseases of the nerve control. However, injury to muscle is very common through accidents or overuse, as are strains or ruptures of tendons.

Left: Muscle power pulls tendons and ligaments, moving the bones and joints which turn thought into action.

OSTEOARTHRITIS

◆

Painful joints caused by 'wear and tear'.

CAUSES

◆

Arthritis, technically called osteoarthritis, is virtually inevitable as people grow older. Although the joints of the body are amazingly resilient, after decades they become worn. The cartilage lining the joint frays, outgrowths of bone form around the joint in an attempt at healing and fragments of bone break off and irritate the joints, which themselves lose their natural lubrication, tending to become stiff and creaky.

Osteoarthritis is hastened by any trauma to a joint, such as accidents, **breaks and fractures** or prolonged overuse through work or exercise such as jogging. There is a strong hereditary tendency, too. Being overweight often hastens osteoarthritis of the weight-bearing joints of the hips and knees. It is a non-inflammatory condition. There is no actual disease process attacking the joint, as is the case with **gout** or **rheumatoid arthritis** (blood tests can be done if these are a possibility).

Although everyone thinks of osteoarthritis as a disease of the bone, it is more a disease of the cartilage that caps bones, which splits and degenerates until eventually bone is rubbing against bone. The deformation of osteoarthritis is caused by overgrowth of bone attempting to repair damaged cartilage. However, research is suggesting that there may be ways in the future to slow down cartilage breakdown, if not reverse it.

SYMPTOMS

◆

The joints most commonly affected are the hips, knees, neck, back and the small joints of the fingers. They become stiff and may creak. It takes time to get them moving each morning and damp weather worsens the pain. As osteoarthritis of the hip progresses, pain in the joint may stop patients sleeping.

The fingers and knees become distorted as bone grows around the joint. It is common to have flare-ups of pain and stiffness from time to time and the joints may swell with fluid.

TREATMENT

◆

Despite mild pain, it it best to keep using the joints, otherwise they stiffen even more. Exercise strengthens the muscles supporting the affected joints, relieving some of the pressure on them. Exercise should be gentle and not put sudden stress on joints such as running. Keeping joints warm also helps reduce pain. Excess weight must be reduced, especially for osteoarthritis of the hips or knees, which take all the body's weight.

Pain relief

It is best to use the mildest painkiller that is effective. For many this will be paracetamol, possibly with some aspirin or codeine. Non-steroidal anti-inflammatory drugs (NSAIDs) are useful for severe pain or to give prolonged relief. Which drug suits which individual is often a matter of trial and error, and previously effective drugs can lose their effect in time.

Heat treatment such as wax baths can be given as part of a physiotherapy programme. Sudden pain in the joint can be helped by a steroid injection.

Surgery

Surgical replacements of the hip and knee can, in selected cases, bring relief of pain and disability. Hip replacement relieves pain and restores mobility in at least 95% of cases. Only in relatively few cases does it make little difference, and rarely makes things worse. At present hip replacements last at least ten years. Less common, but possible, is to replace the shoulder or the small joints of the fingers. These operations are becoming more routine.

QUESTIONS

Is pain a measure of severity?
Severely distorted joints may be relatively pain free and vice versa. Even X-rays may be misleading – hips that look dreadful on an X-ray can cause no pain. Doctors have to go by what patients report to them in assessing treatment.

How safe are painkillers?
Paracetamol or co-proxamol are safe at recommended dosages; high dosages damage the liver. Non-steroidal anti-inflammatory drugs (NSAIDs) often cause indigestion, rashes and diarrhoea. The latest ones do this less but still should be taken as little as possible.

Complementary Treatment

Chiropractic manipulation, mobilization and soft tissue techniques are effective in increasing joint mobility and reducing pain. **Aromatherapy** and **massage** with an oil made up of one of the following can help: black pepper, ginger, frankincense, rosemary, lavender, marjoram or juniper oil (three drops in 10 ml carrier oil). **Acupuncture** is very effective in the early stages of the disease. **Alexander Technique** – see BACKACHE. *Other therapies to try: most have something to offer.*

RHEUMATOID ARTHRITIS

An auto-immune condition, with inflammation and distortion of the joints.

CAUSES

Unlike **osteoarthritis**, rheumatoid arthritis is an aggressive disease, which often leads to destruction of joints and considerable disability. Research points to it being an auto-immune condition, one in which the body's protective mechanisms turn against its own tissues. In rheumatoid arthritis the target tissue is called synovium, a membrane that lines joints and provides a lubricating synovial fluid. The synovium is invaded by cells that normally protect against infections. An array of destructive biochemicals is released, causing the synovium to swell. These biochemicals attack nearby cartilage, leading eventually to distortion of the joints.

Three-quarters of sufferers are women in whom the disease starts in their 30s and 40s. It affects 2% of the population worldwide, often those with a family history. About 10% of people end with considerable disability, but by contrast 40% experience only intermittent trouble; the rest have mild to moderate problems. Progression of the disease can take years, and in any case about 25% of cases eventually 'burn out' for reasons not understood.

SYMPTOMS

Rheumatoid arthritis is an illness that is remarkable for affecting not only the joints but many other organs, too. The disease fluctuates in its intensity. It usually begins in an undramatic form, starting with discomfort and swelling of the small joints of the hands or feet; in 25% of cases only a single joint is affected. Eventually the same joints are affected on both sides of the body with pain and stiffness, which is worse in the morning and lasts for several hours. Gradually deformity and weakness of the affected limbs appears. Often people with rheumatoid arthritis feel generally unwell.

Other joints affected may include the knees, shoulders and hips, but not the back. Over time the joints become deformed in a highly characteristic way: the fingers look spindly and fingers or toes distort away from the midline. The distorted and weakened tendons may snap.

Other symptoms include skin nodules and rashes, fluid accumulations in the lungs, **anaemia**, heart, kidney and nervous system problems, and inflamed or dry eyes.

Rheumatoid arthritis is diagnosed on a clinical picture that includes bilateral pain and characteristic deformity of small

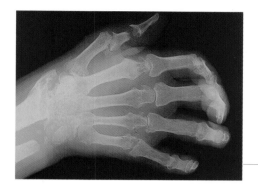

Left: Joints swollen by rheumatoid arthritis, with the fingers displaced to one side.

joints. The disease produces characteristic blood changes – a protein marker (rheumatoid factor) is positive in about 80% of cases, but a negative test does not rule it out.

TREATMENT

Exercise is beneficial at all stages, with physiotherapy encouraging people to use joints and limbs to the maximum.

Non-steroidal anti-inflammatory drugs (NSAIDs) are good for relieving pain and swelling; the choice is a matter of preference. The latest, called cox-2 inhibitors, e.g. rofecoxib, combine power with a lower risk of side effects. Splints are used to support the joints and tendons. Many get by on these methods but some require more powerful medication. In the past the next step was steroids by mouth. These dramatically reduce acute flare-ups but have many potential side effects. The trend is to use other medication that appears to alter the condition fundamentally – not just damp it down. These drugs, which tend to have more side effects than NSAIDs and need careful monitoring, include gold and sulphasalazine. The latest is methotrexate.

Orthopaedic surgeons can repair ruptured tendons, inject steroids into joints to reduce inflammation, replace joints, including finger joints, and operate on bones to reduce pain.

Complementary Treatment

In the early stages of the disease **acupuncture** can produce dramatic improvements, partly by helping regulate the immune system. **Nutritional therapy** – extra B complex vitamins, vitamins C and E and zinc are recommended. **Alexander Technique** – see BACKACHE. **Chiropractic** mobilization and soft tissue techniques can help ease pain and stiffness as part of an overall treatment regime. *Other therapies to try: cymatics; tai chi/chi kung; biodynamics; chakra balancing; healing.*

BACKACHE

The causes and treatment of backache are still a matter of controversy.

CAUSES

The high incidence of back problems in humans is probably a reflection of a fundamental design fault that has not entirely adapted the back to an upright position. There is disagreement on where such a fault may lie, and why pain arises in one person but not in another. The bones of the spinal column, the vertebrae, rest on each other, cushioned by fibrous discs, and join with each other via bony projections called pedicles. Tough ligaments surround the bones. The spinal cord runs through an arch of bone; nerves leave the spinal cord snaking past the discs and running close to the bony projections.

Mechanical causes of backache include any pre-existing malformation of the spine leading to unusual curvature, excess weight, pregnancy and physically demanding work – all put extra stress on the spine. In the not uncommon spondylolisthesis, vertebrae are misaligned on one another.

Bone disease accounts for an important minority of cases of backache. **Osteoporosis**, in itself pain free, may lead to the painful collapse of one vertebra. **Bone cancer** causes pain, although there are usually suggestive symptoms elsewhere. Infection of the spine, notoriously from tuberculosis, is now uncommon. The disease ankylosing spondylitis causes a painful, very inflexible back in young men.

In diagnosis, X-rays are over-rated as they can only show osteoporosis, expected changes from **osteoarthritis** and occasionally features of malignancy. The MRI scan is the best procedure for showing the bone, spinal cord and nerves (see page 351). If bone disease is suspected then doctors may order blood tests of inflammation and calcium balance. At least 30% of all cases will remain undiagnosed. Despite psychological strategies and self-help groups, some people remain unable to work and in constant pain for which little can be offered other than variations of painkillers.

SYMPTOMS

Pain is felt on getting up, bending or lifting, and the individual may limp. Pain radiating into the legs suggests **sciatica**. The pain is often sudden in onset and individuals have good and bad days. Pain that was gradual in onset and steadily worsens, is relatively unrelated to movement and present day and night, suggests a secondary cancer or other bone disease. Examination reveals little apart from restricted movement.

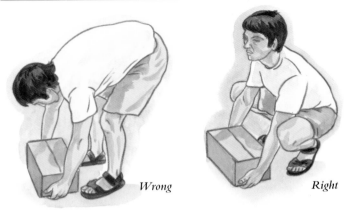

Wrong   *Right*

Above: It is important to lift using the power of your legs and shoulders rather than your back. Keep the object close to your body.

TREATMENT

Severe back pain forces you to rest for a few days but you should start moving again as soon as you can. This replaces the old advice to rest until pain free. Physiotherapy or osteopathy are helpful, encouraging mobilization and showing you correct ways to move. Take the simplest painkillers that give relief – paracetamol alone or with codeine or anti-inflammatories. Muscle spasms can be helped by a relaxant such as diazepam. Do not underestimate the value of a hot bath or a warm pad. Where there is no serious underlying disease, take painkillers for flare-ups and be careful lifting and carrying.

An epidural corticosteroid injection reduces pain and speeds recovery. It is worthwhile in sciatica not responding to routine treatment. Less than 1% of patients with back pain require surgery; procedures range from the removal of the prolapsed disc (microdiscectomy) to a spinal operation to fuse the vertebrae so they cannot move and cause pain.

Complementary Treatment

The **Alexander Technique** leads to release of over-contracted muscles, a freeing up of the joints and a lengthening of the spine, all of which reduce mechanical strain. **Chiropractic** manipulation is particularly useful for general, non-specific back pain. **Osteopathy** is effective and one of the least invasive treatments for backache. **Hellerwork** relieves symptoms by organizing the whole body structure with respect to gravity. **Rolfing** improves spinal alignment and posture. *Other therapies to try: acupuncture; aromatherapy.*

MUSCLE CRAMPS

Benign spasms in muscle, usually in the leg.

CAUSES

Cramps follow vigorous exertion when waste products accumulate in muscle. Although this explains the cramps of a marathon runner it does little to illuminate the night cramps that affect the elderly and others, for instance those who have cramps plus restless legs (Ekbom's syndrome).

Some people have particularly sensitive muscles, with points of more exquisite tenderness called trigger points. This condition is called fibromyalgia. This is not a disease, although the condition can certainly be very distressing.

Only rarely are cramps caused by an underlying abnormality; the most important to consider are poor blood circulation and, less often, disorders of calcium balance.

SYMPTOMS

A muscle, usually in the leg, goes into a spasm of contraction; the toes may be pulled over. The cramp lasts just a few minutes. Pain after exertion which recurs when an individual is re-exercising suggests a blood flow problem.

TREATMENT

Quinine tablets at night are widely used and effective; beware taking excessive amounts as they can affect the heartbeat. Muscle relaxants like diazepam are helpful, as are anti-inflammatory gels rubbed on to the muscles. Exercises and massage can also be tried to stretch the affected muscles.

QUESTION

What is Ekbom's syndrome?
This refers to restless legs – legs continuously moving whether or not you want them to, a symptom allied to night cramps. It is sometimes caused by iron-deficiency anaemia. If anaemia has been treated, other medication to use includes diazepam and phenytoin.

Complementary Treatment
Chiropractic – soft tissue techniques are effective with muscular cramps brought on by overuse and sporting injuries. **Western herbalism** – cramp bark is a muscle relaxant. *Other therapies to try: most have something to offer.*

SOFT TISSUE DAMAGE

Injury to muscles, tendons or ligaments, as opposed to bones or joints.

CAUSES

Soft tissues mean muscle, ligaments (the tough strips connecting bone, for example around the knee joint) and tendons (strips where muscle attaches to bone, for example the tendons of the fingers). Injury occurs through overstretching from sport, exercise and awkward movements and direct blows caused by accidents. Occasionally, other pre-existing illness can cause inflammation, for example arthritis.

SYMPTOMS

The affected structure is painful and tender. It swells, often very rapidly, and as a result there is restriction of movement of the affected limb. Complete inability to use a joint or deformity suggest a more serious rupture or tear of soft tissue.

TREATMENT

Most injuries are self-limiting, settling over a few days or weeks; they require only care in use of the affected limb and rubbing in of an anti-inflammatory gel or taking an anti-inflammatory tablet. More chronic problems often respond to a steroid injection into the tender area and physiotherapy with heat treatment or ultrasound, as well as exercises to restrengthen the muscles around the affected soft tissues. You should also consider changes to sports technique and avoid any repetitive strain.

Complementary Treatment
Chiropractic is effective in the treatment of injuries anywhere in the body. **Osteopathy** techniques effect a maximum rate of healing. **Hellerwork** – see BACKACHE. **Rolfing** is a therapy that aids mobility; this helps new tissues to build and helps joints to function in appropriate alignment.

OSTEOROSIS

Thinning of bone, with an increased risk of fractures.

CAUSES

Whereas osteoporosis used to be regarded simply as an inevitable result of ageing, increasingly it is being targeted for prevention and treatment. There is now recognition of its consequences in terms of fractures, hospital admissions and deaths. The bulk of bone is calcium and phosphorus regulated by an extremely complex system, including parathyroid hormone and vitamin D, which is necessary to absorb calcium. Large amounts of vitamin D are produced by the action of sunlight on the skin; the rest comes from dairy products.

Thin bones
Each year some 20% of the calcium in bone is replaced. For much of adult life this turnover is unimportant, but it becomes a major problem for menopausal women when their oestrogen levels fall. Calcium and phosphorus in bone is lost rapidly up to ten years after the menopause. Men suffer much less from it, but the more it is looked for the more it is also found.

Old age
Bone density, which peaks at the age of 30, continues to fall into the 70s and 80s with immobility contributing to this.

Steroids and other factors
People taking oral steroids for severe **asthma** or **rheumatoid arthritis** risk osteoporosis, a fact that is now more widely recognized. Others are at risk if they have a poor intake of calcium and get little exposure to sunlight. There are also several unusual hormone disorders that predispose to osteoporosis.

SYMPTOMS

Osteoporosis causes neither pain nor tenderness. Often the thin bones are discovered by chance during X-rays for some other reason. Otherwise it reveals itself when a weakened bone fractures. If this happens in the vertebrae there is sudden severe **backache**; the other common sites are hips and wrists. Gradually, the individual becomes shorter through loss of height of the vertebrae and shrinkage of the intervertebral discs, and the back bends into the so-called dowager's hump.

A bone scan called a dexa-scan determines the degree of osteoporosis and is helpful in deciding whether treatment is wise and also whether it is working. Blood tests may be advisable to exclude the rarer causes of osteoporosis.

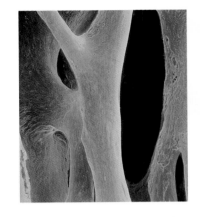
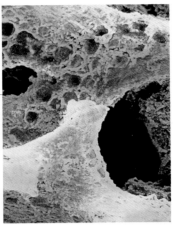

Above: Osteoporotic bone; the many small, round, dark areas are empty, causing brittleness. Left: Normal bone.

TREATMENT

For menopausal women the best treatment is hormone replacement therapy (HRT), which reduces the rate of bone density loss (see page 20). This is even more important for women having an early menopause or who have previously had oral steroids, who are immobile or smoke or drink excessively – all factors further increasing the risks of osteoporosis.

Diet and vitamin D
To build and maintain bones, women should have a diet rich in calcium and vitamin D and stay active throughout their life. Both women and men should take at least 1.5 g a day of calcium, plus vitamin D supplements if they are housebound and getting no sunlight. The same treatment applies to men and women with established osteoporosis of old age.

Medication
Drugs such as etidronate and alendronate improve osteoporosis by reducing activity of the cells in the bones which otherwise remodel it. Though inconvenient to take, they are effective.

Complementary Treatment
Nutritional therapy – as well as lack of calcium, magnesium deficiency can be a contributing factor; zinc supplements could be helpful, together with a daily intake of ground sesame seeds and comfrey leaves. **Chiropractic** soft tissue techniques are frequently used to help ease the pain of spinal problems caused by osteoporosis; there is always muscle spasm in the area of the fracture, which causes pain. *Other therapies to try: chakra balancing; cymatics; tai chi/chi kung; shiatsu-do; Alexander Technique.*

BREAKS AND FRACTURES

There are many causes of bone injuries or malformations.

CAUSES

It is easy to think of bones as inert structures acting simply as girders for the body. However, bones are living things with vital roles in calcium metabolism and in forming the cells that circulate in the blood stream. It is because bones are living that fractures do heal, by regeneration of the broken surface.

Accidents account for most fractures, through either direct trauma or some repetitive stress that causes a bone to shear. In theory, any bone in the body can fracture; in practice it is the longer bones of the arm and thigh that are at greater risk through mechanical reasons. There are one or two small bones that fracture readily because of their shape. For example, the scaphoid bone at the base of the thumb can be fractured by a relatively minor fall on the hand.

Anything that weakens the bone increases the chances of it fracturing under normal stresses. **Osteoporosis**, which is the usual reason for this weakening of bone, leads to fractures of the vertebrae of the spine and the hip.

Many types of cancer spread around the body, or metastasize, and bone is a favoured target. The cancerous deposit weakens the bone, causing pain. It then takes just a little extra stress to make the bone fracture. Sites where this occurs most are the vertebrae and the long bones of the arms and the legs (see BONE CANCER).

SYMPTOMS

Following trauma, a bone feels tender and is painful to use. There may be obvious deformity of the limb and bruising over the site of injury. Less commonly, pain occurs spontaneously in the absence of obvious trauma. This most often happens in the case of collapse of a vertebra through osteoporosis or a stress fracture of one of the small bones of the feet.

A spontaneous fracture of a long bone raises suspicion of underlying bone disease or cancerous spread but it must be stressed that these are relatively uncommon.

X-rays confirm most fractures; sometimes subtle fractures need investigation with repeat X-rays or specialized scans.

TREATMENT

This depends on both the site and severity of the fracture. At the most severe, for example fracture of the hip or skull, immediate surgery is required to remove dead tissues and

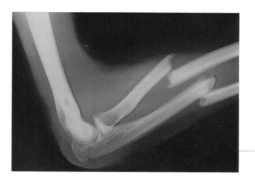

Left: A compound fracture of the forearm, which can be repaired only by surgery.

bone fragments, and to reset bones and fix them in place with screws or artificial replacements, as in the case of a hip joint. More often, bone has fractured in a clean break, requiring only realignment and fixing in position with a plaster cast or firm bandage while healing. Not all fractures need treating: a fractured rib or foot bone can usually be left to heal naturally. Often people need physiotherapy after a fracture in order to recover full use of the muscles around the fracture site.

QUESTIONS

How are fractures categorized?
Simple fractures are partial or complete breaks that just need re-setting without other surgical treatment. Compound fractures are where there are multiple bone fragments, damage to local flesh or opening of overlying skin. These need intensive surgery to reset and in order to avoid infection.

How long does healing take?
Fractures of the upper limbs take three to six weeks to heal; lower limb fractures such as the thigh and tibia take six to twelve weeks. Any fracture may take a year or more to recover full strength.

Complementary Treatment
Alexander Technique – see BACKACHE. A **nutritional therapist** might suggest zinc and vitamin C supplements. **Chiropractic** – soft tissue techniques are often used after a break or fracture has healed to restore movement and help reduce soft tissue swelling, which may remain long after bone damage has healed. **Rolfing** – see SOFT TISSUE DAMAGE. *Other therapies to try: Chinese herbalism; acupuncture; cymatics; healing; Ayurveda; tai chi/chi kung; Western herbalism.*

SCIATICA

Pressure on a nerve, leading to backache and pain in the leg.

CAUSES

Sciatica in younger people probably follows partial slippage of a vertebral disc. The intervertebral discs are made up of a jelly-like core within a fibrous ring; a tear in this ring allows the contents to leak out and impinge upon the nerve roots. These coalesce to form the sciatic nerve, which runs down the back of the thigh into the calf and the foot. In older people the cause appears to be osteoarthritic outgrowths of bone that similarly irritate the nerves (see OSTEOARTHRITIS). The sciatic nerve is particularly affected because the vertebrae at the base of the spine – the lumbo-sacral region – are curved to a degree that increases the chances of a disc slipping. Sometimes there is a clear episode that precipitates sciatica; more often a minor exertion seems to bring it on or it appears out of the blue.

SYMPTOMS

The onset is usually acute with sudden severe low back pain, worse on coughing or straining and flexing the back. The pain radiates down the back of the thigh and calf and ends in the sole of the foot. This is classic sciatica but there are variations depending on exactly which nerves are being affected. For example, pain may radiate more over the side and back of the foot. Along with the pain there may be muscular weakness in a pattern that again reflects which nerves are irritated, for example weakness in pressing the foot down or extending the knee. The ritual of tapping out knee and ankle reflexes further determines which nerves are affected. Your doctor will check your straight leg raising, which means lifting your leg to see how high it can go without severe pain. Anything less than about 45° suggests significant pressure on the sciatic nerve.

Investigations are of little benefit at this stage unless examination suggests a serious disc slippage that might need surgery, or any other worrying symptoms of **backache**.

TREATMENT

Treatment overlaps with that of backache. Rest for a few days, then attempt as much movement as you can. Use painkillers, and muscle relaxants if muscle spasms are a problem. Doctors are reluctant to prescribe the most powerful and possibly addictive painkillers for what they know may be a chronic condition. Physiotherapy helps to mobilize the spine and it is also good for boosting confidence.

On this basis most episodes of sciatica will settle, many within a few weeks, but be prepared for full recovery to take three to twelve months. Persistent pain might be helped by a steroid injection into the spinal canal; this requires a general anaesthetic and the effects are often temporary.

In less than one in a hundred cases, symptoms point to a persistently slipped disc: constant pressure on nerves, paralysis of foot movements, interference with urinary control and unremitting pain. Here investigations with an MRI scan (see page 351) may confirm a seriously slipped disc and surgery might be appropriate. This aims to remove the slipped disc by surgically exposing the vertebrae or, as is increasingly done, by guided microdiscectomy, where fine instruments are guided to the disc through a small cut in the back.

QUESTIONS

Why do doctors ask about bladder control?
They want to know about bladder control even if the sciatica seems otherwise routine because you may lose the ability to control your bladder or your bowels and may require emergency disc surgery.

What investigations are available?
The MRI scan is the best for seeing how badly a disc is slipped (see page 351). Back X-rays are of little positive use, although many people find a normal plain X-ray reassuring. If bone disease is suspected, your doctor may suggest blood tests and a bone scan.

Why is surgery done so infrequently?
Since about 80% of episodes of sciatica recover within a few weeks delay is prudent. Although 95% of selected disc surgery is successful, 5% of cases remain the same or get worse.

Complementary Treatment

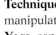

Acupuncture is a very powerful treatment. **Alexander Technique** is also useful – see BACKACHE. **Chiropractic** manipulation is an effective and speedy treatment. **Yoga** can be helpful, but must be undertaken only under the guidance of a suitably qualified teacher. **Osteopathy** can help if the cause is a prolapsed intervertebral disc or other spinal condition. **Hellerwork** – see BACKACHE. **Rolfing** corrects imbalances which can compress the sciatic nerve. *Other therapies to try: chakra balancing; shiatsu-do; naturopathy; cymatics; auricular therapy; Ayurveda.*

BUNIONS

A deformity of the big toe, very common to one degree or other.

CAUSES

A bunion is a 'lump' at the base of the big toe, which bends inward, cramping other toes. The lump is caused by outward displacement of the metatarsal bone in the foot itself. Adding to the deformity is a fluid-filled structure, a bursa, where toe and metatarsal meet, plus bony outgrowths. Heredity is thought to play the major part in this. Bunions mainly affect middle-aged people and, occasionally, adolescents.

SYMPTOMS

There may be none at all. Pain is possible from the pressure of footwear. The bursa itself may become inflamed or infected.

TREATMENT

Well-fitting footwear relieves any pain from the bunion and allows many people to put up with bunions if the appearance does not bother them unduly.

Otherwise treatment is surgical correction of the displaced bones, via one of a number of operations to trim different parts of the bones involved. They are quite successful, although they are rather painful at the time.

QUESTION

Do tight shoes cause bunions?
This is a question on which everyone has an opinion and few have a scientifically confirmed answer. Current orthopaedic opinion is that footwear does not play any significant role, even shoes that are narrow and pointed with high heels. Heredity is more likely to blame. Everyone, however, agrees that cramping footwear is best avoided if only for the sake of comfort.

Complementary Treatment

Chakra balancing promotes relaxation and pain control, and can lessen inflammation and improve healing of damaged tissue. **Cymatics** could help – consult a therapist. *Other therapies to try: chiropractic.*

MUSCULAR DYSTROPHY

Inherited disorders that can affect muscle function.

CAUSES

These disorders alter the way muscle grows, leading to weakness of certain muscles. The most common, Duchenne muscular dystrophy (DMD), affects one in three thousand newborn boys. The genetic defect causes abnormal entry of calcium into the muscle fibres because of lack of dystrophin, a protein in the muscle cell wall. Girls are carriers but are unaffected. DMD can be identified via a heel prick sample of blood from newborn boys. If positive, mothers can be offered screening of subsequent at-risk foetuses and abortion if desired. Female siblings of affected boys should also be tested to see if they carry the gene. There are no easy choices with this disease.

SYMPTOMS

In DMD the boy experiences leg weakness, which hampers normal walking and running; it is usually obvious by the age

of four. The calf muscles often look well developed. Later, other muscles become involved, including the heart muscle. Deterioration is inevitable, ending with heart and breathing problems; survival is unlikely beyond the age of 20. Other types affect the muscles of the shoulders, neck and hands. Most of these, other than DMD, follow a relatively benign path.

TREATMENT

Nothing arrests the progression of DMD, although steroids may slow it down. Physiotherapy helps avoid otherwise inevitable contractures of muscles. It is important to analyse the exact type of muscular dystrophy for an accurate outlook.

Complementary Treatment

Chiropractic treatment is often used as part of the overall treatment regime to help general joint and muscle movement and flexibility. **Ayurveda** oils are very powerful for improving wasted muscles; specific oil massages are recommended.

REPETITIVE STRAIN DISORDER

Apart from a few accepted syndromes, this problem, sometimes known as repetitive strain injury (RSI), is dogged by controversy.

CAUSES

Many tendons run for part of their course through insulating sheaths, which lubricate and guide them. If these tendons swell through excess use, they can 'snag' against the insulating sheath. This is best known in the fingers and thumbs, where it is called tenosynovitis. Different types of tenosynovitis have agreed symptoms and signs and even their own names, for example De Quervain's tenosynovitis of the thumb.

The concept of repetitive strain disorder (RSD) is more controversial, with its combination of non-specific tiredness and discomfort of the limb, especially the hands. This is because, unlike tenosynovitis, there are no identified abnormalities in the limb to account for the symptoms. Latest research is starting to show how pain links with muscle and tendon function.

Nevertheless, in many countries the law has stepped in where doctors fear to tread and it is now accepted as a condition associated with keyboard workers and assembly workers whose jobs involve repetitive wrist and finger movements.

SYMPTOMS

The pain of tenosynovitis overlies specific tendons, for example those of the fingers, often with red inflammation over them. The patient and doctor may feel a grating sensation on flexing those tendons. At worst the tendon fails to run freely at all through the sheath, moving instead in a series of painful jolts as it catches and breaks free. De Quervain's tenosynovitis involves pain on movement of the base of the thumb.

This contrasts with repetitive strain disorder where there is nothing to find on examination and where the diagnosis rests entirely on individuals, who may have overused their muscles and their tendons, reporting discomfort during work, which disappears on rest.

TREATMENT

Doctors first wish to exclude known treatable syndromes that cause hand and wrist pains, for example carpal tunnel syndrome, which is caused by compression of a nerve at the wrist where pain spreads in a characteristic way across several fingers. It may take electrical tests of nerve function to exclude this kind of problem. Carpal tunnel syndrome is treated by surgical release of the compressing band.

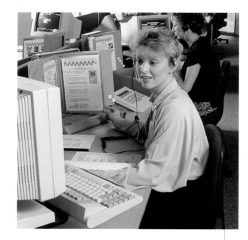

Above: Comfortable working positions are important for everyone, not only people with RSD.

Tenosynovitis responds initially to rest – perhaps aided by a splint on the wrist, the rubbing on of anti-inflammatory gels or taking anti-inflammatory tablets and physiotherapy. The next step is a steroid injection into the point of tenderness. Occasionally there is constant pain and a grating of tendons, for which the treatment is to open up the tendon sheath surgically, although sometimes symptoms recur.

This leaves a number of people with the vaguer complaints of RSD. For these, too, a short period (perhaps a few weeks) off work plus anti-inflammatory treatments may relieve symptoms. Their working practice needs assessing, preferably by a physiotherapist skilled in this area, who will be able to review the timing and length of breaks, and the working position. She might suggest, for example, a better chair or a work desk at a better level, or using a wrist support to help relieve discomfort from typing. Some people, however, still might find they are unable to cope with certain occupations.

Complementary Treatment

Acupuncture is most helpful in the early stages of the disorder. **Chiropractic** manipulation, mobilization and soft tissue techniques, alongside ergonomic advice, is very effective. **Yoga** is sometimes very effective. **Ayurveda** recommends regular oil massage. **Osteopathy** has achieved excellent results. **Rolfing** eases strain on joints and helps you to move them with less effort. *Other therapies to try: chakra balancing; shiatsu-do; Alexander Technique; cymatics; Hellerwork.*

BONE CANCER

Tumours of bone, usually spread there from cancer in other sites.

CAUSES

Cancers shed cells into the blood stream that are liable to lodge and grow in bones because bones have such a high blood flow. This is called secondary cancer. The cancers most likely to spread in this way are breast, lung and prostate cancer, although many others can do so. Tumours arising from within the bone itself, primary bone tumours, are extremely uncommon; they affect mainly children and young adults. Types include osteosarcoma and chondrosarcoma.

SYMPTOMS

The prime symptom is persistent and gnawing pain, often with tenderness over the site. Cancer pain feels worse at night, so night pain is an ominous symptom. That said, there are certain primary bone tumours that are painful but benign, and also other conditions that can cause bone pain, including injury and infection (osteomyelitis), which can be difficult to differentiate from cancer even after detailed scans.

There may be swelling over the cancer, especially with primary bone tumours. Sometimes the first sign of a cancer is when the weakened bone fractures under modest stress. However, many secondary bone tumours grow with minimal symptoms and are discovered only on investigation of cancers elsewhere following a bone scan. This is a routine test before planning treatment because the options will be different if the cancer has already spread into the bones, liver, lungs or brain.

Bone tumours affect the body's calcium balance and they release enzymes into the blood stream, which in turn can cause other symptoms such as excessive urine production, vomiting and **constipation**.

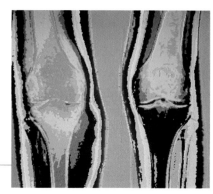

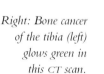

Right: Bone cancer of the tibia (left) glows green in this CT scan.

TREATMENT

In primary bone tumours the exact type of tumour needs to be established by biopsy to plan treatment, which now consists of replacing the diseased bone with metal implants; radiotherapy and chemotherapy are additional treatments (see pages 370 and 371). Secondary tumours are very serious, but something can still be done: radiotherapy can greatly reduce pain and preventive surgery can strengthen a long bone like the femur (thigh bone) that looks as if it might fracture.

Pain relief begins with anti-inflammatory drugs such as diclofenac or ibuprofen, which can be taken together with conventional painkillers such as paracetamol or dihydrocodeine. Eventually it may be necessary to turn to narcotic painkillers. The choice is increasingly wide, with morphine available as a liquid, in tablets and once-a-day preparations.

At the same time, treatment is given to the cancer from which the bone cancer has spread; chemotherapy for the primary may also reduce the pain from the secondary deposits.

The treatment of high calcium may be necessary to relieve excess urine production and constipation. The level of calcium is also a means of monitoring the response to treatment.

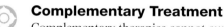

QUESTIONS

When should bone pain in children be taken seriously?
Without a clear history of injury, pain persisting for over a week or so should be assessed, especially if a bone appears swollen. Even so, the chances of it being due to a tumour are extremely low.

Why is bone cancer so difficult to cure?
Cure, even if possible, would require high doses of chemotherapy and radiotherapy, which would eradicate the vital bone marrow. Because the cancer is bound to have spread elsewhere, cure would still be improbable.

Complementary Treatment
Complementary therapies cannot cure cancer, but can make a valuable contribution during orthodox treatment. **Chakra balancing** can promote relaxation and pain control, and offer support during orthodox treatment. **Massage** improves self-esteem and encourages a sense of wellbeing. **Reflexology** and **aromatherapy** can both help cope with the stress and tensions generated by this disease. *Other therapies to try: see STRESS.*

FROZEN SHOULDER

A term covering a variety of conditions that cause pain and limit shoulder movements.

CAUSES

The term 'frozen shoulder' is more a description of the effects of shoulder pain than an explanation of the underlying disease process. The joint is literally frozen in position by pain. Uncertainty about the precise cause is mirrored by the many alternative terms for a painful stiff shoulder, for example sub-acromial bursitis, capsulitis and rotator cuff lesions.

The shoulder joint is between the upper arm (the humerus), the collar bone (clavicle) and the shoulder blade (scapula). These are bound together by joint capsules, tendons and muscles in a way that combines strength with a wide flexibility of movement. Usually, movement takes place in the ball-and-socket joint of the upper humerus (the ball) and the shoulder blade (the socket), stabilized by the clavicle. Several of the shorter muscles which move the arm meet in a fused sheath of muscle called the rotator cuff, which overlies the joints. The actions of the rotator cuff are supplemented by those of many other muscles, including the biceps and deltoids. At a rough count there are ten main muscles acting via a number of tendons and cushioned by two large fluid-filled sacs called bursas, which insulate the tendons from bone.

It is clear that there is plenty of opportunity for muscle fibres to tear through excessive force, for tendons to fray, for the fluid-filled sacs to inflame and for bone to rub. It does not take much effort to damage the shoulder and indeed one possible cause is simply disuse of the shoulder. It is fortunate that frozen shoulder usually affects one side only.

SYMPTOMS

The main symptoms are pain and stiffness of shoulder movements, especially those involving rotation of the arm. Symptoms can vary from a twinge when the shoulder reaches a certain position to the situation where any movement of the shoulder is painful, a true frozen shoulder. Specialized examination can pinpoint reasonably precisely which muscles or tendons are involved by seeing which positions provoke pain.

TREATMENT

There is a natural tendency for a frozen shoulder to heal with time, regardless of treatment, taking nine to fifteen months on average. The value of any treatment therefore has to be judged against this natural recovery time. Anti-inflammatory drugs are the logical first choices, but it is important to choose one that is least likely to cause stomach irritation because it will probably need to be taken for several months.

Having early physiotherapy to the shoulder helps prevent the additional stiffness arising from an individual's understandable reluctance to use it. Heat treatment, ultrasound and exercises should relieve pain sufficiently and give back enough confidence to keep the joint in use. A steroid injection into a specifically painful site can be very effective.

In selected cases of frozen shoulder, an orthopaedic surgeon will need to look into the joint with a fibreoptic endoscope, for example if healing is delayed or if a surgical repair of a tendon is thought necessary.

QUESTIONS

Are X-rays helpful?
These are less informative than people think. They are advisable after major trauma which might have broken a bone, but otherwise their value is limited because they do not show up the muscles or tendons. These structures are demonstrated by an MRI scan (see page 351), which is now the preferred investigation.

When is more urgent treatment needed?
If there is severe loss of function, for example inability to lift or rotate the arm. In this case a tendon may have ruptured and will need urgent repair.

How does movement occur if the shoulder joint is locked?
By rotating the shoulder blade and so lifting up the arm. This is similar to overcoming a stiff knee by swinging the leg from the hip.

Complementary Treatment

Acupuncture increases the circulation of blood and energy, reduces inflammation and pain, and stimulates healing of damaged tissues. **Alexander Technique** – see BACKACHE. **Chiropractic** manipulation, mobilization and soft tissue techniques are very effective. **Ayurveda** recommends regular oil massage and yoga. **Osteopathy** can offer highly specific manual treatments. **Rolfing** restores mobility by lengthening the compressed tissues. *Other therapies to try: shiatsu-do; cymatics; yoga; tai chi/chi kung; Hellerwork.*

Knee pains

The causes of knee pain are many and various.

Causes

The knee joint is formed by the thigh bone (femur) and the shin bone (tibia). The bones are cushioned by cartilage pads called menisci, which have a curved shape. Tough ligaments tether the bones and the joint is further stabilized by the kneecap and strong thigh muscles.

In children, the cause of pain is almost certainly injury from sport or accidents. The resulting pain is more from strain of tendons and ligaments than any damage to the bone.

Adolescents experience growing pains – they really do exist. In relation to knees the classic condition is Osgood Schlatter's disease, with tenderness where the bone is growing, just below the kneecap. Chondromalacia patellae is a common problem in adolescent girls; it is thought to be caused by irregularity of the back of the patella (kneecap) where it rests against the bones of the thigh and lower leg.

In adults injuries are the most likely cause of knee pain. Sportsmen and women are prone to tear the cartilages in the knee; the torn fragment prevents full movement of the joint. **Rheumatoid arthritis** and **gout** are less common causes of knee pain.

In late adult life and old age, **osteoarthritis** is the cause of most knee pain. It is possible for fragments of bone to break into osteoarthritic knees with an effect like that of throwing sand into a watch movement.

At all ages infection must be considered in any acute pain. Knee pain can reflect disease of the hip joint, as in osteoarthritis, or, in children, a slipped cartilage in the hip joint.

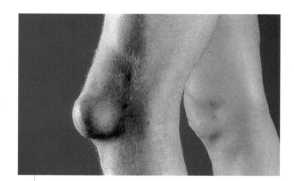

Above: Housemaid's knee – fluid over the kneecap that is caused by constant kneeling.

Symptoms

The knee is painful and may feel unstable. A locked knee that cannot be bent very far is probably due to a torn cartilage or a fragment of bone in the knee. Torn ligaments cause unusual laxity of the knee joint. There may be features of osteoarthritis of the knees or hips. Swelling of the knee is common after injury; immediate swelling or bruising mean bleeding in the joint.

Knee pains plus fever or joint pains elsewhere suggest infection or more generalized joint disease such as rheumatoid arthritis. A red, hot and swollen joint suggests infection, bleeding or an inflammatory cause such as gout or rheumatoid arthritis. In Osgood Schlatter's disease there is a tender prominent nodule below the kneecap. An MRI scan is useful to detect a torn cartilage or a ruptured tendon.

Treatment

Minor injuries settle with rest, support and an anti-inflammatory preparation in either gel or tablet form. Even torn cartilages and tendons will recover with rest, although it can take months. Physiotherapy is essential in order to maintain the thigh power needed to keep the knee stable.

Knee supports are helpful immediately after an injury to reduce swelling and to prevent swelling on further use of the joint. A knee support must be firm, but not so firm that it cuts into flesh or restricts the blood flow.

Orthopaedic surgeons can look inside the joint with arthroscopy to establish diagnosis of the problem, repair tendons and remove torn cartilages and debris. Any suspicion of infection calls for investigation of the swollen knee and infection requires a prolonged course of antibiotics.

Drawing fluid off a swollen knee joint relieves pressure and restores movement. Analysing the fluid aids the diagnosis of infection and gout.

   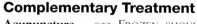

Complementary Treatment

Acupuncture – see FROZEN SHOULDER. **Shiatsu-do** shows excellent results for improving the musculoskeletal system. **Alexander Technique** and **Hellerwork** – see BACKACHE. **Chiropractic** manipulative and mobilization techniques can be very effective, especially if the pain is due to a sporting injury. **Ayurveda** recommends oil massage and yoga. **Osteopathy** offers specific manual treatments. **Rolfing** improves alignment, taking stress off the knee. *Other therapies to try: naturopathy; cymatics; tai chi/chi kung.*

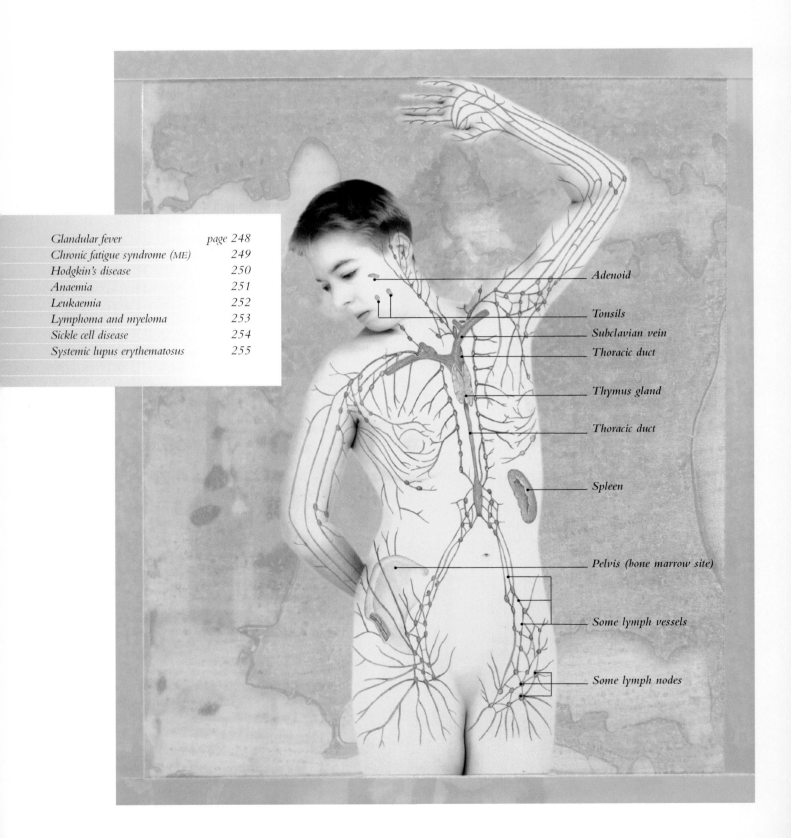

Adenoid

Tonsils

Subclavian vein

Thoracic duct

Thymus gland

Thoracic duct

Spleen

Pelvis (bone marrow site)

Some lymph vessels

Some lymph nodes

Blood and tissue fluids bathe nearly all parts of the body.
Within them float billions of cells and molecules involved in
oxygen transport and fighting infection. Lymph glands, liver,
spleen and bone marrow play fundamental roles in this system.

BLOOD, GLANDS AND THE IMMUNE SYSTEM

BLOOD IS THE MEANS by which oxygen and nutrients are taken to every part of the body and carbon dioxide and waste products are returned to the lungs, liver or kidney, for elimination. The main components of blood are red blood cells, which carry oxygen, white cells, which are defence cells, and platelets, which help the blood to clot. There are also hundreds of other components in the blood stream involved in defence, hormone transport, nutrition and much more.

Blood cells are formed within the bone marrow, at least in adults, although the liver and spleen can assist if needed. Adults have about 5 litres/9 pints of blood in their bodies, each drop of which contains millions of these cells.

Glands and the immune system

Throughout the body there are collections of glandular tissues called lymph nodes whose job it is to deal with infection in the body. These glands can be felt around the throat, at the back of the neck, in the groin and in the armpits. There are many more internal lymph nodes within the intestine and following the paths of the major blood vessels.

The siting of these lymph nodes is not random; it provides maximum protection where infection is most likely to enter the body – the various orifices, the lungs and the intestines. Lymph nodes are connected by the lymphatic system, which is similar to the circulatory system of blood. The lymphatic system collects tissue fluid – fluid that has leaked out of the arteries and veins of the blood circulatory system – and returns it to the blood stream via special ducts in the chest. Other crucial parts of the lymphatic system are the spleen, located below the ribs in the left upper abdomen, and the thymus gland, in the neck below the breastbone. The spleen destroys aged red blood cells and is a kind of filtration plant removing debris from the blood stream. The thymus gland activates lymphocytes, which are attack cells produced in vast quantities by the bone marrow, lymph nodes and spleen.

Defence

The defensive forces of the body are lymphocytes and antibodies – proteins released by lymphocytes which recognize foreign invaders. These primary defences are assisted by a complex array of additional biochemicals such as complement, interferon and cytokines. The cells within the body are continually being challenged to see if they are 'self' or 'foreign', which might include viruses, bacteria and any transplanted tissues. Once foreign matter is detected a cascade of defensive forces swings into action, generating large numbers of lymphocytes from rapidly enlarged lymph nodes, such as the swollen neck glands during tonsillitis, assisted by an assortment of biochemically destructive proteins.

The defence process goes on in the body at a mostly undetectable level but if the system has to meet a major challenge we will experience this as 'feeling ill' with **fever**, sweats, malaise, muscle pains and many enlarged glands.

Potential problems

Considering how complex both the blood and lymphatic systems are, their reliability is high. Where serious problems do arise they are usually due to disease of the bone marrow, cancers of lymph nodes or bone marrow or, commonly, **anaemia**.

Left: A complex fluid based system,
fighting infection and carrying oxygen,
food and hormones around the body.

GLANDULAR FEVER

A viral infection causing a sore throat and enlarged lymph glands.

CAUSES

The virus causing glandular fever was first identified in 1964 and named the Epstein Barr virus, after its discoverers. This virus is a variety of herpes virus and is spread through saliva – giving the disease a reputation as the 'kissing disease' – although cases can happen via spread through the air. The medical term for glandular fever is infectious mononucleosis, which refers to certain types of white blood cell appearing during the illness. People of all ages may contract glandular fever, but it is most common in young adults and adolescents. In children the disease is very mild.

SYMPTOMS

Glandular fever begins with a sore throat, which rapidly worsens and often looks indistinguishable from **tonsillitis**. As the name implies, the glands all around the body enlarge, especially the neck glands, and there is the usual malaise and aching that is typical of any viral illness. The virus often affects the liver, causing a hint of jaundice (see LIVER PROBLEMS). Skin rashes are common, too.

The diagnosis can be confirmed by the Monospot or Paul Burnell blood tests. This is useful because it allows prediction about the long course of the illness and reinforces the futility of changing from antibiotic to antibiotic to cure the sore throat.

A couple of other viruses, such as cytomegalovirus and toxoplasmosis, can cause a similar picture, and are distinguished by blood tests. Although the list of possible complications from glandular fever is long, for example effects on the heart and pain in the joints, most are rare.

TREATMENT

Many people who present at an early stage with a bad throat or tonsillitis will be prescribed an antibiotic in the reasonable belief that they have a streptococcal sore throat. Once the diagnosis is established, however, antibiotic treatment should be abandoned. The body simply has to develop resistance to the virus, which takes several weeks.

A short course of steroids is helpful in severe cases, for example where there is massive enlargement of the tonsils or inflammation of the liver. Glandular fever may make the spleen enlarge and become fragile, so it is advisable not to play any contact sports for three months after glandular fever. For similar reasons it is advisable to cut out alcohol.

The question of post-glandular fever debility is a much vexed one. Many people experience profound tiredness during the illness, which may persist in a few cases for weeks or months after clinical recovery. A very few fall into the category of **chronic fatigue syndrome**, but far fewer than popular wisdom holds. Because glandular fever does have such a reputation it is best to be positive about the outcome from the start, rather than to assume that you are doomed to a year of lassitude. Immunity to glandular fever is lifelong; you cannot catch it twice and if you think you have had it before chances are one of the diagnoses was wrong.

QUESTIONS

What is the effect of ampicillin on glandular fever?
Ampicillin is an antibiotic used for sore throats. It is a curious fact that taking ampicillin in a case of glandular fever will result in a rash in 90% of patients.

How infectious is it?
Glandular fever is so infectious that nearly all children in the Third World contract it, whereas in the cleaner environment of the developed world children miss catching it until they go to secondary school – hence its frequency in teenagers.

How can the spread of glandular fever be reduced?
Ideally, anyone with glandular fever should not kiss others nor share drinking utensils. Since glandular fever has an incubation period of about 50 days, adherence to such rigid isolation would no doubt devastate teenage social life.

Complementary Treatment

Western herbalism – infusions of yarrow or elderflower induce sweating and keep the temperature stable. Rosemary and yarrow tea alleviate persistent tiredness after glandular fever. Cleavers is specific for the lymphatics. **Chakra balancing** – if you are sensitive to touch, you could benefit from the non-touch techniques employed by this therapy. **Aromatherapy** can boost the immune system and help psychologically too – your practitioner will advise. **Ayurvedic** medicine recommends oral preparations and *panchakarma* detoxification. *Other therapies to try: Chinese herbalism; homeopathy; naturopathy.*

CHRONIC FATIGUE SYNDROME (ME)

Profound tiredness in the absence of definite medical diagnosis.

CAUSES

The term chronic fatigue syndrome (CFS) is preferable to the widespread term ME (myalgic encephalomyelitis), which implies an understanding of the condition unwarranted by current research. It is the enormous publicity given to certain high-profile cases that has helped turn the condition from a curiosity into a research topic. This research has yet to bear any significant fruit. Current thinking is that there is no one cause of CFS, although viral infection may trigger fatigue. The **glandular fever** virus is most often suspected, but its role is completely unproven. Research is currently looking at abnormalities of cell metabolism and the hypothalamic/pituitary axis, but with no firm conclusion as yet.

It is clear that prolonged tiredness acquires psychological overtones long after the virus has left the body. In other words, although it may be a physical event that triggers CFS, it is almost certainly psychological factors that prolong it.

SYMPTOMS

Many healthy people feel tired – some people all of the time. Tiredness alone is not enough to establish the diagnosis. The agreed criteria for CFS are at least six months of fatigue associated with loss of ability to function at work or home; there are often muscle aches and irritability. Tiredness alternates with bursts of activity but these have to be 'paid for' by increased fatigue and muscle pains one to two days later. There are often sleep and mood disturbances but not true **depression**.

The diagnosis of CFS cannot be accepted without first having a full medical examination and comprehensive blood tests, including tests for **diabetes**, thyroid disease (see THYROID PROBLEMS) and hormonal disturbances.

TREATMENT

Probably the first step in treatment of the syndrome is acceptance by both doctor and patient that there is a problem, the cause of which is unknown, but which is not life-threatening. No one dies of CFS. While the cause is still debatable, current thinking is that patients must accept that their own psychological approach to chronic fatigue is their key to overcoming the problem. Treatment starts by identifying any possible contributory psychological factors such as work, relationships or general unhappiness about life.

You must accept that effort will be tiring; this does not mean that you must constantly rest. On the contrary, the more you rest the more tired you will get when you do exert yourself, leading to a vicious circle of rest, frantic effort, tiredness and muscle pains and more rest. You need an agreed level of activity – enough to stimulate you a little but not so much as to exhaust you. This should replace the rest/activity cycles otherwise common in this condition. Do not spend the day sleeping or napping; you will then have restless nights and wake unrefreshed. Antidepressants are widely used and worth trying. Also, the modern serotonin re-uptake inhibitors have a slight stimulant effect which is helpful. Whatever the strategy, you must accept that there is no 'quick-fix' and that improvement may take months rather than weeks.

QUESTIONS

How common is chronic fatigue syndrome?
Surveys suggest that up to one in two hundred of the population has CFS; many more have a CFS-type picture but with features of clinical depression. CFS is most common in women who are aged between twenty and forty.

When is tiredness abnormal?
This is a difficult question because the same surveys show that 20–30% of the population feel tired all the time. Probably the diagnostic criterion is when tiredness is profound enough to interfere with home and work performance, but a great deal rests on your own assessment of your degree of tiredness.

What about recovery?
The picture is still bleak. About 70% of people with CFS remain unwell even after a year. Children recover faster than adults.

Complementary Treatment
WARNING: Do not attempt self-treatment – you are likely to be sensitive to all medication, including natural remedies. **Chinese herbalism** uses herbs to clear 'dampness', which is a kind of clogging of the body's functions, producing lethargy, a muzzy head and poor concentration. **Chiropractic** can help joint and muscle stiffness and improve mobility. *Other therapies to try: Western herbalism; tai chi/chi kung; homeopathy; acupuncture; cymatics; chakra balancing; aromatherapy; Ayurveda; nutritional therapy; naturopathy.*

HODGKIN'S DISEASE

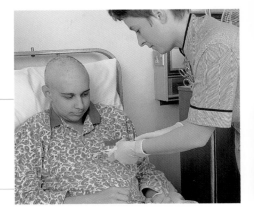

Right: Chemotherapy for Hodgkin's disease may be distressing but cure is highly likely.

A disease of the lymphatic system, the outlook for which has been transformed since the 1960s.

CAUSES

This disease is one of a group of cancers called lymphomas (see LYMPHOMA AND MYELOMA), which involve abnormalities of the lymphoid system, comprising lymph glands, liver and spleen. The trigger for Hodgkin's disease remains unknown. There has been much speculation and research on the possibility of a virus triggering it, especially the Epstein Barr virus which causes **glandular fever**, but the evidence is inconclusive. There is a slightly increased family risk, but it is uncertain whether this implies a genetic risk or whether the family has been exposed to some common hazard or infection.

SYMPTOMS

Peak incidence is in young men, who are affected about twice as often as women. It is more common again in old age. The classic early symptoms are enlarged lymph glands in the neck. These are painless, in contrast to the enlarged glands associated with infection, and have a rubbery feel to them. There are usually other rubbery glands in the armpits and groin and the spleen is frequently enlarged. Additional symptoms include sweating at night, weight loss and generalized itch.

The enlarged glands are highly suggestive of the condition but confirmation has to be made by a biopsy of a gland. As well as confirming the diagnosis, the cells' appearance shows what subtype of Hodgkin's disease is present, which is essential in planning treatment and for predicting the outlook.

Assessment is completed by scans of the interior lymph nodes and spleen. Occasionally an operation might be needed to see how far the disease has spread, but this is increasingly unnecessary thanks to refinements in scanning. The information is put together using an internationally agreed scheme to stage the condition and to decide treatment.

TREATMENT

A choice is made of a combination of radiotherapy (see page 370) and chemotherapy (see page 371), the precise 'cocktail' depending on the type and stage of the illness. The aim is to eradicate the cancerous tissues from all affected sites. The various cocktails are the subject of continuing refinement and increasing sophistication in dosage and in controlling the otherwise unpleasant side effects of therapy such as nausea.

Treatment is given in cycles over several weeks for up to six months, by which time most people are free of active disease. It can normally be given as an outpatient procedure, even though up to eight drugs might be required each time, and some people are able to continue working during part of their therapy. Follow-up has to continue for many years.

The results of treatment have been spectacular. As late as the 1950s fewer than 10% of people with Hodgkin's survived more than five years, whereas now over 80% do so. Even if the disease recurs, there is a high probability of getting it back under control and even of curing it.

QUESTIONS

What does treatment do to fertility?
Now that a cure is likely, attention has turned to the side effects of treatment. In men, subfertility invariably follows from the chemotherapy; they are now offered the chance to donate a sperm sample which is kept frozen for later use. Women are most unlikely to suffer any permanent effect on fertility.

Is there a risk of other cancers?
The more that people are surviving, the more it is found that they have an increased risk of other cancers. These are mainly blood disorders like leukaemia. This is a good reason for continued review and regular blood tests.

Complementary Treatment
Complementary therapies cannot cure this cancer. However, they can offer a great deal during diagnosis, treatment and follow-up. **Chakra balancing** can promote relaxation and offer support during orthodox treatment. **Massage** helps to improve self-esteem and encourages a sense of wellbeing. **Hypnotherapy** – hypno-healing could help. **Reflexology** and **aromatherapy** can both help you cope with the stress and tensions generated by this disease. *Other therapies to try: see STRESS.*

ANAEMIA

A condition of below-normal levels of red blood cells.

CAUSES

Anaemia is a symptom and not a definite diagnosis in itself. The causes fall into three main categories: failure of production of red blood cells, excessive loss of blood, or chronic disease leading to abnormal breakdown of cells.

Failure of red blood cell production

The average adult has 5 litres/9 pints of blood made up of billions of cells; the average life of a red blood cell is four months. Red blood cells are produced in vast numbers by the bone marrow, together with the other essential components of blood such as white blood cells and platelets. This frantic production line requires basic raw materials: protein to make the cells and iron to make the haemoglobin molecule. Various trace elements are needed, the best known being vitamin B_{12}. If these are deficient then anaemia inevitably develops. If it is vitamin B_{12} that is deficient, the cause may be pernicious anaemia. Strict vegans may become anaemic through lack of iron, but there is no reason why vegetarians should, as long as they follow a varied diet including eggs.

The cause of anaemia is usually dietary deficiency but it may be failure of absorption through a bowel disorder such as **coeliac disease**. The other production cause is failure of the bone marrow, which occurs in **leukaemia**, or destruction of the marrow after, for example, chemotherapy for cancer.

Excessive blood loss

The spleen destroys worn out old blood cells; a hormone system matches the rate of destruction and the rate of production. This all goes wrong if blood is lost in excessive quantities. The most common reasons for this are heavy menstrual periods, bleeding from ulcers in the stomach or duodenum, cancers of the large intestine or loss in urine. Several drugs cause leakage of blood from the stomach, for example aspirin and anti-inflammatories used for arthritic conditions.

Abnormal breakdown of cells

Some people have inherently fragile blood cells, including those with spherocytosis or **sickle cell disease**. Many chronic illnesses like cancers and kidney disease cause anaemia for reasons not well understood, and are often difficult to treat.

SYMPTOMS

There is a non-specific tiredness. When blood count falls to half the normal count there is profound tiredness and breathlessness through lack of the oxygen carried by red blood cells. Older people may get chest pain. There may be the symptoms of any contributory conditions, for example the weight loss of cancer or malabsorption or heavy periods. Skin colour is not a good measure of anaemia. It is slightly more reliable to judge pallor by turning down the eye lid yet some people may have normal complexions but profound anaemia and *vice versa*.

TREATMENT

It can take some detective work to discover the cause of anaemia: going over diet, checking for blood loss in the bowels or urine and looking for associated diseases such as **hiatus hernia**, **stomach cancer** or **bowel cancer**, especially in older people. If the cause is obvious, as in a poor diet or heavy periods, immediate treatment is with iron and vitamins. Follow-up blood tests are important to ensure response to treatment.

Pernicious anaemia is treated by injections of vitamin B_{12} plus folic acid supplements. Blood transfusion is reserved for profound anaemia causing serious symptoms.

See also PREGNANCY PROBLEMS for anaemia in pregnancy.

  Complementary Treatment
Nutritional therapy – besides iron, likely deficiencies include vitamins B_6 and B_{12}, folic acid and zinc. Boost your intake of soya beans, green-leaved vegetables, dried fruit, especially raisins, and red meat and liver (if you are not vegetarian – and not if you are pregnant). A **homeopath** could suggest ways of improving your body's ability to absorb iron. *Other therapies to try: tai chi/chi kung; shiatsu-do; acupuncture; aromatherapy.*

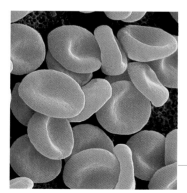

Left: Biconcave red blood cells, packed with haemoglobin. Each drop of blood contains millions of cells.

LEUKAEMIA

◆

Cancer of the bone marrow with abnormalities in the production of the white cells needed to combat infection.

CAUSES

◆

The term leukaemia covers many related cancers, which vary in their degree of seriousness. The disease affects people of all ages but tends to be more common in children and the elderly, and relatively uncommon in adult life.

White blood cells are produced in the bone marrow and are vital in combating infection by bacteria or viruses. The bone marrow also produces red blood cells and the platelets required for the normal clotting of blood. In the condition of leukaemia the bone marrow switches to producing enormous quantities of white blood cells to the exclusion of the other blood components. Far from enhancing the body's resistance to infection, these white blood cells are inefficient.

In the majority of cases leukaemia arises spontaneously with no agreed pre-existing cause. However, it may be due to previous irradiation of the bone marrow causing a mutation to cancerous cells, for example after exposure to radioactivity or as a result of radiotherapy for **Hodgkin's disease**.

Much research has sought a viral cause since there is a form of leukaemia in Japan caused by a virus, but, in general, results have not supported this view; nor is there any definite conclusion about genetic causes except for a variant of leukaemia called chronic myeloid leukaemia.

SYMPTOMS

◆

Childhood leukaemia tends to be of a swift and dramatic onset, with rapid falls in both red blood cells and platelets. The child becomes lethargic through the onset of **anaemia**, breaks out in bruises and bleeds spontaneously from the teeth or nose. The blood count shows large numbers of the characteristic cells of leukaemia. The most usual types are acute lymphocytic leukaemia or acute myelogenous leukaemia.

Older people tend to get more slowly evolving forms of leukaemia such as chronic myeloid leukaemia or chronic lymphocytic leukaemia. They suffer a period of vague ill health, perhaps increased numbers of infections, enlarged lymph nodes, sweating at night and itching.

In all cases diagnosis is confirmed by taking a sample of bone marrow in order to demonstrate the abnormal production of white cells. Leukaemia, although suspected often, occurs rarely. However, a blood test is advisable for someone with prolonged sore throats, bruising or recurrent infections.

TREATMENT

◆

The outlook for childhood leukaemia or other leukaemia of acute onset is very good. It is essential to remember this during the harrowing periods of treatment with radiotherapy and chemotherapy (see pages 370 and 371) with their attendant hair loss, nausea, constant drips and intensive nursing. Out of this comes recovery in at least 90% of cases and ever-increasing numbers remain cured. Prospects have improved even more with the discovery that cells taken from the umbilical cord can be transplanted into leukaemia patients with a high success rate and without needing powerful anti-rejection medication, as is normally needed for transplants.

The prospects in the more chronic adult leukaemia are less good but by no means hopeless. Chronic myeloid leukaemia is treated with a drug called busulphan and increasingly with bone marrow transplantation (see page 363). The average survival is about five years. Chronic lymphocytic leukaemia is an even more benign form, often found incidentally when taking a blood test for some other reason. Even without treatment people can expect many years without problems. Treatment is with chemotherapy such as chlorambucil.

QUESTIONS

How common is leukaemia?
Despite its high public profile, childhood leukaemia is rare. There are under 500 cases a year in the whole of the United Kingdom and about 7,000 adult cases.

Why is the treatment so difficult?
Cancerous cells in bone marrow cannot be eradicated without eradicating other cells made by the marrow, with great risks of infection and bleeding during therapy. Cancerous cells linger within the brain and spinal cord; radiotherapy to these regions is hazardous.

Complementary Treatment
Complementary therapies cannot cure leukaemia and should be used only to support conventional treatment. Any stress-reducing therapy will help both the patient and the family deal with the strains following diagnosis. Many complementary therapies can help the body cope with the effects of aggressive orthodox treatment, particularly **massage**, **aromatherapy** and **reflexology**. *Other therapies to try: see* STRESS.

LYMPHOMA AND MYELOMA

Lymphoma is a cancer of the lymph nodes. Myeloma is a specific type of cancer of the bone marrow.

CAUSES

Lymphoid tissues defend us against invading bacteria and viruses. The system comprises lymph nodes around the head, neck and groin, many internal lymph nodes and the spleen. It responds to infection by releasing lymphocytes, white cells that recognize invading organisms. How do they do this?

Virtually all cells in the body have a protein marker in their cell wall, which in effect says, 'I'm family, back off'. Lacking these markers, germs are recognized as 'non-family' and trigger attack by white cells and antibodies. Antibodies are complex proteins released by lymphocytes, which recognize germs met previously. They latch on to the germs and destroy them directly or release biochemical markers that rally more white cells to help. It is a wonderfully efficient system but the very rapidity of cell turnover paradoxically carries a risk of cancerous transformation, resulting in lymphoma or myeloma.

Lymphoma
It is believed that lymphomas begin when a single cell mutates and proliferates uncontrollably, replacing healthy lymphoid tissues. They are more likely in late adult life but can occur at any age. (**Hodgkin's disease** is a type of lymphoma, considered separately because it is usually confined to a few tissues, rather than spread throughout the body.)

Myeloma
This is a disease of the bone marrow in cells that produce antibodies. It is almost always a disease of the elderly. Again, it appears that a single cell goes out of control and proliferates. The cell continues to produce fragments of antibody, but not complete antibody molecules. Eventually the blood stream is awash with fragments, but short of the useful antibodies – like a factory that changed from producing complete cars to churning out huge numbers of half-finished hub-caps instead.

SYMPTOMS

With lymphoma, as the cancerous cells spread, lymph nodes all around the body enlarge – those in the neck, groin and armpits the most obvious. The individual feels generally unwell and is prone to infections and **anaemia**. Often the diagnosis is suspected purely on examination, but is confirmed by biopsy of the lymph nodes.

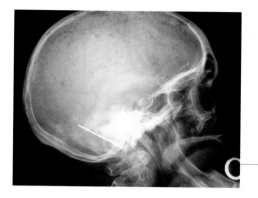

Left: Circular X-ray shadows typical of bone destruction by multiple myeloma.

Myeloma tends to be of less dramatic onset and can be advanced before causing symptoms of pain, from destruction of bone, and anaemia. There are many subtle biochemical changes due to high levels of calcium in the blood stream and kidney function may be impaired, but the resulting symptoms are rather non-specifically those of vague malaise. The diagnosis is made by demonstrating large quantities of abnormal protein in the blood or the urine and abnormal bone marrow.

TREATMENT

There are many subtypes of lymphoma and so treatment is tailored as appropriate, but in all cases involves radiotherapy, chemotherapy or both (see pages 370 and 371). A bone marrow transplant may sometimes be appropriate (see page 363). The outlook depends on the particular subtype; survival can be expected to be measured in years and a significant number of people are cured.

In the case of myeloma, treatment is complex, requiring chemotherapy to damp down the disease, radiotherapy to deal with bone invasion, and kidney support. Bone marrow transplantation is now being used more often, and is pushing up survival times to a number of years.

Complementary Treatment
Complementary therapies cannot cure either lymphoma or myeloma. However, many can offer support during diagnosis, treatment and follow-up. They can also help the body deal with the strains produced by the necessarily aggressive conventional treatments. **Chakra balancing** can help promote relaxation, symptom control and pain relief. **Massage**, **aromatherapy** and **reflexology** can be particularly beneficial. *Other therapies to try: see STRESS.*

SICKLE CELL DISEASE

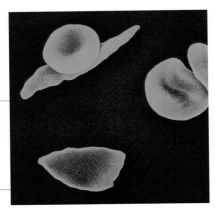

An abnormality of the haemoglobin molecule that alters the shape and stability of red blood cells.

Right: Long, flat sickled red blood cells mingle with normal round red cells.

CAUSES

One of the basic processes of living creatures is to absorb oxygen from the air or from fluids and to transport it to cells where it fuels metabolism. In humans this is achieved by the haemoglobin molecule, carried in millions by each red blood cell. The haemoglobin molecule is like a nest cocooning iron in a special structure, which avidly takes up oxygen but gives it up into the cells. The proteins twist and turn so as to give a particular shape to the molecule, enhancing this function.

In sickle cell disease, there is an abnormality of haemoglobin caused by a single genetic error that substitutes one amino acid for another. This tiny slip makes the haemoglobin molecule less soluble and the red blood cell more rigid. It loses its bi-concave shape and instead looks curved, hence the term sickle cell. For much of the time the red blood cell gets by, but in certain conditions the abnormal haemoglobin becomes even less soluble and the cells more likely to sickle. These conditions include experience of cold temperatures, infection and lack of oxygen at high altitude.

Unlike normal red blood cells, which slip and glide through the narrowest capillaries, rigid sickled cells block small blood vessels and starve surrounding tissues of oxygen. As well as causing pain, this also reduces the life span of red blood cells – normally four months – and causes persistent **anaemia**.

For reasons not understood sickle cell is extremely common throughout Africa and in populations of African origin, for example Afro-Americans. It is not uncommon in Asians and in the Middle East but is rare in Caucasian populations.

SYMPTOMS

The symptoms of sickle cell disease are mainly the result of blockage of blood vessels – pain that can be anywhere in the body, even abdominal pain. Interference with blood flow in the fingers or long bones can lead to stunted growth and irregularly shaped fingers or toes. The persistent anaemia causes tiredness and increased susceptibility to infection. Eventually there may be kidney and brain damage, too.

The severity of symptoms is highly variable, depending on how much normal haemoglobin the individual also has. Those least affected by the disease have few symptoms except in severe infections or lack of oxygen, whereas those most affected suffer constant pain and anaemia.

TREATMENT

Many people with sickle cell disease require no treatment and simply need to be aware of the risks that they face. During any surgical procedures it is important for the anaesthetist to give high levels of oxygen via a face mask. Sickle cell disease may be an explanation of otherwise obscure pains.

People suffering sickle cell crises – acute and severe pain due to blockage of blood vessels, usually in the bones or the spleen – need urgent management in a specialized centre to control pain, infection and dehydration from tissue damage.

The anaemia of sickle cell disease cannot be treated in the normal way with iron. Blood transfusion might be necessary in cases of extreme anaemia. Research may, in the future, find a way of getting the body to switch to production of other more benign forms of haemoglobin.

QUESTIONS

Why is sickle cell so common?
Such a common genetic variant invites questions as to why the disease persists. The best guess is that people with sickle cell trait enjoy some protection against malaria.

Who is at risk?
Anyone of African origin should have a sickle cell blood test, especially if a family member is affected. The test will show how severely affected you are. This is important information to tell doctors during any serious illness and before surgical procedures.

Complementary Treatment

No complementary treatment can cure sickle cell disease so do not abandon conventional approaches. However, many therapies do have a role in helping you cope. If you are sensitive to touch, you could benefit from the non-touch techniques of **chakra balancing**. **Yoga** and **tai chi/chi kung** are gentle forms of exercise that can help.

SYSTEMIC LUPUS ERYTHEMATOSUS

An auto-immune condition, commonly abbreviated to SLE.

CAUSES

The cause of SLE is an attack by the body against its own tissues. The fundamental attack is against the DNA and RNA molecules, which are at the very heart of the cell's structure. (DNA carries genetic information and RNA is involved in protein synthesis.) This explains why SLE affects organs all over the body. It is not known what triggers this auto-immune attack. Research is looking at whether a viral infection could trigger the body to react first against the virus and by extension against its own proteins, but this has not been established.

There is a strong hereditary element; if you have an affected sibling your chances of SLE are about 5% as opposed to one in a thousand of the general population. There are certain racial groups in which it is much more common, for example Afro-Americans. In a few cases SLE follows drug treatment with hydralazine, used for high blood pressure. Women are affected far more than men – about nine to one. The disease is very rare in children and adolescents.

SYMPTOMS

Any body system could be affected but the most common early symptoms are pains in the joints or a butterfly-like facial rash – so-called because of its symmetrical spread across the cheeks. Pain in the joints is of sudden onset and without blood tests could be thought due to **rheumatoid arthritis**. There may be a sensitivity to sunlight, **fever**, odd tender patches on the fingers and Raynaud's phenomenon (see RAYNAUD'S DISEASE). Many other organs are affected, for example the lungs, kidneys and heart, but these rarely cause symptoms at the time of presentation.

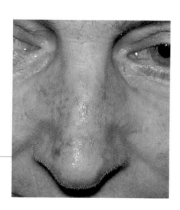

Right: A red butterfly-shaped rash on the face is suggestive of SLE.

The diagnosis is established by showing a certain number of symptoms plus blood tests that reveal antibodies to DNA.

If the disease progresses there is a risk of **stroke**, personality change and kidney damage. However, these represent the most severe end of the spectrum, at the other end of which there are many people with a relatively benign form of SLE.

TREATMENT

People with SLE who become tired and have frequent rashes but are otherwise well need only anti-inflammatory drugs for flare-ups of pain in the joints; for much of the time they need no medication at all. In more serious disease, with increasing kidney damage, steroids are necessary by mouth in a dosage enough to bring things under control. If this is not sufficient chemotherapy is used (see page 371) with drugs such as cyclophosphamide or azathioprine – drugs used to treat cancer that work by reducing the activity of the immune system.

Typically, with SLE there are fluctuations in its severity. Doctors need to recognize a deterioration early enough to begin appropriate treatment while balancing the side effects of the treatment against the damage done by the illness.

QUESTIONS

What is the outlook for SLE?
The liberal use of steroids has improved the five-year survival to at least 95%. There is evidence that if serious problems are going to occur it will be in the first few years of the illness, which thereafter takes a more benign course.

Can I still get pregnant?
Pregnancy can go ahead but with an increased risk of high blood pressure and miscarriage. Taking aspirin reduces the risks of miscarriage. The outcome is good in four out of five pregnancies.

Complementary Treatment

It is important to maintain conventional treatment alongside complementary approaches. **Nutritional therapy** – try switching to a diet rich in fish oil, and supplementing with vitamin E and selenium. Traditional Chinese approaches (**herbs**, **acupuncture**, **tai chi/chi kung**) and **Western herbalism** can help by boosting your immune system. **Ayurveda** might advise detoxification, oil **massage** and specific **yoga** practices.

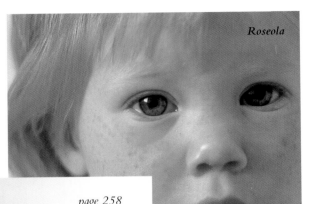

Roseola

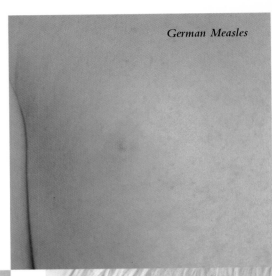

German Measles

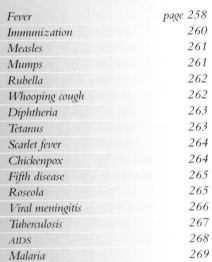

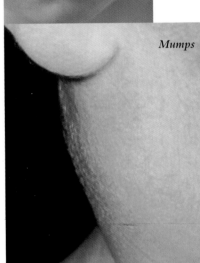

Mumps

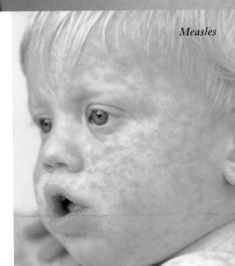

Measles

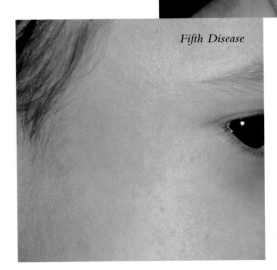

Fifth Disease

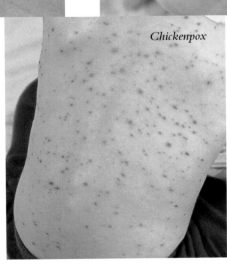

Chickenpox

Infection is the single largest threat to health during much of the human lifetime and the range of infections is quite vast. Old infections change their character and new infections emerge regularly, making infection control a constant problem.

INFECTIOUS DISEASE

THERE IS A MULTITUDE of different types of micro-organisms that can cause infection, and while the body's sophisticated and ubiquitous defence systems can deal with many of them, some are so virulent that medication will be needed to destroy them.

Infecting micro-organisms

Viruses are particles so small that they are only visible through electron microscopes. They contain little other than enough genetic material to make more viruses. They rely on invading another organism to survive, taking over its internal metabolism and diverting it into producing more viruses. Because viruses are so intimately involved in the vital processes of cells, it is difficult to eradicate them with medication, although there are now a few antiviral drugs. The mainstay of defence against viruses is **immunization**. Important viral illnesses are, or were, **measles**, **mumps**, **viral meningitis**, smallpox, herpes and **AIDS**.

Bacteria are much larger organisms, visible under conventional microscopes. They are capable of independent existence and reproduction and cause many major and minor infectious illnesses, such as chest infections, blood poisoning and **bacterial meningitis**. Antibiotics have proved successful in controlling bacteria by poisoning a vital aspect of their metabolism, most often destroying the wall of the bacterium. Bacteria can mutate into forms resistant to antibiotics.

Protozoa are single-celled creatures, often parasitic – meaning that they grow within a host but without necessarily causing disease. They are, however, responsible for several serious illnesses such as **malaria** and sleeping sickness.

Fungi are organisms that grow slowly by throwing out filaments. Many are benign and even useful (penicillin was discovered in fungus). The illnesses they cause are usually more of a nuisance than life-threatening, for example **thrush**.

Other micro-organisms include *rickettsia* and *mycoplasma*, which are responsible for severe illnesses and often respond to an antibiotic.

Defence

The body maintains very complex systems to guard against infection. The mainstays are lymphocytes, a type of white blood cell, and antibodies, which are proteins shaped in a particular way that recognize the outer wall of invading micro-organisms. These components can recruit additional defensive cells and biochemicals to destroy viruses and bacteria, such as interferon, complement, leukotrienes, polymorphs and more.

How infection causes illness

Our bodies are continually being challenged by micro-organisms, most of which are recognized and destroyed rapidly. More established infection causes the release of toxic chemicals by both the invader and the defensive forces, accounting for **fever**, sweating, shivers, muscle pains, falls in blood pressure and fluid loss. Recovery occurs as these micro-organisms are destroyed.

Micro-organisms may cause disease through direct destruction of healthy tissues, such as lungs by **tuberculosis** or blood cells by malaria. Others release poisons called toxins, for example **diphtheria**, diarrhoeal illnesses and **tetanus**. Others destroy the immune system – AIDS is now the major example.

Left: Rashes and skin changes that reflect the ongoing struggle of the body against infecting micro-organisms.

FEVER

◆

A raised temperature is universally recognized as a sign of illness.

CAUSES

◆

The body functions within a narrow band of temperatures, shedding or increasing heat if the temperature strays outside the normal range (see below). Fever is mainly the result of an infection triggering defensive white blood cells to release a substance called endogenous pyrogen. Pyrogen affects the hypothalamus in the brain and turns up the body temperature. Pyrogen may also be released through tissue damage, accounting for some of the more unusual causes of fever.

Infectious causes

Fever is the usual response to invasion by infection for the reasons given above. However fever is only a marker of illness and not a diagnosis. Sometimes it is clear from the outset what is causing fever – a cold, a cough or symptoms of a urinary infection. Therefore, presented with fever alone, doctors go through systematic questions and examinations to determine what the cause may be, moving from the commonplace possibilities to the rare.

Incubation periods

In general, fevers of rapid onset are likely to be due to infection, but it often takes a few days for the infection to identify itself. Fever during those few days reflects the struggle within the body in which defences – white blood cells, antibodies and tissue destruction factors – battle with the infecting agent. If the body wins, the fever abates and you get better. If the infection wins then you eventually exhibit the features of an illness, be it a common cold at one extreme or **malaria** at the other.

The length of this battle varies greatly; the incubation period of common **colds** is two to four days, of **chickenpox** eighteen to twenty-one days. Fever is unlikely for all this time.

Prolonged fever

Unexplained fever lasting more than a week is called pyrexia of unknown origin. It can be a major diagnostic challenge, because the possibilities range through more exotic infections into other generalized illnesses (see below). Possible illnesses are those with a long incubation period – hepatitis A or unusual types of **pneumonia**. After recent foreign travel, malaria, typhoid or leishmaniasis need to be considered.

If fever lasts for weeks, thoughts turn to **tuberculosis**, heart infections, chronic abscesses within the abdomen or non-infectious causes.

Fevers not caused by infection

These bear consideration in someone with prolonged unexplained fever. They include auto-immune conditions such as **rheumatoid arthritis** or **systemic lupus erythematosus**, cancers – especially **Hodgkin's disease**, **cancer of the kidney** or **leukaemia** – and also reactions to drugs. It must be emphasized that these illnesses are unlikely in the case of acute fever and become a likelihood only after weeks if not months of unexplained fever.

SYMPTOMS

◆

Fever makes you feel hot and shivery despite the temperature. You will sweat and you may experience drenching night sweats. Associated symptoms include muscle aches, pains in the eyes, a headache – everything we all understand by saying 'I feel unwell'. Some infections cause rigors – intense shivering plus a high temperature. The symptoms may give the clue to the cause: a cough, a bad throat or a characteristic rash.

Measuring temperature

The glass or electronic thermometer is a good guide in adults; normal mouth temperature is 36.5–37.5°C/97.7–99.5°F. Mouth temperature is affected by hot or cold food for about a quarter of an hour after eating.

Temperature can be measured under the armpit, which gives readings half a degree centigrade lower, or rectally, which is half a degree centigrade higher than mouth temperature. It is often safer to measure temperatures of children in these ways. Increasingly common are heat-sensing thermometers placed in the ear, which give a reliable result in seconds.

Investigations

These are neither useful nor needed in common feverish illnesses where the likely cause is a viral illness, which will be finished by the time the results are back. In some cases a doctor might want to take a throat swab and test a sample of urine, especially in children in whom a urinary infection may cause fever alone (see URINARY PROBLEMS).

The longer a fever lasts the more investigations become advisable. After a week the next step might be a chest X-ray to detect unusual forms of pneumonia, and a blood count. The number of white cells in a blood count indicates whether infection is of viral or bacterial origin; measures called ESR or C reactive protein help indicate the severity of infection.

Further information may come from faecal tests, blood tests for blood infections (septicaemia) or unusual infections such

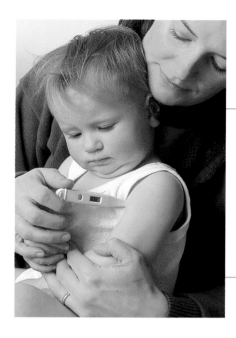

Left: It is safer and easier to measure the temperature of children under the arm or in the ear rather than in the mouth.

as brucellosis and sophisticated immunological tests, which indicate the likely infection, whether viral or bacterial. You will be questioned about medication, as sometimes drugs cause fever. You may require scanning of the heart to detect infection (subacute bacterial endocarditis), the abdomen (for kidney disease or a liver abscess), or CT and MRI scans to search for unexpected cancers or deep-seated infections.

The pace of investigation is influenced by the condition of the individual: a feverish person who is seriously ill with confusion and low blood pressure needs everything urgently. An adult who is able to work, is eating and maintaining weight but sweating at night can have more leisurely investigation.

Many prolonged fevers resolve without anything abnormal being found.

TREATMENT

Even though fever is believed to be beneficial, treatment makes the person feel more comfortable, decreases the aches and aids rest. Fever greatly increases the body's metabolic rate and demand for energy, another reason to get it under control.

Discard excess clothing and do not swaddle children. It is better for them to be naked or at most wear a light vest and be covered with light bedding. Fanning is comforting, especially in summer. Tepid sponging reduces temperature rapidly, which is important in children, even if a little uncomfortable.

Febrile fits

If anyone's temperature rises high or fast enough, there is a risk of provoking a febrile fit. This is a common and potentially serious hazard in children, which is why there is such emphasis on reducing their temperature (see FEBRILE FITS). The risk in adults is extremely low.

Drugs to reduce temperature

The most widely used drug is paracetamol, which is safe for all ages. It is important not to exceed the recommended dosage as damage can be caused to the liver.

Aspirin is an alternative. Although ideal for adults, aspirin must not be used in children under the age of 12 as it can, in rare cases, cause a type of liver and brain damage called Reye's syndrome. Ibuprofen is as effective as paracetamol and safe for children.

Additionally, of course, the underlying cause of the fever should be treated as appropriate.

QUESTIONS

Is it harmful to go out with a fever?
Going into a cooler environment will help reduce fever. Parents often feel that children with fevers must stay at home, but no harm will come to them if they go outside.

Can people simulate a fever?
It is not unusual for puzzling fevers to prove to be due to deliberate deception, for example by putting a thermometer into a hot drink – this is something to consider if blood tests that should support serious infection remain normal.

Complementary Treatment

Western herbalism – catmint will cool you down. Make an infusion with 1 teaspoon per cup and drink freely. Many herbs promote sweating during fever, for example elderflower, ginger, hyssop and yarrow. Echinacea will boost your defences. Many herbs are warming, for example garlic, cayenne and cinnamon. **Homeopathy** – a whole range of remedies are available, for example belladonna and aconite. Their use depends on the specific details of your case and you should seek the advice of a registered homeopath. **Aromatherapy** – a few drops of oil in tepid water can be used to soothe fever. Lavender and Roman chamomile are especially soothing. Antiseptic oils include tea tree, myrrh, thyme. **Ayurveda** encourages regular detoxification to prevent infections attacking the body. If fever strikes, it offers herbal medications. **Nutritional therapy** – during convalescence eat plenty of fruit, vegetables and wholefoods. *Other therapies to try: Chinese herbalism; reflexology; Bach flower remedies.*

IMMUNIZATION

◆

A medical technique that stimulates the body into producing resistance against infectious diseases.

BACKGROUND
◆

There can be few advances in society that have provided so much good to so many people at so little cost as immunization. Less than a century ago infectious disease was a major killer at all ages, especially in childhood. Such diseases are now almost eradicated in the developed world. Other factors have contributed, but immunization is still of great importance.

Infection and the immune response

The 'trick' of immunization is to deceive the body into thinking it is meeting a disease before it actually encounters the real thing. In this way the body is stimulated to produce immune protection ready for when the real germs invade, so that it recognizes and destroys them on first contact.

When an organism invades the body, it is soon recognized as being 'non-self' by proteins that latch on to its unusual protein surface. These proteins, called antibodies, have the ability to call up additional resources to deal with infection. These are white blood cells that have been primed to attack organisms, either through direct recognition or by flowing to where antibodies have pinned down infection. The white blood cells and the antibodies inactivate germs by destroying their surface coating or by engulfing them and digesting them.

It takes a few days for the defences to be rallied, during which time bacteria or viruses may cause great damage and may tip the balance against the body being able to eradicate them. Previous immunization shortens this process by making possible swift recognition and destruction of the infection.

VACCINES
◆

Immunization is achieved by giving the body a vaccine – a substance swallowed or, more usually, injected that is related to a serious infecting organism but has been rendered harmless. In the case of bacterial vaccines, it is extracts of killed bacteria that are enough to generate an immune response. In the case of viral vaccinations, it is usually a strain of the virus made harmless through modification and extended breeding.

Vaccination is given from infancy in order to stimulate antibodies well before the child is at risk of actual infection.

Many countries have vaccination programmes against illnesses such as **measles**, **mumps**, **rubella**, **tetanus**, polio, **diphtheria**, **whooping cough**, haemophilus and **tuberculosis**.

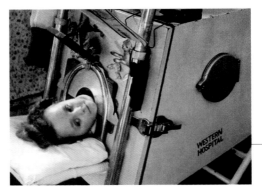

Left: One of the thousands of victims once paralysed by polio, inside an artificial lung.

There are many additional vaccines kept for people at special risk, for example hepatitis A, typhoid and yellow fever for travellers, and hepatitis B for healthcare professionals. It is usual to have a first injection that stimulates a basic immune response and booster injections to trigger the full response. Booster injections may be advisable every few years, the precise details depending on the vaccine involved.

QUESTIONS

What are the overall risks of vaccination?
Before a vaccine enters use it must be shown that its serious risks are enormously less than those of the illness itself. Public concern justifiably pushes for ever safer vaccines, often forgetting that worldwide preventable infectious diseases still kill millions of unvaccinated children each year.

Who should not be vaccinated?
There is a separate list for each vaccine, generally including those with a current febrile illness, or who are on steroids, have reduced immune capability (for example leukaemia patients) or are allergic to components of the vaccine such as egg.

 ### Complementary Treatment

The orthodox position is that there are no alternatives to immunization against the common infectious illnesses, especially those of childhood. However, **homeopaths** claim to offer effective substitutes. If you are considering immunizing your children and are interested in this option, discuss it with your doctor and a registered homeopath before reaching a final decision. **It is the author's opinion that children should be given conventional vaccinations.**

MEASLES

❖

Once a feared childhood illness, now rare in the developed world.

CAUSES

The virus causing measles is in the same family as **flu** and **mumps**. Although measles is not a trivial illness, its effects are greatly reduced if the person is in otherwise good health.

SYMPTOMS

Measles spreads through the air and incubates for up to two weeks. It starts with high **fever** plus symptoms similar to **colds** – a streaming nose, cough and red eyes. After about four days a rash appears on the face, which rapidly spreads to the whole body. The blotchy rash fades to brown over a week, during which time the fever and malaise continue.

TREATMENT

Often a child with measles is put on an antibiotic; although this cannot influence the course of the viral illness it reduces the chances of a serious chest infection. Complications are uncommon in the developed world but are common and dangerous in malnourished people – for example **pneumonia** and heart disease are the main causes of death through measles.

There are rare but tragic instances of permanent brain damage through measles **encephalitis,** but thanks to routine vaccination, measles is now an avoidable disease.

QUESTION

How safe is a measles vaccination?
Even in the developed world, measles kills one in five thousand sufferers – one hundred and thirty children died in a recent epidemic in the United States – and leaves another one in five thousand with permanent brain damage. In Third World children the death rate is up to 15%. The latest estimates of the risks of vaccination are of less than a one in one hundred thousand chance of brain damage and no substantiated deaths.

 Complementary Treatment

It is important to seek a conventional medical opinion. A **homeopath** might be able to help. **Chinese herbalism** can offer formulae for use during recovery.

MUMPS

❖

A viral infection that causes swelling of the salivary glands.

CAUSES

The mumps virus is spread through sneezing or saliva. Mumps has effects throughout the body beyond the typical enlargement of the salivary glands in the cheeks, affecting the pancreas, testicles, ovaries and brain. Mumps is infectious two to three days before the facial swelling appears and for three to five days afterwards.

SYMPTOMS

Mumps incubates for 18 days before producing typical viral symptoms of **fever**, **headaches** and muscle pains. Then there is enlargement of the parotid salivary glands – the ones lying over the angle of the jaws below the ears. The face becomes distorted – hamster-like is as graphic a description as any. The swelling lasts for about five days.

There may be pain in the testicles due to inflammation; girls can experience abdominal discomfort through inflammation of their ovaries. Temporary **deafness** is not uncommon but there is a less than a one in three hundred risk of permanent deafness. There is a small risk of **viral meningitis**.

TREATMENT

Only fluids, rest and painkillers are needed. Even mumps meningitis can be expected to settle within two weeks. The risk of mumps causing sterility is very small. Rarely, **encephalitis** can occur, with a coma lasting months or even permanently. Mumps is preventable by vaccination in infancy.

   Complementary Treatment

Nutritional therapy – supplements of vitamins and minerals can boost your immune system. **Western herbalism** – see FEVER. **Chinese herbalism** can offer formulae to help. A **homeopath** might be able to help.

RUBELLA

◆

Also called German measles, rubella is an infection that is minor for the patient but catastrophic for foetal development.

CAUSES

◆

The rubella virus spreads through coughing or saliva. In a pregnant woman it passes to her foetus. The risk of damage is greatest during the first four months of pregnancy while the organs are forming. The child may be born with **deafness**, heart valve disease, **cataracts** and brain damage.

SYMPTOMS

◆

After two to three weeks' incubation rubella begins with **fever** and enlarged lymph glands, especially at the back of the neck. A brownish rash appears after a few days, soon fading. Short-term joint pain is common; other complications are rare.

TREATMENT

◆

There is no special treatment for rubella, other than taking aspirin or paracetamol to reduce fever or discomfort. For women who are in the first four months of pregnancy, it is essential to have a diagnosis of the illness confirmed by blood tests and then to consider the risks to the baby. These can be as high as a 30% chance of damage, with 20% of babies dying in early infancy. Many countries will offer abortion in these tragic circumstances.

QUESTION

How is rubella controlled?
In the United Kingdom vaccination against rubella is given with measles and mumps vaccinations. All pregnant women are checked for immunity to rubella. Thanks to these measures there were only 12 children born in the United Kingdom with congenital rubella in 1990, while only 10 abortions were needed for at-risk mothers, compared to the hundreds that were done as recently as the 1970s.

  Complementary Treatment
Make sure you and your children are immunized. **Western herbalism** and **aromatherapy** – see FEVER. **Homeopathic** remedies include phytolacca and pulsatilla, but their use depends on a number of variables.

WHOOPING COUGH

◆

Bacterial infection noted for causing a persistent cough in children.

CAUSES

◆

Bordetella pertussis is the organism responsible for this highly infectious illness, once so common in childhood. The incubation period is seven to ten days. Vaccination has rendered the illness rare, with newer non-bacterial vaccines believed to be far safer than getting whooping cough.

SYMPTOMS

◆

In its early stages whooping cough is like an ordinary **cold**, with a runny nose, red eyes and **fever**. The cough begins after a week; it consists of paroxysms of coughing that the child cannot stop until he or she desperately sucks in air, giving the characteristic whoop. In older children or adults, whose airways are wider, whooping is not likely, but they still suffer from the paroxysmal cough.

Complications of whooping cough include the collapse of part of the lung with permanent damage and starvation of oxygen leading to convulsions. The diagnosis is confirmed through swabs taken from the nose and the throat.

TREATMENT

◆

If the illness is suspected within the first week, the infectivity is reduced by taking the antibiotic erythromycin. Once the full extent is known, treatment is with moisturized air, nursing care to keep up fluid intake and vigorous treatment of complications. The cough can last for months afterwards.

Complementary Treatment

   Seek a conventional opinion. **Western herbalism** expectorants include horehound and thyme. Relaxants include lavender and hyssop. **Homeopathy** offers a variety of remedies; seek advice. **Chinese herbs** can be helpful.

DIPHTHERIA

A serious and sometimes fatal bacterial throat infection.

CAUSES

The infection is caused by a micro-organism called *Corynebacterium diphtheriae*; it is spread through coughing, sneezing and saliva. The infection grows in the throat or larynx into a tough membrane that restricts breathing. The bacteria produce a blood-borne toxin affecting the heart and nerves.

SYMPTOMS

A membrane can be seen in the throat and in the nostrils. The child, at first mildly unwell with **fever** and sore throat, soon deteriorates and has difficulty in breathing, becoming increasing blue from oxygen starvation. The effect on the heart is to cause heart failure with increasing breathlessness and collapse of the circulation, carrying a high risk of death.

TREATMENT

This is of the utmost urgency for a child with diphtheria – injections of antitoxins together with high doses of penicillin must be given once the illness is diagnosed. However, even with these measures the risks of the illness are high and may even appear several weeks after apparent recovery.

In the developed world vaccination has rendered the disease extremely rare, but it remains a significant risk in many less fortunate parts of the world. In the United Kingdom a few cases are diagnosed in immigrants who have come from developing countries.

QUESTION

What is the role of vaccination?
There is no substitute for vaccination if you want prevention for your children. In the United Kingdom vaccination is given at two months with monthly boosters over the next two months. Contacts of known cases should have injections of antitoxins. Travellers to countries where diphtheria has re-emerged, such as Russia, should consider having booster vaccinations.

Complementary Treatment

Complementary approaches are not appropriate as treatment. During recovery, **aromatherapy massage** could be very soothing for adults and children alike.

TETANUS

A very serious infection leading to spasms of the muscles, commonly called lockjaw.

CAUSES

Tetanus occurs if spores of the *Clostridium tetani* organism, which lives in the soil, get through a cut in the skin. Tetanus was common until vaccination became routine, and is still an important health hazard in undeveloped countries.

SYMPTOMS

Symptoms begin days or weeks after infection. The first muscles affected are those that close the jaws, which go into a rigid spasm – hence the name lockjaw. Spasm of the back muscles causes arching of the back. There may be **fever** and sweating. Mild cases can recover, but there is a poor outlook if the muscles of breathing or of the heart are affected.

TREATMENT

Any dirty wound is a risk for tetanus and you should have an injection of antitetanus toxin if there is any doubt about your vaccination status.

The illness is treated by intensive nursing care in a quiet environment, since stimuli set off spasms. Muscle relaxants are given to reduce the spasms and also artificial ventilation if needed. Even so the risk of death in serious cases is 20–60%.

In the United Kingdom the antitetanus vaccination programme, which begins in infancy, has made tetanus virtually extinct. Boosters are recommended every ten years for adults, especially those who work with soil (gardeners and farmers).

Complementary Treatment

Complementary approaches are not appropriate for treatment. Any of the therapies discussed under STRESS could help during the recovery period.

SCARLET FEVER

A once notorious bacterial throat infection.

CAUSES

Many throat infections are caused by the streptococcus bacteria, one strain of which is responsible for scarlet fever – now often called scarlatina. However the bacteria, while still causing the same symptoms, has lost its capacity to cause permanent damage, possibly through improvements in general health.

SYMPTOMS

The throat feels painful and there are enlarged neck glands and **fever**. After a day or two a fine red rash spreads all over the skin, from which the illness gets its name. The rash tends to spare the area immediately around the mouth, which looks pale by contrast. The tongue goes from having a white coating with red dots to looking raw. Later, skin may peel from the fingers and the toes. The appearance is typical and the diagnosis can be confirmed by throat swabs and blood tests.

TREATMENT

Penicillin is given for ten days, during which time individuals should use their own utensils; other isolation is unnecessary. Rest, fluids and paracetamol are also recommended.

QUESTION

What was the significance of scarlet fever in the past?
It was associated with rheumatic fever, which led to heart disease, kidney damage and severe infection. These complications made scarlet fever a leading cause of childhood death in the 19th century, whereas now it virtually never has any long-term consequences.

 Complementary Treatment
Chinese herbalism – treatments are offered to ease symptoms and help the body fight off infection. *Other therapies to try: see FEVER.*

CHICKENPOX

A viral infection characterized by a blistery rash.

CAUSES

In childhood, chickenpox is a relatively mild illness. The virus responsible is varicella zoster, which in later life causes shingles. Chickenpox is highly contagious from just before the blisters appear until they are all crusted over.

SYMPTOMS

After two to three weeks' incubation the illness begins with **fever** and aching. Tiny clear-headed blisters appear after two to three days, spreading within hours all over the body, including the scalp and mouth but not the palms and soles.

TREATMENT

The main problem is itching, eased by antihistamines such as chlorpheniramine, and soothing lotions like calamine lotion. It is important not to scratch blisters off or they will leave a scar. After about ten days all the blisters become scabbed and disappear over another two to three weeks. Chickenpox affects the lungs so a worsening cough should be treated with an antibiotic. Adults feel more ill and many doctors give them an antiviral drug such as acyclovir to reduce the severity. Vaccination against chickenpox may soon become available.

QUESTION

Is chickenpox serious?
Complications in children are very rare. About one in a thousand adults develops a form of encephalitis and requires more intensive treatment. In the uncommon event of catching chickenpox in early pregnancy, the mother is likely to have complications and the virus may affect the foetus; urgent medical advice should be sought.

 Complementary Treatment
Bach flower remedies – impatiens for irritability and crab apple for cleansing the skin may both be applied to the skin diluted. All itchy childhood rashes may be relieved with chicory, hornbeam or cherry plum.

FIFTH DISEASE

A benign viral illness, mainly affecting children, and notable for the red facial appearance it causes; hence 'slapped face' disease.

CAUSES

Medically known as erythema infectiosum, fifth disease is caused by a tiny virus, the parvovirus. Parvoviruses are responsible for many non-specific viral illnesses. It is thought to be spread by coughs; the incubation period is up to 18 days.

SYMPTOMS

The illness begins in the usual viral way with **fever** and muscle pains. After a day or two the child's cheeks become bright red with a fine rash, which then spreads elsewhere on the body, but with a more lace-like appearance.

TREATMENT

The only treatment necessary is something to relieve muscle aches and to reduce any fever. Paracetamol or ibuprofen syrups are usually sufficient to do this.

In many cases the child remains well or only a little unwell and may require rest and fluids. The rash may reappear over the course of the next few weeks.

QUESTION

Why it it called 'fifth' disease?
Doctors tend to keep mental checklists for many conditions, including childhood illnesses with rashes. When presented with a patient with a rash, the doctor mentally reviews all of the possibilities. However, what constitutes the first four diseases with a rash varies from doctor to doctor. This author considers the following: measles, German measles, scarlet fever and roseola. This leaves erythema infectiosum as number five.

Complementary Treatment
Bach flower remedies – Rescue Remedy. **Aromatherapy** – bathing and **massage** are soothing, particularly with lavender or Roman chamomile. *Other therapies to try: see FEVER and CHICKENPOX.*

ROSEOLA

Common childhood illness with a rash, often confused with measles.

CAUSES

The virus responsible for this condition was only recently identified as another of the ubiquitous herpes viruses. It is almost always confined to children; most adults are immune.

SYMPTOMS

There is a high temperature, listlessness and runny nose, continuing for several days. In these respects it resembles **measles** before the rash appears. After four to five days the rash spreads, then the **fever** abruptly falls and recovery occurs.

TREATMENT

Treatment is simply a matter of taking fluids plus paracetamol or ibuprofen to reduce the fever. Once the rash has appeared the child will be back to normal within two to three days. It is

highly unusual for the illness to follow other than an uncomplicated course. It is quite probable that the many 'allergic reactions' to antibiotics given for feverish illnesses are actually rashes that are due to roseola or similar viruses.

QUESTION

How does roseola differ from measles?
Measles tends to cause higher temperatures and more illness in the child; also red eyes are common. Otherwise the clinical picture is very similar. The difference is that in roseola the appearance of the rash signals recovery, whereas in measles it signals another few days of high temperatures and misery.

Complementary Treatment
Nutritional therapy – during convalescence children should eat plenty of fruit, vegetables and wholefoods. *Other therapies to try: see FEVER and CHICKENPOX.*

VIRAL MENINGITIS

A form of brain infection caused by a virus. It is relatively benign and rarely causes serious illness.

CAUSES

There is no one virus that causes viral meningitis; the most common ones are those that also cause the routine infections of childhood such as gastroenteritis (see DIARRHOEA AND VOMITING) or upper respiratory infections. Meningitis can accompany other well-known viral illnesses such as **mumps** and **glandular fever**.

The viruses gain access to the brain through the blood stream, having escaped the normally vigorous defences that keep infection away from the brain. Unlike the bacterial causes of meningitis, viral infection does not transmit easily from person to person.

Viral infection of the brain causes inflammation of the fine tissues covering the brain called the meninges, hence the term 'meningitis'. In contrast with bacterial infection, viral infections do not generally spread from the meninges into the brain and so do not often cause swelling nor lead to deposits of pus. These consequences make **bacterial meningitis** very serious and, conversely, make viral meningitis normally follow a much more benign course.

SYMPTOMS

All types of meningitis affect children more often than adults. Early in what appears to be a routine viral illness, the child will start to complain about severe and persistent **headaches**; he may vomit, and grumble about bright light irritating his eyes, and also a stiff neck. The child is feverish and unhappy, irritated at being handled in any way. This is the fully developed illness, but it is probable that many viral illnesses are accompanied by a mild meningitis causing similar, although less pronounced, symptoms.

TREATMENT

Although doctors may feel fairly certain that they are dealing with a case of viral as opposed to bacterial meningitis, it is essential to confirm the diagnosis by hospital admission for investigation. Doctors will be guided by blood tests that show changes more suggestive of a viral cause.

If there is the slightest doubt about any ill child, then a lumbar puncture will be performed to sample the cerebrospinal fluid that surrounds the brain and spinal cord. The fluid is then scrutinized to see if it contains any infection and for changes in the cells in it that reflect the type of meningitis. The identity of the virus responsible is established by further analysis of the blood and cerebrospinal fluid.

If the diagnosis is viral meningitis every one can breathe a sigh of relief, in the virtually certain knowledge that recovery can be expected over the next few days. Should recovery be delayed or the illness worsen, then the diagnosis may have to be reviewed or the child may have developed one of the relatively rare complications. Fortunately, fewer than one in a hundred meningitis sufferers develop **encephalitis**, with drowsiness, worsening headaches and possibly epileptic fits.

It normally takes seven to ten days for full recovery, and hospital care is not necessary once the diagnosis is certain. It is common for headaches to recur for several weeks after the illness and this in itself should not cause concern.

See also BACTERIAL MENINGITIS.

QUESTIONS

How can I recognize meningitis?
The generally agreed symptoms for viral meningitis are as given earlier – abnormal headaches, stiffness of the neck, discomfort from bright lights, unusual drowsiness and vomiting. The more serious bacterial meningitis has the additional symptom of causing a blotchy purple rash. However, the diagnosis of meningitis is not always straightforward and medical opinion should be sought even if it seems to be a remote possibility.

What is the role of antibiotics?
Viral illnesses do not respond to antibiotics. Many doctors would nevertheless prescribe antibiotics even though the diagnosis is viral meningitis – just to be on the safe side.

Complementary Treatment
Complementary approaches are not appropriate for treatment. However, many therapies could help during recovery. If the patient is a child, check that your chosen practitioner is experienced in treating children. Traditional Chinese medicine (**acupuncture**, **herbs**, **tai chi/chi kung**) can be helpful. **Reflexology** supports recovery by giving special attention to areas according to the specific characteristics of the personality and the symptoms. *Other therapies to try: see STRESS.*

TUBERCULOSIS

Slow-growing infection that can spread from the lungs throughout the body. Its seriousness depends on the victim's general health.

CAUSES

Tuberculosis (TB) follows infection with the organism mycobacterium tuberculosis, which gains access to the lungs by close contact with others coughing up the bacteria. In otherwise healthy individuals, infection is unlikely to progress further and will be eradicated by the body's own defence mechanism. Otherwise the bacteria lie relatively dormant causing few if any symptoms.

The disease then becomes reactivated months or years later, when the individual's resistance falls through other reasons such as malnutrition or AIDS. This secondary disease can spread throughout the body, affecting the lungs, brain, bones, joints and more.

Much of the increase in TB in the developed world has been through the spread of AIDS. This illness diminishes the immune response and leaves the individual susceptible to many other infections as well as TB.

SYMPTOMS

If the initial infection causes any symptoms they are temporary vague ill health and a cough that settles in a few weeks. Symptoms from reactivation depend on which parts of the body are affected. The most common are recurrence of cough, which becomes chronic, persistent malaise, weight loss and night sweating. The phlegm often contains blood. At this stage enlarged lymph nodes may appear, typically in the neck.

Aggressive TB

This is called miliary TB and is the result of the spread of the bacterium throughout the blood stream, like a septicaemia. The individual is at first unwell in a vague way but rapidly becomes very ill indeed and may well develop meningitis. Miliary TB is a risk even several years after initial infection, but it is uncommon except in debilitated individuals.

Other effects

These are all fortunately now uncommon in the developed world. Bones are a favourite lodging site for TB and it is still considered in anyone with persistent bone pain. The infection slowly destroys the bone, which eventually collapses. This was previously a common cause for collapse of spinal vertebrae and distortion of the back. Chronic infection of the

intestines can lead to abdominal pain. Other organs that can be affected are the womb, causing pain, heavy bleeding and subfertility, the kidneys, causing chronic kidney infection, and the testicles. Tuberculous meningitis is particularly difficult to diagnose and is a dangerous form of the illness.

The diagnosis of TB depends on seeing typical changes on a chest X-ray, analysing enlarged lymph nodes, identifying the bacterium in sputum and examining tissue biopsies.

TREATMENT

For six months, people with TB need to take daily tablets of the antibiotics rifampicin and isoniazid, and additional antibiotics depending on the individual case. Longer courses are given for bone, brain or gynaecological infection – up to a year. These drugs have proved to be effective and have few side effects. Cure can be virtually guaranteed in those who take the treatment reliably. There is, however, a problem of resistance to these drugs which is a worrying new phenomenon.

Aggressive therapy is required in the treatment of both miliary TB and tuberculous meningitis.

QUESTIONS

Who is at risk of TB?
TB is predominately a disease of poverty, malnutrition, overcrowded housing and self-neglect. Alleviation of these factors was responsible for the virtual eradication of TB in many countries. Immigrants from underdeveloped countries are still at significant risk.

What is BCG vaccination?
This is an inactivated strain of TB given by injection and providing about 70% immunity to TB. It stands for Bacille Calmette-Guérin, the French researchers responsible for this important vaccine.

Complementary Treatment

Remain with your conventional treatment regime and tell your doctor about any complementary approaches you choose to explore. Traditional Chinese medicine (**acupuncture**, **herbs**, **tai chi/chi kung**) can help the body fight off infection, but with TB the effects will be only partial. **Chakra balancing** and **hypnotherapy** can offer support during the long treatment schedule, and help relieve many of the symptoms. *Other therapies to try: see STRESS.*

AIDS

AIDS kills by reducing a person's immune capability.

CAUSES

AIDS (acquired immune deficiency syndrome) is caused by one of two viruses: HIV I, found in most of the world, and HIV II, found mainly in Africa. HIV stands for human immuno-deficiency virus. These viruses probably arose through spontaneous mutation in Africa in the 1950s; some believe they have been around much longer but only recently became aggressive.

AIDS as a specific medical condition was recognized in 1981 and the virus identified in 1983. The virus spreads through semen and blood products and especially through homosexual practices, for example anal intercourse, and intravenous drug abuse. It can be passed from mother to unborn child. Heterosexual spread is far less common in populations with good nutrition, although statistics show that heterosexual sex is becoming the most important means of transmission. The disease has begun to spread rapidly through India and South-East Asia.

SYMPTOMS

On initial infection the virus causes a non-specific viral illness with **fever** and enlarged glands. It continues to live in the body, but causes no symptoms. This is what is meant by being HIV positive. A person who is HIV positive will almost certainly eventually develop AIDS and show symptoms. This may take as little as six months or more than ten years.

The virus damages the immune system so that the later symptoms are from infections – recurrent **thrush**, **diarrhoea**, sweating, shingles, profound weight loss and malaise. Other features highly suggestive of AIDS are chest infections with unusual organisms; characteristic skin tumours such as Kaposi's sarcoma (see SKIN CANCER); **tuberculosis** in a young person and premature dementia. Many other infections and tumours result and, until recently, a progressive decline was inevitable. The illness is diagnosed by the clinical picture and by blood tests demonstrating the presence of the HIV virus.

TREATMENT

The average survival time of AIDS patients has improved from six months to several years, reflecting the progress in treatment. Current treatment is with a combination of three or four drugs which together reduce the activity of the virus – such as zidovudine, saquinavir, ritonavir. This is a highly specialized, constantly changing area of research and treatment. Other infections are treated as appropriate with antibiotics, chemotherapy, antifungal drugs and so on.

Giving combinations of antiviral drugs to HIV positive people reduces their chance of developing AIDS, or of an HIV positive mother passing the virus to her unborn child. This may become the standard treatment for HIV in the future. There are also reports of a promising new anti-HIV vaccine.

QUESTION

How can HIV/AIDS be avoided?
Unprotected casual sex is dangerous; always use a condom, especially if you are having sex with multiple partners. Anal intercourse and intravenous drug use are high-risk behaviour for HIV. Oral sex may carry a risk if you have any sores or cuts in your mouth. If you are travelling abroad, bear in mind that Western standards of blood transfusion may not apply in all countries.

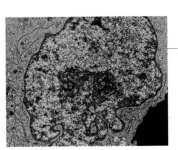

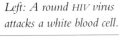
Left: A round HIV virus attacks a white blood cell.

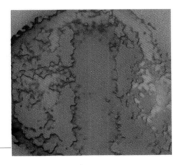

Right: The infected cell produces many more HIV viruses.

Complementary Treatment

Complementary therapies offer support, not cures. **Chakra balancing** – non-touch techniques are ideal and can help with relaxation, symptom control and insomnia, and also stimulate appetite. **Hypnotherapy** can relieve many of the symptoms such as depression and anxiety. Traditional Chinese medicine (**acupuncture**, **herbs**, **tai chi/chi kung**) offers a variety of immune-boosting preparations. **Nutritional therapy** – your practitioner will try to improve your assimilation of food. *Other therapies to try: Ayurveda; Western herbalism: see also STRESS.*

MALARIA

◆

A parasitic infection, spread by mosquitoes. Malaria is probably the most significant and deadly infectious disease in the world.

CAUSES
◆

Malaria is caused by four different types of a parasitic micro-organism, called plasmodium. Each type leads to a slightly different pattern of disease and requires different treatment.

Plasmodium enters humans by the bite of the anopheles mosquito, ubiquitous in hot, humid regions of the world. The parasite's eggs live in the mosquito's salivary glands. When the infected mosquito bites a human, eggs enter the human host and rapidly travel through the blood stream to the liver (see diagram, right). After some time the parasites escape into the blood stream again, this time invading red blood cells and multiplying until the cells rupture. The free parasites then circulate within the blood plasma, awaiting a bite by a mosquito, which sucks up the infected blood ready for the parasite to complete its life cycle, and to infect the next host. A number of parasites remain in the liver; their escape every few days or months accounts for the chronic and repeated nature of malaria.

SYMPTOMS
◆

Depending on the type of infection it takes from ten days to six weeks before symptoms begin. An attack progresses within hours through three distinct phases, corresponding to stages of invasion of the blood stream. First there is sudden intense shivering and feeling cold, despite a **fever**; this merges into several hours of high fever with possible confusion and ends with drenching sweats and feeling better. The pattern repeats itself with variations, depending on which type of malaria parasite is responsible, for example every two days to a more irregular pattern. The illness can become chronic with persistent **anaemia** and ill health. At another extreme it may progress rapidly to **kidney failure**, coma and death.

TREATMENT
◆

The parasite can be seen on blood samples. This is how the diagnosis is confirmed, the type identified and cure monitored.

Once the type of parasite is known, the appropriate drug is given usually by mouth or by intravenous drip in severe cases. The drugs – chloroquine, mefloquine and primaquine – act very quickly even in severe infection, where improvement can begin after just a single dose. Other measures are intravenous quinine, fluids and paracetamol or aspirin to reduce fever.

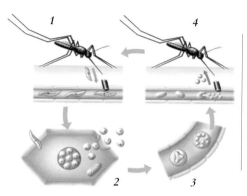

Left: **1)** *Mosquito injects parasite into blood stream.* **2)** *Parasites multiply in liver;* **3)** *invade blood stream and* **4)** *are sucked up by mosquito which later infects new host.*

Preventing infection

Before travelling to a potential malaria zone – especially countries too poor or unstable to maintain the necessary public health measures – get up-to-date advice about the health hazards, including the risk of malaria. There are many help lines and medical publications providing information about the drugs you should take. It is essential to begin the drugs a week before travel, to take them regularly during your stay and to continue for six weeks after you return. Even if your exposure to malaria may only be overnight on a stopover, you should consider taking preventive medication. Additional precautions are to wear clothing that covers exposed skin, use insect repellents, sleep under mosquito netting and avoid going out at times favoured by mosquitoes, for example at dusk.

QUESTION

How dangerous is malaria?
Between two and three hundred million people contract malaria each year, of whom two to three million die, many of them children. Certain forms are extremely dangerous, with collapse of blood pressure, kidney and brain damage and delirium.

Complementary Treatment

It is folly to travel into malaria-infested regions without following conventional medical advice. If you do catch the disease, follow your orthodox doctor's treatment programme, but remember that people living in countries where malaria is endemic traditionally use **Ayurvedic** medications and Chinese approaches, especially **Chinese herbalism**, to treat this disease. Consult the relevant practitioners if you are interested in exploring these options.

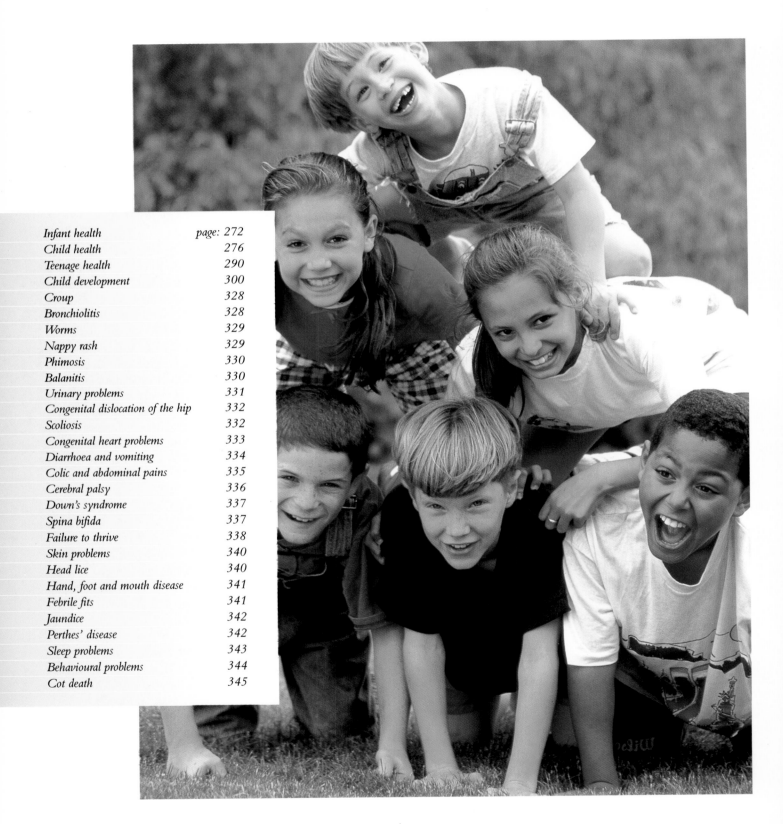

The realization that children are not simply little adults is a relatively late concept in medicine. The illnesses they get, their symptoms and their response to treatment are often quite unlike adult ill health. The speciality of paediatrics only emerged in the second half of the 20th century.

CHILDREN

I F YOU ASK ANY PARENT what they want most for their child they will say health and happiness. All of us worry about the health of our children, partly because we may have little previous experience of babies or young children. We also worry because they can't tell us what is wrong and, even when they have the vocabulary, they may not use it correctly. For example, small children often describe a pain as 'tummy ache', even if it is a headache. With access to so much information nowadays and the support of our families and health professionals, however, we should feel confident that we are doing the best for our children.

After a discussion of child health and development, this chapter covers the common childhood ailments and describes their symptoms and signs, their possible causes and treatments. Viral infections are particularly common in childhood, causing a wide variety of illnesses, from coughs and colds to croup and chicken pox. There is no specific treatment for them, rather it is a case of treating the symptoms to make your child comfortable. In some situations complementary therapies are also suggested, but any qualified practitioner of complementary medicine would agree that certain illnesses must be treated with orthodox medicine.

Childhood illnesses occur during a time of rapid growth and development, and either can be affected if the illness persists. Measuring weight and head growth, particularly during the first year of life, is an important means of monitoring health. As well as growing rapidly in size, infants and toddlers will develop quickly. Some of the developmental milestones, such as learning to walk, show wide variation between individuals while others should occur at particular times. It is always tempting to compare your own child with others, but this can be misleading. If you are concerned it is important to discuss your worries with your health visitor.

There is increasing evidence that our health as adults is affected by what happens in childhood, so it is vital to keep your child healthy. Childhood obesity, particularly if it persists into the teenage years, is likely to be a lifelong problem, predisposing individuals to diabetes. What is worrying is that obesity is now one of the most common problems in children. Establishing a habit of healthy eating for the whole family is something we should all try to do.

Unfortunately accidents are common in childhood. Toddlers have no sense of danger, but there is a lot that parents can do to make the house as safe as possible and gradually teach their offspring where dangers may lie. School-age children are particularly at risk from road traffic accidents, as pedestrians or as cyclists, so teaching them the fundamentals of road safety is essential. As they become more independent, we have to hope that they have learnt the right lessons from us to enable them to remain happy and healthy throughout their lives.

There is no one definition of normality in childhood. Your child's general health and development is of more significance than minor variations in attaining particular milestones. Children born in the developed world enjoy an expectation of health and development unimaginable to children in much of the rest of the world. When reading in the following pages of things that may go wrong, do bear in mind that really serious ill health in childhood is uncommon.

Left: Children carry our hopes; their physical and psychological health is naturally a high priority for parents.

Dr Jane Collins,
Great Ormond Street Hospital for Children

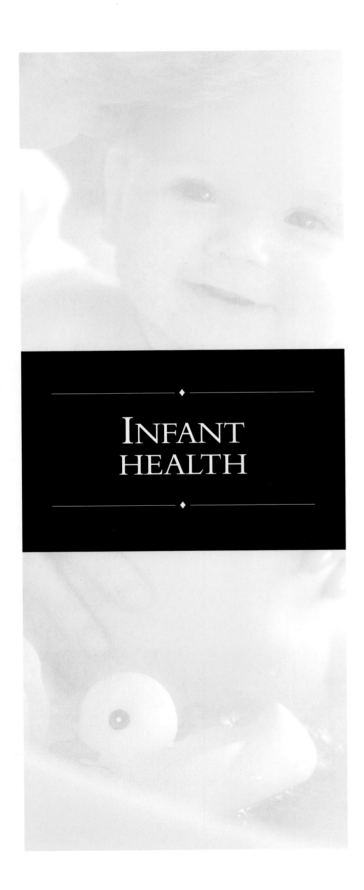

INFANT HEALTH

Fragile and dependent as new infants look, they are actually born survivors. Modern lifestyles and improvements in medicine mean that the newly born now begin life in better health than they have ever done before – and the vast majority of them remain that way. Survival statistics show that, in the United Kingdom, 994 infants out of every 1000 celebrate their first birthdays in good health. Only a generation ago three times as many infants died before they were one year of age, so in the developed countries of northern Europe and North America the prospects for new infants have never before been so promising.

Bonding

For an infant to survive emotionally, bonding is a necessity. Babies do not thrive if only their physical needs are attended to, but as long as their emotional needs are met, most of them develop into caring and empathetic children. What is more, there is evidence that babies who have securely bonded with their mothers develop their innate capacities more fully than babies who do not develop such strong attachments.

What is bonding? Babies need one special person whom they love and who loves them, and initially this is the person the baby spends most time with when awake – usually the mother, but it can be a father, grandparent or a paid carer. (A baby who has more than one special person to care for them – a father and a mother, and perhaps a grandparent as well – is additionally fortunate.) During the first year of life an infant becomes increasingly attached to these special people.

From the mother's point of view, bonding is the process whereby she becomes irrevocably committed to her baby. Some mothers fall in love instantly with their babies. For others the strong feelings of a caring concern and commitment take weeks or even months to flower. The emotional commitment can begin before birth; in fact, in one study almost four mothers in ten reported positive feelings towards their unborn babies. The infant's foetal movements were important to these mothers, perhaps because they encouraged the realization that the bump was a baby. Almost exactly the same number of mothers fell in love with their babies during birth or on the first day, with most of the remaining mothers starting to feel positive about the infant a day or two following the birth. For these mothers, important issues were being able to be alone with their new baby and having the opportunity to hold them.

Unfortunately there are a number of mothers who simply do not bond with their babies, at least in the first few weeks or months. There can be many reasons. Postnatal depression is one, and so is the infant's temperament. Some babies are not responsive. Others have spent weeks or even months in a

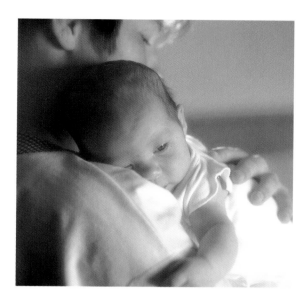

Above: Close body contact calms infant and parent, and makes them feel more attuned. The power of touch in the process of bonding has been under-rated, but is now widely acknowledged: one study showed that blindfolded new mothers could identify their babies by touching their hands.

neonatal intensive care unit where the opportunities for the simple activities known to promote bonding – holding the infant, communicating with them – are not possible or are limited. One mother of a very premature baby, born at 26 weeks, found that she didn't dare love her baby daughter in case the baby died. She hoped that once she got her baby home and she no longer had to ask permission to hold her, her love would flower. However, this failed to occur. Then, when she was two years old, the toddler slipped as she was coming downstairs. 'I suddenly felt an overwhelming surge of love for her. I couldn't stop loving her. I'd always loved her, but you know when you have really bonded. Now I just love her to bits.' This is an excellent illustration of the fact that it is never too late.

Safety equipment

Over half the accidents that happen to children under five years of age occur at home, and while the peak age for accident-prone behaviour is around two, babies enter the danger zone at about nine months, when they become mobile. In the early days your baby will need complete protection. A watchful, caring eye is essential, but safety equipment both helps to protect infants in high-risk areas, such as a sitting room or kitchen, and gives parents peace of mind.

Research suggests that, in the United Kingdom, every year around 15,000 under-fives are injured in accidents involving

nursery equipment. Safety equipment that is bought second-hand, or is not repaired or replaced when worn or faulty, can itself cause accidents. Second-hand equipment does not usually come with fitting or assembly instructions and may only conform to out-of-date safety standards. It may also have worn or missing components. To keep young babies safe, it is best to buy new equipment that conforms with national or international safety standards, or to use equipment handed down by a relative or friend, the origin and history of which is well known.

Car safety seats in particular must always be replaced after a crash because of the risk of unseen structural damage to the shell or the harness. If replacement is not possible, parents should check that the seat conforms with safety standards, using information from the Child Accident Prevention Trust (see Directory for details).

The first few months Equipment needed for a baby initially includes the following: a non-slip bath mat for a baby bath; a safe cot; a safe pushchair with a five-point safety harness; a car safety seat; and a highchair with a five-point safety harness.

Pushchairs suitable from birth must be fully reclining to allow babies to lie flat until they can sit unsupported. They must have good brakes and a safety locking device to ensure they don't fold up unexpectedly. They must also have a safety harness, and should have a guard or shopping tray behind the footrest to stop trailing feet reaching the ground. They should have a deep hood to protect a baby from direct sunlight as well as a place where you can attach a parasol. A lightweight buggy is suitable after a baby can sit up straight: a lie-back buggy is suitable after three months.

Right: A safety gate is a priority purchase for parents keen to protect their mobile and inquisitive toddler from danger. From the stage when children are just walking until the point where they are able to clamber over it, the safety gate enables parents to keep their child out of the most hazardous danger zones in the home.

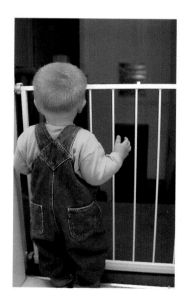

There are two suitable types of child car safety seat for babies under one year of age: a rear-facing seat with an integral harness for babies up to 10–13 kg/22–29 lb, and a forward-facing seat with integral harness, secured by a fitting kit or a lap belt with or without a diagonal belt. The latter are suitable for babies weighing between 9 and 18 kg/20 and 40 lb. All seats should now comply with a new European safety standard and be marked ECE R44.03.

The highchair should have a wide, stable base. Make sure it does not have any sharp edges or places where babies can trap their fingers. Don't leave a baby in a highchair near a table, as they can reach out for dangerous objects or food.

Additional equipment Once a baby is mobile, much more equipment becomes necessary. However, before you spend any money, lie down on the floor to put yourself at the baby's level, so you can see unexpected hazards and observe your baby's environment.

At the age of 11–12 months you will probably need: safety gates to block access to stairs and high-risk rooms; corner protectors to stop your child from banging itself on furniture; electricity socket protectors; a fireguard to protect a mobile baby from coming close to a fire; cupboard, door, fridge and video locks to discourage unwanted inquisitiveness; safety film on low level glass tables, doors and windows.

Some families find playpens useful. If you use one, look for a design with deep sides – more than 60 cm/2 ft high – and safe spacing between any bars. Don't tie strings across the playpen, as anything over 20 cm/8 inches can strangle a baby, and only keep small toys inside – resourceful babies can easily climb out. Baby walkers are popular because they allow a baby who is not quite walking to move around. However, they can cause accidents if the baby is able to reach higher objects and, for example, pull down a tablecloth. They can also tip a baby down the stairs. If a baby spends too long in a walker and their feet only just touch the ground, this encourages tiptoe walking. To be used safely, a baby in a walker has to be constantly supervised.

Warmth
Every human's body temperature is controlled by a thermostat in the brain. Infants also control their temperature in this way, but they differ from adults in that they lose heat through their skin quickly because they are thin, have little insulating fat and their skin area is large compared with their body mass. Young infants need to be kept warm, and are usually comfortable at around 16–20°C/61–68°F, a temperature that is also comfortable for an adult in light clothing. However, once undressed, babies cool down quickly, particularly if their skin is wet; so heat the room before you bath your baby.

In winter you should wrap your baby warmly when you go outside, and pay particular attention to the head and hands. The head has a large surface area and therefore loses heat rapidly. Even on a summer's day, winds can chill. Once babies come inside, however, their outdoor clothing should be loosened or taken off immediately. In this case, inside includes getting into a heated car or going into a shop.

In many homes, an infant is, however, more likely to overheat than become cold. An overheated infant looks flushed and sweaty. Cool by first removing a layer or two of clothing and offering a drink – a breastfeed or cooled, boiled water.

Outside, babies' skin is extremely vulnerable to the sun's ultraviolet rays, so use a shade on a pushchair to protect from direct sunlight. An infant under six months should never be left in the sun, and an older baby should be dressed in a wide-brimmed hat and light clothes to cover most of the body. Protect the baby's skin with a suncream that has an SPF (sun protection factor) of at least 15. Inside a car, glass filters some of the ultraviolet rays, but use a blind for shade.

Smoking
In spite of all the evidence against smoking in pregnancy and around small children, one of the few groups of people who are actually smoking more today is young women. Of those women who are persuaded to stop while pregnant, the majority start again as soon as their baby is born. Yet one of the most protective steps anyone can take on behalf of children is to keep them well away from cigarette smoke. The toll of diseases suffered by the children of smokers rises almost annually.

Not only do pregnant women who smoke run a greater risk of complications and miscarriage, but it seems that their daughters do too, while their sons have an increased chance of minor abnormalities such as undescended testicles.

Infants exposed to cigarette smoke during pregnancy are more likely to be born underweight or premature than infants born to non-smoking mothers, and they are more likely to grow slowly. It is possible that they are also more likely to be born with a limb abnormality. They run a greater risk of sudden infant death syndrome (formerly known as cot death) and, in the first six months, they are more likely to develop respiratory problems such as breathlessness and wheezing. In the longer term, these children are more prone to asthma. All of these respiratory effects stem from the fact that their airways are smaller. The children of fathers who smoke may also run an increased cancer risk, possibly because smoking can cause genetic damage to the sperm.

Smoking in the presence of infants and young children only makes matters worse. Children who grow up in smoking households are more likely to get coughs, asthma, and ear and chest infections.

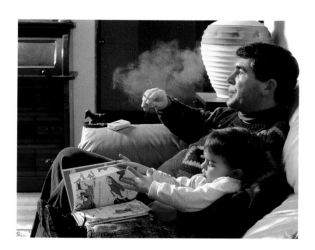

Above: The effects of smoking on the pregnant woman and foetus are perhaps better known and accepted than the effects of passive smoking on children, but they are just as serious. It is now thought that fathers who smoke may also harm their child's health through genetic damage to their sperm.

The family bed

Toddlers and young children often creep into their parents' beds at night. Some parents start the trend by bringing a colicky infant into bed with them for a breastfeed or for the rest of the night. Estimates put the rate of family bedsharing on an occasional basis at 75%, but it is still a controversial practice.

Advocates of co-sleeping argue that young babies who have not differentiated themselves from their mothers are too young to be left alone. They say that an adult lying close to an infant will sense if the baby's breathing falter. Further, the baby will be stimulated to breathe by the movement of the adult's chest. Some research suggests that mothers who are close to their babies are quicker to notice potential danger signs like unusual breathing. Advocates also point to the breastfeeding benefits. Co-sleeping makes night feeds part of the natural continuum. What is more, levels of the milk-producing hormone prolactin are highest at night.

There are, however, strong arguments against bedsharing. Aside from the psychological arguments – that children want to come between their parents and bedsharing allows them to do so, interfering with their sexual relationship; that young children can be exposed to the realities of sex; and that co-sleeping spoils the child and leaves parents with the eventual problem of moving them out – there are physical arguments.

These are clear: a child who sleeps on the edge of the bed can fall out; an infant can suffocate in adult bedclothes; adults can roll on to babies; warm parents' bodies and bedclothes can combine to overheat a baby; long hair can wind round a baby's neck. Most serious is the concern that co-sleeping is a factor in sudden infant death syndrome. However, this only holds true if the mother or her partner are smokers.

Current official advice in Britain is not to bedshare as usual practice with infants under six months old. There are times when parents should certainly not co-sleep, when either parent smokes or is extremely overweight; when the parent is ill, drunk or drugged; when the bed is deep and soft. Also if the infant is feverish or unable to move freely.

Vitamin K

Everyone needs vitamin K to help their blood clot. All babies are born with low levels of vitamin K and in a tiny number this can cause a serious illness – haemorrhagic disease of the newborn – where the baby develops life-threatening bleeding, sometimes into the brain. Fortunately, the disease can be prevented by giving newborn infants vitamin K.

All babies are given vitamin K just after birth. Some infants have their dose by mouth, others by injection. General opinion is that injected vitamin K offers better protection. However, important studies suggested a possible link between injected vitamin K and childhood cancers, although this was later disputed. For some time most infants had vitamin K by mouth. A first dose at birth was followed by a second within a week. Subsequent research revealed a small number of infants who developed the disease later, despite having been given vitamin K by mouth. Most recent studies have again failed to find any link between injected vitamin K and childhood cancers, so most hospitals are reverting to injection, which is also the method for preterm infants and those born by Caesarean section or forceps.

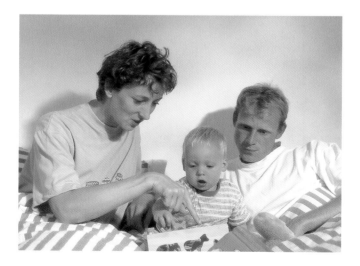

Above: Bedsharing is the natural sleeping arrangement for many families and can solve children's sleep problems. Advocates insist a child needs no prompting to leave the parental bed – when they are ready.

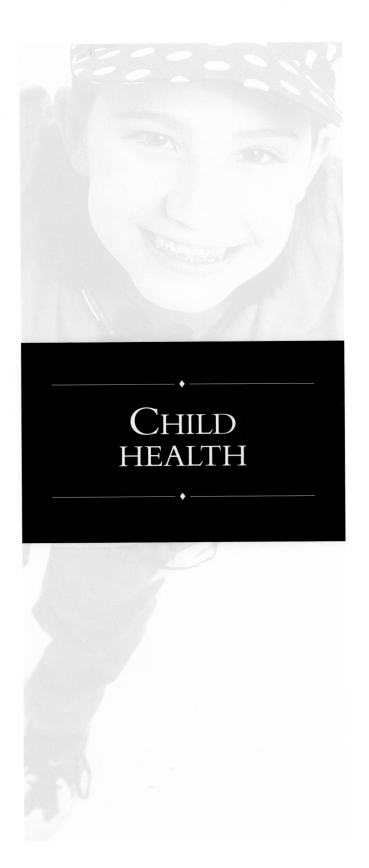

What does being healthy mean to you? Being fit enough to bound up two flights of stairs without feeling breathless? Having a clear skin and a sheen to your hair? Waking up in the morning and springing out of bed, ready to take whatever the day brings? Feeling good about yourself? Since becoming a parent, the chances are that these feelings are a distant memory, but they will come back. In the meantime, nearly everyone agrees that being healthy means much more than not being ill.

It is just the same for children. A healthy child is not just a 'not-sick' child. A healthy child has energy to spare, is eager and maddeningly inquisitive and enjoys life. Healthy children sleep well and eat as much as they need – even if their appetite seems bird-like to you. Their lives show a balance between spells of intense, quiet concentration and equally intense activity.

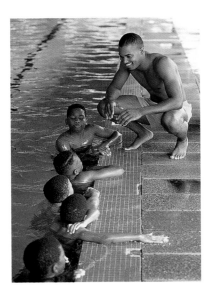

Left: Swimming is an important skill for young children to acquire. As well as increasing their self confidence it provides a moderate to vigorous form of exercise that many will continue. Surveys show that a quarter of young men and women under 25 choose to swim as a leisure activity.

CHILD HEALTH

Promoting mental and physical health Children need to be in very good physical health because they are already laying down the foundations for a healthy adulthood and old age. We know that many adult health problems originate in childhood (or even earlier, in pregnancy) but by endowing children with the best possible health, many of them can be prevented. Children who are physically robust also stand the best chance of throwing off the inevitable infections of childhood without developing serious or unpleasant complications. Diseases that have only mild effects in a healthy population play havoc in undernourished children living in poor conditions.

As infections have become less of a threat in childhood, so diseases that relate to our way of life have increased. All the diseases of atopy (allergic conditions such as asthma, eczema and hay fever) are on the increase, as are nutritional diseases. These are not diseases of want, but of plenty. An increasing number of children are now overweight, and while being a podgy pre-schooler does not predict an overweight adult, being overweight as an adolescent does. Overweight predisposes to a wide range of diseases: respiratory infections are more common in childhood, and asthma and diabetes are harder to control; in adulthood high blood pressure, coronary thrombosis and heart failure are more common, as are diabetes, menstrual problems, certain sex hormone-sensitive cancers and osteoarthritis of the weight-bearing joints.

Emotional health is also important in childhood. What good is it to be bounding with unbridled energy if you are consumed with self-doubt? Many factors play a role in determining emotional health. Not all of them are amenable to change, but some of them are.

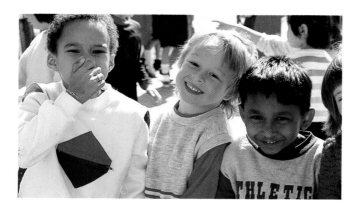

Above: Friendships are especially important to schoolchildren, whose days are spent in a socially demanding group environment. While boys will often make group friendships, girls more typically pair off and feel jealous if they are abandoned for a new friend.

Mental health is now a key issue in child health. Children are as subject to stress as adults, and many children no longer enjoy the supportive family structure that in the past acted as a buffer. Children increasingly need to be taught to relax and to adopt behaviour that keep them and others around them as stress-free as possible.

The seeds of much addictive behaviour – smoking, drinking too much, abusing solvents – that is more common in the teenage years are sown in childhood. However as these assume greater prominence in adolescence, they are considered in the section on Teenage health (see page 290).

Parents have a unique power to influence positively their children's health. Pregnancy is a time when women are more open to messages about good health than at any other time, yet it is easy to let good habits slip. Many families eat well and

exercise well until their children reach school age, when peer pressure combines with the power of the commercialized media to corrupt the messages. Yet it is those early habits that are most important. Good – and bad – health habits are taught, not caught. The best way we can teach our children to lead healthy lives is to do so ourselves.

The importance of family position

What difference does it make to a child to be one of a large family, one of a pair or an only child? We know that there are immediate effects on health for children with older siblings. They tend to catch common cough-and-cold-type infections earlier than first-born children because their older brothers or sisters pick up these infections at school or nursery. This is not necessarily a bad thing. While it is sensible to keep very young infants away from toddlers with streaming noses, there is no reason to protect an otherwise healthy infant over six months of age from the inevitable upper respiratory tract infections. In fact there is a suggestion that early exposure to infection may protect against allergy. One plausible explanation for the recent increase in asthma and eczema is that catching viral infections when young may exert a protective influence. The argument is that as children are increasingly protected against infections so the incidence of allergies rises.

Most concerns about family position centre on the child's social relationships. Will an only child suffer? Or, conversely, what are the effects on the child of belonging to a large family? Here there is some evidence. Most recent research shows that the major differences between families are between those with one or two children and those with several children.

Only children Only children do not, as prejudice suggests, grow into spoilt and lonely misfits. Research shows that, on a range of personality and behaviour tests (evaluating factors such as maturity, anxiety, happiness and self-control), only children are much the same as children with siblings. They are different in that their parents tend to expect a lot of them, but this can work in their favour as, on average, only children talk early and have advanced reading skills throughout their school career.

However, while children with brothers and sisters cut their social teeth in the privacy of their own homes – learning the painful lessons about sharing, taking turns and seeing the other person's point of view – only children have to do this in public, at mother-and-toddler groups, playgroups and at school. There is also a certain amount of evidence that because only children have missed out on the rough and ready lessons that sibling rivalry teaches, an unease and an anxiety may later on underlie relationships that appear superficially straightforward.

First children First children start life as only children. They receive more social interaction, stimulation and play with their parents than any later children, although at the same time their parents tend to be more anxious about them and more controlling, and to apply more pressure. This means that they tend to achieve more both academically and professionally, that they are at the same time more intelligent and less confident in their own abilities and that they are more traditional and conformist in their outlook than subsequent children in the family.

In terms of their anxieties and insecurities, the way the second child is introduced to the family plays an important role (see Jealousy and sibling rivalry, page 319). There is a tendency for first children to be more bossy and dominant in their relationships with younger brothers and sisters, and to use their superior power or understanding, and this tendency may remain throughout life.

Middle or second children Middle or second children tend not to achieve as highly as their older brother or sister or, if they do, to choose a different field. They are more radical – even rebellious – and more free-thinking in their attitudes. When they grow up they tend to be less anxious and more easy-going.

Youngest children Youngest children tend to be the most confident family members of all, and they tend to be tough. However a large age gap can make them less independent. Boys in particular tend to be resourceful in terms of finding

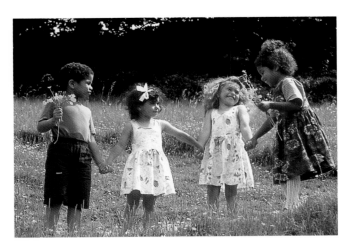

Above: Whether or not a child has brothers and/or sisters can have important consequences for their future social development. It appears that those children who grew up with one or more siblings may be more realistic and relaxed in their dealings with other children. Conversely, children without siblings may find it more difficult to socialize.

ways around difficult situations, and girls tend to be more tomboyish and less concerned with appearances than are their older sisters.

Children of multiple births

Families with twins and other children of multiple births (triplets, and so on) are becoming increasingly common. Since the early 1980s, when infertility treatment became more widespread, there has been a steady rise year-on-year in multiple births.

The first sign of a multiple pregnancy may be a high level of alpha-fetoprotein (AFP) when a woman is tested for a neural tube defect, or an ultrasound scan shows two amniotic sacs. An ultrasound performed by a skilled operator can detect more than one heartbeat in the seventh week of a pregnancy.

It is very likely that twins will be born early; on average, a twin pregnancy lasts 37 weeks and a triplet pregnancy 34 weeks. Starting maternity leave early and avoiding excessive tiredness may help to prevent an extremely early birth, but apart from that there is little you or anyone else can do to prevent prematurity in a multiple birth.

Breastfeeding is the best way to feed all babies, and breast milk is especially important for premature infants. It is perfectly possible to breastfeed twins and triplets, but it is hard work, especially if the babies do not suck strongly at first. Contact with a mother who has succeeded in breastfeeding twins or triplets is the most useful form of support (see breastfeeding, page 142).

Behaviour Behaviour problems are common in twins and particularly in identical male twins. A twin whose behaviour improves when they are alone with one parent may be sending a signal that they need more one-to-one adult attention, and the routine needs to be reorganized to allow each twin to spend some time alone with a parent every day.

Twins – especially identical twins – need to know that they are different. They need to look different from each other; if they have to wear the same school uniform, individual hairstyles can set them apart. Other people should be encouraged strongly to call each child by their name, and not to refer to them as 'the twins' or 'the boys'. As they mature it becomes increasingly important that they have some private space, even if it is only the corner of a room.

Development Proper speech and language development requires regular adult input, which is not easy to organize with children of multiple birth. Forty per cent of twins develop a private language; this does not matter, provided they also develop speech that others can understand. Research shows that mothers of twins use particularly short, simple phrases and answer questions fully when the first twin asks them, but only briefly the second time around. To help twins' speech develop well, parents need to spend time every day playing and talking with each of the children separately, and need to make an effort to answer questions from each child in detail.

When twins start school, parents need to decide whether to keep them together or to separate them. It is important to consider whether, on the one hand, the twins very obviously have different ability levels or if, on the other hand, they make very similar progress; whether they egg each other on to behave badly; and whether one twin is very dependent on the other. Children who are very dependent on each other can find it helpful to start school together. If they have to separate it can be even more traumatic than for a single child who has to leave their mother for the first time.

Once the children start school, it can be tempting to make comparisons. However comparisons between children who achieve at very different levels are destructive to both children. Should such comparisons arise, the children may do better if they attend different secondary schools.

Emotional health

It is impossible to underestimate the importance of looking after children's emotional health. To be fully healthy, children need more than a balanced diet, a safe and unpolluted environment and immunizations to protect them from physical illness. Yet it is a sad truth that behavioural and emotional disorders and mental health problems in children are increasing. What can parents do to protect their children?

First, children need parents who not only love them unconditionally, but are in a position to show it. Parents should be available when they are needed – in the very early months and years, at times of transition, at bedtimes and when children are ill. This can be inconvenient for full-time working parents and needs negotiation with a sympathetic employer, but in the end it is in the child's best interests.

Temperament Temperament differences make some children more vulner-able than others. From the start, some infants are easy to handle, cheerful and adaptable. Others dislike change, are slow to adapt and seem to need constant reassurance and comfort. The type of child you have is very much in the lap of the gods, although once you have worked out your child's temperament you can usually see which traits are inherited – and from whom. If you do have a difficult infant you should pay particular attention to their emotional health as the child gets older.

Children need their parents' undivided attention. 'Quality time' is all very well, but it is lost on a child who is hungry, tired or plain grumpy. Any relationship needs accommodation on both sides and that may mean giving your attention when the child needs it rather than when you want to give it. As children grow older, shared interests and activities can bring them closer to their parents.

Consistent boundaries Children also need a positive atmosphere at home, with plenty of praise when they do things right. However parents need to set clear boundaries for their behaviour and be prepared to restrain them when they go too far. Parents need to agree these boundaries between themselves so that they give consistent messages. It is best to avoid criticism: children who are criticized themselves tend to have critical relationships with others. As long as they feel good about themselves they will be able to make friends outside the home. In the early years they need to try a wide variety of different activities, partly because this builds up their base of skills and self-confidence, and partly because in this way they can discover what they are good at. And every child is good at something.

Children thrive on consistency and routine. When they know what is expected of them they find it much easier to conform. Young lives are already full enough of change without having to cope with unnecessary inconsistencies. A change of school or home, or a change in carer, for example, are major events in a child's life and need to be sensitively prepared for. A sameness that adults may find boring can often provide a healthily supportive atmosphere in which growing children thrive.

Hygiene and food hygiene

Many bacteria and other germs are spread directly from person to person, but by teaching your children some simple steps you can help to keep them healthy. Teach them to use a tissue rather than a cloth handkerchief when they sneeze or blow their noses; to turn their head away from other people to blow their nose, sneeze or cough; and, whenever possible, to wash their hands afterwards.

Children should be taught to wash their hands thoroughly, washing both sides in soap and warm water, rubbing between the fingers and round the nails before rinsing in clean water. Everyone should do this after going to the lavatory, and each family member should have their own towel. If anyone has a stomach upset or diarrhoea, handwashing is especially important and contact surfaces – the lavatory seat, the flush handle, the taps and the door handle – should be wiped down daily with antiseptic.

Once children are active, especially outdoors, they should wash daily. It is easier to give young children a bath, but once they are steady on their feet and do not mind being splashed with water, showers are better. If you do not have one, fit a shower attachment to your bath taps. Frequent washing with soap or using bubble bath may dry out sensitive skin; use a mild cleansing lotion instead or smooth moisturizing lotion into a child's skin after a bath. There is no need to wash hair more than once a week.

Food hygiene Food hygiene is extremely important. Always buy food as fresh as possible and if you are buying chilled or frozen foods in warm weather, buy them last and transport them in a coolbox or frozen food bag. Your freezer should be kept at –18°C or less and your fridge should be between 0 and 5°C. Use a fridge thermometer to check that the temperature is not too high. Store the most perishable foods, such as cooked meats, in the coldest part of the fridge, and wrap each food item separately or put it in a plastic container. Store uncooked meat and defrosting foods in a drip-proof, covered container at the bottom of the fridge. Keep eggs in the fridge and throw away any that are cracked or broken. If you are putting cooked food into the fridge, let it cool for about an hour first.

Before cooking, and after handling rubbish or emptying the bins, wash your hands and dry them on a hand towel or kitchen paper. If you have an open wound on your hand, cover it with a waterproof plaster before cooking. Wash work surfaces frequently and clear up spills immediately, and use separate chopping boards for bread, cheese, vegetables and meat. The most hygienic way to wash dishes and cutlery is to use a dishwasher, but if you do not have one, wash them in hot water and washing up liquid, rinse and leave to dry.

If you are cooking food taken from the freezer, let it thaw fully first, then make sure it is cooked right through. If you use a microwave or reheat food, make sure the food is piping hot right through. For infants, or a child who is ill, eggs should be cooked until the white and yolk are solid, and children should never be given dishes made with uncooked eggs. Wash all salads, fruit and vegetables before use, especially if they are to be eaten raw. Throw away any milk drinks left outside the fridge for more than an hour, and don't eat food after the 'use by' date.

Some foods contain natural poisons. For example, raw kidney beans contain substances called lectins, which can cause stomach ache and vomiting, but are destroyed when the beans are soaked overnight in cold water for 12 hours and then boiled in fresh water at a vigorous roll for ten minutes or more. The green and sprouting parts of potatoes contain high levels of substances called glycoalkaloids. These parts should be cut out and the whole potato thrown away if it still tastes bitter. Damaged or mouldy apples can contain a toxin called patulin, especially near the damaged sections of the fruit, and

should not be eaten. It is also unwise to eat food that shows any sign of mould.

If you use canned food, wipe the top of the can before opening it. Don't leave any food in the can once it is opened, and always wash the can opener after use.

Road safety

From the age of about eight, many children are allowed out alone on the roads. What are the principal hazards that await them and what can parents do to make sure their children behave as safely as possible on the roads?
Here are some facts:
- Children cannot safely cross any road alone, even under the supervision of an adult standing on the sidelines, until they are about 8–9 years old
- Over 95% of all child pedestrian accidents take place in urban areas
- Most accidents to child pedestrians happen while they are crossing a road. A large number occur when a child crosses a road where there are parked cars
- Boys have more accidents than girls. Although boys and girls behave in a similar way when approaching roads, boys may react more slowly to unexpected events
- Most accidents happen when children are coming to and from school, particularly in the summer
- Three out of five accidents involving pre-school children occur when the child is playing in the street

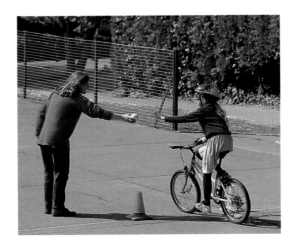

Above: The objectives of cycling proficiency schemes is to teach young riders about the rules of the road, basic road skills and the control of the bicycle, as well as simple bicycle maintenance. Cycling awareness programmes develop the young rider's skills in recognizing, assessing and responding to road dangers. Children attending these programmes are therefore more likely to be safe riders.

Knowing this, what should you teach your child about road safety? First, discourage a child from using or crossing main roads. Where possible, a child should use a bridge or under-pass. Once children have been taught how, they can use pedestrian crossings. When you are out walking, even with a young child, tell them what you are doing: stopping at the edge of the pavement; looking and listening for traffic; wait-ing for a gap in the traffic before you cross; looking for safe places to cross, such as a pedestrian crossing or an underpass.

When children reach five or six years of age, teach them to use the right procedure for crossing a road. Teach the key points of the Green Cross Code: Stop! Look! Listen! Practise first on quiet roads near your home. Show your child what to do, then let them lead you across. Finally, let them cross while you watch. At this age, never let a child cross a road without an adult watching. When children are seven to nine years of age, you can teach the full Green Cross Code.

The Green Cross Code
1. Find a safe place to cross, then stop
2. Stand on the pavement near the kerb
3. Look all around for traffic and listen
4. If traffic is coming, let it pass. Look all around again
5. When there is no traffic near, walk straight across the road
6. Keep looking and listening for traffic while you cross
   Practise this with your child on quiet roads near your home

By the time children are ten years old, they may be ready to walk to school alone. Walk the route with them until you are certain they are safe. Make sure they wear light or bright clothing, or carry a bright or fluorescent bag. If they have to walk after dark, they will need reflective clothing.

Cycling It is estimated that, in the United Kingdom, 150,000 children every year attend hospital following a cycling accident. Boys are more likely than girls to be seri-ously injured. One reason children have cycling accidents is that their bicycles are not properly maintained. Brakes or tyres in poor condition or riding a bike of the wrong size increases the likelihood of accidents. Some children simply lack the necessary skill to ride their bicycle safely or are unable to judge potential hazards, either because they are

inexperienced or because they are just too confident. Motorists often do not see cyclists, particularly children, in the road ahead of them, partly because the cyclists are not wearing bright or reflective clothing. It is unwise to allow children to cycle at night or in the rain, but if they have to, they should use front and rear lights.

The most effective step that parents can take to prevent serious injury is to ensure that their children wear a properly fitting helmet; eight out of ten child cycling deaths are caused by head injuries. Children under the age of nine should never be allowed to cycle on the road, and they should take a cycling proficiency course or follow a cycling awareness pro-gramme before they do. Parents should always accompany their child on the road until their child is fully competent. They should also plan cycle routes so that children do not need to make risky right hand turns: some three-quarters of all cycling accidents in traffic involve a turn at a junction.

Healthy eating
Healthy eating for children means a lot more than balancing a list of essential and desirable nutrients. Eating is both a social activity and a focal point of family life. Providing food is a way of expressing care and love, and meals are times that should be enjoyable.

The United Kingdom Department of Health recently pub-lished *Eight Guidelines for a Healthy Diet**. The first piece of advice is, enjoy your food. The other guidelines are as rele-vant to young people as they are to adults.

The healthy diet
- Eat a variety of different foods
- Eat the right quantity to be a healthy weight
- Eat foods containing lots of starch and fibre
- Don't eat too much fat
- Don't eat sugary foods too often
- Pay attention to the vitamins and minerals in your food.
  The eighth guideline concerns sensible drinking (see page 298)

Once infants have been weaned there is no reason why they should not eat the same food as the rest of the family as long as it is a healthy diet. By the time children have reached school age, their diet should follow the same pattern as that

*Reprinted with kind permission of the Health Education Authority

of adults, with carbohydrates providing 50% of their energy, fats providing 35% and proteins 15% of energy. But what does that mean in practice?

Food groups Imagine an empty plate. Put on a good helping of starchy food (pasta, cereals, rice, bread, potatoes); add an equally good helping of vegetables and fruit, with as much variety as you like; next add a smaller helping of a food that is high in protein (fish, eggs, meat, poultry, nuts, pulses); and finish the plate off with a helping of a dairy food (cheese, milk, yoghurt, fromage frais). The plate now contains a healthy, balanced meal. The only foods that are missing are foods that should be eaten sparingly: fatty, oily and sugary foods.

Good proportions Many children do not eat large platefuls of food. Instead, they skip meals and snack, or 'graze'. In terms of nutrition, this probably does not matter, provided the daily proportions of foods on the imagined plate add up as follows: starchy, carbohydrate-rich foods, five to eleven helpings; vegetables or fruit, five to nine helpings; protein, three helpings; and dairy produce, two to three helpings.

Snacks may actually be beneficial for young children because they need higher energy and nutrient levels than adults to fuel their rapid growth. For pre-school children the snacks can be relatively high in fat: fingers of cheese, whole-milk yoghurts or a glass of full-fat milk or, for children over the age of two, semi-skimmed milk. Children over the age of five do not need such high-energy foods and can drink skimmed milk and eat low-fat dairy produce.

Within the four broad food groups no single food is healthy or unhealthy. It is the combination of foods that is important. Children who eat a wide variety of foods are likely to get all the minerals and vitamins they need. Foods that do not appear in the four groups, such as sugary and fried foods, are not essential and should be kept to a minimum.

Children's food choices The question is, will children eat this sort of food? The evidence shows that they will, as long as they are not presented with high-fat, high-sugar alternatives and they don't fill up on drinks. Young children may drink too much if they are not weaned from a bottle by the age of 12 months. Once a child is eating a range of solid foods, 600 ml/1 pint of milk (including the milk used in cooking) is enough to meet daily needs. Drinking large quantities of squash or fruit juice fills a child up while providing few nutrients, apart from sugar.

Young children tend to eat the same foods as their parents, but as they grow more independent their choices are influenced by their friends, by school meals and by commercial pressures such as television. Advertisements shown in children's prime viewing time frequently feature food that is far from healthy – most often confectionery, highly sweetened breakfast cereals and fast food – and only rarely promote healthy food such as fruit and vegetables.

Partly as a result of these commercial pressures, in the United Kingdom children's diets are not as healthy as they ought to be. They tend to be high in fat and sugar, and low in certain nutrients. There are gender differences too, with girls eating more fruit and drinking more fruit juice, while boys eat bulkier foods, such as breakfast cereals, baked beans and chips, as well as drinking more milk.

Food and health From a physical point of view, healthy eating has obvious immediate benefits. Children who eat a good diet have better teeth, a better build, suffer less anaemia and may possibly be more intelligent. The links between poor thinking ability and poor nourishment are disputed, and while for most children there is no evidence that the ability to learn is limited by the quality of their diet, there is concern about a minority of children with subclinical vitamin and mineral deficiencies.

Preparing for a healthy adulthood Attitudes and behaviour towards food are established in childhood, and diet in childhood plays a vital role in determining health in adulthood. The process that leads to coronary heart disease starts no later than childhood, with evidence that weight, blood cholesterol levels and blood pressure carry through into adult life. Both high cholesterol levels and high blood pressure are important risk factors for coronary heart disease, and as eating fat-containing food has a strong influence on cholesterol levels, children can protect their future by eating a diet that is low in fat.

High blood pressure tends to persist from childhood into adult life, and as blood pressure is affected by sodium intake, establishing a taste for foods without added salt helps to keep blood pressure in the normal range in adulthood. Children who are overweight in middle childhood are likely to stay overweight as adults. Obesity in adults contributes to a range of modern diseases, including high blood pressure, hyperlipidaemia and insulin resistance.

The disease processes that lead to osteoporosis and cancer may also start in childhood. Osteoporosis is affected by calcium intake and levels of exercise, so to protect against bone-weakening and fractures in old age, children – particularly girls – should eat a calcium-rich diet. Diet is believed to be involved in around one-third of all cancers, and diets that are rich in fruit, vegetables and salads seem to be linked with a lower chance of developing cancers of the lung, bowel, stomach and oesophagus. It is the antioxidant vitamins C and E in these fresh foods that are accepted as exerting the protective effect.

School dinners Once children are at school their main source of nutrition each day may be their school dinner, which contributes one- third of their average daily energy intake. But how nutritious is this meal? What is provided depends on the education authority, the caterer and the school, and although school meal providers follow general guidelines, they may not have to conform to set nutritional guidelines. Schools that have a cafeteria system may actually supply unhealthy meals. One British survey has shown that among teenagers, school meals were the source of over half their weekday consumption of chips.

School meals are not compulsory, and around half of all parents send their child to school with a packed lunch instead. Unfortunately the traditional British packed lunch (sandwiches made with white bread, crisps, chocolate bar, sugary drink) is high in fat, sugar and salt, and low in vitamins and micronutrients. However it is much easier for parents to improve the quality of packed lunches than to improve the quality of school meals.

What about beef? Many parents in parts of the Western world are increasingly worried about letting their children eat beef. New variant Creutzfeldt–Jakob disease – an extremely rare but incurable neuropsychiatric disorder that is eventually fatal – has probably been transmitted from cows infected with bovine spongiform encephalopathy (BSE). The disease develops inside the brain for an estimated 10–15 years, or even longer, so it does not appear in young children. although it is possible to come into contact with the infectious agent in childhood.

The government of the United Kingdom is clear in its statements that current practices in slaughterhouses should have made new variant Creutzfeldt–Jakob infection acquired in this way a thing of the past, and that beef, cows' milk and gelatin derived from beef are safe to consume. However as the agent behind the disease has not yet been identified, some parents are cautious about allowing their children to eat beef, gelatin or even to drink milk. Schools provide a choice of dishes so no child should have to eat this meat if they do not want to eat it.

Vegetarian children

For adults, a vegetarian diet offers wide-ranging health protection benefits against diabetes, obesity, high blood pressure and bowel disease. In addition, vegetarian adults have a very

significantly lower rate of heart disease and cancer than meat eaters. But should a vegetarian diet start in childhood?

The answer is that there is no reason why children should not be brought up as vegetarians. As long as they eat dairy products and eggs and their diet is planned with care, it will meet all their nutritional needs, whether they are infants

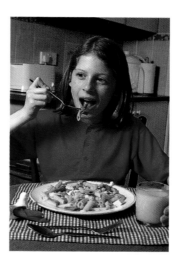

Left: A healthy plate of food for an adult is a healthy plate of food for a child. However girls in particular can be encouraged to eat dairy foods to maintain their calcium intake as well as fortified cereals and lean meat as sources of iron. Vegetarian children should eat plenty of dark green vegetables, wholemeal bread and dried fruit in order to obtain iron that they do not get from eating meat.

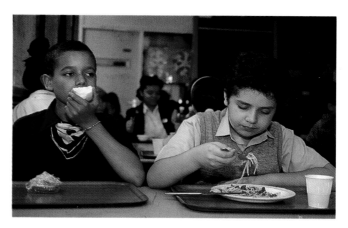

Above: Compulsory nutritional guidelines for school meals should improve the nutrient intake for the chips-with-everything generation. However in the United Kingdom only an estimated one child in three now eats a school dinner; others rely on local shops or a packed lunch.

being weaned, children or teenagers. Even a vegan diet, which excludes all dairy produce and eggs as well as meat, can meet virtually all a child's nutritional needs, although it will call for greater ingenuity on the part of parents, and the child may need to take dietary supplements.

In general, some children brought up on a strict vegetarian diet may be smaller and lighter than average in their early years. When infants are weaned on to a vegetarian diet, they may grow more slowly than meat eaters, although most catch up in the end, and many vegetarian children grow at the same rate as meat eaters. The slowed growth rate is caused by the low ratio of energy to bulk of a typical vegetarian diet, and is best handled by serving high-energy and protein foods first during a meal. This is especially important for picky eaters and children with small appetites. High-fat foods, including nut products, cheese and avocado, are important, and vegetarian children should not be given semi-skimmed or skimmed milk until it is quite certain that their diet is providing ample energy for their needs. Nor should they be given bran or very high-fibre cereals that provide bulk that is low in nutrients, and can impair the absorption of important nutrients such as iron and calcium.

Variety in vegetarian food Vegetarian children – just like other children – need to eat a wide variety of food. Their daily diet should include food from each of the four main food groups: cereals and grains (four to five helpings); fruit (one to three helpings) and vegetables, including leafy green vegetables (two helpings); pulses, nuts and seeds (one to two helpings); and for non-vegans, milk, dairy produce and eggs (three helpings). They also need to eat a small amount of vegetable oil, margarine or butter, and a little yeast extract. Vegetarian children need to combine foods to ensure they get enough essential nutrients, particularly protein.

Protein Protein is found in a surprising range of foods, including breakfast cereals and porridge oats, and, provided these sources are combined, vegetarian children easily get enough protein. Children who do not eat eggs, milk or cheese must eat a combination of pulses, nuts, cereals and grains. Grains and cereals should be eaten together or during the same meal. Grains are incomplete proteins – they lack the essential amino acids lysine and isoleucine; pulses, which lack the amino acid tryptophan, are also incomplete proteins. When eaten together they make a complete protein. Nut creams, seed spreads, tofu and soya yoghurt are also good non-dairy sources of protein.

Calcium To ensure they get enough calcium, vegetarian children need to drink milk (600 ml/1 pint a day) or soya milk enriched with calcium. Yoghurt, cheese, tofu and a range of plant sources including treacle, broccoli, celery, soya, sesame seeds and nuts, particularly almonds, all supply calcium.

Iron and vitamin C An adequate iron intake is important, and vegetarian children need to eat plenty of non-meat foods containing iron, such as fortified breakfast cereals, wholemeal bread, dried fruits and dark leafy green vegetables. Vegetarian diets usually provide high levels of vitamin C and it is important that they should do, as vitamin C is crucial in

helping the absorption of iron, particularly when it is taken at the same time as the iron-rich food.

Zinc Zinc is another essential mineral, and is available in sunflower seeds, soya beans and doughs that contain yeast.

The vegan diet Vegan diets tend to contain even less energy than other diets and vegan children may be both lighter and smaller than their peers. However there is no reason why they should be any less healthy, as long as plant foods are chosen carefully to provide the full range of amino acids, and the diet contains enough fat. There is a risk that vegan children will be deficient in calcium and vitamin B_{12}. Vitamin B_{12} is not available in plant foods, so children on vegan diets need to eat supplemented foods, such as breakfast cereals, soya milks, yeast extracts and specific vegetarian products such as veggie burgers, or they must take a supplement.

With thought and commitment, a vegetarian or vegan diet can be quite suitable for children. However what is not suitable is the diet of a child in a meat-eating family who declares unilateral vegetarianism by simply missing meat out of meals. Should your child do this, you need to discuss alternatives.

A family pet
Having a family pet is beneficial for children's emotional and mental health. Looking after a pet develops a sense of responsibility and interdependence and can help when social relationships are going through a difficult patch. Experience with pets in children's hospitals has shown that children sometimes communicate better with pets than with people, perhaps because pets are accepting and non-judgmental.

Training a pet provides a good lesson in behaviour for children, while riding a horse develops skills of balance, judgment and confidence in able-bodied children as well as those with a disability. Pet therapy has been shown to reduce aggression in disturbed youngsters, and a classroom guinea pig can bring out caring qualities in very young children. Accompanying a pet to the vet's for regular treatments, such as worming or vaccination, is an important lesson in preventive medicine for young children.

The disadvantages While there are benefits to be gained from keeping a pet, there are also a few disadvantages. Pets need to be kept away from food and all areas where food is being prepared or cooked. Children should learn not to feed animals at the table, and small children must be kept away from pets' bowls. When doing the washing up, be sure to either wash the pet's bowls separately or do it after washing everything else.

Children need to learn to respect animals or they risk being bitten or scratched. It is natural for children to cuddle ani-

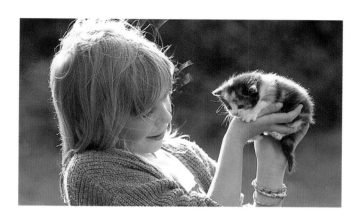

Above: Pets play a very important role in children's emotional health. As they keep secrets so well, children can confide in them with absolute trust. Pets also frequently present children with their first personal experience of death and its healing rituals.

mals, but they should not kiss them and they should not allow an animal to lick their face.

Both dogs and cats carry fleas that can survive for months in a carpet and then jump in response to the vibration of passing feet, usually biting the legs around the upper ankle. If the animal shares a child's bed, the child can be bitten anywhere on the body.

One of the most common sources of allergen (a substance that initiates an allergic reaction) in the home is pet dander found in the fur of cats and dogs. It is so ubiquitous that it is even found in homes with no resident furry animals, but it is present in much higher quantities in homes with pets. This means that any family where an allergic tendency has already shown as asthma, eczema or hay fever should think carefully before acquiring a furry pet.

Research now suggests that it is possible that babies are sensitized to cat allergen when they are in the uterus. Highly susceptible people should therefore think hard before acquiring a cat during a pregnancy.

Infections Cats may also carry infections, and to prevent picking up these infecions, children should always wash their hands after handling a pet and before cooking, handling food or eating. The organism *Toxoplasma gondii* can be carried in cats' faeces, and causes the illness toxoplasmosis, which is rather like glandular fever. It can have serious consequences for the unborn child if women catch it during pregnancy. A bite or scratch from a cat may cause a rare illness known as cat-scratch fever, in which a lymph node near the scratch swells up, and a blister may appear near the site of the scratch. Children with this condition may also go on to develop a fever, a rash and a headache.

Both cats and dogs can also carry the roundworm toxocara. To protect children from infection, with its occasionally very serious consequences, dogs and cats should be wormed regularly, pet owners should clear up after their animals and places where children play, such as parks, sandpits and playgrounds should be protected from dogs and other animals that might carry the infection, such as foxes.

Children should not share a bedroom with a caged bird. Psittacosis is a risk for anyone who keeps a bird. Dusty particles from the bird's droppings can be inhaled and transmit a type of chlamydial infection, which usually appears either as an unusual type of pneumonia or a general infection. It can be treated with antibiotics.

Children can also pick up infections when visiting farms. The organism *Cryptosporidium* can pass from infected animals to children who cuddle them. It causes watery diarrhoea that can last for up to a week. An infected child can pass the organism on to other children. Children should always wash their hands after playing with farm animals.

Healthy teeth

The latest national survey shows that one pre-school child in three has tooth decay. By the time children start school, 45% have some tooth decay, and by the age of nine this figure has risen to 60%. Less than one-third of 15-year-olds have perfect, undecayed teeth. What is going wrong?

Children's eating habits have changed dramatically over the past generation, with much more grazing – snacking between or instead of meals. Unfortunately eating frequently is particularly damaging to teeth, as is regular consumption of sweet fizzy drinks. After any meal, snack or drink containing sugar, the chief ingredients of enamel – calcium and phosphate – start to dissolve into the saliva in a process known as demineralization. This can last for anything up to two hours before the teeth start to reabsorb the lost minerals, but if another snack is eaten during this time, the essential process of restoration never has a chance to start.

The case against sugar Children are also eating more sugar, which is well known to cause tooth decay. In the United Kingdom the average daily intake of sugar is around 90 g/3 oz. Some of this sugar is visible or obvious, but much of it is hidden. For example, many 'plain' and savoury foods contain sugar. Weight for weight, nearly one-tenth of plain cornflakes is sugar, while a supposedly healthy breakfast cereal such as sultana bran has a total sugar content of almost one-third. Labels saying 'reduced sugar' or 'low sugar' sadly do not mean no sugar.

To discover what your children – and you – are eating, scan the labels on food packaging for hidden sugars; the most damaging are sucrose, glucose, fructose and maltose, but you will also find maltodextrin, invert sugar and hydrolyzed starch. Look carefully where you least expect to find added sugars. Soya milks and infant soya formula are sweetened with sugars capable of causing tooth decay.

Tooth erosion Tooth erosion, which is caused by acid drinks and occurs regardless of the presence of sugar, is another common problem. Even a mildly acidic drink such as carbonated water can be damaging, while pure fruit juices and other carbonated drinks have a high acid content. It is not just teenagers with a three-can-a-day habit whose enamel is being etched away by these acid drinks; levels of erosion are almost as high in pre-school children as they are in 13-year-olds. In some children the enamel completely dissolves to reveal the sensitive layer of dentine beneath.

Solutions The first step is to limit the habit of snacking. Young children find this rather difficult, so choose tooth-friendly snacks and train your children to drink tap water. It is almost free, and it is harmless to teeth. If your child needs to take prescription drugs, ask your doctor to prescribe a sugar-free elixir.

Sugar-free chewing gum is not harmful to teeth: rather it is considered to be positively beneficial; the extra saliva it stimulates helps to neutralize the acid content of plaque (the sticky film that constantly builds up on teeth), and if it is sweetened with xylitol it may even suppress acid-producing bacteria in plaque.

Cleaning teeth The next step is effective dental care. Parents should start cleaning their children's teeth the day the first tooth comes through. Cleaning teeth has two purposes: the first is to spread fluoride toothpaste on to the teeth, and the second is to remove any plaque that has built up.

The ideal is to brush twice a day, in the morning and at bedtime, taking two to three minutes at each session. In practice your target should be a thorough brush at bedtime and as thorough a brushing as your child can manage in the morning to get the fluoride on to the teeth.

Most people brush the visible parts of the teeth better than those teeth and parts of teeth that remain out of sight. The most neglected danger zones are the insides of the front teeth, both top and bottom, and the teeth at the very back of the mouth. Until the child reaches the age of seven, parents should do the brushing for them to make sure the teeth are getting the thorough clean they need. The child can then take over, but with adult supervision and help in getting at inaccessible surfaces until the age of ten. Only a small pea-sized blob of fluoride toothpaste is needed.

What does fluoride do? Fluoride is a natural mineral that helps to restore tooth enamel. For perfect healing, however, the amount of fluoride must be just right. If there is too little of it, fluoride is not effective at restoring the enamel. If there is too much fluoride, there is a risk that the teeth might become mottled and stained.

For maximum tooth protection the ideal level of fluoride in tap water is around one part per million; this ensures that fluoride is both incorporated into the developing teeth and stays in contact with the tooth surfaces after they have come through. However most drinking water in the United Kingdom does not contain anything like this amount. To discover the level in your area, telephone your water authority or ask your dentist.

Children who have special difficulties cleaning their teeth, or particularly vulnerable teeth, may have fluoride drops or tablets prescribed or recommended by the dentist. Most children should get enough fluoride from brushing twice a day with fluoride toothpaste.

Children under the age of six and children who cannot gargle or spit out properly may swallow toothpaste or gel. They need a low-fluoride toothpaste as long as their teeth are

> **Fluoride protection**
> For the best possible fluoride protection:
> • Start brushing with a low-fluoride toothpaste. Some homeopathic brands contain no fluoride
> • Use only a small pea-sized blob of toothpaste
> • Brush twice a day – no more
> • Don't wet the brush, as this causes froth, which the child tends to spit out. After cleaning, don't rinse, but spit out or brush again with a little water
> • Once the child is six or more and can spit out reliably without swallowing the toothpaste, switch to a medium fluoride brand

in good condition, they brush regularly and well, and they live in a fluoridated area. Many children's brands are low-fluoride. Infant gels have a very mild flavour and some have only tiny quantities of fluoride. Children over six who can spit out can use a medium-fluoride toothpaste, containing around 1000ppmF. to avoid your child swallowing toothpaste, work it first into the brush with a little water. High-fluoride toothpastes contain about 1500ppmF. Children have no need of such high levels.

Right: Orthodontic treatment to move or straighten teeth produces more than a bright, even smile. It also improves the way the teeth bite and makes them much easier to clean. Without treatent, prominent front teeth are also at risk of damage.

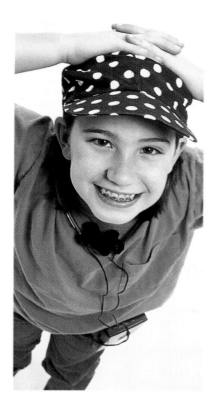

Children should visit the dentist regularly twice a year, but your dentist will tell you if your child needs to attend more often.

Straightening teeth Orthodontics is the branch of dentistry dedicated to straightening teeth using braces. Straight teeth not only produce a nicer, more even smile, but they are also much easier to clean. Depending on when the permanent teeth appear, orthodontic treatment can start between the ages of 11 and 13. There are two main types of brace: removable appliances that are suitable for simple corrections, and appliances that are bonded to the teeth during treatment. Some use small elastic bands that have to be changed every day. Most treatments are completed within two years and some in considerably less time.

Safety in the sun

Warnings about the dangers of exposure to sunshine can appear unnecessarily doom-laden. It is hard to believe that the most natural source of light and warmth can be so deadly that we need to protect ourselves – and especially our children – from it. Awareness that sunshine is good for you also goes against the health promotion messages that children need clothing, adequate shade and appropriate sunscreens to protect them from bright sunlight.

Yet the facts are these: to synthesize enough vitamin D (which is important for both absorbing calcium from the intestine into the bloodstream and for regulating the balance between calcium in the skeleton and in the blood) children need to spend no more than half an hour a day outside in moderate sunshine in summer; and only their lower arms, legs and face need be unclothed to synthesize the amount of vitamin D they need.

Ultraviolet rays and skin cancers Overexposure to the harmful ultraviolet rays of sunlight during childhood is, meanwhile, taking its toll. The latest figures from Australia show that over 2% of people who were surveyed in Queensland had the skin cancer squamous cell carcinoma and that painful sunburn in earlier life had made them more prone to the disease.

Six episodes of painful sunburn made people three times more likely to develop squamous cell carcinoma. Basal cell carcinomas, or rodent ulcers, are also on the increase.

In the United Kingdom over 4000 people a year are developing the fast-growing and most serious type of skin cancer, malignant melanoma, and 1500 a year are dying of it. There are over 40,000 new cases of skin cancer every year (malignant melanomas as well as the more easily treated squamous cell carcinoma and rodent ulcers, or basal cell carcinomas).

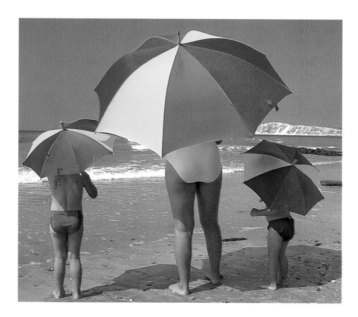

Above: Sensible sun protection measures taken now by most families not only guard against potentially cancerous radiation, they also protect the skin against damage to collagen and elastin. Collagen and elastin maintain firmness and flexibility in the skin and shield it against a premature fragility and thinning of the skin.

These are preventable cancers and children and teenagers should be protected from them.

Protecting your child On an individual basis you can easily make sure your family acts sensibly in the sun. This means wearing wide-brimmed or legionnaire-style hats, and clothing with a dense weave (one that will not allow light through when you hold it up to the sun) that covers the whole body apart from the lower arms, legs and face. It means taking to the shade between 11 am and 3 pm – even in northern latitudes. Infants under six months of age should never be exposed to the sun, and outdoor activities should be sited in the shade.

Unless there is ample shade, children should not take part in heat-of-the-day outdoor activities such as watching sports, picnics or beach trips.

Sun bathing, which is particularly prevalent among teenage girls, should be discouraged. When you cannot avoid the sun, for example on visits to the seaside, you should always use a sunscreen with a minimum sun protection factor of 15, or a higher protection factor, such as 25 or more, for children who have blue eyes and fair or freckled skin.

On a community basis you can form alliances to ensure that there are enough shaded areas in your children's school playground for all the children to play in the shade at midday, that the design of their school uniforms protects children against the sun's rays and that children are encouraged to use sunscreen at school during outdoor sports and outings. You should also lobby your local council to plant extra trees to shade the children's playgrounds.

Television, computers and videos

The flickering screen is as much a part of children's lives today as the library book was a part of yesterday's childhood. Between them, television, videos and computers offer an unrivalled round-the-clock entertainment and information service, and it is not surprising therefore that, on average, children spend two or three hours in front of the television every day. Some children spend longer watching television than they do in the classroom at school.

Effects on health Is there a health price to pay for so much screen-watching? It appears there is. The latest national diet and nutrition survey in the United Kingdom showed that children are becoming overweight not because they are eating more, but because they are taking less exercise. One of the chief reasons for this is because they spend much of the time watching a television or computer screen.

Another finding is that a noticeable delay in language development in children right across the social spectrum is often caused by excessive television viewing. Even infants that are exposed to too much background television are now also experiencing language delay .

Certain types of personality appear to be more likely to become addicted to television. The more time they spend in front of the screen, watching television or videos or playing computer games, the less time they have available to develop creative or interpersonal social skills. There is a real risk that these children may become social loners. But how long is too long? It is any time when the child is not actively engaged in what they are watching, but either are lost in their own world or positively bored.

Possible dangers A number of medical conditions can be triggered by the flickering of a television screen. In a small number (about 5%) of children with epilepsy, flickering light can trigger seizures. Children are often first affected between the ages of six and eighteen, and the seizure occurs when light

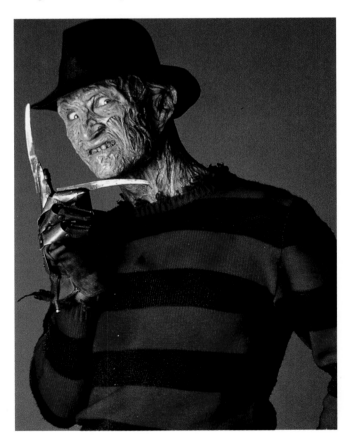

Above: At an age when children find difficulty in distinguishing fact from fantasy, images of violence such as this can be harmful – although they can also be helpful in embodying, acknowledging and ultimately reconciling forceful emotions.

flashes or flickers at a certain frequency. Children with photo-sensitive epilepsy should therefore not sit too close to a television screen and should preferably stay at least 2.5 m/8 ft away from it. Covering (not simply closing) one eye while viewing may be beneficial to some, as may using a screen measuring less than 35 cm/14 in. As further protection the brightness can be turned down and children should view the television in a well-lit room (although some children cope better if it is dark).

Computer screens rarely trigger photosensitive epileptic seizures, but as vulnerable children may be sensitive to sequences in certain video games they should only play using a computer monitor (not a television screen) or hand-held console, and should not play when they are tired. A good, but unfortunately expensive, solution to the problem of flickering screens is to use a television or computer that has a liquid crystal display screen.

Effects on behaviour Many parents' concern over television centres on its effects on children's behaviour. In addition to fostering demands for advertized products, it is believed to make children aggressive. There is no doubt that children do sometimes imitate the violence they have seen recently on television and that children who are already aggressive are most affected. Large numbers of research studies have established that there is an association between television violence and levels of aggressive behaviour, but a causal link has not been established. It is also possible that television violence can exert longer-term effects, and that even after ten years, children who prefer watching violent programmes remain more aggressive than children who prefer to watch less aggressive programmes. However it is important to keep a sense of balance. Occasional viewing in a family where aggression is not used as an approach to solving problems is unlikely to harm children, while unsupervized and frequent viewing of violent films in a home where children see, enact or are the victims of aggression is likely to be very much more harmful to them.

Parenting for positive health

The way parents manage their children's behaviour has a significant effect on their health. Health attitudes matter, too, and are caught rather than taught. So parents who shrug off a cold or a tumble are likely to have children who have a similar matter-of-fact approach. In the same way, parents who reach for the medicine chest (whether to get orthodox or complementary remedies) or the telephone and the doctor's telephone number at the first sign of illness are likely to have children who are equally unsure of their own natural capacities for self-healing.

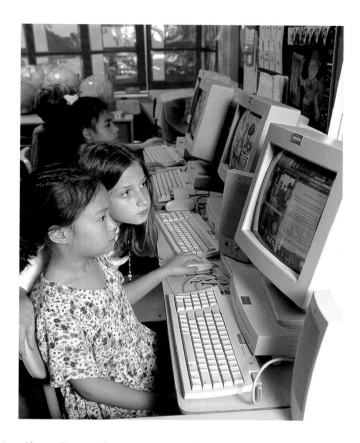

Above: Computer literacy is an essential part of children's primary school education. Commonsense suggests that using computers for positive and investigative purposes helps to protect children against screen exploitation.

Parenting for good health involves attitudes that boost self-esteem and self-confidence, a trust in one's own judgement and an awareness of its limitations. How do parents breed these balanced, health promoting attitudes?

Self-esteem first develops in children from the discovery that their parents like them and spend time with them, trust them and respect them. It comes also from knowing that there are limits – bedtimes, a rejection of any aggression – and that these are applied consistently. This type of parenting, called 'authoritative', rather than its contrasting styles authoritarian or permissive, not only produces children with a high self-esteem, but also children with a high level of self-control and self-reliance, who are able to form their own judgements and have a well developed sense of right and wrong.

In early childhood parents take health decisions on behalf of their children. As their children mature and enter the upper primary school years, they take more and more of these decisions themselves. Those children who have authoritative parents are most likely to take decisions that will be to their lasting benefit.

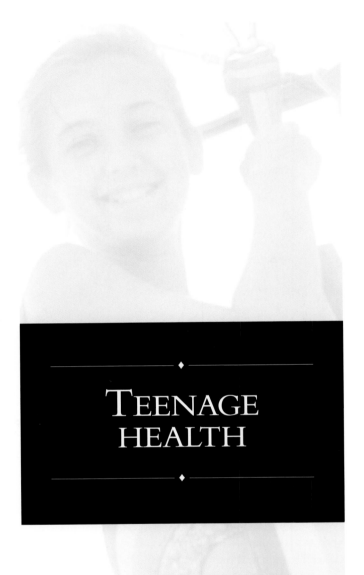

TEENAGE HEALTH

Ask a group of teenagers what their major concerns are, and they are extremely unlikely to mention health. Adolescence is a time when young people are concerned with finding out who they are and where they fit in with the world, with achievement, getting on and enjoying themselves. Health only comes into the equation when it holds them back from what they want to do.

Surveys confirm that the vast majority of adolescents consider themselves to be in excellent health. They may take painkillers for headaches or have fillings in their teeth, but they view these as minor disturbances rather than signs of ill health. If young people do think about health, they realize by the teen years that they are responsible for themselves. In most cases they have had enough health education at school to know that the way they lead their lives has a strong influence on their future health.

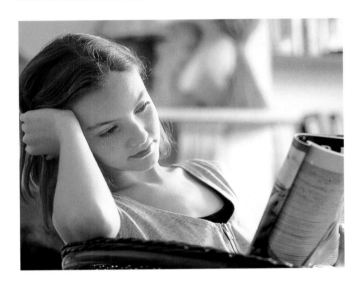

Above: Adolescence is rarely a period of unbroken serenity. Teenagers are prone to turbulent and confusing emotions, which can expose them to the risks of mental health difficulties. Depression and distress are common and in teenagers suicide is a leading cause of death. There is hardly an age when reassuring parental support is more needed.

Yet when things do go wrong who do they turn to? Reassuringly, perhaps, the evidence points to the fact that most teenagers first turn to their parents for health advice. Despite appearances, parents matter to teenagers. The way parents behave and what they believe in has a strong impact. Approval and disapproval are important. Research shows that teenage children of parents who strongly disapprove of smoking are seven times less likely to smoke themselves, and as there appear to be strong links between smoking and drug-taking, parental disapproval acts as a strong health incentive.

Of course parents are not the only reference source for health information. Teenagers also find out about health from their friends, from school, from television, and from books and magazines. But the importance that teenagers attach to their parents' attitudes puts parents on the spot. How much do parents know about the health issues that teenagers might raise? How much up-to-date information do they have? Parents need more and better information on the health risks their teenagers are likely to run – on alcohol and smoking, on illicit drugs and underage sex. When things start to go wrong – as they well may, because teenagers need to experiment just as their parents once did – parents need help recognizing the signs and knowing what to do.

Teenage eating

Teenagers, especially girls, are notorious for eating an inadequate diet. However the blame does not lie entirely with the teenagers themselves. Many school cafeterias provide what young people will buy, rather than what is necessarily nutritious; television commercials advertize what will sell. At an age when appearances and peer-group pressures are at their peak and health concerns are at their lowest, it is hardly surprising that image matters more than intrinsic healthiness. What teenagers care about is not long-term health gains or postponing the onset of chronic illnesses in old age, but weight loss, body shape, complexion and the environment. When it comes to exercising food choices, adolescents consider friendships, group identity, image and the amount of money to which they have access.

Surveys show that teenagers eat food that is high in fats and sugars, and that as they get older they drink less milk and more canned drinks, tea and coffee. By and large they get enough calories from their food, but these are likely to come from high-starch and/or high-fat foods, such as chips, milk, biscuits, meats and puddings. Three-quarters of all 10–15-year-olds eat more fat than they need. A large number of girls go short of calcium or iron, although boys, because they drink more milk, usually get enough calcium. Intake of some micronutrients, such as vitamin B_6, folate, magnesium and zinc, is low in both girls and boys. There is also clear evidence that teenagers do not eat enough of the non-starch polysaccharides, better known as fibre.

However in some ways at least, the situation is improving. While it is true that teenagers often go short of micronutrients, they usually get enough of the major nutrients – carbohydrate, protein and fats – and enough energy. Growing children do need extra energy, but actually not as much more than an adult as you might imagine; even at the peak of their growth spurt, it has been estimated that young people only need an extra 70–120 calories a day.

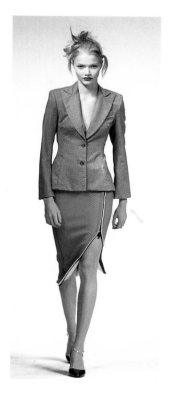

Left: A constant media bombardment of catwalk images of unnatural thinness can seriously undermine the fragile self-esteem of a teenage girl. Schools and families have a duty to present children with a balanced image of good health at a normal weight.

With their interest in weight loss, teenage girls eat more healthy foods, such as fruit and vegetables, and drink more fruit juice than boys. This is reflected in television commercials, which are as likely to promote 'healthy' foods, such as fruit products, high-fibre cereals, wholemeal crispbreads and low-fat butter substitutes, as they are to promote high-fat burgers and ice cream.

Problem areas A general survey of teenagers' food choices will point to a number of problem areas:

- *Weight-reducing diets that are too strict* By the age of 15, more than half of all teenage girls have tried to lose weight. Obsessive weight control can leave youngsters undernourished, and in girls this can delay the start of menstruation or make it erratic. By cutting certain foods, such as potatoes, out of their diet, young people not only lose bulk and starch, but risk upsetting their balance of vitamins and minerals as well. Equally, if they cut out milk or dairy products there can be effects on bone density leading to problems with osteoporosis later in life

- *Too little calcium* Around 45% of the adult skeleton is laid down during adolescence, so teenagers need a substantial calcium intake. Traditionally, boys have drunk enough milk to meet their calcium needs, but girls have not, although the wider availability of low-fat milk products may be changing this. The two periods in life when calcium requirements are highest are, first, in infancy and young childhood, and second, in adolescence. Although adolescents absorb calcium more efficiently than adults, they still need calcium-rich foods to ensure that the skeleton is properly formed. Apart from milk, other dairy foods are the best form of easily absorbable calcium for most teenagers. For children who are vegans, calcium-enriched soya milks and vegetable sources (for example, broccoli, sesame seeds, almonds, spinach and watercress) are also important

- *Anaemia* This is common among teenagers, partly because their rate of growth means that they need more iron and partly, in girls, because of blood loss through menstruation. One-fifth of all adolescent girls are thought to be anaemic. Eating fortified breakfast cereals, red meat and green, leafy vegetables will boost iron intake

- *Poor quality, low-budget food eaten away from home* Many teenagers rarely eat family meals at home and snack instead. Food provided at school is extremely important both in terms of the nutrients it provides and the health promotion example it sets. Meals at many schools follow a cafeteria system, providing popular high-fat foods as well as fruit and salads. A recent survey found that over half the weekday intake of chips for 14–15-year-olds was eaten at school. Many schools also have vending machines offering additional unhealthy foods and drinks

- *Skipping meals* In terms of overall food intake this does not matter, provided the equivalent amount of food is eaten over the course of the day, but many girls miss breakfast and some skip lunch as well, then make up by eating less nutritious break-time snacks

- *A low folate intake, inadequate to protect a baby should a teenage girl become pregnant* Foods that naturally contain folate include dark green leafy vegetables, such as broccoli and sprouts, as well as enriched foods, such as many breads and breakfast cereals. In the United Kingdom the recently introduced symbol on food packaging that identifies folate-enriched foods should help girls to make healthier choices

Improving teenagers' diets

Healthy eating for teenagers is little different from healthy eating for other age groups. Teenagers should eat a variety of foods every day, with at least four helpings of starchy foods (some of them high-fibre); five helpings of fruit and vegetables; three helpings of meat and/or other protein alternatives, such as fish, pulses and grains (see Vegetarian children, page 283) or eggs; and three helpings of low-fat dairy foods. Whether these foods are eaten as snacks or as meals is much less important than the fact that they are eaten every day. Teenage girls should make sure they include foods that are high in calcium (low-fat yoghurt, fromage frais) and iron (for-

tified breakfast cereals and lean meat). Teenagers should eat enough food to maintain a healthy weight, but no more, and they should not eat too many fatty or too many sugary foods. It is also important for teenagers to enjoy their food and to establish eating habits that will have a positive influence on their future adult health.

Parents can have a considerable influence on what teenagers eat. While home economics has been removed from the curriculum in many schools in the United Kingdom, there is no reason why parents cannot teach simple cooking skills. In a society where people are becoming less and less skilled, there is every reason that they should. Shopping can be a joint undertaking, with young people taking the chance to exercise their food choices. If school meals are nutritionally inadequate, make a simple packed lunch and, if your income allows, give the teenager the cost difference as extra spending money. Share the cooking at home, so that each teenager takes responsibility for one family meal a week.

Exercise and sport

One of the biggest lifestyle changes for today's children is the lack of exercise naturally built in to their daily life. The number of parents who drive their children to school has reportedly risen by 60% in the past ten years. In the 1970s, 90% of junior school children walked to school; now, fewer than one

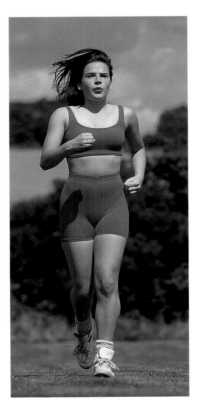

Left: Physical fitness among teenagers is a growing concern. Recently almost half the potential British army recruits had to be rejected because they were unfit. Laying emphasis on general fitness activities, such as running, instead of competitive team sports is more likely to take lasting fitness into adult life.

in ten does. Fewer teenagers are cycling to school – although 90% of children own a bicycle, only 2% of journeys to school are made by bicycle.

In school, sport no longer commands the central position it once held in the curriculum. Over half of all children spend less than two hours a week in school on physical education and fewer children are taking part in sport outside school hours. What is more, the activities that children do pursue in school, especially competitive team games, tend not to be continued outside school or past childhood. At home, children's opportunities for free, active play are limited by parents' concerns for their safety. The result of all this is that children are less fit than they used to be.

The benefits of exercise

Regular exercise is one of the best ways of keeping healthy. It controls fat deposition and is associated with stronger bones. It not only makes the heart and lungs work more efficiently and strengthens muscles, but it keeps joints moving well and helps children to relax and sleep better. Exercise promotes a good appetite, lowers the risk of illness, and makes children livelier, more energetic and more alert. It improves a child's self-confidence and sense of well being. And children who are active are much more likely to be active adults.

For the keen and well-motivated there are organized sports activities. A recent survey has shown that nearly two-thirds of all boys aged 14 and 15 play football outside school lessons, over half of them ride a bicycle, and more than one in five plays basketball or tennis or goes jogging. The figures for girls, however, are less reassuring: almost a quarter undertake no organized sport at all outside school, and the only activity undertaken by more than one girl in five is riding a bicycle.

Exercise for non-sporty teenagers If you have a child who can't catch a ball, can't kick straight and is always the last to be picked for the team, how can you ensure that they stay active and fit throughout their childhood years and retain an enthusiasm for activity that they will carry them through into adulthood?

Non-sporty teenagers need non-competitive sports. Girls can work out to fitness videos in the privacy of their homes. Many prefer aerobics and weight-training to traditional forms of activity, although the benefits of aerobic exercise in terms of fitness have been questioned. Swimming is an excellent whole-body activity of moderate intensity. Most swimming pools run their own clubs and in the early stages at least, they are not particularly competitive. Walking can be either a sociable, whole-family activity or strictly functional. Try to walk with your children at least three times a week, making each walk at least 3 km/2 miles long.

Cycling is another good form of whole-body exercise. Whether your children are able to cycle safely depends largely on your local road conditions. However, they should always have road safety training (see page 280) and wear a properly fitted helmet.

Equipment and safety Appropriate clothing and protective equipment are particularly important for children. Trainers should fit well and be shock absorbent. Headgear should be of an approved standard and correctly and regularly maintained. It is also important to make sure that sports-mad children do not overdo it and do not take up inappropriate activities, such as boxing. Although there have been no definitive studies, many adult cases of arthritis and back pain are thought to derive from excessive exercise in childhood, and not allowing enough time to recover after sports injuries. International studies show that children are sustaining more sports injuries, some of them quite serious. Some specialists believe that injuries occur more frequently after a growth spurt, and believe that children should concentrate on exercise for flexibility at these times. If a child does sustain an injury, activity levels should be minimized until they are fully recovered.

Drug and substance abuse

The use of illicit drugs among teenagers has increased in recent years and is now alarmingly common. The United Kingdom arm of a recent Europe-wide survey covering 7700 15- and 16-year-olds in 70 schools revealed that drug use in this age-group is more common than cigarette smoking. The most commonly used drug is cannabis: around four teenagers in ten had experimented with it and one in ten use it frequently. One teenager in five had sniffed glues or solvents; one in seven had used LSD; and one in eight had used amphetamines. Ecstasy was used by around one teenager in fifteen.

Drugs are part of the scenery for today's teenagers. Most will be offered them, often by friends or schoolmates. They take them because they are curious; because everyone else is doing it; because they are bored; and because they like the thrill of doing something dangerous.

Another finding of the Europe-wide survey was the link between cigarettes and cannabis. Very few non-smokers tried cannabis, while most teenagers who smoked ten or more cigarettes a day had also smoked cannabis. Most young people who use cannabis do not go on to use other illegal drugs, but it may bring them into contact with the criminal underworld.

Recognizing the signs For parents, one of the problems with illicit drug use is that they may have no personal experience on which to draw. Children are unlikely to volunteer the

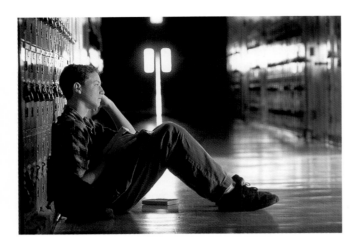

Above: All children can be tempted to experiment with drugs and solvents. School, family income or background and intelligence make no difference. Drugs are usually bought in clubs or pubs, or even on the street, so parents who want to protect their children need to know where their spend their leisure time.

information that they have been taking drugs or sniffing glue, and it can be difficult to recognize the signs. Some of the signs are similar to normal adolescent behaviour, so it is important not to jump to conclusions. However it helps if parents are alert to any changes in their patterns of sleep, unexpected mood swings and unusual behaviour, secretiveness, loss of money from home, loss of appetite, irritability and aggression, loss of interest in their friends and pastimes, poor memory and concentration, and a deterioration in school performance.

If you notice an accumulation of the signs listed above, bring up the subject. If your teenager is taking drugs, tell them you disapprove and explain why. For many teenagers, drug-taking is a single experiment that can be put down to youthful curiosity, but if it has been going on for some time it would be sensible to contact a family support group for advice and information.

Protection against drug dependency

The factors that protect young people from going beyond the experimentation stage are difficult to categorize, because every case is different. However a stable, happy family life is a strong protective factor. Parents need to be available to listen and talk to their teenage children, and they need to do things together – even if it is only watching television. It helps if they can meet their children's friends and invite them home. And it also helps to set a good example with their own drugs of dependence – alcohol, cigarettes and even medicines. For the teenager, it helps to have clear goals in life, and also to acquire

certain social skills – knowing how to be assertive without being overbearing, how to cope with stress, how to stand up to social pressures and how to solve or at least weigh up their own problems.

In Britain it is illegal to possess, sell or give away an illicit drug, or to allow anyone to sell, give away or produce a drug in the home. A parent who finds drugs in their home can hand them over to the police or destroy them to prevent an offense being committed.

Types of drug The following is a necessarily brief description of the main types of drug to which children may be exposed. Parents may wish to obtain further information from the wide range of organizations and agencies specializing in the subject.

Street amphetamine (speed, whizz, sulphate, billy) is usually sniffed or mixed into a drink. It induces feelings of energy, exhilaration and self-confidence and reduces appetite, but these feelings are followed by a bad hangover effect. Speed can also bring on tantrums, irritability and mood swings. Long-term use causes insomnia and mental problems, as well as debilitation caused by the lack of food and sleep.

Barbiturates (barbs, downers, blues, reds) are usually taken as tablets. They are sedative drugs and although their first effect is one of relaxation, they then produce an effect like drunkenness, which is compounded by drinking alcohol. It is easy to overdose on barbiturates.

Cannabis (marijuana, dope, hash, shit, grass, weed, pot) is the most commonly used drug. Within a few minutes of smoking it, or longer after eating it, cannabis lifts the mood to a feeling of calm and well being. It also makes the user dreamy and relaxed, slows down reactions and affects coordination and concentration. These effects last for a few hours. Larger doses can provoke a state of panic or other unpleasant effects. In the longer term, heavy users can become dependent. Cannabis smoke contains more carcinogens than tobacco and because the smoker inhales more deeply, four 'joints' may well do as much damage to the lungs as 20 cigarettes will do.

Cocaine (coke, snow, charlie) is a stimulant drug and an anaesthetic that is usually sniffed, but can be injected intravenously or prepared in smokable form as freebase. Crack is a form of smokable cocaine. Cocaine makes the user feel energetic and euphoric, but it causes dependence and regular users may become excitable and paranoid.

Ecstasy (E, diamonds, doves) is often used as a party drug. It comes in tablet form and induces a feeling of calm, alertness and well being. However the hangover is unpleasant and high doses can induce panic or anxiety attacks. When combined with dancing for many hours, Ecstasy can contribute to a rise in body temperature and dehydration. Users of Ecstasy who are dancing need to take sips of water, but drinking too much water can be fatal.

Heroin (smack, H) can be smoked, sniffed or injected. It is a painkiller similar to morphine and produces an effect of warmth, drowsiness and calm. However heroin is taken, it is addictive, and sudden withdrawal triggers very unpleasant side effects. Injecting drugs is not common among school-children but is particularly dangerous because of the risk of infections such as hepatitis or HIV from shared needles. Accidental overdose of heroin can be fatal.

LSD (lysergic acid diethylamide, acid, trips, tab) is an hallu-cinogen that is supplied on small squares or as pills that pro-duce a 'trip'. It can trigger 'bad trips' in which the user feels panicky, agitated and may experience terrifying hallucina-tions. Spontaneous flashbacks can occur months or even years after the drug was taken.

Magic mushrooms (Liberty cap mushrooms) have an hallu-cinogenic effect which is similar to that of LSD. The mush-rooms can be eaten raw, cooked or infused as a tea. Apart from the risk of causing unpleasant hallucinations, magic mushrooms may be confused with other, poisonous, species of mushroom.

Solvent sniffing is most common among groups of young teenagers. Solvents are not illegal and there are around 30 dif-ferent types commonly found in the home – for example, sol-vent-based glues, aerosols, butane gas and nail varnish remover. Sniffing solvents quickly makes youngsters feel 'high', happy and carefree. This can be followed by a feeling similar to a hangover. They can cause heart failure if sprayed directly into the nose or mouth, and young people can hurt themselves while intoxicated or may suffocate while inhaling from a plastic bag. Youngsters who lose consciousness may die from inhaling their own vomit. Empty aerosol or glue cans in the house, spills and stains on clothes, a chemical smell on the breath or clothes, and obvious mood and behaviour swings are all signs that a teenager may be misusing solvents.

Tranquillizers (Valium, Librium, Ativan, temazepam) are commonly prescribed sedative drugs used to treat depression, anxiety and stress. At first they lessen feelings of anxiety, but in higher doses they have a sedative effect. Tranquillizers are addictive and withdrawal effects are unpleasant. In high doses tranquillizers can be fatal, especially if they are taken with alcohol.

Who can help? Most countries have at least one organiza-tion that parents can contact for help and advice about drug abuse. They will usually also offer support and information to families and friends of drug users. See the Directory for further details.

Teenage sexuality

During their adolescent years teenagers develop a growing awareness of their individual value and uniqueness, and of their sexual identity. Although they may have developed phys-ically, their emotional development may not have prepared them to meet fully the consequences of their sexual behav-iour. Schools attempt to address these issues in sex education. Pupils learn the basics of the biological processes in science lessons, while relationships, HIV and AIDS, and other sexually transmitted diseases are discussed outside the core curricu-lum against a background of moral considerations and the value of family life. However parents also need to address the issues of sexuality with their children.

Surveys show that far from getting all the information they need from school, young people want their parents to talk to them more about sex. They want them to talk about it early, before they need to know. Some parents worry that their chil-dren know everything already. Although this is not the case, teenagers may well know more about school-taught topics, such as HIV and AIDS, and it is up to parents to discover what is taught at school and when. What does their child think of what has been taught? Were there issues that were not cov-ered? Talking about sex education given at school can be a good starting point for discussing it at home.

Discussing sexuality Depending on the experience and skill of the teacher, sex education at school is likely to impart facts rather than discussing feelings, relationships and indi-vidual preferences in an intimate way, which can be more eas-ily discussed at home. Talking about sex has to be balanced

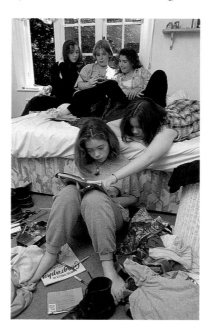

Left: Teenagers are often more likely to discuss their concerns and worries with their friends than they are with their parents, particularly their concerns about personal relationships and sexual matters. A social get-together with peers will usually elicit lively discussion and debate.

against the young person's need for privacy and confidentiality, and it is best to be ready to respond openly to a young person's tentative questions. Talking about sex more will not, as some parents worry, encourage young people to become involved in sexual activity at a younger age. On the contrary, evidence shows overwhelmingly that, if anything, more information tends to lead to a delay in the start of sexual activity, especially for boys.

One aspect of developing sexuality that boys find particularly embarrassing is getting an erection, especially if it happens in public. It may not be easy to discuss this at home, but it can be reassuring if you do. Both girls and boys worry about masturbation, not realizing how common it is, partly because most parents feel inhibited about talking about it as well. Almost all adult men have masturbated at some time, while two in three women have done so, although people vary greatly in how often they masturbate. Knowing that masturbation is a perfectly normal and healthy activity can come as a relief to a guilt-wracked teenager.

Many young people feel attracted to members of their own sex as well as the opposite sex. For most this is a transient phase. Some young people remain bisexual, while others pass through a phase of homosexuality and eventually settle for heterosexuality or vice versa. The early teen years are frequently an uncertain time, and the parents of a teenager who thinks they may be homosexual are often the last people the child will tell. Public attitudes towards homosexuality are still largely unaccepting and these young people often find very little support; one thing they do need is their parents' continuing love.

Starting a sexual relationship Far from being sexually precocious, many girls and boys are extremely self-conscious about their bodies around puberty, and are positively embarrassed by signs of their own sexuality. Later, many young people are uncertain about whether they are ready for sexual activity. Figures for the United Kingdom show that currently around one young person in four has had their first experience of sexual intercourse before the age of 16, with figures higher for boys than girls.

Many young people are acutely aware of peer pressure to start sexual activity. There is a lot of peer-group bragging about prowess, although only one girl in five is sexually active before the age of 16. Despite the images created by the teenage media, adolescents who do have early sexual intercourse usually have it in the context of a lasting relationship. Issues that parents can helpfully discuss with their adolescent children should include whether their child has a relationship in which they trust their partner; whether they feel under pressure and if so how they can say no; whether the couple

have discussed contraception; how ready they are for the emotional experience; whether they are sure they will be completely protected from sexually transmitted diseases.

The law also protects children who may not be old enough to decide for themselves whether to enter into a sexual relationship. In England, Wales and Scotland the age of consent (when a young person can make decisions about sex for themself) is 16; in Northern Ireland it is 17. Any man or boy having sex with a girl under this age is committing a criminal offense. The age of consent in homosexual relationships is 18 throughout the United Kingdom.

Contraception Discussing contraception can be difficult for young people, which may explain why half of all young couples having sex for the first time are unprotected. This lays them open to the risks not only of unwanted pregnancy, but also of sexually transmitted diseases. The advice and knowl-

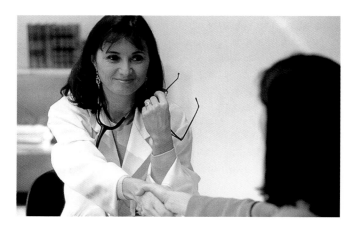

Above: Every year in the United Kingdom about 100,000 teenagers become pregnant. While some want to, for most the pregnancy is unwanted. Free and confidential contraceptive help is available from a doctor or family planning clinic regardless of age or parental permission.

edge of a tactful adult can be especially valuable here. Parents' worries that, by talking about contraception, they may appear to be condoning underage sex are misplaced: teenagers who are told about contraception are more likely to be able to say no.

Contraception is a joint responsibility and in the young the usual options are using a condom (male or female), the pill or a diaphragm. In the United Kingdom condoms can be bought from pharmacies, supermarkets and vending machines, while other methods of contraception are available only from a family planning clinic or a doctor. If a young person under the age of 16 consults a doctor about contraception, they are entitled to free and confidential advice. Doctors are not obliged to tell the young person's parents, although they will usually encourage the teenager to tell them.

For many young people sexual intercourse is not premeditated, which helps to explain the high rates of unprotected first-time sex. To ensure a girl does not get pregnant emergency contraception (after intercourse) is available from family planning clinics or doctors. This can be a pill that is taken within 72 hours of intercourse. Alternatively, a doctor can fit an intrauterine device within five days of unprotected sex.

Despite these efforts, there are 40,000 pregnancies a year in girls who are under the age of 16, and this rate is not falling significantly. The most common reasons for hospital admission for 15–16-year-old girls are termination of pregnancy and childbirth.

Sexually transmitted diseases HIV and other sexually transmitted diseases can be transmitted by unprotected sex, and the best way to reduce the risk of contracting them is always to use a condom and to limit the number of sexual partners. The most common infections today are nonspecific urethritis, gonorrhoea and herpes, but there are many others, all of them more common in teenagers and young adults than in older people. Condoms provide the best safeguard against sexually transmitted diseases, but they do not provide 100% protection. A teenager who develops any of the following symptoms should see a doctor: painful urination; itchy, burning or smelly discharge from vagina or penis; inflammation, sores, lumps or irritation in the genital area. All sexually transmitted diseases can be treated, and treatment at a special clinic for sexually transmitted diseases or genito-urinary medicine clinic is free and confidential, and the service is often a walk-in one.

Who can help? For details of organizations who can provide help and/or support. counselling and contraceptive advice for young people and parents see the Directory.

Smoking

Unlike other activities that can damage teenagers' health, smoking is harmful from the very first puff or drag. Children learn about the dangers of smoking from a young age, so why, by the age of 15 or 16, have over two-thirds of teenagers tried a cigarette, and why does one in three smoke regularly? The answer is that teenagers do not care about the long-term health risks. What does lung cancer, coronary heart disease or emphysema mean to an 11-year-old – the age at which most children start experimenting with cigarettes? Nor do the immediate health problems (shortness of breath, lack of fitness, nicotine cravings, reduced skin temperature, raised blood pressure and heart rate) matter compared with the

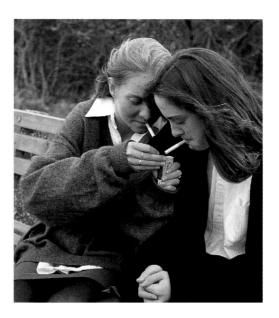

Above: Smoking among teenage girls carries enormous health risks that transcend generations. In Scotland more women now die from lung cancer than from breast cancer. Teenage girls who smoke and who take oral contraceptives are ten times as likely to have a heart attack or a stroke.

perceived benefits of being one of the crowd and looking older than you are.

It is only once they are smoking that teenagers realize it does not achieve this, that it may put some people off and that it costs a good deal of money. But by then many are hooked. A recent survey showed that eight out of ten teenagers do not want to be smoking by the time they are 20; but almost the same number expect that they will be. Fifteen per cent of the calls to the Quitline – the helpline in the United Kingdom for smokers who want to give up – come from people who are aged16 or under.

Prevention What can parents do to help? Researchers have found six key factors that help to protect adolescents against smoking. First, parents' attitudes and behaviour: children in smoking households are twice as likely to smoke as those in non-smoking households, but parental disapproval (even if the parent smokes) is a strong disincentive. What is more, a recent survey found that over 80% of young people thought their parents were among the best people to talk to them about smoking. Second, peer pressure: friends who do not smoke and disapprove create a non-smoking culture. Among girls in particular, smoking appears to be linked with their position in the teen hierarchy. Third, not having a brother or sister who smokes. Fourth, wanting to do well at school. Fifth, being involved in a sport, and sixth, having a good self-image and self-respect.

The anti-smoking message should start in infant school, and parents should reinforce it at home. Even if you are a smoker, make it plain that you disapprove of the habit and tell your child how difficult it is to give up. Stress a healthy life style at home. Teenagers who do not smoke often cite fitness for sport as a reason. Keep young children busy: research reveals that a key reason for taking up smoking is boredom. Accept that your child is likely to experiment with cigarettes, and when they are around the age of 11, raise the subject. If you ignore it you risk conveying to them the message that you do not care.

Talk about the associated issues – tax on cigarettes, advertizing, how easy it is for underaged children to buy tobacco products. Open up a dialogue, but do not be disappointed if your child does not feel like talking to you about is. They may think you are prying into their private, adolescent life. And they may be right. However you also have rights: a right to know where your child gets the money from to buy cigarettes; a right to know who sells them to your child, because they are breaking the law.

The facts Smoking is now more common among teenage girls than boys, and some of the reasons they give for smoking are rather revealing. They say that smoking puts them in a better mood; they feel better socially if they have a cigarette in their hand; and they worry that if they do not smoke they will eat more and put on weight.

Girls also develop a psychological dependence on smoking, which they believe makes them more socially competent. Psychological dependence is quickly followed by physical dependence. Within seven seconds of drawing on a cigarette, the effects of nicotine are felt in the brain. In habitual smokers it boosts the heart rate and raises the blood pressure, and causes the capillaries under the skin to constrict. Once the level of nicotine in the bloodstream falls, the unpleasant symptoms of withdrawal are felt: craving, irritability, anxiety and difficulties in concentrating. Smokers quickly learn to top up with another cigarette.

Cigarettes are well-known to be harmful to health. Stress the dangers, and give teenagers the facts. Of over 4000 chemicals in cigarette smoke, 43 independently cause cancer. Carbon monoxide in the smoke displaces oxygen in the blood, so there is less oxygen available to the tissues, and tar irritates the lungs. In the long term smoking is linked with coronary heart disease, atherosclerosis, bronchitis, emphysema, peptic ulcer and, possibly, infertility. The longer a person smokes, the greater are the risks.

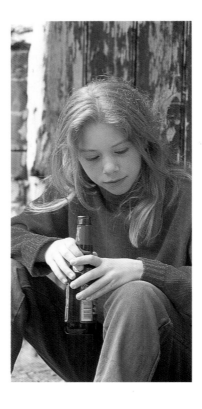

Left: In recent years there has been a spectacular growth in the sale of fruit-and-alcohol drinks, which have a particular appeal to teenagers and young children. Many people believe that these products have largely contributed to the rapid growth in underage drinking.

Giving up Even if a teenager is smoking regularly, do not despair – teenagers' attitudes and behaviour are not as fixed as they appear. Stress the benefits of giving up: the smell of smoke on clothes, breath and hair will vanish; the lungs will go back to being as efficient as before; the sense of taste and smell will improve; breathing and being able to cope with sudden exertion will improve; and they will save money. Warn a teenager not to expect instant success, as giving up is a process rather than a single event, but tell them there will be a well-earned feeling of pride once they have stopped.

Alcohol Critics say alcohol is a legalized drug, and if it was discovered today, it would probably be banned immediately. Yet 90% of the population drinks alcohol, and most drink it safely as a normal social activity.

Within minutes of drinking, alcohol passes into the bloodstream and is carried around the body to the brain and other major organs. The concentration of alcohol in the blood depends on a person's body weight. Alcohol has a more pronounced effect on younger people, partly because they are usually smaller and partly because their bodies are not used to dealing with alcohol. Girls tend to be affected more than boys, again because of their smaller size and also because boys have a higher water content in the body than girls, so the alcohol is diluted further.

In the brain, alcohol acts as a depressant, slowing reactions and thoughts. Its first effects – relaxation and disinhibition – last for around an hour if just one unit (a glass of wine, single measure of spirits or half a pint of beer) is drunk. The alcohol is then broken down in the liver and its effects pass. If more is drunk, however, the toxic effects mount up, causing nausea and vomiting, dehydration, headache, lack of coordination, loss of control and sleepiness.

Because alcohol undermines judgement it can be difficult even for an experienced drinker to be sure when the early pleasant effects are starting to become unpleasant, and it is little wonder that around 1000 children under 15 are admitted to hospital every year with acute alcohol intoxication. All of them need emergency treatment and some of them need to be looked after in intensive care.

There are laws to protect young people from the harmful effects of alcohol. In the United Kingdom no child under 14 may go into a bar; and no one under 18 is allowed to buy alcohol, apart from 16- and 17-year-olds who are permitted to buy beer, cider, porter or perry to drink with a meal in a restaurant or dining area.

Starting to drink alcohol Children over five are allowed to drink alcohol at home, and all the evidence suggests that this is where many children have their first taste of alcohol. Most children have their first drink between the ages of 9 and 14; by the age of 11, 16% of children have at least one drink each week. Over half of all 15–16-year-olds drink regularly, and almost all have had a drink at some time.

Many teenagers drink too much: in a recent report more than one in five 13-year-old boys and more one in eight 13-year-old girls said they had been very drunk once or more in the previous year. By the age of 15, the same report revealed, one in three boys and one in five girls had got into fights or arguments after drinking. A significant number will have drunk more than the recommended safe weekly limit of 14 units of alcohol for women or 21 units for men.

Alcohol education Alcohol education is taught in most secondary schools; pupils learn how alcohol affects body processes and are advised about the risks of alcohol abuse. Yet for most young people the first experience of drinking alcohol is at home. It seems sensible, therefore, for parents to teach their children about alcohol when it is relevant or when the subject arises naturally. It is also a good idea to allow them to become aware of the effects of alcohol under parental guidance at home.

Parents should set a good example, and can encourage sensible drinking by teaching simple social skills, such as how to refuse a drink politely. They can explain the strengths of different drinks, so that young people are better able to make an informed choice.

Parents should also discuss the downsides of drinking too much: behaving inappropriately, talking too much, being boring, losing control and falling asleep in a social setting. Losing control and becoming unattractive to the opposite sex are potent messages to teenagers. Pointing out that alcohol is frequently involved in suicide attempts, accidents involving severe head injuries and criminal damage will also help to illustrate the dangers.

Who can help? For organizations and agencies offering advice for children and teenagers with drinking problems see the Directory.

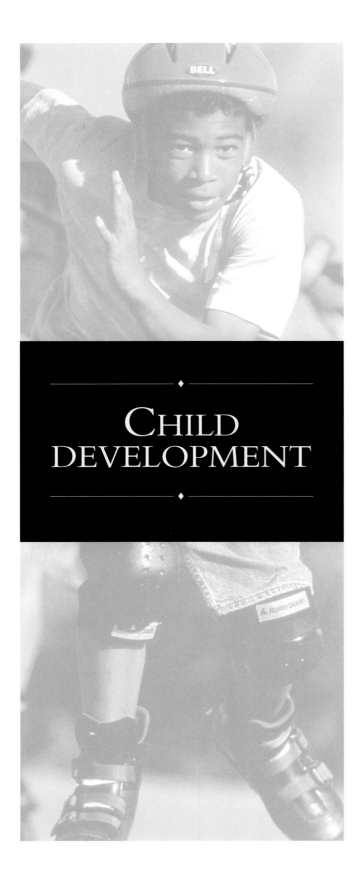

CHILD DEVELOPMENT

Babies and children are naturally programmed to develop in a reasonably orderly sequence. They put on weight, grow, smile and laugh, recover from colic and their first cold, develop teeth, learn to sleep through the night and then become risky little people as they start to crawl and walk around the furniture. In the early years children's achievements and milestones come thicker and faster than ever again. Parents may feel tempted to take the credit for these achievements – and so they should. In the nature-nurture debate, no one denies the impact that a stimulating, loving and opportunity-rich home life can have on children.

Children's experiences mould them from birth, and in all probability prior to birth. Babies who are at the receiving end of much chatting and talking from adults frequently grow into children who talk early and fluently. Children who live in homes with a flight of stairs learn to negotiate them earlier than children who live in flats. Children who are taken outdoors on foot as toddlers learn to walk further and more robustly than those who are always ferried by car or push chair. The best two-year-old walkers I ever came across were twin boys, just two years older than their twin sisters. With four children under two-and-a-half, their mother could simply never carry them. They walked everywhere.

However experience is not everything. Personality makes all the difference between the child who grasps an opportunity, learns from the experience and moves on to the next stage, and the child who needs endless coaxing and repetition before they can feel confident.

The pace of development

Children develop and learn at different speeds – some faster, some slower. The pace at which a child can take on a new learning experience depends partly on their personality, genetic make-up and environment, and partly on any particular difficulties they may have. For example a baby who has a visual problem will smile later than a baby who can see their mother's face from birth. A child whose hearing is impeded by bouts of glue ear may well speak late. One of the main reasons for the development reviews regularly offered for your child is that the doctor can identify any particular problems your child may face and help to overcome them.

Parents instinctively know their own child best and health professionals are aware of this. In many places parents are given a child health record to keep throughout their baby's childhood. You should be encouraged to record your observations in it and share these with your health visitor or doctor. In this way everyone keeps track of your child's medical progress and physical development. Whenever you take your child to the clinic, either at the doctor's surgery or at the hospital, take the child health record with you.

Assessing child development

When assessing a child's development, health professionals now tend to ignore rigid tests and charts. Instead, by talking to you and carefully watching your child play, they can form an idea of the child's level of development. It is undoubtedly true that parents are the first people to spot any problems, but health professionals have a better idea of what is normal for a child at any particular age.

Before a health review, let the doctor or your health visitor know if your child has been under the weather recently, as this will affect how the child behaves. If the child was born prematurely, remind your doctor or health visitor of this. The rule that children develop at very different rates holds particularly true of children who were premature babies, and allowances are usually made until they are two years old. If you are still concerned about your child's progress at the end of the review, ask if a second review is necessary or if a referral to a specialist can be arranged.

The neonatal examination The doctor or midwife who performs the neonatal examination will ask about the family history and any problems during pregnancy or birth. They will also ask you if you have any particular worries, so this is an opportunity to express any concerns you may have.

The infant is examined for any obvious physical abnormalities. The heart is checked, as well as the infant's general colour and breathing rate. A male infant's genitalia are examined to see whether the testes have descended. The infant is weighed and, if possible, measured, and the head circumference noted. The fontanelles – those areas where the skull has not yet fused – are felt.

The doctor or midwife will test the baby's hips to see if they are dislocated or can be easily dislocated. The eyes are checked for major structural problems, such as a cataract, and the inside of the mouth is checked to make sure there is no cleft in the palate. In some health areas the baby's hearing is also checked.

The health review at six to eight weeks The infant has a second examination at six to eight weeks. The doctor or health visitor weighs and measures the infant and their head circumference. This gives helpful information about how the infant is feeding and growing, as most infants lose some weight in the first few days following birth.

The infant has a thorough physical check, which will include assessing whether the hips can be dislocated and possibly checking the legs and arms for muscle tone. Even in such a small space of time, the baby's muscles will have started to strengthen. The doctor may well show this graphically by gently pulling the infant from a lying to a sitting posi-

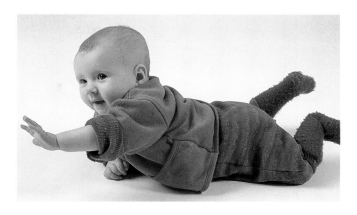

Above: Now that parents are advised to lay their infants on their backs to protect against sudden infant death, it is important to allow infants to play on their stomachs. The front-down position allows infants to develop strength in the neck, shoulders and trunk, ready for crawling.

tion and watching how the head no longer flops back, but follows the movement of the back.

The eyes will be examined and checked for any signs of a squint or other abnormality, which might have been missed at birth. The doctor will test to see if the infant can follow a moving toy to right and left and back again; to see if the infant is interested in looking at brightly coloured objects, that the eyes move smoothly; and the infant has started to smile.

The doctor will want to know about the infant's hearing, and will ask if your baby responds to your singing or talking voice, is quiet when talked to. and whether the baby reacts to sudden loud noises or soothing sounds. The infant's heart and, in male boys, genital area are checked again, and if the baby's testes have not yet descended, the doctor will arrange a referral to a paediatric surgeon. Babies who are exclusively breastfed may be given an extra dose of oral vitamin K.

The health review at six to nine months By the time infants have their health review at six to nine months, they are very different individuals. Your baby will be starting to eat real food, sitting up and taking notice of the world and may be babbling. At this review the infant can be weighed if you are concerned that your baby is putting on weight too fast or not fast enough, and measured if you are not certain your baby is growing at a normal rate.

The baby's hips and legs are checked again for any signs of dislocation, as hip dislocation occasionally develops after the neonatal period. The baby's eyes are assessed for any squint (which, if present at the last check, should have disappeared by now) and to see that the infant focuses well when a toy is held some 3 m/10 ft away, and that the infant can follow with their eyes a toy moving at a distance of around 3 m /10 ft.

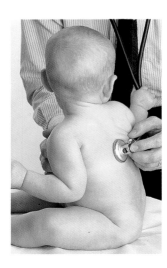

Right: Between six and nine months of age most infants acquire enough muscle control and balance to sit up straight while turning their head. Suddenly the world is a more interesting place in which to live.

The doctor will usually perform a distraction test to assess the baby's hearing. A sound is made from a position beyond the baby's field of vision to see if the baby turns towards it. An infant who has a cold or is tired – or can't hear – will have a second assessment, and if they can't hear on that occasion they will be referred to a specialist in children's audiology.

The infant's sounds are noted (at this stage the infant may well be making *a-ga*, *dada* sounds). The doctor or health visitor will also notice how interested the infant is in listening to parents speak, and how the infant manages to attract their parent's attention.

Balance will be checked to see if it is good enough for the infant to sit alone. There will also be a check to find out what attempts the infant is making to become mobile, and to see if they can bear weight on the feet when you hold their hands.

You may also be asked questions about how your baby is getting on. Concerns that can loom large in the second half of the first year often include feeding, manipulating finger foods, holding a cup and sleeping, as well as the baby's general health, including any episodes of wheezing.

The health review at 18 to 24 months By the time of this health review the erstwhile infant has probably turned into a mobile toddler who is into everything. The health visitor or doctor will check that the child is walking properly and ask about general development and speech. They will explain that at this age understanding and being interested in making social contact is more important than talking. By now a toddler's vision is mature, so they can see fine detail. Health professionals will be able to judge from the child's behaviour and from asking questions about books, pictures and television whether there are any serious difficulties.

If the child had any earlier problems with slow growth the child may be weighed and, if necessary, measured.

The health visitor may well ask about play and activities such as walking up and down stairs, running and jumping. Your toddler may not have mastered these skills yet, but by now they will have good control over muscles and will be making steady progress with hand-eye coordination. The idea is to spot any problems early.

The doctor or health visitor will also talk about toilet training, eating and the child's behaviour – if major problems are to arise this is usually when they will happen.

The pre-school health review This review is carried out to check that the child is well and able to benefit fully from education at school. It may be done at the same time as the child is given pre-school booster immunizations: diphtheria, tetanus, polio, measles, mumps and rubella.

The health visitor or possibly doctor will discuss any worries you may have about the child's eyesight and might ask your child to perform a simple task, such as threading bricks, in order to check hand-eye coordination. In some health regions the child may be asked to do a simple test, during which each eye is covered separately to check for any signs of a latent squint.

The health visitor will ask whether the child can now speak clearly enough for anyone outside the home to understand them. The child will only need a hearing assessment if they have problems with speech or if parents are concerned about their speech or hearing.

The doctor or health visitor will measure the child and plot their height on a chart, but they will only weigh your child if you want them to, or if there has been any concern in the past about growth. If your child shows signs of clumsiness or falls frequently, this is an opportunity to mention it.

By this age most children are dry by day although some, especially boys, are still wet at night. This is a good opportunity for parents to air any concerns they may have.

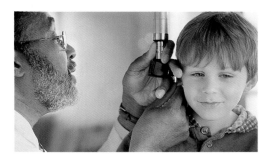

Above: Most children will be given a hearing test when they start school, but they will only need a thorough examination of the ears and further tests if the doctor finds that there is a problem.

STAGES OF DEVELOPMENT

It is fascinating to see how babies develop. The guidelines given below, which indicate the various stages of achievement, can serve as a basis for developmental activities that parents can enjoy with their children. However parents should remember that each baby is unique and, within a broad span of 'normal', will develop at their own pace.

The one-month-old infant *Moving* If you pull your baby into a sitting position, the back will curve and the head will need support to stop it from flopping forwards or backwards. When lying on the stomach, your baby will turn the head to one side or the other. However you should only lay them on their stomach to play when you are with them. If you hold them under the arms over a hard surface such as a table, your baby will press down with their feet and make apparent walking movements. This is not real walking, however; it is one of the reflex actions with which babies are born. Another one is stepping; if you hold your infant with the top of their foot held against a table edge, for example, they will step up on to the table.

Hearing and speech The month-old infant responds to loud noises by appearing startled, blinking or stiffening. When they are at peace they may make tiny throaty or cooing noises, especially if they are 'talking' to you.

Seeing At this age infants blink in response to light and turn their head towards a source of light. They are interested in the difference between darkness and light and can stare at lights for a long time. However your baby will be most interested in your face, which they will watch intently as they feed. From around four to six weeks they start to smile.

The three-month-old infant *Moving* Lying on their back, infants wave their arms symmetrically and kick with both legs together, or 'cycle'. If you pull them up into a sitting position, they will hold their head still for a few seconds before it wobbles forwards. Do lay them down to play on their stomach; by now your baby can lift his or her head and chest up to look around them.

Hearing and speech As long as the baby is not crying, they will quieten and appear to listen when they hear your voice or an interesting sound such as a bell or a rattle. They make noises when you speak to them and when they are alone. If the baby is trying to discover where the sound is coming from, they may move their eyes or even roll their head from side to side.

Handling objects At first your baby could not hold an object without letting it go, but by now, if you place a toy or rattle in

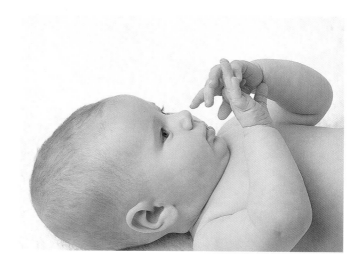

Above: By three months of age a baby will be able to focus on close objects, such as her hands, and, fascinated, will begin to play with them. At this stage of development she will be able to hold a small object for a short time and also have control over her head movements.

their hand, they can hold it for a few moments and may move it towards their face, often hitting themselves. Your baby is starting to reach out for objects and starting to put their fingers into their mouth. Everything else also goes into the mouth for investigation. Dribbling becomes obvious.

Seeing Babies are very interested in human faces at this age and follow them constantly. They can perceive colours as well as shades and variations in shade. If a ball or brightly coloured toy is held and moved about 20 cm/8 in away from the face, the baby can follow its movement. Soon they start to watch their own hands and to recognize the activities that precede a feed.

The six-month-old infant *Moving* Lying on the back, your baby can lift their head to look at their feet. As long as the baby is supported in their cot or chair, they can sit up and turn their head from side to side to see the world around them. Their back is straight and they can support their head well. Your baby has probably learned to roll over by now – from front to back or back to front. Hold them under the arms and you will find that their feet press down on the surface you hold them above, and they may start to bounce up and down.

Hearing and speech Your baby turns when they hear your voice. Soon they will be able to turn to a quiet noise made on either side of them, as long as there is not something more interesting to attract their attention. They will sing to themself and laugh and chuckle while playing. A child who is annoyed or frustrated can scream.

Handling objects Your baby can grasp a toy and pass it from hand to hand.

Seeing Your baby can see across a room and follow activities with interest. They are aware of depth and distance and can see in 3-D; this is important because your child is about to become more mobile. Once they can sit up they can be offered finger foods.

The nine-month-old infant *Moving* At nine months infants can sit on their own on the floor for quite a few minutes and lean forward to pick up a toy without toppling forward. They may be on the move, either crawling or commando crawling across the floor, and may be strong enough to pull themself to a standing position, but then fall backwards with a bump.

Hearing and speech At this age infants babble in long strings of tuneful sounds, such as '*dadada*' or '*mumumum*'. They can also imitate other sounds such as coughing or smacking their lips in a pretend kiss. They know the meaning of words such as 'no' and 'bye bye'.

Handling objects Babies can stretch out to grasp a toy or other object if offered, then let go to give it to you, but can't put it down yet. They can also pick up small objects between their finger and thumb. They can poke at something close to them, and are starting to point at objects a little further away from them.

Seeing If something falls off the high chair, the baby will be able to watch the direction in which it falls.

The one-year-old infant *Moving* The one-year-old infant can sit on the floor for as long as they want, crawl, bottom-shuffle or bear-walk on their legs and arms. When they pull themself into a standing position they can let themself down gently or side-step around the furniture, still holding on for support. However if you hold their hands they may be able to step out across the floor. Some babies can walk by now, others can just stand alone, while others are ready to learn to crawl upstairs.

Hearing and speech The one-year-old knows their own name and chats, although you may not understand a word. They can understand a simple instruction or words that are familiar to them in their context. They may even be able to give you a named object such as a shoe or cup.

Handling objects They can pick up small objects and feed themself competently with finger foods, throw objects and can point to things that interest them. They will soon start to feed themself with a spoon – which is extremely messy at first – and take off clothes such as socks.

Seeing At this age infants can look in the right direction for things that roll out of sight or disappear from their view. They

are beginning to enjoy looking at pictures, so you can spend some time looking at picture books with them.

The two-year-old toddler *Moving* The two-year-old can run without falling over and have a go at kicking a large ball. They can walk up and down stairs using two feet to each step, as long as they steady themself on the wall or banisters. They can squat on the floor and climb on to furniture, sit on a tricycle and push themself forwards with their feet on the floor, but they are not able to use the pedals yet.

Hearing and speech The two-year-old's vocabulary has grown to around 50 words and they can link two words into a meaningful phrase. They ask what things and people are called and can join in with songs, jingles and nursery rhymes. The toddler can now point to parts of the body on request and, depending on their mood, can obey commands such as 'Go and pick the letters up'.

Handling objects At this age toddlers can grip objects and may hold a pencil correctly between the thumb and first two fingers. Their drawings are becoming more interesting – they can imitate a vertical line and their scribbling becomes more circular. When they are looking at a book, they can turn the pages one by one by themselves. If something interesting such as a wrapped sweet is placed in front of them, they will unwrap it without too much difficulty. Hand preference is usually clear.

Seeing They can appreciate the fine detail in the pictures in their favourite stories. They may be able to recognize themselves in photographs.

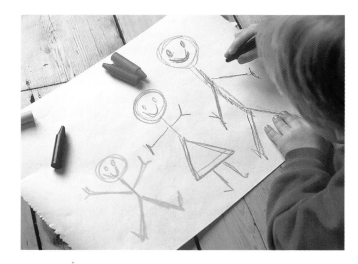

Above: Children usually start to draw people with a circle to which eyes, mouth and later a nose is added. Legs come next, followed by arms sticking straight out of the head or halfway down the body. Eventually the child reaches the separate gender sophistication of this drawing.

The three-year-old child *Moving* Three-year-olds can walk upstairs one foot to a step and down again two feet to a step. When they reach the bottom they can jump off the bottom step. They love climbing frames and slides and are usually perfectly confident using them. They can use the pedals on a tricycle and, given enough space, can steer it around corners. They can kick a ball, stand on tiptoe and stand just for a second or two on one foot. They can also throw a ball and catch a large one with both arms.

Hearing and speech People outside the family can understand what a three-year-old says, although some of their sounds are still not quite adult and they make regular and endearing grammatical errors. At this age children adore stories and have their own repertoire of nursery rhymes and rote learning, such as numbers up to ten.

Handling objects Children are fairly manually dexterous by now. They can eat with a fork and spoon and wash their hands, although they may still need help with drying them. They can pull their own pants up and down, but may need help with buttons. They can thread wooden beads on a lace and play competently with different construction toys. They can use (round-ended) scissors and can hold a pencil correctly and use it to draw a circle, a V-shape, imitate a cross and simple letters such as H. They can draw a man with a head and usually some other body parts as well, and can paint with a large brush.

The four-year-old child *Moving* Four-year-old children can walk up and down stairs quite well, climb ladders and trees, ride a tricycle with ease, hop, stand and run on tiptoe and sit with their legs crossed, and are quite expert with a ball and even a bat.

Hearing and speech By now children speak clearly although they still make mistakes with certain sounds. They ask many questions, make up long stories and enjoy jokes.

Handling objects Four-year-olds can draw quite expertly, often choosing to draw people and houses. They can use a knife and fork.

The five-year-old child *Moving* The five-year-old child can walk steadily down a line, skip on alternate feet, hop on each foot and play all sorts of ball games.

Hearing and speech The only sounds which children may still have problems with are usually *s*, *f* or *th*. They can tell you their full name, age and address as well as their birthday. They love stories and often act them out.

Handling objects At five years of age children are able to thread needles and to sew. They can write and draw with pencils and brushes, and the people they draw have a large number of features.

SPEECH AND LANGUAGE

◆

Children who have a good mastery of speech and language have experienced many interesting conversations with adults at home. However it is true that there are factors outside a parent's control that can interfere with a child's fluent acquisition of speech and language – for example a physical problem such as glue ear or an unusual speech disorder. It is also true that genetic influences play an important role in deciding how fast a child will acquire and use language, and that in speech as in all other areas of development, some children mature more quickly than others. Yet the greatest contribution parents can make to their child's speech and language development is to speak to their child.

It is neither necessary nor desirable to make conversation a special event. Talking as often as possible to children about what interests them at that moment is more helpful. Speak clearly, using short sentences and simple but not babyish language. Making two-way conversation encourages babies and young children to participate, especially if the noises they make are interpreted as real speech. Busy parents who do not have time to sit down and talk face-to-face can give a running commentary on what they are doing.

You should limit the background noise from the video, television and radio so that the child can hear speech clearly. Draw their attention to other noises around them – a bird in the garden, traffic or even silence. Listening, like speaking, is an acquired skill.

In an important recent study researchers found that a large proportion of nine-month-old babies showed signs of delayed speech. The researchers suspected that babies in homes where the television or video was on all the time were likely to be at greatest risk of speech delay, and their evidence proved them right. When parents were advised to reduce the time the television was on, and to set aside half an hour a day to play and talk to the child, the results at the age of three showed a great improvement in performance. Children whose parents had followed the advice were at least a year further ahead in their language development than the children of parents who did not follow the advice.

This does not mean that the television has to be turned off permanently. It depends on your circumstances at home, although the study found the greatest progress in the children who not only benefited from extra adult attention but also had the television off during the day. The problem with continuous television is thought to be two-fold: it makes it difficult for children to distinguish background noise from speech, and it reduces the number of times children interact in a social way and have conversations with adults. However sitting down to watch a programme with a child and talking about it can increase the child's vocabulary, while watching a video (usually the same video) again and again can help young children to appreciate the way in which events follow on from each other.

Specific types of language, such as nursery rhymes, help the child to develop an awareness of sounds. This acuity can then be helpful in learning to read.

The bilingual family Increasing numbers of children in many parts of the world are brought up in bilingual families, and some parents worry that coping with two languages will slow down the child's acquisition of speech, as well as lead to problems with their speech. However there is absolutely no evidence that this is the case. Until the child is three or four years of age the parents should use their mother tongue or the language with which they feel most comfortable to express emotions. It is easier for children if the parent uses only one language with them or if certain situations are linked with certain languages.

Childhood speech problems The most common speech problems that occur in childhood are the following.
The child's speech cannot be understood Either the child cannot hear the differences between sounds or cannot say them. The most common reasons for being unable to discriminate between sounds are a hidden hearing loss, frequently caused by glue ear, and a lack of clear one-to-one conversation at home. If adults outside the family have difficulty understanding a three-year-old child, an assessment by a speech therapist may prove helpful.

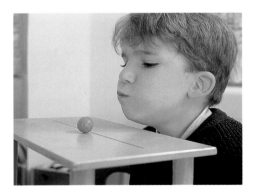

Above: Speech therapy should be fun. This five-year-old boy has had a cleft palate repaired and is practising blowing to increase his control of air pressure inside his mouth. Speech therapy sessions are held individually or in small groups.

The child cannot hear properly In children under the age of five the most common cause of deafness is glue ear. Children vary enormously in their ability to compensate for the fluctuating hearing loss that glue ear brings. If speech is clearly immature or unclear there is often an additional factor or the glue ear is severe. Children with glue ear should be spoken to face to face, using language they can understand and without background interference from television or radio. They should also have a hearing test and possibly treatment with grommets (see page 204).
The child lisps By the time children reach their first birthday they have learned to discriminate between all the sounds of their mother tongue. However every language has its stumbling blocks and in English these are the sounds *s, f, th, w* and *y*. Many children do not sort these out until the first or second year of primary school, but the lisp is endearing rather than worrying. When a child pronounces a sound in the wrong way, just say it correctly, in an approving tone of voice.
The child has started to stammer As children gather speed with their speech – frequently around the age of three or four – it is amazingly common for them to pause, repeat themselves or get stuck midway. Speech therapists call this nonfluency, but it is stammering to everyone else. Listen to what the child is trying to say, give them your full, patient attention and resist any temptation to finish the sentence for them. The stammer often dies away in a month or two. If other people in the family stammer, or if the stammer lasts more than six weeks or is very severe, ask for a speech therapy assessment.

Complementary treatment
Music therapy has proved to be particularly beneficial in cases of specific speech delay, and speech and language therapists will sometimes recommend it. It can explore psychological causes, build confidence and establish rewarding patterns of nonverbal communication, as well as encourage verbal communication at a developmentally appropriate level. Music therapy may also offer help and support in cases of stammering that arise from anxiety. Emotional causes of stammering may be helped by the **Bach flower remedies**: Mimulus for shyness; Larch for lack of confidence; Centaury for inassertiveness; Vervain for over-excitement; and Impatiens for impatience. Both **play** and **drama therapy** can be beneficial in cases of speech and language delay, and play therapy for stammering.

How speech develops

- Soon after birth infants may make quiet breathy sounds such as *heh*
- By four to eight weeks infants may respond by starting to coo if you leave a gap in your speech
- At three to five months infants often enjoy making a variety of different noises when spoken to and may start a 'conversation' themselves
- By six months infants can squeal, chuckle and scream. Tuneful babbling starts soon, at first with single sounds such as *goo* and moving on to double sounds such as *ama* or *uduh*
- By 12 months infants often make sounds that could be words and even conversations. Listen carefully and you will hear most of the consonants and vowels
- By 18 months toddlers can say between five and twenty words or more, and understand many more. They try to sing and join in nursery rhymes and can point out parts of the body
- By two years of age children use 50 or more words and understand far more. They string them together in at least two-word sentences, ask constant 'What's that?' questions and understand instructions such as 'See why the baby is crying'
- By three to three-and-a-half years of age children can build complex sentences and stories linked by 'and', and ask endless questions. However many sounds are still childish, as are speech forms such as 'I bringed it.'
- By four to four-and-a-half years of age children are sophisticated communicators with an active vocabulary of over 1000 words and a wider passive vocabulary. They still muddle sounds (*r* and *w*, *l* and *y* or *p* and *th*, *s* and *f*, or *t* and *k*). They can talk about the past and the future
- By five years children are fluent, using nearly all the correct sounds except for *s*, *f* and *th*. They understand abstract words and jokes and can tell stories using subordinate clauses
- Beyond the age of five years children learn to connect their speech fluently using linking words such as however, for instance, perhaps and really. They learn different registers of language for school, home and the playground. By late primary school, children have a vocabulary of 10,000 to 20,000 words – still a mere fraction of the million and more words in the English language

LEARNING DIFFICULTIES

A child with a learning difficulty is a child who has significantly greater difficulty in learning than most children of the same age, and/or has a disability that prevents or hinders them from making use of the educational facilities available to children of the same age.

Some children with a learning difficulty find learning most things difficult. They may have been slow to sit up and walk and they are very likely to have been late talkers They may be quite unresponsive to noises and speech, so there are early concerns that they may be deaf. Parents are usually the first to notice their child's difficulties and this usually happens when they compare them with other children of the same age. Sometimes a health visitor or a doctor who sees the child for a development review notices the learning delay before the parents.

Many children with learning difficulties have physical difficulties as well. Children with Down's syndrome (see page 337) or fragile X syndrome (see page 309) all experience some degree of learning problem. Some, although not all, children with cerebral palsy also have difficulty in learning. Babies born prematurely, in particular babies born with a very low birth weight, may have a general or specific learning difficulty that may be accompanied by cerebral palsy. Damage to the brain before, during or after birth can leave a legacy of learning problems, although the brain has a remarkable ability to compensate when even large areas are damaged. However no cause is ever found for 50% of children who have difficulty in learning.

What to do Discovering that a child has a learning difficulty is upsetting for all parents, particularly if the discovery follows months or years of uncertainty. In the initial stages parents require a good deal of information, which is sometimes not easy to obtain. Many parents report that parents of children with similar difficulties are the best source of information. Voluntary organisations can also provide advice, information and support.

Children with a learning difficulty are entitled to assessment and help. As a second problem, for example, with hearing or vision can compound their problems, they should receive regular checks. Therapy depends on the cause but parents are always kept closely involved.

Once it comes to schooling, some children can attend a mainstream school with additional one-to-one support, while others thrive better in a special school. In the school population of the United Kingdom, one child in five needs some level of extra help to cope with the curriculum. These children are held to have a special educational need (SEN), which in many cases can be met in school by the teacher, with support where necessary from outside bodies. Some children catch up quickly when given specialist help and are able to keep up with their classmates. Others continue to need help and support.

Predicting the outlook for children with learning difficulties is not easy for specialists or parents. Children generally improve, although some have a problem in a particular area for the rest of their lives.

Dyslexia

This is one of the most common of the specific learning difficulties. Dyslexia represents a disorder in processing symbolic information. People with dyslexia have difficulty making sense of different words and symbols, getting them in the right order and recalling them afterwards. This can lead to difficulties with reading, spelling and writing. Number and organization skills and coordination may also be involved in some cases. However it is important to remember that dyslexia is not related to intelligence, culture, class or socio-economic background.

Dyslexia is thought to be four times more common in boys than in girls and can often be inherited. In fact, genetic markers for dyslexia have been found on two chromosomes, numbers one and fifteen. The condition may have its roots in slight differences in brain structure and organization of sufferers. Neurobiology has shown that in some people with dyslexia the right and left hemispheres of the brain are unusu-

Right: A number of children with dyslexia have additional visual problems that contribute to difficulties with reading and writing, and make schoolwork extremely frustrating. Detailed eye tests are vital and the use of coloured overlays on reading text can result in unexpected progress.

ally symmetrical. A dyslexic's fundamental difficulty is usually with the sounds that spoken words make (the phonology), so that the child has difficulty breaking words into syllables and in knowing whether they rhyme or not. Typically, a child with dyslexia has most problems with verbal short term memory; finding the right word; and distinguishing similar sounds such as *t* and *d*.

Children who are thought to suffer from dyslexia should always have an eye examination, because subtle defects of vision may contribute to the condition, although they are not the primary cause. For example, visual problems with focusing over a wide range of distances, and with eye coordination, are more common in dyslexics than in other children. Some experience eyestrain and visual distortions when reading, a condition known as scotopic sensitivity syndrome (also known as Mearles-Irlen syndrome), which can be helped by using coloured filters.

Dyslexia usually becomes obvious when a child is struggling with reading and writing at school. However there are early signs to watch out for. When present on their own they are not evidence that a child is dyslexic, and many children who are not dyslexic show some of the signs. However a pre-school child with many obvious and persistent signs deserves observation. This is especially true if someone else in the family already has dyslexia.

You may notice
Pre-school:
- *The child is markedly better at some things than others. They may be good with construction toys and craft activities, but have no interest in pre-reading and pre-writing activities and skills*
- *The child is late in talking clearly. They confuse the names of objects and directions (in/out; up/down) and have difficulty in remembering nursery rhymes*
- *The child cannot clap in time and may be clumsy*
- *The child cannot remember easily more than one instruction at a time*

At school:
- *A child eight years of age or less may show particular difficulty learning to read or write, may persistently reverse letters and numbers and/or find it hard to remember information sequences, such as multiplication tables, the alphabet or days of the week. Concentration may be difficult and frustration may lead to behavioural problems*
- *A child aged nine to twelve years may still make mistakes reading and spelling, take longer than expected over written work and have difficulty copying from the blackboard or taking down oral instructions. There may be increasing frustration and a growing lack of self confidence*

♦ *A pupil over the age of 12 years may read inaccurately, spell inconsistently and have difficulty planning and writing essays. They may have difficulty with verbal instructions and foreign languages. Self-esteem may be low*

What to do If your child shows most of the signs above, ask his or her teacher whether the child needs extra support at school and whether there are any helpful activities that can be done at home. If the school agrees with you that your child has a special educational need, an individual education plan may be drawn up describing their difficulties, the action to be taken and the support the child can expect, as well as targets to be reached in a given time. This may be enough for the child to keep up with classmates. If it is not, the child may need a full assessment, followed by help from special educationalists. There are many approaches to dyslexia, but children learn best from a structured programme to literacy that uses a variety of senses, ideally taught by a teacher with a special qualification.

You should also make arrangements through your doctor for your child to have a detailed vision and hearing assessment, and make arrangements through the school for an educational psychologist to assess the child.

At home, put emphasis on the things your child is good at and praise them for it. Avoid drawing attention to their failures, as children with dyslexia experience enough of that at school.

Never accept diagnosed dyslexia as an excuse for not trying. Success just takes longer and is harder to achieve. Be patient and remember that trying hard is stressful.

Who can help? For organizations that offer an information and referral services to local associations see the Directory.

Complementary Treatment
Musical activities devised by teachers may support specialized teaching methods. The **Bach flower remedies** may be helpful in dealing with emotional problems associated with the condition.

Fragile X syndrome Fragile X syndrome is a common inherited cause of learning disability. As accurate tests have only recently become available, the incidence is not yet agreed, but it is thought to affect approximately one boy in four thousand. It has remained a hidden cause of learning disability because people with fragile X are often not immediately identifiable, although they do have typical physical characteristics. In the same way, the amount of learning disability and behaviour problems fragile X causes vary widely from child to child.

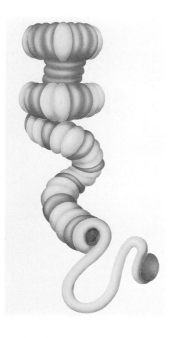

Left: If you examine under a microscope the X chromosome of a boy with fragile X syndrome, you will see that the end of the chromosome seems to be breaking off, as reflected in this illustration.

The fragile X condition is transmitted on the X chromosome, one of the chains of genetic material that control inherited characteristics. Examined under a microscope, the tip of the X chromosome appears to be breaking off. This occurs at the site of a particular gene, FMR 1, where a genetic change has resulted in a small segment of the gene being repeated many times. Some people have a large change (a full mutation) in the gene and consequently have fragile X. Others have a small change (a pre-mutation) which does not usually cause symptoms, but is likely to increase, possibly into a full mutation, when the gene is passed on by a woman to the next generation. Pre-mutations in men do not increase in size when passed on.

Males have one X and one Y chromosome: females have two X chromosomes. A woman with a fragile X chromosome is likely to have a second, normal X chromosome, and it seems that the normal chromosome protects her from some of the effects of the fragile X chromosome. Therefore the woman will have no fragile X symptoms. However such women still have a 50% chance of passing the condition on to their children.

Fragile X can be diagnosed accurately from a blood sample, which can identify both affected children and carriers. The condition can usually be detected prenatally at 11–12 weeks of pregnancy by chorionic villus sampling. However a full discussion with a genetic counsellor who specializes in the emotions and realities of such conditions is recommended before becoming pregnant.

Children with fragile X may show only some of the following symptoms, and to an extremely varied degree.

You may notice

♦ *Learning difficulties, such as specific difficulties with number work, thinking in 3-D and processing sequential information*
♦ *Speech may be rapid, with poor rhythm control and may be difficult to understand*
♦ *Difficulties concentrating, and the child is easily distracted*
♦ *Impulsive behaviour*
♦ *High activity levels, restlessness*
♦ *Babies may be noticeably floppy*
♦ *Some people with fragile X develop epilepsy*

Strengths Some children with fragile X syndrome can understand words surprisingly well and have excellent memories. In terms of behaviour, these children may combine being happy, friendly and likable with certain autistic-like features such as avoiding eye contact, hand-flapping and speech and language delay.

What to do Early diagnosis does help children with fragile X syndrome, because appropriate support and therapy – particularly speech therapy and, later on, special educational support – can be given. As many children take in what they see better than what they hear, a demonstration is often more helpful than instruction, and a practical, concrete teaching approach helps.

Behaviour modification – rewarding desired behaviour and ignoring undesirable behaviour – helps. Preparing children gently for change is important, and supporting them with social skills is beneficial.

The family should receive genetic counselling so that the risks of future children being affected can be explained and the implications discussed.

 Complementary Treatment
The Bach flower remedies may be helpful in dealing with the emotional problems that may be associated with the condition.

Attention deficit hyperactivity disorder
All children are sometimes overactive, restless and difficult to handle. However children with attention deficit hyperactivity disorder (ADHD) are so inappropriately impulsive, overactive and/or inattentive for their age that their behaviour impedes their social activities, development or educational progress. ADHD is not a fixed syndrome but a rather contorversial evolving concept, therefore ideas about it are constantly changing as more is discovered about the causes and most effective treatments.

Current thinking holds that ADHD can have many causes. Genes play an important part and brain scans of affected children have shown underactivity in areas of the brains, particularly in the frontal lobes, the command centres for self control, among other things. Usually a variety of different factors add up to a final picture of hyperactivity, commonly including a restless and impulsive temperament and a delay in developing the ability to concentrate. For a small number of children allergies to certain foods or ingredients also seem to play a

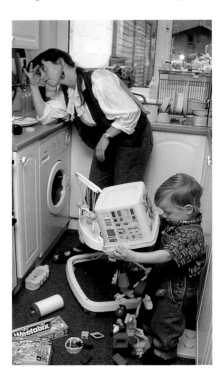

Left: Behaviour that is appropriate in a young child can signal an attention deficit disorder in an older child. Unceasing and sometimes purposeless activity is an early indication that the child's behaviour may need to be looked at by a professional.

role in the disorder. Three to four times as many boys as girls are affected by Attention Deficit Hyperactivity Disorder. In the United Kingdom one child in two hundred is thought to suffer from the disorder, while in the United States as many as one child in twelve has been diagnosed with attention deficit hyperactivity disorder. It is believed by many specialists that the disorder is overdiagnosed in the United States and underdiagnosed in the United Kingdom.

The outlook is fairly good for these sufferers. Affected children do usually improve as they mature and learn ways of coping. However, they may grow out of the overactivity and impulsiveness associated with the disorder, while the inability to concentrate may be more difficult for them to overcome and could accompany them into adult life.

Although ADHD is diagnosed most frequently around the age of seven when educational demands on young children increase, some symptoms may be clear from earliest years of childhood. The following list includes some of the most common features.

You may notice

♦ *Frequent disorganized and aimless activity. Pointless, forbidden and even painful actions are repeated*
♦ *Constantly changing activities*
♦ *Constantly waking in the night*
♦ *Difficulty acquiring self-control. Possibly aggressive play*
♦ *Difficulty following instructions, learning to cope with a new situation or fitting in with a group*
♦ *The child is clearly different from their unaffected brothers and sisters*
♦ *Possibly extreme temper tantrums*
♦ *Some children show signs that commonly accompany the hyperkinetic syndrome – a severe type of hyperactivity. These may include being slow to talk and clumsiness*

Diagnosis Many of the typical features of ADHD are common and normal in young children so the diagnosis needs to made carefully. A paediatrician, psychologist or psychiatrist diagnosing ADHD or the hyperkinetic syndrome will look for clear signs before making a judgement. These include six of the following symptoms denoting lack of concentration, all six lasting for more than six months and being inappropriate for the child's age. The symptoms are: often being careless and failing to pay attention to detail; losing concentration quickly at play or work; not appearing to listen to what is said; not following instructions or completing tasks; not being very good at self organization or organizing activities; an avoidance or dislike of tasks that need a sustained mental effort; losing things that are needed for work or games; being easily distracted; and being frequently forgetful.

The doctor will also look for signs of overactivity or impulsiveness in the child, including frequent fidgeting or squirming when sitting down; getting up and leaving the seat when expected to stay still; frequent running or climbing about; being inappropriately noisy; being unable to hear the whole question before blurting out the answer; and having difficulty waiting in turn.

What to do Children who cope best with the disorder are often the children of coping parents. Try to encourage self control, establish and adhere to clear house rules and plan structured days.

Be positive, encourage and reward good behaviour, including small achievements such as sitting still at the table. Use the child's best time of day to teach new skills.

Ask for help when the child's activity levels become too much for you to bear.

Treatment No single treatment works for all children and doctors often combine different approaches. A small number

of children respond to changes in diet. Some children with attention deficit hyperactivity disorder are thought to suffer from food allergies, while others cannot metabolize certain substances in food or drugs, especially artificial colours, some preservatives and salicylates. Cows' milk, chocolate, fizzy drinks and food additives are believed to be common culprits in the disorder. A few children improve in their behaviour when they avoid a wide variety of manufactured, processed and frozen foods. Others respond to a diet that does not contain caffeine. However, the dietary connection is still not scientifically proven although many parents find they can make differences by changing the child's diet.

Drugs used for severely affected children include stimulants, such as methylphenidate hydrochloride (Ritalin), which appear to increase concentration. However this is not a cure and is not suitable for children under the age of six. The drug is thought to help nerve cells in the brain carry messages to other cells, allowing children to filter out unwanted information. Medication does not help all children and can have adverse effects, including headaches, appetite and weight loss and poor sleep. However when it is effective the child is able to concentrate, learn and behave sociably and respond to the behaviour or cognitive therapies that should always accompany drug therapy.

Other approaches to hyperactivity in children include psychological treatments. Behavioural and cognitive therapy are the most common; treatment plans are drawn up individually for the child and are tailored to his or her needs. Behavioural therapy includes reward schemes and positive encouragement. Cognitive therapy can help children manage their own reward schemes, control their impulses and solve problems in an ordered way.

Who can help? For organizations offering help and advice, see the Directory.

Complementary Treatment

Children with mild to moderate symptoms of ADHD may benefit from **music therapy**, developing better concentration and commitment through musical activities when they are unable to tolerate educational ones. Severe cases may benefit from receptive music therapy to encourage relaxation. The **Bach flower remedy** Vervain is often useful for over-excited, over-enthusiastic children who cannot switch off, wind down or relax. Cherry Plum is helpful if there is a tendency to lose emotional control and Impatiens for those who become impatient, irritable and do everything in a hurry. **Play** and **drama therapy** can also be beneficial.

Autism

Autism is a developmental disorder that interferes with a child's social and communication skills. Four times as many boys as girls are affected and most, although not all, have learning difficulties. The cause is not yet understood, although events before, during or shortly following birth may be involved. Genetic traits appear to be an important factor in many children; however the sites of any relevant genes have yet to be identified.

Children with autism live in a world of jumbled fragments of information, which means they cannot assess other people's feelings or reactions. This makes their behaviour and responses appear bizarre, unsociable and at times unpredictable. In a child affected by autism, patterns of behaviour will already be strange enough for a diagnosis by the age of about three years. Sometimes the typical lack of response is visible right from the earliest days of infancy. All children with autism show the following three features. First, they ignore other people or approach them but pay no attention to their response (some children want to be sociable but don't know how). Second, they have difficulty communicating using either words or gestures and expressions, and they do not listen to others. Third, they have difficulty developing pretend or imaginative play.

You may notice

- *Your baby turns from your gaze, dislikes being picked up and prefers to be left alone*
- *They appear deaf and you are left with an uneasy feeling that something is wrong*
- *They are probably slow to reach their milestones and are not only late to develop speech but respond inappropriately to sounds. However, as they develop they may be good at certain tasks such as jigsaws and sorting shapes*
- *As a child they insist on a precise routine and find it extremely difficult to accommodate change*
- *Other signs shown by some, but not all, children with autism include: looking past people rather than straight at them; a tiptoe walk; flapping hands; indifference to pain; laughing in the wrong situation; erratic sleeping; and seemingly uncontrollable behaviour problems.*

What to do A health visitor or doctor may refer your child to a psychiatrist or psychologist for assessment. Autism cannot be cured, but careful education, care and support can improve behaviour and develop life skills. A range of approaches is used when working with people with autism, but as the disorder is both complex and quite individual in its effects, there is no single definitive treatment. Children should be assessed and regularly reviewed at a child develop-

ment centre. By school age a child will need appropriate education and support. Some people with autism lead successful working lives, often in areas requiring a particular attention to factual detail.

Asperger syndrome Asperger syndrome is a type of autism in which children often have average or above average intelligence, but in other ways share many of the characteristics of children with classic autism. Language skills tend to be better developed and children may have a tendency to talk at people whether they are interested or not, as well as to be over precise and very literal in their understanding of language.

Children with this syndrome often have a narrow range of obsessive interests and dislike even small changes in their lives. Some children with Asperger syndrome are clumsy and find it difficult to learn skills requiring coordination, such as riding a bicycle.

Because of their intelligence and language skills, some children with Asperger syndrome may go undiagnosed for many years. Others are educated in special schools. With appropriate support and education, children can go on to lead full and fulfiling adult lives, and may be especially valued for their reliability and their dedication in a sympathetic and informed workplace.

Who can help? For organizations who can offer advice, support and help, see the Directory.

Complementary Treatment

The **Bach flower remedies** would be helpful in a supportive role when chosen to suit the personality, mood and temperament of the child. **Drama** and **play therapies** can be helpful. **Music therapy** can be particularly beneficial, as music is a dynamic language rich in emotional nuance, and requires no understanding of verbal language. The child may become more accessible, manageable and contented.

THE PRE-SCHOOL CHILD

♦

During the pre-school years children develop from infants who are dependent on others for their very survival into children who have practised at home all the skills they need to launch themselves into the world beyond the family. How do they manage it?

For their physical and psychological survival infants have one overwhelming need: the committed, loving care of an adult. They need care to survive physically, and love and commitment to survive psychologically. A child who is deprived of this relationship in the earliest years, before the age of three, is very likely to grow into an adult who cannot make relationships with other people.

An overview

Initially infants see themselves as a single unit with the mother. Only in the second half of the first year does the awareness of their separateness dawn, and for the first two or three years children's security is tied in with the constancy of their care. Learning to separate is a key experience of the pre-school years and one that many children find hard to handle. However as children approach school age, they do get better at it. They still need a replacement for the mother, and the social grouping they find easiest to cope with remains an enlarged substitute family. Many pre-school children – and quite a few school children – need a prop when they are without their habitual emotional support. The cuddly or transitional object stands for the absent caretaker, whether it takes the form of a well-sucked thumb or a silky blanket.

During the pre-school years this simple, fundamental need for a securely anchored emotional life is increasingly counterbalanced by the child's desire for independence. This powers the drive to acquire the simple but basic skills that turn a baby into a child – self-feeding, attending to daily tasks, toilet training. It takes time to learn these skills and this, together with an unbridled impulsiveness, can lead to the frustrations, moods and tantrums that can characterize two- and three-year-old children.

Emotions in very young children are extremely strong. Prey to jealousy, anger, love, fear and excitement, they have neither the words to express how they feel nor the understanding that others feel as they do. This can leave them open to quite marked fears and anxieties at an age when the demarcation between reality and fantasy is not yet clear.

Perhaps the single most important skill pre-school children acquire is language. Once their language blossoms they can use words to think. Words and stories help children give their emotions shapes and names and teach them that others have felt as they do. By the age of four, some children are using language to grapple with the larger issues of death, love and eternity in a way that is unthinkable in the pre-verbal child.

Threading through the pre-school child's career is the unfolding of their personality. Discernible from the earliest days, it is clear by the age of two whether a child is outgoing and confident or adopts a more tentative and thoughtful approach to life. While early childhood experiences can moderate differences – by boosting the child's self-esteem, for example – watching the child's unique individuality develop is one of the most exciting rewards of parenthood.

Attachment and separation

The earliest bonds infants form with people around them will serve them for life. Their early attachments – to their mother, their father and a range of other important people in their world – provide the secure basis for their emotional development. Their first experience is dependence, and from this they learn whether or not their needs will be attended to.

In the early years children may venture towards independence, but only with a backwards glance to be sure that their mother (or other attachment figure) is still there. A well-known piece of research showed how a one-year-old in a new environment would venture 7 m/23 ft from their mother and a two-year-old 15 m/50 ft. With each succeeding year the distance would grow.

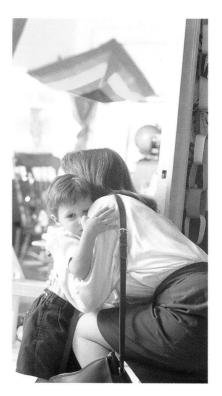

Left: Separation can be difficult for parents as well as children, but a confident and loving farewell is more helpful than wavering uncertainly. And it is usually the case that, once the mother has left, the child very soon forgets his unhappiness at separating and becomes immersed in an absorbing activity.

By the second year forces are already tugging the child in contrary directions, as the need to depend intertwines closely with the wish for independence. As demands on toddlers increase – for appropriate behaviour or even skillful performance – toddlers start to assert themselves. Excessive demands can lead to defiance, and even reasonable requirements often meet negativity and refusal. This is the age of food fads and manipulation, followed swiftly by the demand 'I want mummy'.

Inevitable separations have to be handled sensitively. Young children need to be told of them in advance, and they need to know that the parent is returning. At first their separations need to be very short – just minutes. Ideally, during separation from the parents, they should stay with a person who is one of their attachment figures, so that their experiences are reassuring.

Even so, not all children respond positively to separation. Children who are clingy may be too young to separate. After the age of three, children start to cope better with separation and there is plenty of evidence that spending time away from home in a group nursery environment helps the child's development. By the age of four most children no longer need physical proximity, although throughout childhood they continue to fear losing one of their prominent attachment figures.

At each stage of transition it will be easier for the child if they are accompanied by someone or something familiar. If they start school with a friend, they will cope better. Other factors that make separation easier are: a secure mother-child bond; an harmonious atmosphere at home; the child's growing awareness of past and future; their use of language to explain and express their emotions; and good experiences.

Complementary Treatment

Music therapy is highly recommended where separation presents particular problems, as the relationship with the therapist can re-enact the damaged or delayed process of separation from the primary carer without substituting a new dependency. **Play therapy** can also be very helpful. Recommended **Bach flower remedies** are: Chicory for the clinging child; Walnut for adjustment; and Mimulus or Rock Rose where there is fear.

Temper tantrums

Temper tantrums are usually a feature of pre-school behaviour, often triggered by frustration, tiredness or by over-excitement. Although they are extremely common, not all children develop them; personality and home circumstances are important underlying factors. The peak years are 18 months to 3 years of age.

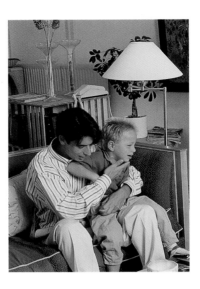

Left: A child having a temper tantrum can become very frightened, especially if the adult also loses control. Remaining calm and holding the child firmly helps him to feel secure and confident. Be sure to cuddle him as soon as his body relaxes.

The following strategies appear to be the most effective methods of coping with tantrums.

Prevention Prevent a temper tantrum in a supermarket by providing an apple for the child to eat, rather than have a fight beside the sweet display. Give your child as much loving attention as you can spare when they are behaving well.

Distraction When a temper tantrum is brewing, try to draw the child's attention to something interesting.

Ignoring the tantrum Try not to explode yourself; when your child has a temper tantrum in public, ignore any comments or disapproving looks from other people.

Time out Either leave the child somewhere safe but boring for a short while so they can calm down, or remove yourself. Between three and five minutes is usually enough. This approach is known as 'time out from positive reinforcement'. As an alternative to time out, hold the child firmly but calmly until they have calmed down.

The response to guard against is changing your reaction because of the temper tantrum. This merely teaches the child that they have only to throw a tantrum whenever they want their own way.

Note that tantrums may be more severe in a child with a hidden difficulty – such as glue ear or speech delay – that affects their ability to communicate.

Complementary Treatment

Rescue Remedy, a **Bach flower remedy**, can be useful in relieving some of the frustration and tension, but other remedies, chosen on an individual basis, may be more effective. They include Vine for very strong-willed children; Holly for tantrums that develop as a result of jealousy; Willow for the self-pitying, resentful element; and Chicory if the tantrum is used to manipulate or gain attention. **Music therapy** will have a dual function where tantrums are a response to a genuinely frustrating situation, either internal or external. It provides an alternative and creative method of expressing frustration and offers fulfiling and less frustrating activities to build confidence. Both **drama** and **play therapy** can also provide support.

Fears and phobias

Fears in children are common. All children are afraid of being abandoned by a parent or of a parent simply walking out. Young children typically fear darkness and shadows; animals and insects; monsters, witches and ghosts. Older children's fears are more obviously rooted in the challenging experiences they face at school. They may be fearful of teachers, tests and coping with their schoolwork. They also learn to fear social rejection – for example, being the last child to be picked for the team. During the teenage years fears become more similar to adult fears – of closed or open spaces and of social situations such as losing their role in their peer group or being the subject of ridicule.

Some children are born more fearful, while others learn fearful ways of behaving from their parents. Pre-school children are particularly prone to insecurities because of their lack of knowledge and experience of the world; they also have powerful imaginations, which can transform everyday events into terrifying ordeals; and they have very little control over events. The things of which they are frightened – insects, animals, darkness, abandonment – are all quite logical if one remembers that it is not long since humans lived in a far more hostile environment than they do today.

With an unclear dividing line between reality and fantasy, pre-school children are particularly prone to imaginary fears – of ogres, monsters and witches. Some psychologists believe that such creatures embody children's powerful emotions at an age when rage, jealousy or hatred is intense. The embodiment helps young children to give shape to their feelings and to imagine them as separate from themselves. In this way, they learn to cope with what would otherwise be overwhelming emotions.

What to do Some parents belittle fears, try to distract their children's attention or make allowances for them. If the child is afraid of the dark, for example, they turn on the light rather than exploring with the child gently and gradually how safe darkness is. It is important to respect a child's fear and consider how best to approach it, agreeing a planned approach in which the child stays in control. Reflective listening is helpful, opening the subject with a statement such as 'I know it seems hard to get into the water . . .'. Once children with these fears

have realized that nothing awful will happen to them when they confront their fear, it will soon fade. Another technique is to give children something they like to do – such as eating crisps or sweets – at the same time as they confront their fear, so that the child is being rewarded for confronting it and learning to associate something pleasant with a previously frightening situation. Role playing the frightening situation (with people, toys, drawing or writing) helps to desensitize the child in advance or to rework the situation afterwards. Many children do this instinctively themselves through play, repeating an experience again and again until they get used to it. For older children who can acknowledge and talk about the fear but still cannot control it, simple breathing exercises and relaxation techniques are helpful.

A phobia is a fear that is so intense that it prevents the child from doing normal things. A child who is afraid of the dark, for example, won't get out of bed in case something grabs them. A child with a phobia about darkness sleeps in full light and starts to fear even small shadows. As it is possible to prevent their fears from developing into phobias by judicious intervention, it is important that parents are sensitive to a child's developing fears.

The phobias that unfortunately do develop in children and teenagers follow certain patterns. In older children phobias about their appearance are relatively frequent and can sometimes become extreme, as can social phobias, school phobia (see page 322) and the phobias common in adults, such as agoraphobia and claustrophobia. If you are aware that your child's fears are becoming more intense, your doctor can refer the child to a child or adolescent psychiatrist or a clinical psychologist.

Complementary Treatment

Music therapy can be an effective alternative or possible adjunct to verbal forms of psychotherapy where phobias result from traumatic stress disorder or other forms of anxiety. A child may be supported in the exploration and resolution of the anxiety in musical terms, with or without words. **Drama** and **play therapy** may also help in this way. The **Bach flower remedies** offer Aspen for fear of the unknown, Rock Rose for terror and terrifying dreams, and Rescue Remedy for combined elements of panic, fear and shock.

Comfort habits

Children's comfort habits often leave parents feeling guilty. Are they a sign of insecurity or of unmet emotional need? Should parents wait until the child grows out of the habit – even if that seems to take forever – or should they help the child to move on by intervening in their dependence on the comfort object or habit? And will one bad habit just be replaced by another?

While it is not clear why some children develop comfort habits when others do not, it is reassuring to know that, within reason, comfort habits seem helpful to children, acting as an emotional crutch at times of transition. There are thought to be only three times when they are not advantageous psychologically: when a normal, moderate dependency becomes acute; when the child persistently turns to the comforter while rejecting the mother; and when an older child suddenly takes up a comfort habit.

Comfort blankets These are the pieces of cloth that usually originate in the cot, and on which young children become passionately fixated. They are a middle-class phenomenon, and the association for the child is with a comforting permanence while the mother is not there. Over the years they become unrecognizable scraps or rags, or the attachment is transferred to another object, so that silk ties, large underwear labels, powder puffs and cuddly toys become the child's constant companion. Although children are most dependent on their cuddlies between the ages of two and three, especially at times of stress or change (such as bedtime or starting nursery school) the passion can last until the teenage years.

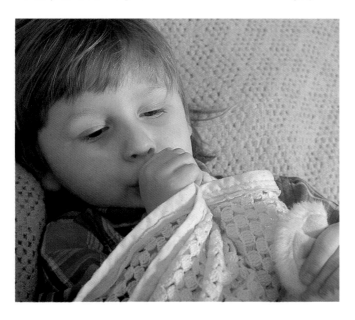

Above: There is a surprising consistency in the comforters that children take to bed with them. Blankets and soft toys are the universal favourites of many, including this girl. Dummies, rags, sheets, clothing and fluff that has been fiddled from clothes are all popular. Parents should be reassured that the comforter is a useful emotional tool; they therefore should not discourage their child from making use of them.

Boys of 11 have been found with terry nappies under their pillows, and toy shops do a steady trade in soft toys to university students. Eventually the scorn of their peers usually puts a stop to the dependence, but meanwhile research shows that children who have had a transitional cuddly in their pre-school years are better adjusted and more sociable later.

Sucking habits: thumbs, fingers, bottles, dummies
Even in the uterus, foetuses show a difference in their wish to suck. Later, some suck hard and strong while others are happy to be spoon-fed. Such differences may be innate.

Individual differences apart, virtually all babies need to suck for sustenance in the first six months and many need extra comfort in the early weeks. Sucking objects, like cuddlies, stand in for an absent mother, and it is easy to encourage the habit in babies. Some children give the habit up without difficulty; others need persuasion. Research suggests that a persistent sucking habit may not be quite as supportive as a persistent cuddly. Four-year-olds who were still regularly sucking thumbs or fingers were found in one study to be more awkward and moody as teenagers. However, reassuringly and perhaps surprisingly, they were not any more likely to have started smoking.

Holding something like a dummy in the mouth for years rather than months is thought by some psychoanalysts to hold children in the infantile oral phase of development and to discourage the development of speech. For example, as a dummy fills the front of the mouth, it is impossible for children to make the sounds *t* or *d* properly. Beyond this, some dentists believe that dummy-sucking children are more prone to tooth decay because at night the saliva, which normally acts as a mouthwash, dries out if the child's mouth is open, allowing plaque to build up more quickly. As persistent and strong sucking really does pull teeth out of alignment there is every good reason to encourage a child of seven or eight to stop thumb or finger sucking.

For thumb and finger sucking, the most successful strategies involve motivating the child (telling them they will look more grown up); choosing a good time, such as school holidays; and providing a big reward and a 30-day star chart with smaller rewards at the end of each week's unbroken nonsucking. To encourage a child to give up a dummy, keep it for sleeping only and pay special attention when the child is talking, because they will not be able to talk properly with a dummy in their mouth.

Nail-biting There is reassurance for parents of nail-biters: there is no evidence that children who bite their nails are more poorly adjusted than others, although it is true that children do bite their nails under stress. It is an extremely com-

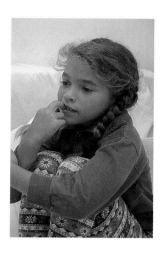

Right: Nail biting may very well be a sign of stress, but it does not indicate any deep-seated emotional or psychological problem. There is a genetic component to the habit, with identical twins more likely to bite their nails than non-identical twins.

mon childhood habit affecting one school-age child in three. The tendency is probably inherited and children often stop and later relapse.

Masturbation Very many pre-school children discover the pleasure that touching their genitals bestows. In one study, researchers found that over half the pre-school boys and one in six girls masturbated. However at this age there is no sexual connotation. For many children the activity is no more than a reassuring habit at a time of stress. Others discover the pleasures of rhythmic stimulation – even babies have been known to rub against cot bars so frantically that they appear to be having a fit. Tell a child who is old enough to understand that this is an activity to keep private. Otherwise turn a blind eye.

Head banging Rhythmic head banging frightens parents, who fear either that their child is disturbed or that the banging will eventually lead to brain damage. In a normal child with no other diagnosed difficulties, neither is the case – the

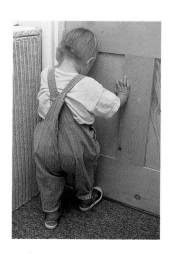

Right: Children who headbang towards the end of the day may be acting to release a build-up of tension. Spending time quietly with the child before they are over-tired may successfully avert a storm or frenzied behaviour.

child is usually having a massive tantrum or is bored. If the head banging is part of a tantrum the child may hurt themself and never try again, or they may continue to get whatever they want as a result of a tantrum (see Temper tantrums, page 314). Ignore it.

Sleep

Infants and children need anything from ten to sixteen hours sleep. The amount of sleep they need drops as they grow older, until by puberty they reach adult levels. At first infants sleep in snatches varying from a few minutes to five hours, regardless of day or night. By the age of three months they have often developed a pattern of a longer sleep at night as well as having three or four periods of sleep during the day. By six months of age babies no longer need to have a night feed, and with luck and encouragement they may even sleep through an abbreviated night. At this stage parents choose between late nights and early mornings – but some unlucky ones get both.

How well young children sleep is culture-dependent. Recent research from Pennsylvania State University established that Kenyan babies who are expected to wake several times a night do, while babies in Los Angeles do what their parents expect and sleep through the night from the time they are a few months old.

Average sleep requirements
Note that there are enormous individual variations.

Age	Number of night hours spent sleeping	Total number of hours in 24 spent sleeping
6 months	10-12	14½
1 year	11	14
2 years	11	13
3 years	11	12
4 years	11½	11½
5 years	11	11

Night waking Parents do not need to be told that problems in settling the child down to sleep and night waking are the commonest sleep difficulties. Night waking is strongly conditioned by what parents do in response. There are three basic strategies: checking that the baby is all right but disturbing them as little as possible, and repeating this as often as it takes until the baby settles; lifting the baby out of the cot and doing what the baby appears to want – feeding, nappy change, cuddle – before putting them back down; and taking the baby into the parental bed (see The family bed, page 275).

A good night's sleep

The following tips can help to get your child to sleep through the night.

- From the earliest days, feed the baby, then lay them in the cot to sleep while they are still awake. Try not to allow your baby to fall asleep while feeding
- Create a suitable sleep environment and set up a daily bedtime routine, such as tea or a feed followed by some quiet play, a bath, story, drink and, finally, bed
- For a period of two weeks write down when the child sleeps, what wakes them and what their response is. This will make you more aware of what is really going on
- Use behavioural methods to train a child who is mature enough to sleep through the night to do so. When the child wakes one of the parents goes in, checks the child is all right and then leaves. If the child continues to cry or comes out of their room, they are taken back and the parent checks that they are all right every five minutes. The intervals may extend to 10 or 15 minutes until the child finally goes off to sleep
- A doctor may prescribe a sedative such as promethazine (Phenergan) or trimeprazine (Vallergan) that is suitable for children and encourages them to sleep for a few nights to give parents a rest

Night terrors Night terrors occur during deep sleep and most often affect young primary school children. The child behaves as if they are really terrified, screaming, shouting, sweating and even running away from the imagined danger. They remain asleep throughout the experience, which usually lasts between 10 and 30 minutes. During the terror the child cannot be woken, and in the morning remembers nothing about it.

Night terrors are quite unconnected with emotional problems. If they recur at a predictable time, as they often do (usually in the first three hours after falling asleep) try waking the child 15 minutes beforehand. Alternatively, wake the child

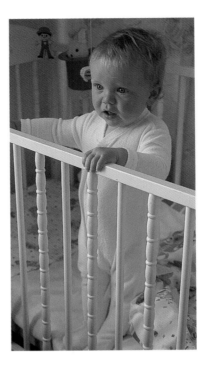

Left: All babies wake at least occasionally at night, but their persistence in staying awake varies. For some families the only workable solution is the family bed.

when they appear restless. If the terrors arrive at unpredictable times, stay with the child as the night terror occurs. Switch on a light or turn on a favourite tape. It is best if the child remains in bed, but if they get out do not stop them. Night terrors usually fade quite quickly.

Sleepwalking Sleepwalking often happens during the first hours of deep sleep. A sleepwalking child has their eyes open but is clearly asleep and can walk around the house, up and down stairs, opening and closing doors. Many sleepwalking children take themselves back to bed. If they do not, lead a sleepwalking child gently back to bed and stay quietly with them until they fall asleep again. They probably won't acknowledge you or wake. For the future, secure the bedroom windows and the stairs. Sleepwalking is most common between the ages of five and ten years, and children eventually grow out of it. It does not indicate emotional disturbance, although your child may start to sleepwalk during a particularly anxious time.

Nightmares Nightmares are very common, particularly in pre-school children. They usually occur during light dream sleep. When the child wakes up, or if you decide to wake them, remain with them and let them talk if they wish.

Nightmares can be triggered by experiences that are frightening to a child, if not to an adult. One three-year-old had nightmares when his baby sister developed an eye condition in which her eyes moved uncontrollably.

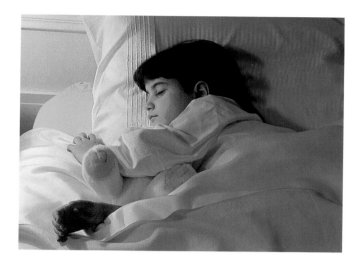

Above: A child who has enjoyed a full and active day, followed by a quiet, familiar bedtime routine, may well reward her parents with an unbroken night's sleep – for herself and them. Making the bedroom as comfortable and welcoming as possible may well persuade the child to remain there, rather than get up to enjoy the company of her parents.

Other children may react to frightening videos and films, so it is wise not to allow young children to watch videos or television programmes that stimulate the imagination an hour or two before bedtime. Soothe the child in their own room so that they learn to associate their bedroom with stillness and calmness. The nightmares will reduce in intensity as the child's anxiety levels fall, but in some vulnerable children they will linger well into adulthood.

Complementary Treatment

Music therapy can be an effective alternative or possibly an adjunct to verbal forms of psychotherapy where nightmares and night terrors result from traumatic stress disorder or other forms of anxiety. A child may be supported in the exploration and resolution of the anxiety in musical terms, with or without the use of words. **Drama** and **play therapy** may also help in this way. The **Bach flower remedies** offer Aspen for fear of the unknown, Rock Rose for terror and terrifying dreams, and Rescue Remedy for combined elements of panic, fear and shock.

Jealousy and sibling rivalry

For many young children the three most stressful life events are separating from their mother, starting full-time education and the birth of a brother or sister. Given that a young child views their relationship with their mother as similar to that of a married couple, the arrival of a baby might be seen as tantamount to an extra-marital affair, in which the girl or boy friend is brought into a ménage à trois. From this inauspicious beginning a loving sibling relationship is expected to develop. Parents should not be surprised when it does not, but instead leads to intense jealousy and rivalry for parental affection that can thread through childhood into adult life.

Certain children are especially vulnerable to jealousy. They include: children with low self-esteem and lack of confidence; children with intense emotions; the eldest child; and children who feel under threat from more than one direction – for example, if the arrival of the new baby coincides with a time when they are having particular difficulties with their own friendships.

What to do It is sensible to anticipate these events and let a young child, particularly an only child, down gently. Children need to know about the birth in advance, although telling a child under five around the sixth or seventh month is enough for their needs. Involving your child in preparations may help to stop them feeling excluded. Throughout the preparations you need to take the child's level of understanding into account. A very young child who is told that they are going to have a brother or sister to play with can only be bitterly disappointed at the outcome of childbirth. Using their own baby book, or photographs spanning their own babyhood to the present, will help the child to realize that the baby will eventually become a playmate.

It is also important to protect children from other major sources of stress. This is not the time to move the child from a cot to a bed, to enrol the child in a playgroup, to start potty-training, to have the child admitted to hospital for any procedure that could be delayed, to spend nights away from home, nor to start school.

Once the baby is born you should continue your daily routines as normally as possible, respecting the older child's individual needs rather than projecting on to them a new role as the older brother or sister of the new baby. It is one thing to be a big boy or girl; quite another to be a big brother or sister. Big boys and girls do, however, sometimes require compensatory privileges, such as a later bedtime or special outings. It is also sensible, if for no better reason than self-preservation, to avoid blatantly provocative actions, such as breastfeeding the new baby in front of your older child in the first few weeks until the child has had time to get used to the idea.

Preparation will not sanitize a young child's feelings; it will just soften the blow, as will developing the child's relationship with the father. Your child's feelings of jealousy will almost inevitably come out: early reactions may include aggressive or clingy behaviour, desperately seeking attention or regressing to infantile behaviour. Behind all these is a fear of exclusion, so being angry only increases the child's insecurities. Research shows that jealousy tends to persist where parents punish children for behaving meanly or aggressively.

What else? Encouraging the child to talk about their feelings helps – even children as young as three can be helped to find words to express what they feel. Tell them how jealous you used to feel as a child. Read children's books that reflect their experiences.

Set aside a special time every day for each child in the family. Fifteen minutes when the child knows that no one will interrupt may be all that is needed. Protecting the child's possessions and space matter as well.

A natural emotion Despite all parents' endeavours, a certain level of jealousy and rivalry will persist. It is natural, and part of growing up. Troubled teenagers can feel as threatened as toddlers and may be barely more articulate. In one study, one-third of five- and six-year-olds said they would prefer not to have a brother or sister.

Two-thirds fought or came to blows regularly. Jealousy may produce superficial discord, but psychologists tend to view it as helpful, as quarrels that are played out in the safety of the family home are rehearsals for coping with rivalries in the outside world. Jealousy only becomes harmful if it reflects a situation where one child is always more successful, competent or preferred to another.

Complementary Treatment
Interactive **music therapy** offers the enriching experience of being noticed, valued and competent, as well as addressing any anxiety, and can help to compensate for any actual emotional impoverishment in the child's past or present experience. The **Bach flower remedies** Holly is useful for jealousy and hatred, and Chicory for the desire for attention. **Drama** and **play therapies** may also be particularly beneficial.

Dealing with a jealous child
- Parents need to be even-handed with their children, but this does not mean giving them all the same thing, the same privileges or responsibilities. Some children need more cuddles, others need more challenges. Children understand if privileges and responsibilities are consistently applied and can be justified
- Particularly avoid comparing the jealous child with other (less jealous) children. Nothing is better calculated to increase the jealous child's sense of insecurity than believing that their parents think they are inferior
- Above all, avoid direct comparisons between children. It is tempting to try to get one child to behave better or do better at school by pointing out how well the other child does, but these comparisons usually misfire. In any case, children know perfectly well how good their brothers and sisters are, and this may be the cause of their disaffection. It is better to use the one child's superior abilities to bring on the other child, so, for example, the child who dances beautifully can teach the less able child the steps
- Notice and praise the times when the children cooperate. It is terribly easy not to notice when they are getting on well, but praise in the end works better than being told off when children area at odds with each other

THE SCHOOL YEARS

◆

The early years in school mark a gradual transition from the secure protection of the family to the more challenging world outside. At the same time, those basic infant skills that were built on in the pre-school years are fine-tuned and differentiated. Latent aptitudes, parental encouragement and dogged perseverance contribute to the widening skills and differences in ability that develop between children in their early primary school years.

The early school years: four to seven From a social point of view, classes in the early years of education are organized so that children can identify the teacher as a safe parent-substitute, which helps those children who are still experiencing difficulties separating from their mother. (How many young schoolchildren have inadvertently called the teacher 'Mummy'?) At the same time children now have to cope for the first time with being one of a very large group of children.

Parent participation in the school can be very helpful in breaking down large groups into more manageable units, and in easing the child's transition from home to school. It can also help children with another new task that faces them: integrating what may be two quite different worlds – school and home – with possibly different languages, accents, expectations, attitudes and beliefs. In this atmosphere of change, children like to know what is expected of them. They like clear rules, which make them feel safe.

Coping with new situations As children settle at school, academic demands increase, and at this age subtle or specific learning difficulties begin to become evident. Success and failure loom large in the child's life, and it is important for parents to maintain a balance. If a child is experiencing unavoidable difficulties at school as they try to grapple with new concepts, parents need to provide compensation. Can the child swim? Are they good with animals? Can they join a football course?

A few children react to increasing pressures, or stress at home, by exhibiting a reluctance to attend school. At this age reluctance is not entrenched, and if you can spend time listening to whatever is worrying your child, it can usually be managed. You may need to liaise with the school to make sure your child still attends (see School phobia, page 322).

The friends of pre-school children are still in part chosen by their parents, but once at school children start to forge their own friendships. Most children have at least one best friend at this age, but friendships can be fickle and sometimes change almost daily. It is unusual for a child between four and seven years of age to be unsociable, so the child who appears to spend all their school playtimes alone may need sensitive observation by school staff. Solitary pursuits with pets, on the computer or watching television can compensate, but do not help the child to practise their social skills.

As they mature children learn to stand up for their own point of view. This can lead to quarrels with friends and siblings and parents have to decide whether to intervene. It is usually better to allow equally matched children to sort their quarrels out themselves, but watch for rough fighting or any actions that could hurt a younger or weaker child.

Four- to seven-year-old children are still avidly curious, asking endless questions and unable at first to cope with the notion that the parent or teacher does not know all the answers. As their widening vocabulary enables them to think in an abstract way, their still unfettered curiosity prompts deep abstract questions about death and eternity. This is the age when you should encourage your children to search for knowledge themselves and give them the means to find it.

By the age of seven children can be amazingly competent. They can usually cook simple meals, play an instrument and look after the needs of a younger brother or sister for hours on end. However their competence depends on opportunity. Parents in a position to offer their seven-year-olds a chance to pursue their interests do them a service. Many activities will be dropped later, but the skills remain, as does the self esteem that comes with their acquisition.

The middle school years: eight to ten The years of increasing independence are now beginning. For many children this is symbolized by having pocket money, sometimes earned, which they have the freedom to spend according to their own judgement. The judgement of children at this age is quite refined; they know the rules of the activities that fill their lives and they can believe fervently in right and wrong. At this age it is not unusual for a passion for good causes to emerge. Children of this age like rules and following them may underpin favourite activities, such as playing board games and joining in team games.

By the age of eight years many children have the perseverance to learn and practise a musical instrument, and while they will not, on the whole, become professional or even talented musicians, they acquire self confidence by having a skill that they realize other children do not necessarily possess.

The more stable friendships often become extremely important at this age, and clubs assume a new role. Many children organize their own, partly to formalize their own alliances but also partly to exclude other children – even if it is only a tiresome three-year-old sister. Children of this age also like to join organized activities and to wear uniforms and badges as marks of achievement.

By the middle school years most children have the confidence to stay away from home overnight, in a group such as Brownies or Woodcraft, or with a special friend. Children's friendships develop quite independently of family intervention, but home is still vitally important for support and continuity. The more home remains the same as ever, the better.

At this age some children appear to be quite independent and secure, although in fact they are not. They need back-up when things go wrong – when they forget their pencil case for school or on those days that they come home feeling completely friendless.

Once children reach the age of ten they have acquired an impressive range of abilities that can help to support their independence. Many can cycle safely on a road, others can be allowed to undertake short, familiar journeys – to school and back, for example – alone. With supervision they can try out dangerous activities, such as abseiling and canoeing, on adventure holidays organized in the school holidays or during term-time. Their physical skills are now advanced and quite complex; if you watch any team game organized within a primary school you can see children's acute awareness of justice and fairness.

By now children are aware that home and school may have very different rules. As children become increasingly conscious of differences between themselves and other children, they may use them to create stereotyped images. At best, and with a little prompting from adults, children will learn to celebrate differences. At worst, they use them as a means to single out victims for bullying (see page 323).

Puberty By the age of 11 many girls have entered puberty, while the majority of boys have not. Girls may be growing taller, leaving boys of the same age behind. As breasts begin to develop, periods start and, eventually, hips widen, girls are more likely to be upset by body changes than are boys. Research suggests that on the whole boys experience fewer problems at the onset of puberty.

By the time these changes begin children are quite independent within the family. They are able to look after themselves and to choose and regulate their own friendships. They can play a part in the running of the home, and in many families are expected to shoulder quite considerable responsibilities. Yet they are not old enough to be completely independent. Eleven-year-olds can still be immature; they are only just old enough to coordinate the many skills required to reliably cross a road safely. They have not had enough experience of life to know the right thing to do at all times. Therefore they still need a firm, consistent and supportive home.

Such a home is particularly important, as at the age of 11 most children begin secondary school, with the less family-

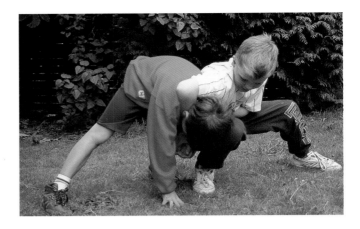

Above: Children frequently fight – physically or verbally – to sort out arguments and problems. Before intervening, adults should observe and decide whether the children are in fact play-fighting and have no intention of hurting each other, or are engaged in a real fight.

centred and more challenging environment that accompanies it. School children of this age need to be able to organize themselves and to cope with the stresses and extra work that are imposed on them by matters such as regular exams and homework.

Friendships may now take the form of gangs. Many friends of this age have known each for years, and the groupings no longer change as much as they did in the past. At this age children sometimes make friends for life.

Members of certain groups can be extremely unkind to outsiders, to newcomers, people they wish to exclude and members of other groups. Boys in particular can be competitive and argumentative and resort to physical fighting to sort out their differences.

School fear or phobia At some point during their school years many children decide that they do not want to go to school. They may claim to be ill or may appear unhappy and afraid. They may simply refuse to go or, if dragged to school, try to run away or hide. This is school refusal and, when it is taken to extremes, it can become school phobia.

There are two chief triggers for school refusal, circumstances at home and circumstances at school. Children sometimes fear leaving home for school if they feel unsure what to expect when they return; if past separations have been stressful or upsetting; if they are very dependent on protective parents; or if a parent is depressed.

Children who are afraid of going to school may be being teased or bullied; they may have specific difficulties with work, playtimes, other children, friends, physical activities, school dinners or even the toilets.

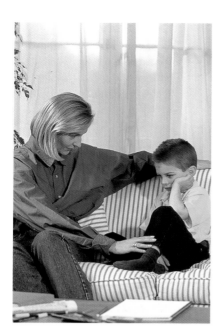

Right: Studies show that a disinclination to go to school is more common in boys, especially if they feel that they are failing there. With patience and persistence the reason behind the reluctance usually becomes clear.

What to do It is worth trying to get the child to continue attending school so that any fears are not magnified. You may have to talk to someone at the school so that you can work out a combined strategy. Forcing a child to attend instead of examining the underlying issues will simply make matters much worse.

Helpful strategies include keeping the atmosphere at home secure and calm; maintaining a regular morning routine; arranging for someone at the school to welcome the child and, if necessary, take the child into the building. Make an arrangement with the school to have someone contact you if the child turns out to be genuinely unwell (which is always a possibility). Going to school with another child can also be helpful, as it avoids the need for the fearful child to arrive alone at school. Alternatively, you could ask another parent, neighbour or educational social worker to accompany the child. The child who does go to school should receive a positive reward.

Solving the underlying difficulty usually means spending time discovering why the child is frightened. The class teacher or the assistants who supervise lunchtime play may have some ideas. Listening to the child and believing what they say is important.

If your child refuses to go to school you will need to liaise with the education social work service. A gradual approach involving activities for you and your child, such as meeting children from school at home, helps to expose the child to the experience of school without increasing their anxieties by actually going there. Other school children can be told that the child who is refusing to go to school has been ill, in order to spare the child embarrassment when they return. You will almost certainly need some support from an outside agency such as a child and family consultation unit.

  ## Complementary Treatment
In **drama** and **play therapy**, specific phobias might be successfully dramatized or played out and then gradually resolved. Useful **Bach flower remedies** include Mimulus for known fears, and Aspen where the child is frightened of something, but does not know what. Red Chestnut is useful where the child is anxious for the safety or health of others, such as their parents, siblings or pets.

Bullying

Bullying is aggressive behaviour consistently and deliberately directed towards another child. It can start in the early years at primary school but is more likely to start in the final years, in children aged between nine and eleven. Common types of bullying include: name calling and teasing; threats to injure the child; threats to exclude the child from a group of friends; hitting, hair-pulling and scratching, kicking and throwing things; stealing; demanding money or (with younger children) toys; and racial or sexual harassment.

The bullied child tends to be physically weaker than others their own age and is different from other children in an obvious way. For example, they may be overweight, have the wrong accent or a different skin colour. They tend to be sensitive, intelligent children who have little experience of conflict at home and are unprepared to deal with it at school, and they experience bullying as confirmation of their inadequacies.

Signs of bullying may include any of the factors in the list below.

You may notice

♦ *An unwillingness to go to the playground or take a certain route home for fear of meeting the bully*
♦ *Your child makes excuses to avoid attending school*
♦ *Their possessions, clothes or books are damaged. Victims may be scratched or bruised themselves*
♦ *The child loses confidence and becomes withdrawn, or they become aggressive, anxious or distressed*
♦ *The child cries easily and has nightmares*
♦ *The child begins to bully other children*

What to do Bullying is never acceptable. Addressing it requires an atmosphere of openness and trust between adults and children, which enables children to feel free to tell adults about it and to know that their worries will be dealt with discreetly but effectively. Victims usually feel ashamed and unwilling to admit to being bullied, so the enquiring adult needs to be clear and direct, making a statement such as 'I think you are being bullied and I am worried about it. Let's talk about it.'

First, believe what the child says, and if the bullying is taking place at school talk to a teacher or head teacher. All schools should have a written policy on bullying that parents can read and of which children are aware. Some schools operate a system of counsellors – adults or older children to whom younger children may turn with their worries.

Second, work out ways you can protect your child. You can meet them discreetly on the way home from school; if the bullies have been identified at school, they can be kept in until other children have arrived home. Parents can help by making the home more secure, warm and friendly during a spell of bullying.

Victims can sometimes be helped by being encouraged to act self-confidently so they do not invite trouble. KIDSCAPE (the UK children's charity dealing with bullying) suggests that they can practise assertiveness techniques – saying 'No' or 'Leave me alone'. They can be encouraged to stay in a group, to avoid places where bullying often occurs and to ignore the bullying or defuse it with humour.

Bullies can sometimes be helped if they are encouraged to excel at something. The younger the child is when the problem is addressed, the more likely they are to improve.

What makes a bully?
KIDSCAPE has found that bullies often share the following characteristics.
- They often feel inadequate
- They are bullied at home within the family
- They come from families that accept or even praise bullying types of behaviour
- They are victims of some types of abuse
- They are unable or not allowed to show their feelings and have low-self esteem
- Some bullies are self-confident and spoilt children who are prepared to bully to get their own way

Who can help? For organizations and agencies offering help, advise and support, see the Directory.

Complementary Treatment
Drama and **play therapies** may help the child face up to their antagonist. The **Bach flower remedy** Mimulus is useful for victims who are shy and nervous, Centaury for a child unable to stand up for themself; and Larch for the child who lacks confidence. Holly is useful for a child who bullies because they are envious, and Vine for a child who bullies because they are full of hate. Children who bully may also benefit from **music therapy**.

Handedness
Handedness is a clear preference for using one hand rather than the other for skills needing fine coordination, such as writing or using scissors. It is related to the division of the brain into two hemispheres, each of which controls sensation and movement on the opposite side of the body. A preference for one hand or the other may be obvious when an infant is 15 months old, and is usually clear by the age of two. However children up to the age of 12 who suffer damage to the dominant side of the brain can change their preference for which hand they use.

Almost nine children out of ten are right-handed, while the rest are left-handed or ambidextrous. Left-handedness is more common among boys, twins, and babies born before 32 weeks of pregnancy. Of children with a clear hand preference, some are very strongly left- or right-handed, while others are

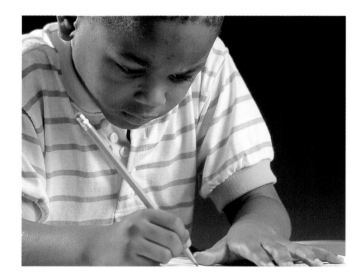

Above: Handedness only becomes obvious when a child is faced with a manually demanding task, such as writing or drawing. For simple actions such as pointing, either hand may be used, while more difficult tasks such as writing demand that the child uses his more skillful hand, whether it is his left or his right.

more confident about using either hand. The preferred hand is often linked with the preferred foot – the one that kicks the ball or presses the pedal first – but not necessarily with the preferred eye. Around one-third of left-handed children have a left dominant eye, and this is usually associated with a preference for the left ear for listening.

The left side of the brain usually relates to language ability and logic and the right side to emotions and spatial awareness. However attempts to infer from this that right-handed children are more logical or have better language abilities, while left-handed children are better at appreciating and understanding art and architecture, are disproved by reality. In 70% of left-handed people, the speech centre is on the right side of the brain.

What to do Handedness has the following main effects. Children who are very strongly right- or left-handed have difficulty acquiring skills that need two hands, such as playing the piano, or catching, but not throwing, a ball. Left-handed children need to cut with left-handed scissors or to be taught by someone who is also left-handed how to use right-handed scissors. They also need to be taught the most efficient way to cut food with a knife and how to position their hand and paper when learning to write.

Complementary Treatment
In rare cases where there has been damage to the dominant hand, **music therapy** might provide motivation for free and specific exercises to develop skills in the unaffected hand. Musical activities might also be useful in the early identification of handedness.

Depression
In children depression usually occurs as a reaction to severe emotional stress, and frequently takes the form of pure misery, rather than the more complex set of symptoms exhibited by adults. Depression is particularly common in adolescents, in whom it combines with feelings of self depreciation, creating inner turmoil. Sadness is of course part of everyday life and learning to cope with it is part of growing up. However sadness that cannot be overcome or which interferes with the child's normal activities could be a warning sign of depression.

The following are among the common reasons for children and adolescents to feel depressed: the loss of a special person, a parent or a pet; bullying at school or elsewhere; changing school or moving house; living with a parent who is depressed; family tensions, such as rows, a new baby, divorce or joining a step family; academic or social problems at school; and physical, sexual or emotional abuse.

You may notice
In very young children:
♦ *Being unresponsive and finding it hard to settle*
♦ *Tearful, clinging behaviour*
♦ *Nightmares and waking at night*
♦ *Appetite loss*
♦ *Very demanding behaviour or temper tantrums*
All these signs are common in perfectly well adjusted children. The difference to watch for is a change in the child's behaviour. The length of time the symptoms last is also important.
In school-age children:
♦ *Difficulty concentrating, possibly school refusal, irritability or hard-to-handle behaviour*
♦ *Lack of confidence*
♦ *Negative or destructive behaviour, for example stealing or playing truant*
In teenagers:
In teenagers who are often moody, the difference between feeling depressed and teenage moodiness is important. Distress and feeling depressed are common in teenagers, and these are possible signs:
♦ *Extreme moodiness and irritability*
♦ *Social withdrawal. Losing interest in school and in outside activities; losing touch with friends*
♦ *Not looking after themselves; a change in eating pattern*
♦ *Low self esteem*
♦ *Sleeping too much or not sleeping soundly*
Teenagers may act out their feelings by living dangerously, taking drugs or drinking too much. They may contemplate suicide and, if they are very depressed, they may attempt it or try to harm themselves.

What to do If the feelings of depression do not lift in a couple of weeks, speak to your doctor, or encourage your child to do so. The doctor can discuss treatment options and possible referral to a child and adolescent mental health service. Counselling for child and family can be helpful. Many psychiatrists prefer to reserve antidepressants for severely depressed children.

Who can help? Children who are depressed need to talk to someone about their unhappiness. If they cannot talk to a person they know they may be able to use a confidential telephone helpline. See the Directory for details.

Complementary Treatment
Music therapy may alleviate some of the distress of acute depression.

Stealing

Stealing is extremely common in young children, partly because they do not have the rigid rules about property that adults do. Very young pre-school children do not have fully developed ideas of possession, particularly when it comes to shared property such as nursery crayons and toys. When they are found in a child's pockets at home they should just be returned openly to the nursery with an explanation that it was a mistake. This will also be a good opportunity to explain to the child very clearly, but not in a punitive manner, the rules about not taking other people's property home.

Later in childhood more serious types of stealing may develop. Comfort stealing affects children who do not feel sufficiently loved. They may steal from their parents or from outside the home, taking comfort in possessions or in the particular objects of which they feel they have been deprived. This may be the motive behind stealing at home, rather than outside. This type of stealing is sometimes also seen in children whose parent has died, and who are trying to adjust to a new step family.

Older children may steal in groups, partly as a dare and partly to gain status among their peers and guarantee themselves a place in the gang. Such children are frequently boys and tend to come from families without a consistently enforced code of moral conduct.

What to do If you find your child has taken something by mistake or stolen it, say quite simply but clearly that it must go back.

Give your child pocket money so that they learn to value and manage resources. Point out how bad they would feel if someone stole from them.

Set a good example. Adults rarely steal, but they often keep things they find or keep the wrong change at the supermarket. Give it back and explain your reasons to your child.

Complementary Treatment

 If psychological investigation suggests an emotional cause (in addition to any faulty socialization) **music therapy** might be one element in a programme of correction. **Bach flower remedies** may be helpful in dealing with any underlying emotional issues. Both **play** and **drama therapy** may also be beneficial.

Lying To suggest that a child who is too young to distinguish fantasy from reality is capable of lying is not reasonable. To lie, a child needs to intend to deceive, and this is not something that children under the age of three or four can do. The two perfectly normal and largely universal types of lie that come later are boastful lies and lies to get out of trouble.

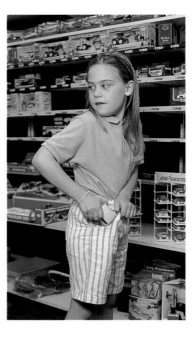

Left: A child who steals when she self-evidently knows it is wrong may be acting as part of the gang, or may have been put up to it by an older child or a teenager. Alternatively, she may steal as a form of compensation for love she feels she is not getting – a type of behaviour known as comfort stealing.

Boastful lies are lies to the outside world that make a child's life, home or background seem more interesting than it really is. Later on in childhood, children of demanding parents develop a variant of the boastful lie in recounting their school exploits. As virtually all children tell these lies, it is inappropriate to suggest that they stem from low self-esteem. However they are best countered by stressing what the child is good at and has to be proud of.

Lies to get out of trouble and avoid punishment are by no means the exclusive province of children. Virtually all adults are also capable of abandoning their moral principles if the punishment seems too threatening. Parents who punish severely tend to reinforce lying, particularly if they punish a child who is found out. This will usually lead to the child becoming a more skillful liar. Parents should always stress the importance of trust and respond warmly when a child confesses to having lied.

Complementary Treatment

 If psychological investigation suggests an emotional cause (in addition to any faulty socialization) **music therapy** might be one element in a programme of correction. **Bach flower remedies** may be helpful in dealing with any underlying emotional issues. **Play therapy** may also be beneficial.

Stress

Stress is a fact of modern life, and although it can be harmful it is not always bad. A certain amount of stress helps to prime both children and adults for challenges. It only becomes a problem when it is excessive, clouding a child's entire life or making them focus on a single activity, such as taking exams.

Children respond to the same stressful pressures as adults, and in much the same ways. Family rows, starting school, the death of a loved relation or friend, not doing well at school, and rejection are all stressful. So are events that might seem on the surface to be pleasant, such as joining a club or going on holiday. Personality, age and experience all play a role in determining what is experienced as a stressful situation, so that a situation that can seem crushing to one child may be insignificant to another.

Studies show that children subjected to a string of stressful events are more likely to catch minor infections and may also be more accident-prone. However other studies have shown that children who cope with minor stressful experiences are strengthened by the experience and better able to manage major stressful experiences.

What can parents do to get the stress level just right and help a child feel that they can cope?

What to do Avoid stressful situations when the child is young, such as leaving your child alone in an unfamiliar environment, and try to avoid more than one stressful experience occurring at the same time. Parents who arrange for a separation or divorce just before a major exam are certain to create unnecessary problems for their children.

Anticipating events and discussing with your child the feelings they may cause will help, and so will devising problem-solving approaches. For example, if the child feels homesick while they are staying with their best friend, discuss what they can do to alleviate the stress. The options will most likely be to telephone home regularly, to tell the friend's parents, or to come home. Knowing the options and finding different ways to manage the new experience will help your child take control of the situation.

Listening to your child and reflecting on what they tell you will help the child cope with a stressful situation after it has taken place. Comments such as 'You must have felt awful when . . .' are a useful technique. So is acting out stressful situations at home in order to investigate different approaches to the problem.

Encouraging the child with gentle praise when they have coped well offers the child an extra reward in addition to the flush of pride they will feel knowing that they have managed. And it is just as important to ignore situations in which your child fails to cope.

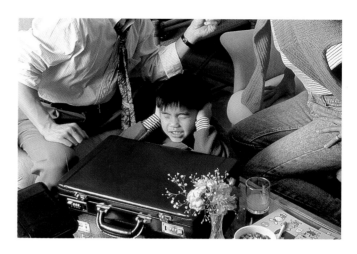

Above: Family rows, particularly those between parents that occur in front of the children, can be extremely stressful for the child. Stress that is experienced over a long period can have adverse effects not only on the child's emotional health, but also on their physical well being, causing minor infections and even making the child accident prone.

 Complementary Treatment
Relaxation techniques can be very helpful in dealing with stress, as can massage allied with **aromatherapy**. **Drama** and **play therapies** can also help to relieve the condition.

Common causes of stress in children
- Starting school full-time
- Changing schools – especially from primary to secondary school – and having to make new friends, especially if the child has to integrate into an existing friendship group
- Preparing for school tests and exams
- Family rows
- Divorce or separation
- Parents arguing about money, employment and, for young children, politics
- Parents needing reassurance from the child, rather than the other way round
- Death

If you are aware from your child's difficult behaviour that they are under stress but can't pinpoint the cause, keep a two-week diary, noting your child's behaviour as well as potentially stressful events. A pattern may emerge.

CROUP

Infection that narrows the airways, causing characteristic noises.

CAUSES

Many viruses can invade the upper respiratory tract and make the lining of the larynx and trachea swell, hence the medical term for croup – laryngo-tracheo-bronchitis. This swelling obstructs the smooth flow of air and leads to the croup sound when breathing out and stridor, which is noise on breathing in. Infection often spreads further down into the lungs. Croup mainly affects children between one and three years of age.

SYMPTOMS

Starting as a **fever**, cold and cough, croup worsens into hoarseness and a cough like a sea lion's. Serious deterioration is relatively uncommon but is suggested by an increasing rate of breathing, increasing stridor, lethargy and pallor.

TREATMENT

Treatment involves ensuring that the child stays quiet and rests, because any increased effort will increase the airways' obstruction. Make the child comfortable in a warm moist atmosphere such as a steamy bathroom or kitchen. This will rapidly give relief from the croup. For severe cases, steroids may be given in a nebulized mist. The worst of croup usually goes within 24–48 hours.

QUESTION

Why might children suffering with croup occasionally be admitted to hospital?
This may be necessary in a case of severe airway obstruction when the child is very breathless, increasingly lethargic and exhausted. Sometimes the diagnosis of croup might be in doubt and some other reason is suspected for obstructing the airway. For example, a foreign body might in fact be the cause of abrupt stridor in an otherwise well child.

  Complementary Treatment
Aromatherapy – try dispensing lavender oil via a room humidifier. **Homeopathy** – a variety of remedies is available, including aconite, spongia and hepar sulph; their use depends on the details of your child's condition. See also BRONCHIOLITIS.

BRONCHIOLITIS

A viral infection in babies that causes coughs and wheezing.

CAUSES

Of several viruses causing bronchiolitis, the most common is respiratory syncytial virus (RSV), which provokes inflammation throughout the lungs and is highly contagious.

SYMPTOMS

Bronchiolitis mainly affects babies aged two to six months and begins as **colds** do, with a runny nose and wheezy cough. Many children remain only modestly unwell, but in some the illness becomes rapidly worse over a few hours. The child becomes lethargic. Breathing exceeds 30 breaths a minute; the ribs appear to suck in with each breath and the child is too breathless to feed. Blueness around the lips suggests severe lack of oxygen and needs immediate medical assessment.

TREATMENT

Mild cases need fluids and rest, and protection from smoke and fumes. It helps to put the child in a warm moist atmosphere such as a steamy bathroom or kitchen. Since the illness can deteriorate rapidly, doctors send any but the most mildly affected children into hospital for oxygen and close nursing.

About 10% of children develop **pneumonia**, so antibiotics are usually prescribed, even though the basic viral infection will not be affected by an antibiotic. The illness lasts three to five days. There is some evidence that children who keep getting bronchiolitis may later develop **asthma**.

   Complementary Treatment
WARNING: Tai chi/chi kung is not suitable for children under ten. Children respond well to **acupuncture** (some acupuncturists specialize in treating children), **shiatsu-do** and **Chinese herbs**. See also CROUP.

WORMS

Threadworms (Enterobius vermicularis) are the likeliest worm infection in temperate zones, where other worm infections are rare.

CAUSE

Children playing may pick up soil containing the eggs then suck their fingers, as children do. The swallowed eggs hatch inside the large intestine and appear on the motions.

SYMPTOMS

At night worms congregate around the anus to lay eggs, provoking intense itching. Itching leads to scratching, scratching leads to eggs under the fingernails, fingers are sucked and the cycle is repeated. The worms may crawl into the vagina, causing itching there, too. The worms and tiny white eggs can be seen around the anus or on the motions, the former looking like strands of white thread, 0.5 cm/¼ in long and very thin.

TREATMENT

Suitable drugs include piperazine or mebendazole (the latter also kills several other types of worm apart from threadworms). Usually a single dose is enough but a repeat treatment after two weeks is advisable. Ideally the whole family should take treatment at the same time. However, do not treat children under two without taking medical advice on safety. The risk of re-infection is reduced by keeping fingernails short and by encouraging frequent handwashing. Since eggs are laid at night, a morning bath or shower will wash these away.

QUESTION

Are threadworms serious?
They hardly ever cause problems other than itch. In very rare cases, large numbers live within the appendix, discovered if the appendix is removed. The unpleasantness of the itch should not be underestimated as it can drive children (and adults) to distraction. Therefore they are well worth treating, especially in families and close communities where threadworms spread rapidly.

Complementary Treatment
Nutritional therapy – raw garlic is toxic to worms, but it can be difficult getting children to eat it; carrots and pumpkin seeds also help clear infection. *Other therapies to try: Western herbalism; Ayurveda; homeopathy.*

NAPPY RASH

Raw red rashes in the nappy region affect all infants at some time.

CAUSES

The warm and wet conditions under a nappy favour colonization by **thrush**. Urine irritates the skin, creating **eczema** and letting in infection. A rubbing nappy may cause rawness. Children with **diarrhoea** are likely to get a rash.

SYMPTOMS

The skin is red and inflamed across the nappy region and raw in places. The edge of the rash is quite sharp. Thrush is likely if the rash extends deep into all the skin creases. A rash sparing the skin creases is typical of inflammation from urine, which has not penetrated the creases. The baby may be mildly irritated; parents are usually more upset by nappy rash than the infant. Considering the unhygienic conditions prevailing under nappies, the risk of serious skin infection is extremely low. In theory, a nappy rash might cause serious ulceration of the skin, scrotum and vagina but this rarely happens in practice unless the rash has been grossly neglected.

TREATMENT

Nappy rash is less common in this era of disposable nappies, which should be frequently changed and should contain no detergent to sensitize the skin. The many creams available contain an antifungal, an antiseptic and substances that protect the skin from urine. Ideally, the nappy should be left off.

Complementary Treatment
Homeopathy – use calendula cream. **Aromatherapy** – add one drop of one of the following to 15 ml of carrier oil and apply to the affected area: Roman chamomile, lavender or yarrow.

PHIMOSIS

An unusually narrow opening of the tip of the foreskin.

CAUSE

Boys may be born with this slight abnormality, or the foreskin might be scarred by repeated **balanitis**. Ill-advised attempts to roll back the foreskin can traumatize it and lead to narrowing.

SYMPTOMS

There may be no symptoms; the boy's parents simply notice the small tip. The foreskin cannot be rolled back, but this is quite usual in boys until three to five years of age anyway. In significant phimosis the foreskin balloons out when urinating and urine dribbles out rather than exits in a stream; this needs a medical opinion. Balanitis under the phimotic foreskin is common and it can be hard to decide which is cause or effect.

TREATMENT

Treatment may not be necessary, in the expectation that the foreskin will stretch as the boy gets older. Where there is clear obstruction or repeated balanitis, surgery is appropriate. It may be enough to dilate the foreskin under anaesthetic. Afterwards the parents should show the child how to roll back the foreskin regularly to prevent renarrowing. Circumcision, if requested by the parents or advised by the surgeon, will of course cure the problem for good.

QUESTION

Is circumcision a good thing?
Opinion on this vexed question predates modern medicine, with views going back to biblical times. There is good evidence to suggest that circumcised men are much less likely to get cancer of the penis. Since non-ritual circumcision requires an anaesthetic, most surgeons try to avoid it in children unless recurrent infection or phimosis make it unavoidable.

 Complementary Treatment
Homeopathy – to reduce itching, bathe the foreskin and head of the penis with a solution made from five drops each of mother tincture of hypericum and calendula in 300 ml/½ pint of cooled boiled water.

BALANITIS

Infection under the foreskin, a problem closely related to phimosis.

CAUSES

Almost inevitably, sweat and secretions get under the foreskin and can become infected. Whereas adults can roll back the foreskin and clean beneath it, in children it is natural that the foreskin will not roll back until the boy is about five years old and attempts to do so may lead to scarring and **phimosis**. The latter adds to the problem in a chicken-and-egg way.

SYMPTOMS

The tip of the foreskin becomes reddened and inflamed; it can swell alarmingly, but harmlessly, because the skin is so lax. Infection often spreads to around the penis, the tip of which becomes inflamed. There is a discharge of pus from under the foreskin. After repeated attacks the foreskin becomes thickened, cracked and phimotic.

TREATMENT

Early mild infection is helped by bathing the penis in warm salty water and gently irrigating under the foreskin. More severe infection requires medication: creams that usually combine an antifungal and an anti-inflammatory agent as well as an antibiotic. This is because **thrush** often invades balanitis and adds to the inflammation. The very soreness and narrowness of the foreskin makes it difficult to get the cream inside, which is why oral antibiotics are often necessary, too.

Repeated balanitis is very uncomfortable for the boy and will cause the narrowing of phimosis. In such cases surgical dilation may be advisable, if not circumcision.

  Complementary Treatment
Children do generally respond extremely well to both **acupuncture** and **Chinese herbs**. Some acupuncturists specialize in the treatment of children. **Homeopathy** – see PHIMOSIS.

URINARY PROBLEMS

Malformations and infections of the urinary system occur quite frequently and predispose to kidney trouble in adult life.

CAUSES

The urinary system comprises the kidneys, where urine is made, the ureters (the tubes through which urine flows to the muscular bladder), the bladder itself and the urethra, through which urine exits in front of the vagina, or via the penis.

Malformations

There are many anatomical abnormalities, the most serious of which occur in boys, some of whom have posterior urethral valves. These are flaps of skin within the urethra which impede the outflow of urine from the bladder. They lead to great back pressure of urine into the kidneys and permanent damage. Many urinary system malformations are detected only on investigation of urinary infection.

Infection

In girls the urethra is short enough to allow bacteria to ascend fairly easily from the perineum into the bladder. As a result of this about 5% of girls get urinary infections during their first two years. Bacteria find it much more difficult to gain access via the penis and the infection rate in boys is correspondingly lower at 1–2%.

Infected urine may ascend (reflux) from the bladder into the kidneys, causing permanent damage, which in later life increases the risks of **high blood pressure** by 20%. Furthermore, about one-third of cases of **kidney failure** are believed to originate in kidney damage due to childhood infection. The risks are not huge – kidney failure is rare – but it may be partially avoidable (only partially, because a tendency to reflux is probably genetically determined).

SYMPTOMS

Childhood urinary infection is rarely accompanied by the classic symptoms experienced by adults – burning when passing urine and needing to go frequently. More likely, the child is simply feverish or 'off colour'. A child previously dry at night might become incontinent again and might also complain of stomach ache. Boys with posterior urethral valves tend to dribble urine rather than pass a proper stream.

It can be difficult to confirm urinary infection because it is so awkward to obtain a good sample from children, who do not obligingly 'pee to order' into a specimen bottle.

TREATMENT

Any infection is treated with an antibiotic. Many specialists recommend further investigation after even a single proven infection. Investigation has been greatly simplified by high-definition ultrasound and scans of the kidney, which display many malformations and existing kidney scars.

It may be necessary to have specialized X-rays in order to see whether urine is refluxing into the kidney and scarring it. If this is the case, the child needs to have both long-term antibiotics to reduce the chances of further infection and regular checks of kidney function. It is possible to reduce reflux by re-implanting the ureters into the bladder in a position that is less likely to reflux. The value of such surgery is debatable and is done only where infection is not controlled by antibiotics and where there is clear evidence of progressive scarring of the kidney.

QUESTIONS

Should all ill children be tested for urinary infection?
This is an unrealistic ideal. However urinary infection should be considered in any child who remains unwell or feverish for more than a few days.

How serious is a first infection?
It is not actually known how often infections go undetected; they may be more common, and therefore of less significance, than believed. On present evidence they should be taken seriously.

Can problems be detected before birth?
Many can be detected from just 18 weeks, including posterior urethral valves. A drainage tube can be inserted into the bladder before birth and the abnormality fully corrected surgically after birth. It is not known whether all abnormalities are a problem in later life.

Complementary Treatment

Treatment depends on the specific details of your child's problem. Always check the practitioner is experienced in treating children. **Western herbalism** works on the urinary system and reduces tension. Children respond well to **Chinese herbalism** and **acupuncture**. A **homeopath** will build up a picture of your child and should be able to help. **Chakra balancing** improves the immune response.

CONGENITAL DISLOCATION OF THE HIP

An abnormality at birth, which if undetected in infancy may cause the child to have a permanent limp.

CAUSE

The femur (thigh bone) should fit securely into a socket of the hip bone; in congenital dislocation of the hip (CDH) the femur is dislocated or slips out easily. Girls are affected six times more than boys and there is a higher incidence in breech-born babies. CDH is probably due to failure of the hip socket to grow normally; it affects about one in five hundred children.

SYMPTOMS

A baby should have symmetrical skin creases around the buttocks; in CDH these are asymmetrical. With time the affected leg looks shorter and turns outward. Doctors check for CDH at birth and again at six to eight weeks of age. They twist and press the hips to see if they will dislocate. Also they look at the skin crease around the buttocks with the baby lying on its front. If there is doubt, the child should have an ultrasound scan of the hips. Any hip that feels 'clicky' or fails the test should be assessed by an orthopaedic surgeon.

TREATMENT

The child has to stay in splints for some months to keep the top of the femur pressed into the cup of the hip, so encouraging the socket to grow properly. The few children who do not respond to this may need surgery to fix the femur in place.

QUESTIONS

Why is CDH missed despite examination?
The standard tests miss at least 30% of CDH. Evidence is also increasingly suggesting that the condition can develop in hips previously passed as normal. There is an argument for screening for CDH using ultrasound scans of the hip. Otherwise it may be detected only when the child limps when she starts to walk.

Complementary Treatment

Rolfing can improve the muscular balance around the hip joint. **Chakra balancing** can help relax an irritable child and reduce pain. *Other therapies to try: cymatics; shiatsu-do; Alexander Technique.*

SCOLIOSIS

A permanent side-to-side curvature of the spine.

CAUSES

For unknown reasons, scoliosis in the developed world is mostly congenital, i.e. an abnormality present at the time of birth. Occasionally disease of the muscles around the spine causes the twist. Poliomyelitis used to be a common cause.

SYMPTOMS

Scoliosis often only becomes apparent with the growth spurt of puberty, especially in girls. From behind, the spine should look almost straight. In scoliosis a sideways twist throws the ribcage on one side into prominence. If muscle imbalance is the cause, there may be weakness down one side of the body. Poor posture may resemble a fixed scoliosis but the abnormal curve goes when the child straightens or bends forward. In true scoliosis the curve remains however the child moves.

TREATMENT

It takes great judgement by an experienced surgeon to decide whether and when to treat scoliosis. Repeated review and measurement of the degree of scoliosis aid this judgement. The decision is more straightforward if the scoliosis is severe enough to compress the lungs or heart.

The surgery, called spinal fusion, involves fixing a number of vertebrae together so no further twist is possible. Other measures include wearing firm frames (braces) or inserting a rod into the vertebrae to prevent progression; the value of these techniques is more controversial.

Complementary Treatment

Chiropractors can advise on good exercises to do. If there is back pain, the child can be treated using specific manipulative and mobilizing techniques. **Rolfing** allows the spine to lengthen by relaxing both it and the soft tissues around it.

CONGENITAL HEART PROBLEMS

Abnormalities of the heart, many of which are minor, affect 1% of children at birth.

CAUSES

The heart develops by a rather beautiful series of twists that transform an initially straight tube into the complex heart, but with a high risk of malformations. Before birth the heart does not have to pump blood around the lungs, oxygen instead being supplied via the placenta. At birth all this changes as the lungs expand for that first cry. This is a time when many serious abnormalities first show themselves.

Heart problems are generally divided into those that cause a blue baby (cyanotic heart disease) and those that do not. In cyanotic heart disease the abnormality allows blood that is low in oxygen, and therefore blue, to mix with blood from the lungs. In non-cyanotic conditions blood circulates through the lungs in the normal way, but problems arise through leaks and abnormal pressure of flow. Both types may end in **heart failure** or in disease of the lungs.

Common congenital heart defects

There are a number of common congenital heart defects (congenital meaning an abnormality present at birth). While most serious ones are apparent at birth, a few cause minimal symptoms and may not be apparent until later in childhood.

Ventricular septal defect (VSD): There is a hole between the right and left ventricles – the larger beating chambers – of the heart. When the powerful left ventricle pumps, it squeezes blood through the hole into the right ventricle.

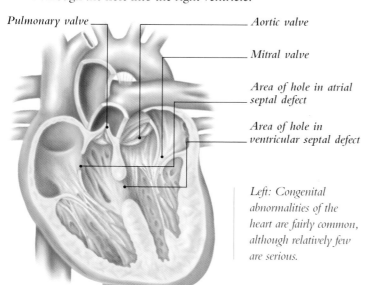

Pulmonary valve

Aortic valve

Mitral valve

Area of hole in atrial septal defect

Area of hole in ventricular septal defect

Left: Congenital abnormalities of the heart are fairly common, although relatively few are serious.

Atrial septal defect (ASD): There is a hole in the wall between the atria, smaller chambers that hold blood before it passes into the powerful ventricles. The effect is similar to a VSD.

Fallot's tetralogy: This is a cyanotic heart condition where there is gross malformation of the heart with a large VSD and a narrowing of one of the heart valves.

Hypoplastic left heart: In this serious condition the whole of the left heart has failed to form properly. The baby cannot survive more than a few days without major surgery.

Coarctation of the aorta, patent ductus arteriosus, pulmonary stenosis: These are abnormalities of major blood vessels around the heart, the significance of which varies.

SYMPTOMS

Some conditions cause symptoms at or around birth, for example cyanosis (blueness), breathlessness and a variety of murmurs over the heart – unusual sounds heard through a stethoscope and caused by turbulent blood flow. Badly affected babies rapidly go into heart failure, unable to feed properly and requiring resuscitation. Less badly affected children have heart murmurs but are otherwise reasonably well, although they may get breathless easily. Congenital heart disease is a major reason for **failure to thrive**.

The majority of minor heart conditions are detected as a murmur, the exact diagnosis defined by echocardiography and possibly angiography (see Modern investigations, page 46).

TREATMENT

Many congenital heart conditions will correct themselves during the first few years of life, for example 50% of cases of VSD, or require no surgical treatment at all. Some extreme forms require immediate surgical treatment and even a heart transplant (see page 363). Several other serious conditions can be corrected in a number of operations spread over a few years.

Complementary Treatment

Complementary therapies cannot correct congenital heart problems. They can have a supportive role, but always check the practitioner is experienced in treating children. A sick child may benefit from the sense of wellbeing generated by **aromatherapy** with **massage**. **Reflexology** can also be supportive.

DIARRHOEA AND VOMITING

Usually minor illness caused by stimulation of the gastrointestinal tract by viruses and bacteria, acquired by chance or by food poisoning. Also called gastroenteritis.

CAUSES

Among children in the developed world, most diarrhoea and vomiting episodes are caused by viruses, usually rotaviruses, which irritate the gastrointestinal tract. Here it is rarely more than an inconvenience and few children become severely ill. Globally, however, gastroenteritis is a major killer of debilitated young children who lack access to simple but effective treatment. Breast-fed babies are less likely to contract gastroenteritis, thanks to the inherently sterile milk supply and the protection from antibodies within the mother's milk.

Vomiting

Initiated by a vomiting centre within the brain, vomiting is a non-specific reflex reaction to many infections or pains. It has presumably evolved to get a possibly poisonous substance out of the stomach as soon as possible. Children and babies vomit readily since it is under less conscious control than in adults.

Diarrhoea

The intestinal tract normally absorbs fluid very efficiently; diarrhoea occurs because infection irritates the lining of the intestines so they fail to absorb carbohydrate. This has the effect of retaining excessive quantities of fluid within the bowel, hence diarrhoea. Another influence may be toxins from infections that paralyse the normal activity of the bowel.

SYMPTOMS

The child often has a cough and cold, suggesting a viral origin for the gastroenteritis. Food poisoning is suggested by abrupt vomiting in a previously well child, diarrhoea soon following. Vomiting frequently precedes diarrhoea and ends before it. Diarrhoea can begin without forewarning. Abdominal cramps are common but diarrhoea and vomiting with severe pain suggest an abdominal problem that needs urgent medical assessment. Most gastroenteritis settles within three to seven days.

TREATMENT

Gastrointestinal upsets are a normal feature of childhood and need cause no immediate alarm. The treatment principle is to replace fluid in small but frequent amounts, using electrolyte mixtures containing salt and sugar in concentrations similar to the natural fluids within the body. These widely available drinks are better absorbed than plain water and are pleasant to drink. Do not give the child sugary drinks, which tend to make diarrhoea worse. There are no recommended anti-diarrhoea drugs for children.

Once the vomiting phase has passed the child can eat if he wishes. Do not be alarmed if eating provokes a bout of diarrhoea. This is not 'food going straight through' but simply a reflex bowel action, which is normal after eating. Give the child bland food like rice or eggs, not milk or dairy products, which may worsen the diarrhoea.

It is important to monitor the child for dehydration (see box below). Most children can be managed at home unless dehydration becomes apparent, when they may need hospital treatment with intravenous fluids. This is more likely with babies, who become dehydrated much more quickly than older children.

WARNING SIGNS WITH GASTROENTERITIS IN CHILDREN

- *Blood or mucus in the diarrhoea*
- *Persistent or severe abdominal pain*
- *Vomit stained yellow with bile*
- *Reduced urine output – dry nappies for several hours*
- *Increasing lethargy*
- *Sunken eyes, sunken fontanelles (soft spots in the baby's skull)*
- *Pallor and cold skin*
- *In children below the age of one, symptoms continuing for more than 24 hours*

These suggest significant dehydration or another serious cause for the symptoms.

Complementary Treatment

Complementary therapies have much to offer, but do check the practitioner is experienced in treating children. **Western herbalism** – peppermint or blackberry tea may help shorten recovery time. Several **homeopathic** remedies are available; the one to use depends on many variables. Diet – rest the digestive system by offering only liquid for a while; a **naturopath** could give specific advice. *Other therapies to try: acupuncture; Chinese herbalism; shiatsu-do; Ayurveda.*

COLIC AND ABDOMINAL PAINS

Abdominal pain in children has physical and emotional origins.

CAUSES

Children do get pains for serious reasons but frequently their pains are recurrent, non-specific, less easily categorized and settle without treatment. In an otherwise well child, maintaining weight and eating, a serious cause is unlikely and emotional problems at school and at home should be explored.

Colic
Colic means pain due to distension of a hollow internal organ, typically the intestine, to which children are especially prone. Colic rises to a crescendo then diminishes, the process repeating every few minutes. For some reason, babies aged between one and three months commonly go through a phase of recurrent colic at night, despite being well for the rest of the day.

A **hernia** in the groin will cause colic if it becomes trapped. Other causes in older children may be **constipation** or worry.

Inflammation of an internal organ
This is always the number one worry for both parents and doctors. The most common serious inflammation is appendicitis. Children occasionally get general inflammation of the bowel called colitis, **indigestion** or even a peptic ulcer. Boys may have a **twisted testicle**. Inflammation caused by **urinary problems** is notorious for causing abdominal pain in children. Diarrhoea is frequently accompanied by abdominal pains (see DIARRHOEA AND VOMITING).

Mesenteric adenitis/abdominal migraine
These are efforts at explaining the many abdominal pains where other causes are excluded. A sore throat is thought to cause painful glands within the abdomen as well as the neck, which accounts for many pains. Headaches in children are often accompanied by abdominal pains, as they are in adults.

SYMPTOMS

Older children complain of pain. Babies cry, appear distressed, curl up their legs and may vomit. More serious is pain accompanied by vomiting yellow bile or bleeding from the back passage. Other serious accompanying symptoms are **fever**, a raised pulse and coated tongue. Doctors look for another infection – **tonsillitis**, **ear infection** or chest infection.

Appendicitis usually starts over the belly button, shifting within hours into the lower right abdomen, plus fever,

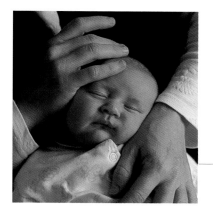

Left: Babies with colic often respond well to gentle cranial osteopathy, which is very calming.

vomiting and great abdominal tenderness. It can, however, present without these symptoms and even in the lower left abdomen. It may be diagnosed only by exploratory surgery.

The examination of the child's tummy is an art, assessing tension of the abdominal muscles, pain on releasing the abdomen, the sounds from the intestines. Doctors also check for a hernia or twisted testicle and test urine for infection.

TREATMENT

For babies suffering from colic, ensure they are well winded. If you are bottle feeding, experiment with changing the milk and timing of evening feeds. Paracetamol syrup can be given.

Suspected appendicitis, twisted testicle or intestine, trapped hernia and other serious internal problems require surgery. Exploratory operations are not undertaken lightly as surgeons prefer to operate with a definite diagnosis in mind.

Pains apparently due to infection elsewhere, such as tonsillitis, should settle as the infection goes. This leaves many instances where there appears not to be a serious cause for pain. Then it is reasonable to give a painkiller such as paracetamol and plenty of fluids and await spontaneous recovery, always being prepared to reassess the child if pains persist.

Complementary Treatment
Complementary therapies have much to offer, but do check the practitioner is experienced in treating children. **Homeopathy** – see DIARRHOEA AND VOMITING. **Aromatherapy** compresses and inhalations can help; oils are chosen according to the case. **Osteopathy** can be extremely helpful, especially some of the cranial techniques. *Other therapies to try: Western herbalism; acupuncture; shiatsu-do; Chinese herbalism; chakra balancing; naturopathy; cymatics; Ayurveda.*

CEREBRAL PALSY

Brain damage at the time of birth or occurring soon thereafter.

CAUSES

The natural hazards of birth can, in a few cases, damage brain cells enough to cause cerebral palsy. Prematurity is a major risk: about 10% of premature babies are affected. Infection after birth may damage the delicate brain.

At least half of the cases are due to developmental problems within the womb or infection during pregnancy such as **rubella**, although the latter is now very rare. For many children with cerebral palsy there is no obvious explanation and the assumption is that the child's brain simply failed to develop properly within the womb. Cerebral palsy affects one to two children per thousand in the developed world but is a much larger hazard in the underdeveloped world where pregnancy and childbirth are more dangerous.

SYMPTOMS

Children affected with cerebral palsy have some degree of weakness and abnormal stiffness of the muscles down one side of the body, called a hemi-paresis, or of all limbs – a quadriplegia. Symptoms can range from stiffness and clumsiness to complete paralysis of one side. There is an increased risk of **epilepsy**. Because of the muscle imbalance these children often develop distorted backs (**scoliosis**) or limbs.

At the worst extreme the baby may clearly be abnormal at birth, unusually floppy, breathing badly, not moving its limbs properly – all symptoms that are suggestive of major brain damage. The worst-affected children may never become continent or indeed capable of independent existence. At the other extreme there may be just a barely detectable difference in strength between the two sides of the child's body or slight developmental delays.

Many cases are recognized because the child fails to reach the 'milestones' of development, for example there is delay in sitting, walking, talking and social development. The diagnosis in mildly affected children often is not considered until rather later as a result of queries over school progress, unusual clumsiness or difficulty in reading.

It is important to review the pregnancy: perhaps the mother contracted rubella or **chickenpox** or had **high blood pressure**. Was the birth difficult? Was the child premature? Did the child have **jaundice** or a severe infection soon after birth? Further investigation would most likely include genetic analysis and tests for a biochemical abnormality.

TREATMENT

Although the diagnosis of cerebral palsy is a parent's dread, it is important to remember two things. First, a baby's brain can overcome brain damage that would be permanent and devastating in an adult. Although the baby may not ever fully recover, her final abilities may be much better than thought at the time of diagnosis. Second, cerebral palsy does not necessarily mean that the child's intelligence is affected.

Great changes have been made in treatment in recent years, aiming to help all children suffering from cerebral palsy make the most of their abilities, with physiotherapy to keep all muscle groups working, speech therapy to aid articulation, aids for speech or walking and constant stimulation. Operations may be advisable to correct twisted limbs.

Most children with cerebral palsy can attend a normal school and only a minority need special schooling or are too badly affected to benefit at all.

SEE ALSO CHILD DEVELOPMENT, PAGE 300.

QUESTIONS

Do children develop at the same rate in all areas of learning?
No, it is quite normal for a child to be advanced in one area and to lag in another, but a generalized delay in development should be further assessed medically.

What is the real outlook?
It may not be until the child is ten years old or more that the full extent of their abilities is clear. Unfortunately this is often a period of enormous strain on the parents, not knowing if their child will ever lead an independent existence.

Complementary Treatment

Programmes providing intensive stimulation have received much publicity in recent years, and it is now accepted that increased stimulation improves development. **Arts therapies** could have a role here. Any therapy that works the tissues – **osteopathy**, **chiropractic**, **rolfing**, **Hellerwork** or **massage** – could be beneficial. **Chakra balancing** could be supportive. The entire family could benefit from stress-reducing therapies such as **yoga** or **aromatherapy**.

DOWN'S SYNDROME

A genetic fault that causes heart and brain abnormalities.

CAUSES

Chromosomes that carry the genetic information normally exist in pairs. In Down's syndrome chromosome 21 exists as a triplet, hence the condition's alternative name trisomy 21. The defect arises when the fertilized egg begins to divide but the fundamental reason is unknown. There are other rarer genetic reasons for the defect.

Down's syndrome affects one in seven hundred children who are born live, the risk rising according to the mother's age: for example about one in three hundred and fifty at the age of thirty-five and one in twenty-five to thirty by the age of forty-six. Many affected foetuses die pre-term.

SYMPTOMS

Among numerous Down's syndrome features there is a prominent fold in the eyes as is found normally in Asian races, which accounts for the old term 'mongolism'. The tongue is large and the skin coarse. Heart abnormalities are common and 10% have **epilepsy**. Intelligence is invariably reduced but the range is wide. Since the baby will show the typical Down's syndrome features at birth it is unusual for there to be a delay in making the diagnosis.

TREATMENT

The condition cannot be reversed. The child is prone to chest infections that need vigorous treatment, as may heart disease. Some are intelligent enough to lead a semi-independent existence eventually and hold down a simple job, while others require constant monitoring. Few Down's syndrome adults live beyond 50 but their life can be a relatively happy one.

QUESTION

What screening is available?
Parents are offered a combination of blood tests and a scan at 16 weeks – an unusually thick neck suggests Down's. Amniocentesis is needed to confirm a suspicion; this is drawing fluid from the womb, for genetic analysis of cells shed by the baby and a check for biochemicals associated with the condition. As amniocentesis may provoke a miscarriage, expert guidance is needed as to when this risk is outweighed by the risk of an affected baby.

Complementary Treatment
Down's syndrome children could benefit from any **massage**, including one with **aromatherapy**. Check the practitioner is experienced in treating children.

SPINA BIFIDA

Failure of the foetus's spinal bones to fuse, associated with damage of the spinal cord and brain.

CAUSE

In embryonic life the bones of the vertebral column fuse together, enclosing the delicate spinal cord. This fails to happen in spina bifida, leaving part of it exposed. It is associated with hydrocephalus, increased pressure in the fluid surrounding the brain. It now affects about one in six thousand births.

SYMPTOMS

The child may be born with an obvious opening at the base of the back. The skull swells because of hydrocephalus. There are many degrees of spina bifida, all of which are serious.

TREATMENT

The spine must be immediately protected or surgically covered against infection. If there is hydrocephalus a tube is fitted within the skull to drain fluid from the brain to the heart, keeping pressure down. People with spina bifida are often paralysed below the waist and subject to urinary infection, **incontinence**, pressure sores and reduced life expectancy. Yet the top half of the body is normal, as is intelligence.

The risk of spina bifida is greatly reduced if the mother takes 0.4 mg folic acid daily, before and in early pregnancy.

Complementary Treatment

If you are planning a baby, a **naturopath** or **nutritional therapist** could advise on preconceptual diet, focusing on your intake of vital nutrients, including folic acid.

FAILURE TO THRIVE

A concept unique to paediatric practice, this means failure to gain weight and is a sensitive indicator of serious illness or of emotional deprivation in children up to about two years of age.

CAUSES

Children differ fundamentally from adults in that they are growing constantly. Growth continues throughout childhood, although there will be times when it is imperceptible. During the first two years of life growth should be especially rapid and sustained. Any serious illness interrupts growth by diverting the energy that would go towards growth into fighting the disease. Failure to thrive is therefore a challenge rather than a diagnosis and all aspects of the child's physical and emotional health need to be examined to discover the causes.

What counts as failure to thrive? Even a trivial illness interrupts growth briefly; babies' weight in particular may swing alarmingly. These brief perturbations are normal and should only raise concern if growth is interrupted for several weeks.

Inadequate nutrition
The rapid metabolic rate of children demands adequate energy input, lack of which is one of the most common reasons for problems. It is often a matter of mismanagement rather than deliberate misfeeding, for example a teat that is too narrow to let milk out or continuing to feed a baby solely on milk beyond the time when it is ready for solid food. Many babies do go through periods of faddy eating, if not food refusal, and their weight may fluctuate wildly at such times.

Emotional mishandling
It may come as a surprise to learn that children fail to grow if they are unhappy but this is certainly the case. The emotional neglect has to be severe – not being allowed to watch a certain programme on TV does not count. Emotionally deprived children are likely to be delayed in overall social and emotional development as well as in growth.

Intestinal disease
Constant vomiting will lead to weight loss for obvious reasons. This happens in pyloric stenosis, where an abnormal band narrows the duodenum, preventing food from leaving the stomach. That said, many babies vomit both small and large amounts of food without having any underlying physical abnormality. Other gastrointestinal possibilities are malabsorption through **coeliac disease** and chronic parasite infection, for example with hookworm.

Heart and lung disease
Serious **congenital heart problems** such as cyanotic heart disease cause failure to thrive through chronic oxygen starvation. Similarly, chronic lung diseases – severe **asthma**, cystic fibrosis or chronic lung infection – make the child constantly breathless, starve the body of oxygen and take energy. Ordinary coughs and **colds** are negligible but severe **pneumonia** or **bronchiolitis** might reduce growth for a few weeks.

Metabolic conditions
This covers a range of disorders in how the body handles energy. They range from the relatively uncommon such as **kidney failure** or an underactive thyroid gland (see THYROID PROBLEMS) to the downright rare, for example glycogen storage disease or liver disease.

Miscellaneous
Children born with **cerebral palsy** tend not to grow as well as normal children. The same applies to children born with genetic disorders of any type, **Down's syndrome** being the most common. Failure to thrive is unlikely to be the first indication of a problem, as these children will either be diagnosed at birth or will exhibit generalized delay in development of which failure to thrive is just one aspect, for example delay in language, manipulation or walking.

Certain premature babies remain small and fail to thrive throughout childhood, presumably because of permanent disruption of their potential for growth.

SYMPTOMS

While no one individual child grows at an average rate, by following large numbers of children average growth rates have been established to produce growth charts. These are not single figures but show a range – for example by six months it is normal for a child to weigh double its birth weight, but this could be anywhere from 6 to 9.5 kg/13 to 21 lb. These growth charts are specific for particular populations – the expected growth of affluent European children is quite different from that of children in the developing world. Moreover, the average changes over time, as children have tended to grow bigger and heavier, and also rates are different for boys and girls. Height and weight are the fundamental measures of growth. Babies also have head circumference measured.

It is important to realize that a single abnormal reading means very little – unless it is grossly extreme. This is because the weighing process may be affected by such things as wear-

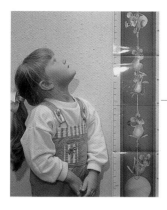

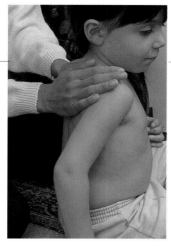

Above: Height gain is a basic measure of health in children. Right: Massage helps children to feel loved.

ing different clothes, or even whether the child has a full bladder or not. What is important is to take several measurements over several weeks or months in order to plot growth curves.

Patterns of abnormal growth

Two types emerge: there is the child who was growing normally but whose growth then declines. This suggests a new and serious problem. Then there is the child whose height or weight start abnormally low and remain low, the implication being a congenital problem interfering with growth from the start. Most children have rather zigzag curves, with minor variations reflecting minor childhood illnesses.

Tests

A careful full examination is essential, when the doctor will look especially for signs of heart or lung disease, malnutrition (for example loose skin folds and thin buttocks), bruising or parental attitudes suggestive of emotional and physical abuse.

Blood tests establish the state of health of the kidneys and liver and detect whether there is **anaemia**, vitamin deficiency or the abnormal results that accompany malabsorption and **diabetes**. Additional basic tests might include a chest X-ray and testing a urine sample for infection. Many additional tests are available, depending on the suspected problems, for example a biopsy of the bowel might be used to establish **coeliac disease** or stool samples examined for malabsorption, chronic parasitic infection and metabolic diseases.

Measuring emotion

The paediatrician needs an insight into the usual emotional climate surrounding the child and so takes note of how you handle her. Does the child appear at ease with you or does she appear wary or apprehensive? Some parents truly interact with their child and respond to them; others pick them up and put them down like playthings. Is the child appropriately

dressed and reasonably groomed? This said, however, dirtiness or old clothes no more indicate neglect than a pristine child in designer gear signifies parental concern.

TREATMENT

Reasons for serious failure to thrive are generally rapidly established and treated. This also applies to the child growing normally but who then loses weight rapidly. More difficulties surround the child who is not severely unwell but whose growth is unsatisfactory without being disastrously bad. Many paediatricians, having established the child has a reasonable diet, will keep a watching brief, weighing and measuring the child monthly while waiting for a pattern to establish itself.

QUESTIONS

Can growth recover?
Most children will catch up after illness at up to three times the normal rate. The exceptions are chronic illness, for example kidney disease, or children suffering prolonged severe malnutrition, who may always remain smaller and lighter.

What about height?
Many of the influences on weight affect height, too. Investigation and treatment are largely the same except that the influence of heredity is greater and problems may not become apparent until the child is much older.

Complementary Treatment

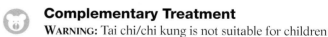

WARNING: Tai chi/chi kung is not suitable for children under ten. Complementary therapies can have a useful role here, especially if the failure to thrive is a consequence of emotional or psychological upset. Details of any treatment programme will always depend on the specifics of your child's case. Always check that your chosen practitioner is experienced in treating children. **Play therapy** could be of significant benefit, enabling children to come to terms with emotions through structured play. **Massage** – any type of massage will help build the child's feeling of being loved. Children respond extremely well to both **acupuncture** and **Chinese herbalism**. A **homeopath** will build up a picture of your child, and should be able to offer help. **Reflexology** can offer much support to your child.

SKIN PROBLEMS

Problems in young skin – mostly eczema or minor infections.

CAUSES

The newborn baby's skin is virgin territory for germs and irritants, which invade from the instant of birth. This is not through lack of cleanliness but is a natural and inevitable process. **Eczema** often causes rashes from an early age. Birth marks are extremely common (see box right). Other causes, for example **psoriasis** and **acne**, are unusual in children.

SYMPTOMS

Most babies get a few spots after birth, usually around the face, from germs picked up from family members. Some babies have milia, tiny shiny dots around the nose due to blocked sweat glands, that go spontaneously. Few babies escape **nappy rash**, just as few older children escape **warts**. Older children have **boils**, **impetigo** and eczema, too.

TREATMENT

The principle of treating skin problems is to use the mildest skin preparation that controls the problem. Many, especially eczema, respond to simple moisturizing creams and emollient bath oils, keeping steroid creams for more resistant cases. Antibiotic creams are sufficient for minor infections and only occasionally are antibiotics by mouth required for such problems. (See WARTS for treatment details.)

QUESTION

What are birth marks?
Birth marks are coloured patches and lumps that are persistent, unlike the temporary bruises caused by the trauma of birth. Strawberry naevi are deep red raised lesions, which enlarge for a year or two before nearly always disappearing by the time the child is about five years old. Although many birth marks require no treatment, a few do. See your doctor for an opinion.

Complementary Treatment

Ayurveda is a therapy that is very successful with skin problems; treatment is through *panchakarma* detoxification. **Chakra balancing** promotes healing of the skin and pain control. *Other therapies to try: homeopathy; shiatsu-do; acupuncture; aromatherapy.*

HEAD LICE

Small insects that thrive in hair, whether it be clean or dirty.

CAUSES

Head lice are 3–4 mm/⅛–³⁄₁₆ in long and feed on the rich blood supply of the scalp. A typical infection involves only five to ten lice, each laying up to three hundred eggs during its four- to six-week lifetime. The eggs are cemented to the hair shaft; the lice may similarly cement themselves or go roaming. Infection spreads through close contact and the sharing of combs or brushes. There is evidence that lice prefer longer hair and warmer weather.

SYMPTOMS

Itching is the main symptom, caused when the lice feed. You may notice the white eggs, called nits, adhering to hair shafts or spot a louse on an excursion. It is uncommon for any additional infection to enter the scalp unless the skin is greatly damaged by scratching. Itchy scalps are common so do not automatically assume head lice without definite evidence.

TREATMENT

The nit comb, used to comb out nits, is effective in recurrent infection. Standard medication includes malathion, carbaryl and permethrin in a wide range of brands and applications. A single treatment is highly effective; it is essential to treat all members of the family together and to follow the instructions for use precisely. Some treatments affect asthmatics so do check the label.

Complementary Treatment

Aromatherapy – add one drop of one of the following oils to your child's shampoo: lemon, rosemary or tea tree. Use the shampoo in conjunction with a nit comb.

HAND, FOOT AND MOUTH DISEASE

A viral infection, typified by a rash covering the above areas.

CAUSE

This is not to be confused with foot and mouth disease, which is a different illness and caught from pigs, sheep or cattle. The virus responsible for hand, foot and mouth disease is called Coxsackie, although occasionally other common viruses may cause a similar picture. The illness is mainly confined to children and occurs in outbreaks in all parts of the world.

SYMPTOMS

The illness begins with mild **fever** and a sore throat. The typical rash appears after a couple of days as tiny red painful spots on the tongue, gums and lining of the mouth. A day or two later a rash consisting of tiny fluid-filled spots called vesicles appears on the palms of the hands and the soles of the feet.

The rash is uncomfortable and the child may go off her food because of discomfort and even be reluctant to walk because of the pain from the rash on the feet. The illness lasts seven to ten days and has no long-term health consequences.

TREATMENT

All that is needed is to give painkillers as appropriate, for example paracetamol syrup, and drinks. Avoid acidic fruit juices as these will make the mouth sting.

Complementary Treatment
Ayurveda treatments are available, according to the details of the case. Ayurveda believes this disease could be linked to faulty digestion, and offers appropriate dietary advice.

FEBRILE FITS

Convulsions triggered by high temperatures, affecting about one child in twenty-five.

CAUSES

Anyone whose brain is heated rapidly and high enough will eventually have a fit. The brains of babies and children are more sensitive to modest rises in temperature, whatever the reason for the **fever**, hence the febrile fits. The chances of **epilepsy** in later life are higher than in unaffected children, but only very slightly.

SYMPTOMS

The hot child suddenly becomes unresponsive and begins to twitch. The child's eyes roll up and the limbs jerk rhythmically, which may last for several minutes. After the fit the child is drowsy but otherwise normal.

TREATMENT

Try to prevent a fit in a very hot child by reducing his temperature by removing clothing and with paracetamol, fans and tepid bathing. During a fit place the child on his front but otherwise leave the child until the fit ends. Call for help if it is a first fit or if the fit is prolonged and the child remains unresponsive. Hospital admission is advisable for a first fit and also in babies to exclude conditions such as meningitis. Thirty to forty per cent of children have recurrent fits; their parents can give diazepam rectally to stop them.

WARNING SIGNS

Children with these features need urgent medical attention:

♦ *A first fit (to confirm the diagnosis)*
♦ *A fit occurring in a child less than six months and more than five years (febrile fits are unlikely)*
♦ *A non-feverish child (other causes are likely)*
♦ *A fit lasting more than ten minutes (needs sedation)*
♦ *A fit following a head injury (possible brain damage)*
♦ *Associated with headaches and aversion to light (meningitis)*

Complementary Treatment
If your child has a persistently high temperature, or a fit, he should quickly receive conventional medical attention. Many complementary therapies give advice on lowering transiently high temperature. See FEVER.

JAUNDICE

A yellow tinge to the skin caused by liver problems.

CAUSES

'Normal' jaundice is when, for one to two weeks after birth, the immature liver fails to handle fully the yellow pigment bilirubin from the normal breakdown of red blood cells, which therefore leaks into the skin. High levels of bilirubin may cause permanent brain damage.

Also, before the mother's milk flows plentifully, a newborn baby may get slightly dehydrated, which is believed to account for jaundice. The child remains lively and well.

'Abnormal' jaundice is jaundice occurring within 24 hours of birth, probably from destruction of blood cells through rhesus incompatibility, although this is now rare. This is when a rhesus negative mother carrying a rhesus positive baby produces antibodies that destroy the baby's red blood cells. The mother's liver handles the resulting bilirubin during pregnancy. After birth, however, the baby's liver cannot cope, resulting in jaundice.

Jaundice persisting beyond two weeks may reflect abnormal drainage in the liver, called biliary atresia, or an underactive thyroid gland (see THYROID PROBLEMS). Other causes include severe general infection or hepatitis (see LIVER PROBLEMS).

SYMPTOMS

The jaundiced baby looks tanned and the whites of the eyes turn yellow. The blood level of bilirubin indicates whether treatment is necessary or not. In 'normal' jaundice, the baby remains well; in 'abnormal' jaundice the baby is often feverish, breathing rapidly, and has other signs of illness as well.

TREATMENT

The treatment in the case of 'normal' jaundice that does not improve spontaneously after a few days is to put the baby under ultraviolet light; this breaks down bilirubin in the skin. Give extra drinks to a slightly dehydrated breast-fed baby who is otherwise well, unless blood levels of bilirubin rise high, which is relatively uncommon.

In severe or 'abnormal' cases the baby needs blood transfusion plus treatment of the basic cause.

Complementary Treatment
Let your child sleep by an uncurtained window, to receive maximum light. A **Chinese herbalist** will be able to offer help. During the recovery period children may respond to **shiatsu-do**.

PERTHES' DISEASE

Abnormal growth of the hip joint leading to pain and a limp.

CAUSES

This is a problem caused when growing bone outstrips its blood supply, so that some of the bone dies. Perthes' disease involves the head of the thigh bone (the femur) and affects mainly boys between the ages of five and ten. Several similar disorders affect bones elsewhere in the body and are generally the scientific explanation for 'growing pains'.

SYMPTOMS

With Perthes' disease pain in the affected hip begins mildly but becomes constant. The child starts to limp. X-rays will show the typically abnormal appearance of the hip joint in Perthes' disease. (Although hip pain is common in childhood do not ignore it, especially if accompanied by a limp.)

TREATMENT

Usually the blood supply will re-establish itself enough for bone to regrow, although it may take two years before the final result is clear. Should this fail to happen, the affected child is likely to have a permanent limp and a higher risk of developing **osteoarthritis** of the hip later as an adult.

During the painful period, the child has to rest in bed but generally no other treatment is necessary. If the deformity is permanent, then surgery is performed in order to set the head of the femur in a better position in the hip joint.

Complementary Treatment
Do not abandon conventional approaches here. **Rolfing** can improve the muscular balance around the hip joint. **Chakra balancing** can be beneficial by helping relax an irritable child and reducing pain. *Other therapies to try: Alexander Technique.*

SLEEP PROBLEMS

Children refusing to sleep or waking at night cause great stress for parents and solutions are rarely easy or perfect.

CAUSES

The newborn baby sleeps most of the time, reducing to two or three sleeps by the age of one year. By three years old many children have two sleeps, having dropped an afternoon nap. Children tend to wake naturally between 5.00 and 6.00 am. It is also normal for children above 18 months to lie awake at night talking or amusing themselves.

Refusal to go to bed or frequent waking interferes with parents' peace after a day of mayhem and with their full night's sleep before another demanding day. Common contributing factors are: too much daytime sleep, which reduces the need for sleep at night; a poor routine for getting the child off to bed; fears on the child's part about being alone or separated from her parent, feelings which are at a maximum between 18 months and 2½ years; and disturbances, which might include traffic noise, loud television and parental arguments.

SYMPTOMS

The child cries at night or sleeps only briefly before waking and crying or attempting to get up. This behaviour might be constant or might have appeared very recently. Older children may wake early and talk or cry. The child may be sleepy in the day but still doggedly refuses to go to bed at night.

TREATMENT

First review the child's physical comfort. Check whether the child is hungry or thirsty, too hot, too cold, damp, dirty or irritated by noise. These are more relevant in the young baby, less so in children above about one year old.

Sleep patterns and bedtime routines
Try to keep the child awake during the day or keep any nap brief. Help the child to know bedtime is coming and, by implication, what is expected of him. Instill a routine such as a bath, a cuddle, reading a story and settling into bed with favourite toys.

Controlled crying
Babies normally cry for a few minutes on settling. You must resist the temptation to go back to give another cuddle. Older children, being cunning, will extend their crying until a parent

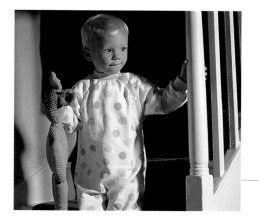

Left: Dealing with children's sleep problems calls for firm though caring handling.

reappears. Resist this also for five to ten minutes, then briefly enter to reassure the child and leave. Let the child cry for ten minutes, re-enter, reassure and leave, repeating as long as you can and letting the child cry for longer each time.

There is no reason to believe that crying can do psychological harm. Most experts agree that it is better to attempt to discipline children within a loving and consistent environment, rather than give inconsistent messages in an atmosphere of resentment from parental sleep deprivation.

Crying during the night should be handled in a similar way, checking first on physical discomfort, then leaving the child to cry. How long can this go on? As long as your nerves hold. Most experts agree that the worst will usually be over after four days, although individual children may stay difficult and go on much longer and louder. Be reassured that sleep problems rarely extend past about five years of age.

Medication
There comes a point when medication is reasonable to give the parents a break, for example when on holiday. Medication available includes chloral and trimeprazine. It should be seen as a last resort used for only a day or two at a time.

Complementary Treatment
Bach flower remedies depend on the cause of the problem, for example agrimony for children who keep their worries to themselves. If the problem follows change such as a new school, try walnut. Olive can help overcome tiredness. **Aromatherapy** – try one drop of Roman chamomile or lavender in the pre-bedtime bath or on the pillow. **Play therapy** could be of benefit if the problem has an emotional cause. *Other therapies to try: most have something to offer.*

BEHAVIOURAL PROBLEMS

The child is capable of better behaviour but seems driven to act otherwise. The diagnosis and management is complex.

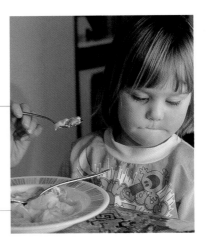

Right: Children will eat if they are hungry. Remember this before turning meals into battlegrounds.

ADHD

Causes: Attention deficit hyperactivity disorder is thought by some to be a genetic abnormality of neurological development in which the brain nerve transmitters are disordered. There are associations with low birth weight, pregnancy complications, or the mother smoking or drinking during pregnancy. Others cannot accept that a genetic disorder could become so common so fast – 1% of UK and 5% of US children being diagnosed. Though diet is often blamed, there is little evidence for this. Controversy will remain while there is no clear cause.

Symptoms: A short attention span, impulsive behaviour, overactivity, variable school performance and an inability to follow rules. There is often a delay in speech or physical co-ordination. Symptoms usually appear at 2–3 years of age and affect all areas of the child's life. Symptoms persist into adult life in over 50% of cases.

Treatment: Exhausted parents and the unhappy child both need sympathetic support to try to structure the child's life with clear rules. Increasingly the drug methyphenidate is used in children over 6 and improves 80% of cases. Alternatives are anti-depressants such as imipramine.

FEEDING PROBLEMS

Causes: Many young children are faddy eaters and refuse foods. Some simply dislike the taste and texture of solid food.

Symptoms: These include outright refusal, sticking to one food, throwing food and spitting it out.

Treatment: With a thriving child there is little harm. Offer varying textures and flavours, praising 'good eating'. Remove food left after 20 minutes but do not allow sweets or snacks.

TEMPER TANTRUMS

Causes: Tantrums are normal, but likelier in children from disturbed families, neglected children and those with chronic illness, especially **cerebral palsy** and speech disorders.

Symptoms: Shouting, biting, scratching and breaking things in response to frustration. Tantrums beyond four are abnormal.

Treatment: Ignore the tantrum – if possible by leaving the room. If this is impossible and, for example, you are in the middle of a supermarket, attempt to distract the child or hold the child tightly. Do not give in with a reward.

HYPERACTIVITY

Causes: This is controversial in diagnosis and cause; dietary factors are unproven. Theories include children on the edge of normality, inappropriate learnt behaviour or slight brain damage.

Symptoms: The child is impulsive, rapidly switching activity, fidgeting and running around. It rarely lasts beyond adolescence.

Treatment: Rule out neurological damage, **epilepsy** or hearing disorders. Behavioural techniques ignore unacceptable behaviour and reward 'good' behaviour.

Avoid food colouring, though there is no good evidence for extreme diets. Medication is used infrequently in the UK.

BED-WETTING (ENURESIS)

Causes: There are emotional and strong hereditary influences.

Symptoms: The child wets the bed when deeply asleep.

Treatment: Rule out urinary infection. Resolve family or parental tension. Restrict drinks before bed. The drug desmopressin reduces urinary output during the night.

INCONTINENCE OF FAECES

Causes: This is often **constipation** with leakage of faeces. Deliberate incontinence suggests psychological disturbance.

Symptoms: Leakage of faeces with embarrassment typify constipation with overflow or other physical problems. Deliberate soiling typifies psychological causes.

Treatment: Constipation with leakage requires laxatives for regular motions. Other causes need specialist psychological help.

Complementary Treatment
Bach flower remedies depend on the cause, for example cherry plum for loss of control. **Homeopathy** can succeed in overcoming school phobia. **Hypnotherapy** can help the child express the underlying issue. **Play therapy** is useful for emotional problems. *Other therapies to try: most have something to offer.*

COT DEATH

Sudden death of apparently healthy baby for no obvious reason.

CAUSES

The term cot death covers all unexpected infant deaths. Of those, a number will eventually be explained on post-mortem, when a few babies are shown to have a previously unsuspected abnormality of their heart or lungs and some may have a rare metabolic disorder. Those that remain unexplained are technically called sudden infant death syndrome (SIDS).

It is likely that SIDS is caused by a number of factors, rather than by one single cause. Some current theories are that babies are being kept too hot, that viral infection suddenly halts breathing or that allergic reactions are produced by environmental stimuli.

Following an unexpected infant death the police must be involved and invariably the possibility of deliberate harm must be considered, although this accounts for less than one in twenty-five cases in the United Kingdom.

Children at greatest risk of SIDS are between one and six months old; it is a little more frequent during winter, in boys, in babies of low birth weight, in babies living in poor socio-economic circumstances and in babies whose parents smoke.

SIDS is the most common reason for infant deaths after one month of age. In the United Kingdom about ten children a week die from it. This apparently high incidence is because other causes of death in infancy are now so rare, for example infections, accidents and **leukaemia**. Cot death is extremely uncommon after the age of one year.

SYMPTOMS

In most cases the child appeared well, fed normally and slept normally. Sometimes they had a minor infection. Children have been known to die just after being settled down, just after feeding or even in their parents' arms on a routine day.

TREATMENT

Every effort should be made to revive the baby, looking especially for food stuck in the throat. If efforts fail, the police and coroner must be informed and a post-mortem carried out.

Twins and other siblings

It is a sad but important fact that the surviving twin is at great risk of sudden death and a period of observation is recommended after one twin has died through cot death.

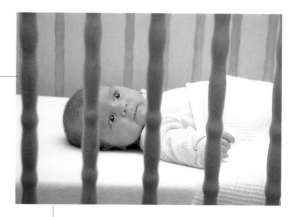

Above: Babies should be placed to sleep on their backs on a firm mattress, with their feet to the foot of the cot. Do not use pillows, duvets and cot bumpers.

Other siblings have a very slightly increased risk, too small to require any action, although it is understandable to be extra vigilant about minor illnesses until they reach one year of age.

Counselling

After such a tragedy parents have to cope with guilt, anger, fears about the health of remaining children and apprehension about another pregnancy. Such unresolved emotions can and do lead to the disintegration of the family. Parents experiencing a cot death should seek specialized counselling and consider joining one of the excellent support organizations.

Prevention

The 'Back to Sleep' campaign has been very effective in reducing the incidence of cot death worldwide. The simple message is to let babies sleep only on their backs. Other steps are not to smoke near a baby and not let the baby get over-hot (keep bedrooms within a degree or two of 18°C/65°F). Also, ensure the baby's head cannot be covered by bedding by making up their bed with their feet at the foot of the cot, which prevents them from wriggling down under the covers. Campaigns based on these messages have contributed to reducing by two-thirds the number of cot deaths since 1988 – decreasing in the United Kingdom from 1500 a year to 500 and still falling.

 ### Complementary Treatment

No complementary therapy can prevent a cot death. Ensure you follow the preventive advice above. During mourning deep relaxation techniques can help parents and other children. See BEREAVEMENT; also STRESS and ANXIETY. If you decide to try for another baby, **hypnotherapy** could help reduce anxiety about the progress of the pregnancy, and the health of your next baby.

DIAGNOSIS IS AT THE CORE of medicine, for without it it would be impossible to plan treatment. Diagnostic tools include everything from simply looking at your tongue to more complex studies using high-tech equipment to monitor the blood flow around your heart. This section covers many diagnostic procedures you may come across or undergo yourself, what they are used for, how they are performed, any risks they may have and likely future developments.

Low-technology medicine

Glancing through a textbook of medicine, you may be struck by the many entries named after doctors from the 18th and 19th centuries. These include Paget's disease, Heberden's nodes, Broca's area and Parkinson's disease to name just a few. Although these great doctors lacked modern diagnostic tools, they used their acute powers of observation to name the parts of the body and to recognize patterns of symptoms signifying specific diseases. They had nothing to go by but touch, smell and listening to the patient.

High-technology medicine

Modern medicine tries not to overlook the importance of observation in arriving at a diagnosis. There is still a great emphasis in medical training on teaching the skills of both history taking and physical examination (see pages 358 and 359), but this is increasingly being overshadowed by sophisticated investigations.

Investigations

At the simplest, an investigation might mean testing a sample of urine for sugar (glucose), and at the most complex having an MRI scan (see page 351). With easy access to investigations, doctors find it tempting to test for many things almost routinely, rather than thinking of probable diagnoses and doing the relevant tests. Since many tests are automated, it is relatively easy to do this.

However, there is a balance between the risks or discomfort of an investigation and the benefits that are to be accrued. The area most often involving risk is X-rays (see page 348). Although the risk is small, an X-ray is still a dose of radiation, which is why doctors may try to avoid them in circumstances where the X-ray is unlikely to make any difference to treatment, for example in uncomplicated lower back pain (see page 236).

Other tests carry disturbing implications. Antenatal tests for foetal abnormality fall into this category, posing a possible decision about terminating the pregnancy. This is why

DIAGNOSTIC TECHNIQUES

counselling is used before certain tests to be sure that you understand the decisions you will be faced with if a test proves abnormal. Genetic testing (see page 357) will certainly become one of the most controversial areas of medicine in the next few years.

Interpreting results

The more tests are done, the more likely an abnormality will appear, requiring a decision about further investigations. In arriving at this decision the doctor takes account of your general health, other symptoms and the pattern of abnormality as shown in the test. Unfortunately, this uncertainty is bound to generate anxiety on the patient's part, but without investigations there would be even more anxiety about illness.

Normal and abnormal Few investigations are absolutely 'normal' or abnormal; more often there is a large grey area of results ranging from possibly abnormal to probably 'normal'. Once again the interpretation has to take account of the history, the examination and the results of other tests. For this reason doctors will often repeat tests, especially the simple blood and urine tests, until the results become more definite. Interpreting the results from all of the diagnostic tests takes up a great deal of a doctor's thinking in order to come to an accurate diagnosis.

Right: Observation, touch and analysis are the fundmentals of diagnosis, helped by increasingly powerful investigative tools. The Physician's Visit by Jan Havicksz Steen (1625/26–79).

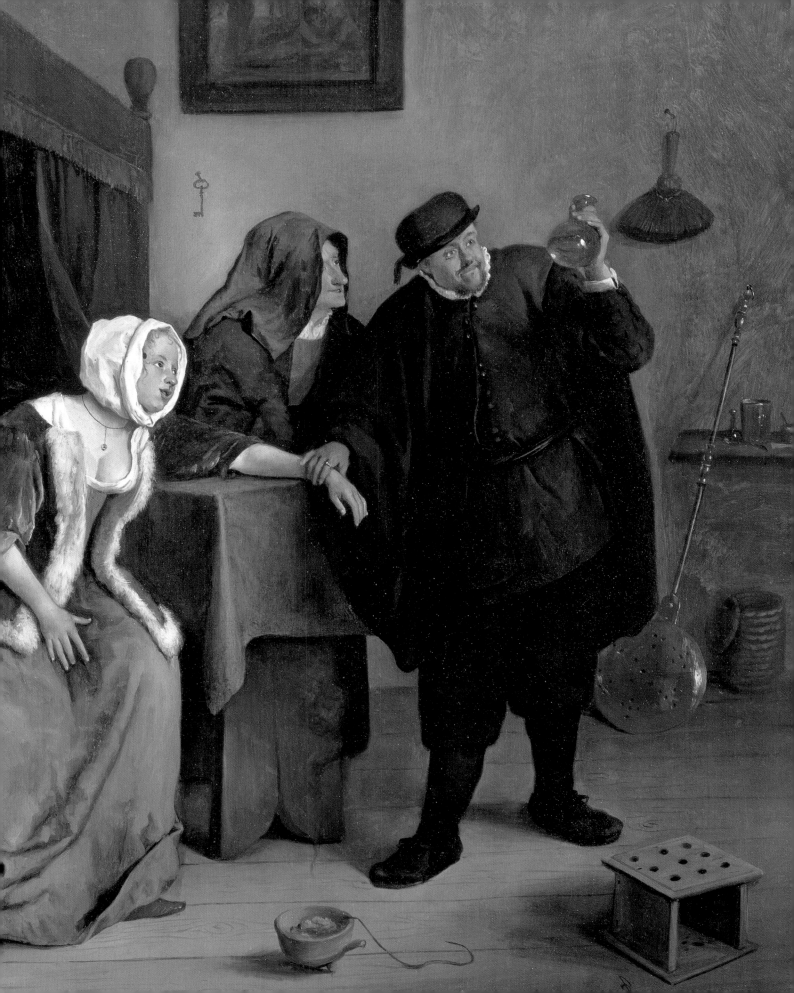

X-RAYS

Discovered by chance by Roentgen in 1895, X-rays are waves of electro-magnetic radiation that are in the same family as light and radio waves. Their very short wavelength (much shorter than visible light) lets them penetrate solid material. Variations of density within the material show up as X-ray shadows similar to light shadows. X-rays are captured on photographic plates as negative films. They are taken by radiographers, skilled in positioning patients to get the most informative views and calculating the exposure needed. The interpretation of X-rays is done by radiologists, doctors who also perform a wide range of investigations using X-rays.

What X-rays can detect

X-rays are good for detecting abnormalities in bones, especially fractures (see page 239), and problems in the lungs. They are not good at detecting abnormalities in soft tissues, for example in the brain or the intestines. This is because X-rays penetrate these parts too well to show much detail and because everything they pass through casts shadows on the photographic plate, thereby blurring the image. X-rays can detect gross changes, such as whether the heart is enlarged or there is paralysis of the bowels. They may not give the precise diagnosis but they are enough to show that something is seriously wrong.

How an X-ray is performed

The X-ray equipment is brought close to the part of you being studied while you stay very still for the fraction of a second required. Some studies call for a series of photos, such as X-rays of the kidney, or a continuous film as in coronary artery angiography (see below). It takes a minute or so to develop the film.

X-ray films are nearly always photographic negatives where dense material, such as bone, shows white, and less dense material such as muscle shows grey.

Other forms of X-ray

By using materials that appear white on an X-ray, radiologists can improve how well soft tissues show up. For example, dyes can be injected into the blood stream to show blood flow within internal organs. When used in the kidneys, this is called an intravenous pyelogram; in the heart it is called coronary angiography (see below).

Barium studies Barium liquid is another material that is widely used, since barium does not dissolve in water and passes harmlessly out of the body. A barium swallow or barium meal outlines the gullet, stomach and intestine, and is used to detect ulcers, cancers and narrowing of these organs. A barium enema involves pumping barium into the rectum, then manoeuvring the patient around to coat barium on the walls of the bowels. A barium enema is used to investigate abdominal pains and bleeding from the back passage and for detecting cancers, diverticular disease and inflammatory bowel disease (see page 176).

Coronary artery angiography A very thin tube called a catheter is fed to the heart via a large artery or vein, usually in the groin. Under X-ray control the tip is brought close to the heart's own arteries, the coronary arteries. A harmless dye is pumped into the blood stream, while taking a rapid series of X-rays showing how blood flows around the heart. This will detect blockages and determine whether a person should have coronary artery bypass surgery (see page 41). A similar

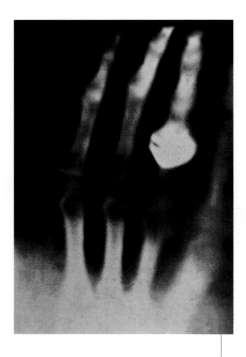

Above: An X-ray by Roentgen of his wife's hand. X-rays are among the most important diagnostic aids ever invented.

technique can demonstrate blood flow through the arteries of the abdomen and legs, if arterial disease is suspected.

Safety

X-rays can burn in overdose, which is why the early specialists, not knowing this, frequently developed cancers of their hands. Modern X-rays are very low dosage, thanks to finely focused equipment and sensitive photographic plates. For example, a chest X-ray involves a dose of radiation similar to that received naturally during a transatlantic plane journey. Legal guidelines limit the annual exposure to medical X-rays to an amount equivalent to six months' natural exposure to radiation. They should be avoided altogether during pregnancy unless essential to protect life.

ULTRASOUND

This is a technique in which high-frequency sound waves penetrate the body, casting sound shadows, which are then analysed. It is called ultrasound because the sound frequency is much too high to hear (the frequencies are well above 30,000 cycles per second). Each time the sound beam passes through a different material (blood, water, flesh and bone) the signal changes slightly. These tiny variations in the transmission and reflection of sound are detected by sensitive microphones. The pattern is further analysed by computer to generate a picture of the internal organs as grey shadows on a TV screen. The display is a continuous one, unlike most X-rays (see opposite), and reveals a world of internal movement and structure.

How ultrasound is performed

A watery gel is rubbed on to the skin in order to improve the transmission of the ultrasound beam. The source of ultrasound, shaped like a flat probe, is held against the skin. The operator focuses the ultrasound beam and moves it around. The resulting echoes are electronically analysed as pure sound, such as the baby's heartbeat, or into pictures showing structures, which is technically called echosonography.

What ultrasound can detect

Ultrasound is good at showing hollow internal organs. This has made it the method of choice for monitoring the growth of the unborn baby by taking measurements of the diameter of the skull or the baby's length (see page 130). Other uses for ultrasound are in looking at the kidneys or bladder and abdominal organs

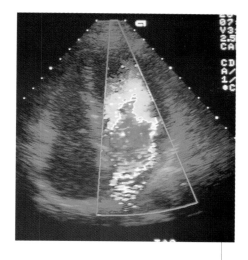

Above: An ultrasound view across the heart. The colours reflect the speed of the blood flow through one of the valves — red for slowest, blue for fastest.

such as the liver and gall bladder. Ultrasound is also helpful for detecting disease in the prostate gland (see page 118) or the breasts.

Gynaecological uses of ultrasound include detecting disease of the ovaries, such as cysts, and diseases of the womb, such as fibroids (see page 158). Ultrasound has made the diagnosis of an ectopic pregnancy (see page 134), where the fertilized egg settles in the Fallopian tube rather than the womb, much more reliable. It is also used in investigating bleeding in early pregnancy to see whether the foetus is still alive or has miscarried (see page 144).

Ultrasound images look rather like a television picture with a lot of interference. It takes a trained eye to see the detail, but with modern equipment the degree of it is remarkable.

Echocardiography

Ultrasound examination of the heart has become one of the most important applications of the technique and is revolutionizing the understanding of heart function and heart disease. The ultrasound beam is shone between the ribs (a constant nuisance in imaging the heart) to focus on

each chamber of the heart (the atria and the ventricles) and the heart valves (the aortic, mitral, tricuspid and pulmonary valves). Measurements can be electronically analysed to give the work capacity of the heart, to show how efficiently the valves are performing, whether any of them are leaking and whether the heart muscle is healthy. Ultrasound is now the best way of confirming whether someone has heart failure, valve disease and aneurysms (abnormally swollen blood vessels with fragile walls). What ultrasound cannot yet do is to show actual blood flow around the heart. For this you will still require X-ray coronary artery angiography (see opposite).

Other forms of ultrasound

Some other applications of much higher energy ultrasound make use of its heating effect, as applied in sports physiotherapy. Similarly, lithotripsy (see page 369) is a means of shattering kidney stones by employing sound waves at a much higher and more focused level of energy.

Safety

Ultrasound has been exhaustively tested for safety. There is no evidence that the doses used in ultrasound imaging do any harm at all, even to the unborn baby, which is why it is used so extensively.

CT SCANNING

Computed tomography (CT) is a means of using X-rays (see page 348) plus powerful computing to generate images of the interior of the body. When X-rays pass through the body, the shadows from everything they pass through lie superimposed on top of each other. The result is a flat image of the actual three-dimensional structure of the body, just like a television picture is a flat image of reality. However, if an X-ray is taken from a slightly different position (called an X-ray cut) all these shadows shift slightly and they shift once again when another 'cut' is taken. The breakthrough of CT scanning was in harnessing computers to analyse the tiny variations in each of the X-ray cuts in order to reconstruct an image of the interior of the body.

The technique was not entirely new. It was called tomography, but the results were a blurred image of one part of the body and not much else. In CT scanning the computers allow a reconstruction of any part of the body caught in the X-ray beam. Thus for the first time it was possible to see details of soft structures of the body, especially the brain and the abdomen, without painful or hazardous injections or operations. Indeed, the technique revolutionized the investigation of brain disorders, which until the 1970s had often been extremely unpleasant and not very revealing. CT scanning was an amazing advance in X-ray technology, for which the inventor Godfrey Hounsfield was awarded a Nobel Prize.

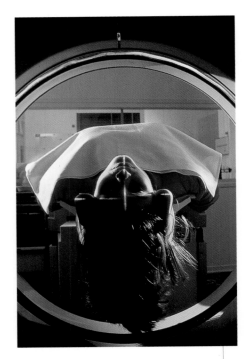

Above: A patient lying still within a CT scanner. Newer CT machines are not so bulky and intimidating and take less time to perform the scan.

How a CT scan is performed

All the work is carried out by the X-ray apparatus; the person being scanned just lies there as still as possible. Every few seconds the equipment takes a fresh X-ray cut through the body, moving on a few millimetres before taking the next cut. The process takes between ten and twenty minutes depending on how much is being scanned. The images can be improved by giving an injection of a contrast material which shows up better on X-ray; this is particularly useful for images of the brain. The very latest scanners take their photos much faster and are able to cope with moving organs such as the heart.

Safety

The total X-ray dose is larger than an ordinary X-ray but is still very small and no important side effects have emerged. Some people get claustrophobic in the apparatus or they cannot lie still enough for good images so it is not useful for people who cannot cooperate or for children, unless they are sedated beforehand.

What CT scanning can detect

Modern CT scans can detect abnormalities of less than 1 cm/⅜ in diameter. When scanning the brain, CT can investigate headaches, confirm strokes and detect brain tumours and features of multiple sclerosis. Another major application is in scanning the abdomen to investigate abdominal pain and possible cancers, in particular cancer of the pancreas, which is otherwise difficult to diagnose.

A further application has been in imaging the spinal bones and the spinal cord to investigate back pain or slipped discs. CT scans – and MRI scans even more so (see opposite) – are shedding new light on disease of bone (see page 243) and joints elsewhere, replacing exploratory surgery.

High-speed CT scanners can be used to investigate the heart, providing high-quality images and giving useful information about the muscles and valves. However, the scans do not give such good information about blood flow or atherosclerosis (see page 40), although research may improve this application. Other invaluable applications of CT scans are in investigating lung, liver and kidney disease.

MRI SCANNING

The letters MRI stand for magnetic resonance imaging, the latest and so far the most spectacular way of showing images of the interior of the body. The concept behind MRI is basically simple, although the physics and computers needed are very complex.

The technique relies on the fact that atoms in certain circumstances behave like tiny magnets. Hydrogen atoms are the best ones to show this property and are found throughout the body in fluids, fat and soft tissues such as the brain. Placing someone in an extremely powerful magnetic field makes many of their hydrogen atoms line up in relation to the magnetic field. The next step is to push those atoms out of alignment using a beam of radio waves. When that beam is switched off, the hydrogen atoms realign in the magnetic field, emitting a radio signal as they do so. By analysing that radio wave it is possible to build up an image of the hydrogen-rich parts of the body and turn this into photographs.

How MRI is performed

To achieve the very high magnetic field, you have to lie inside a bulky apparatus during the 20–30 minutes it takes to perform the scan. Some people find this claustrophobic, much more so than with CT scans (see opposite). Because of the magnetism, you must remove all metal objects such as jewellery from your body. People who have implanted metallic objects such as heart pacemakers or metallic clips from surgical operations cannot therefore be scanned.

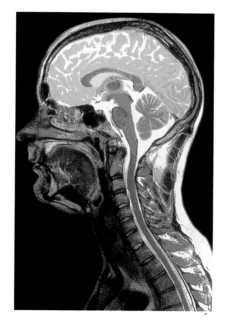

Above: An MRI scan showing the brain and spinal cord in anatomical detail.
Above right: A section through the brain and eyeballs.

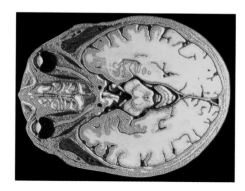

Safety

Intense magnetic fields and radio waves produce temporary changes in the body but so far none that appear to cause any serious effects. Until this is certain, there are restrictions on how long people are exposed to the magnetic fields. Scanning appears to be safe during pregnancy, but under current guidelines it is not routinely used until more research has been done.

What MRI can detect

The scans provide brilliant images of the brain for diagnosing tumours (see page 92), strokes (see page 80) and multiple sclerosis (see page 82). They show up slipped discs and narrowings in the spinal canal that may be the cause of back pain (see pages 236 and 240). So successful and reliable is MRI scanning for these conditions that it is gradually replacing CT scanning, even though it is still much more expensive.

Joint problems are another success story for MRI scanning, whether in the neck, shoulder or, especially, the knee, where MRI can reveal whether the internal ligaments are damaged and various other causes of knee pain. In all of these joints it shows muscle damage and bruising far better than any technique hitherto available. Probably MRI scanning will replace arthroscopy (looking inside the joint under anaesthetic) in the near future as a means of diagnosis, although arthroscopy will continue as a means of treatment.

Scans are also performed on the abdomen and the heart. Using rapid scanning, it is becoming possible to image the abdominal organs in detail to investigate abdominal pain or possible cancers, for example in the liver, pancreas, womb, ovaries and gall bladder. Scans of the heart can visualize the valves, the muscle of the heart walls and blood clots from previous damage, such as a heart attack. It is now possible to see blood vessels well enough to tell if they are narrowed with atherosclerosis (see page 40), a valuable use of MRI that will eventually transform the ease of investigating coronary artery disease.

The future

This is a rapidly evolving technology, still under 15 years old. Exciting future prospects are to improve the images of blood vessels in the heart and brain and to focus on the activity of the brain by giving injections of materials taken up by its active parts.

NUCLEAR MEDICINE
AND PET SCANS

Although viewed by many with suspicion, radioactive techniques have a long-established role in medical investigation and treatment.

What is radioactivity?

Atoms are usually stable particles that do not break down. Radioactive atoms are unstable; they break down into their component parts, such as neutrons, protons and electrons. Many substances contain a small percentage of naturally radioactive forms called isotopes, which are therefore unavoidable in the environment, whether in food, water or the rocks and atmosphere around us. These contribute to what is called background radiation. For the purposes of nuclear medicine, isotopes are selected which are rapidly excreted from the body and which pose minimal risk of radiation damage. Radiation techniques are not used in pregnancy and are avoided in people of reproductive age unless it is essential.

Safety

Safety has to be uppermost in using radioactive substances. The dosages used are carefully regulated and there are maximum annual amounts that can legally be given. While it is true that there is no absolutely safe minimum dose of radiation, the risks are much lower than the risks of other investigations that they can replace, for example bone biopsy under anaesthetic or coronary artery angiography, and are actually comparable to the natural background radiation to which we are all exposed.

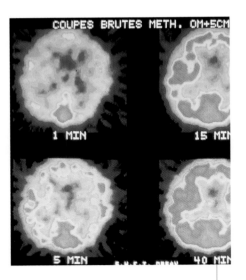

Above: Consecutive PET *scans; the red marker spreads to areas of high brain activity.*

How radio scans are performed

The idea behind radio scans is to label with a radioactive isotope something that is concentrated in the part of the body to be investigated. To do this, a few days or immediately before scanning, a radioactive substance is either taken by mouth or injected into the body. In the case of the thyroid gland this is radio-labelled iodine; for the heart it is the elements thallium or technetium, which are absorbed by the heart muscles. The radioactivity given off is measured by detectors and the results can be shown as a scan.

Heart Radioactivity scans are much less detailed than CT or MRI scans (see pages 350 and 351), but they do give important information on whether particular organs are working and how efficiently. For example, radio scans of the heart show whether there is a problem with blood flow during exercise which is serious enough to justify going on to the more detailed but more hazardous coronary artery angiography (see page 348).

Lungs and bones Radioisotopes have an important role in detecting disease in lungs and bones more quickly and safely than taking biopsies.

The main use in lung disease is to detect a pulmonary embolus (see page 67). This is done by intravenous injection of a liquid isotope or by breathing in a radioactive gas. The resulting scan shows whether blood is reaching all parts of the lungs or is blocked by a blood clot.

Scanning is particularly used to see whether bone pain is from secondary deposits from cancer. This is an important investigation before starting intensive treatment, for example in breast cancer (see page 146), which may not be advisable if a bone scan shows that the disease is already widespread in the skeleton.

PET scanning

Positron emission scanning (PET) is a relatively new type of scan using isotopes that emit particles called positrons and gamma rays. The main use has been in brain scans. An injection is given of an isotope, usually absorbed into glucose (sugar), which is the brain's main fuel. By detecting where the glucose goes, the PET scan shows the levels of activity of different parts of the brain. This is useful in detecting brain damage.

As a research tool PET scans show what parts of the brain are involved when performing mental activities such as speech as opposed to mental arithmetic, when smelling something or performing a particular task, such as writing. Such scanning may eventually lead to more precise knowledge of how the brain is organized.

BIOPSY

A biopsy means taking a sample of living body material. This is often the only way to make a definite diagnosis for some conditions.

Types of biopsy

Even a simple blood test (see page 354) is a type of biopsy, since the blood contains living elements, but more usually two other types of biopsy are performed. The first involves cutting out a section of a tissue such as skin or muscle for analysis under a microscope. This is most commonly done with skin problems such as coloured lumps, the nature of which is not clear to the naked eye (see page 225).

Other forms of biopsy are taken with a specially designed needle. These are used to diagnose suspicious breast lumps (see page 146) and to take samples from the liver, kidneys or bone marrow. The needles are inserted under local anaesthetic and pick up a core of the material desired. After being withdrawn the core is pushed out into a preservative solution.

Biopsies can also be taken from the stomach, intestines and even the brain.

When is a biopsy performed?

Not every condition can be diagnosed by appearance alone, yet important decisions on treatment require a precise diagnosis. Rather than subject someone to an unnecessary major operation, it is more practicable to obtain a small sample of tissue first. This is common practice in dealing with coloured skin lumps and with lumps in or under the skin that have a suspicious feel to them. It is also carried out on the cervix after a suspicious smear test (see page 148).

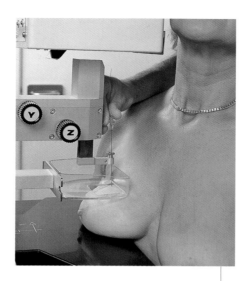

Above: A breast biopsy, using a frame to guide the needle precisely.

Persistently swollen lymph glands are one of the most common diagnostic dilemmas. Lymph glands in the neck or armpit are only doing their job if they swell up temporarily when there is an infection, but persistent swelling is abnormal and may be a feature of types of leukaemia (see page 252) or Hodgkin's disease (see page 250). In these cases, a diagnosis can only be arrived at by taking a biopsy of the gland.

At other times biopsies are taken as a kind of fishing expedition, for example, in investigating unusual bleeding from the womb or changes of bowel habit. In the case of bleeding from the back passage, although the lining of the bowel may look normal, a biopsy may indicate features of inflammatory bowel disease (see page 176). Certain obscure illnesses affecting nerve or muscle may prove a complete mystery until a sample of muscle can be analysed.

Lastly, after surgery for cancer, it is common to take a sample from the margins of the tumour that has been removed to make quite sure that none has been missed at the very edges of the growth.

How the material is analysed

Normally the tissues or cells are analysed under the microscope. To be seen well a biopsy usually has to be stained to show the cells, the nuclei of the cells and other tissue components. Staining takes time, after which the material has to be carefully cut into thin fragments small enough to be spread on a microscope slide. Interpreting the slides is done by a pathologist, skilled in recognizing different types of tissues and deciding what is normal and what is abnormal.

Healing after biopsies

Often so little material is taken during a biopsy that you need nothing more than a protective plaster for a couple of days; sometimes you need a stitch or two. The linings of the stomach, bowels and womb heal extremely rapidly without the need for stitches.

Getting results

Having a biopsy generates unavoidable anxiety, and because doctors are aware of this they try to get results back rapidly. Ordinarily it takes a couple of days to perform the analysis, but occasionally biopsies are taken during surgery to guide the surgeon on whether he has completely removed a tumour. In these cases a pathologist will stand by to report on the tissue immediately.

BIOCHEMISTRY AND BLOOD TESTS

The blood is one of the most easily accessible parts of the internal workings of the body and at the same time one of the most informative. Just a few millilitres of blood is all that is needed for even the most sophisticated blood tests.

What blood contains

Blood comprises red and white blood cells and platelets, which all float in a pool of liquid called plasma. Plasma contains hormones, proteins, sugar and many other chemicals essential to the working of the body.

Taking blood

For routine tests, blood from a vein in the arm is acceptable. The large antecubital vein lies in the fold of the elbow and is prominent enough for easy access. A cuff is placed around the arm to make the vein swell, then a hollow needle is passed into the vein by the doctor, nurse or technician (phlebotomist). The operator draws back on a syringe to get the amount required, although some syringes are vacuum sealed and fill automatically. The cuff is released, the needle withdrawn and a swab kept over the site for a few minutes to stem any bleeding.

The blood is transferred into a sample bottle – there are various types depending on the tests required. Some have fluid at the bottom to stabilize components of the blood until it can be analysed.

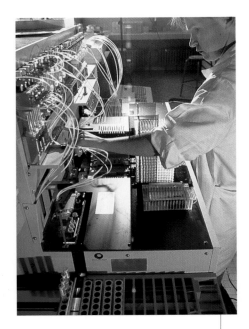

Above: Many blood tests are performed using sophisticated automated analysers.

Types of test

Blood chemicals The common ones measured are sodium, potassium, calcium and iron. These are fundamental to nerve and muscle function. Less often measured are magnesium, copper, zinc and many others that are important in rare medical conditions.

Biochemicals These more complex molecules are formed by the body, for example sugar (glucose), uric acid, ferritin, creatinine, albumin, alkaline phosphatase and many more. The commonly requested ones are grouped according to the organs most responsible for making them: liver function tests, kidney function tests, bone function tests and blood fats (cholesterol and lipids).

Hormones These are not measured as routinely. Examples are prolactin, thyroid-stimulating hormone, insulin, progesterone, testosterone and growth hormone. Frequently the test must be taken under more precise conditions – for example at a specific time of day, at rest, or mid-menstrual cycle.

Blood cells Tests analyse the quantities, types and appearance of the red and white blood cells and the platelets. Such information reveals anaemia or types of infection or explains unusual bleeding, among many other possibilities.

Miscellaneous Numerous proteins are tested if particular diagnoses are in mind, for example C reactive protein is a measure of inflammation within the body. The commonly requested ESR (erythrocyte sedimentation rate) is another measure of inflammation within the body whether from infection, arthritis or cancers and is measured by seeing how long it takes for a thin column of blood to settle into its component parts. Commonly measured vitamins include B_{12} and folic acid.

Arterial blood This might be analysed to measure oxygen concentrations for people with acute heart and breathing problems. The blood is taken by a more complex technique from the radial artery in the wrist or from the femoral artery in the groin.

Analysis

Most blood tests are now analysed through automatic blood sampling machines capable of working on very small quantities of blood. The analysis actually starts in the tube(s) the blood is put into, which are selected according to the tests required.

The analysis comes out of the analyser as a string of values, which can be compared to the normal range for that item, for example a normal level of blood protein can be 62–80 g per litre.

For haematology tests, as well as counting cell types it is also important to know the sizes and shapes of cells. Much of this can be also be done automatically, but sometimes a technician has to physically grade a sample of cells by examining them under the microscope.

ENDOSCOPY, COLONOSCOPY AND BRONCHOSCOPY

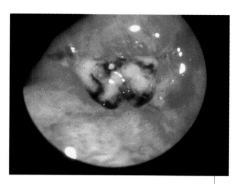

Above: Endoscopy of a stomach ulcer, showing black clotted blood and red fresh blood. Right: An endoscope being passed down the throat into the oesophagus and stomach.

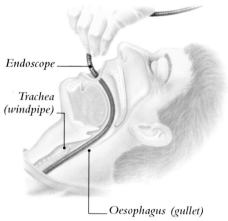

Endoscope — Trachea (windpipe) — Oesophagus (gullet)

Endoscopy means looking inside the body through tubes in order to investigate abnormalities. The technique relies on narrow fibre tubes called endoscopes, which carry light efficiently and are highly flexible. A bright light source plus miniaturized operating devices allow both biopsies (see page 353) and manipulation of flesh. In electronic endoscopes fibre-optic bundles are replaced with tiny colour-sensitive electronic chips displaying a television image, which can be recorded and reviewed.

Endoscopes have flexible tips in order to get the best view and devices that squirt water and suck or blow air – also important for obtaining the best possible view.

The purpose of endoscopes

One of the major uses is in the examination of common intestinal symptoms, ranging from indigestion and stomach pains to bleeding from the back passage, constipation and chronic abdominal pains. Endoscopy has greatly simplified the exploration of these problems, for which the only earlier techniques were barium meals and barium enemas (see page 348), although these are still useful. One enormous advantage of endoscopy is that it allows the lining of the intestines to be seen and samples to be taken. Another important use of the technique is bronchoscopy, which looks inside the tubes of the lungs (bronchi) to investigate lung symptoms such as breathlessness and coughing blood.

Endoscopy

This is done under light sedation and after spraying a local anaesthetic on the back of the throat. The thin flexible tube is guided down the gullet and beyond. The operator twists the tip so as to inspect the walls of the gullet, then the stomach and as far as the duodenum, taking samples from suspicious-looking areas.

Instruments attached to the tip of the endoscope can be used to stop bleeding from veins in the gullet and to pass tubing up the ducts connecting the gall bladder to the duodenum. This latter technique is very important for visualizing the flow of bile from the gall bladder, to remove gall stones that are stuck (see page 180) and for investigating disease of the pancreas. The technique is called endoscopic retrograde cholangiopancreatography (ERCP). It is necessary to rest for an hour or two after undergoing an endoscopy.

Colonoscopy

Colonoscopy is done to inspect the lower bowel, from the anus through the rectum and along the large intestine. It may also be possible to reach as far as the caecum, where the small intestine joins the large intestine – an important region for cancerous growths and other diseases.

For a proper examination, bowel contents have to be cleared a day before examination by laxatives and possibly an enema. Patients are given a sedative plus a painkiller and drugs to relax the bowel. The flexible instrument is passed through the back passage and guided right around the large intestine. As with endoscopy, the operator sees the walls of the bowel and can sample suspicious-looking areas. Growths, called polyps, can also be removed. Because of the higher sedation, patients have to rest under observation for at least two hours after colonoscopy.

Bronchoscopy

This procedure is also done under sedation. The bronchoscope is passed via the nose down the trachea and bronchi, and biopsies are taken from the walls of the bronchi or the lung itself, which is more hazardous. The examination takes about 15 minutes.

Safety

The main risk is pushing the endoscope through the wall of the bowel; this is a very rare complication, estimated at one in every hundred thousand colonoscopies. In bronchoscopy, where a lung biopsy is taken, there is a risk of causing a pneumothorax (the collapse of one lung) so a postoperative chest X-ray is done routinely. The instruments are of course fully sterilized to eliminate the risk of cross-infection.

ANTENATAL TESTS

Increasingly sophisticated techniques are giving ever more information about the health of the unborn child. These possibilities are also raising ethical dilemmas about handling the results, which is why it is routine to offer counselling beforehand. This is so that parents understand the risks of the test, its reliability and what recommendations apply if an abnormality is detected. These tests are changing all the time; below are the currently used ones. Others are being developed using urine samples.

Blood tests

Rubella (German measles) This infection has devastating effects on the developing foetus if contracted during the first four months of pregnancy. A blood test in the first 16 weeks of pregnancy shows whether the mother is immune, in which case exposure to rubella (see page 262) carries no risk. If blood tests show no immunity, the mother must avoid exposure to rubella and ensure she is immunized after the baby is born well before any future pregnancy.

Alpha fetoprotein This is a substance released by a foetus with spina bifida (see page 337), which is detectable in the mother's blood stream. Finding high levels of alpha fetoprotein suggests either twins or a risk of an affected baby. The diagnosis must be further checked by detailed ultrasound scans (see page 349) and by amniocentesis (see below).

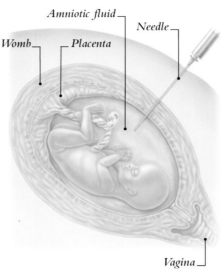

Above: Amniocentesis – a sample of amniotic fluid being withdrawn at 16–18 weeks.

Labels: Amniotic fluid, Needle, Womb, Placenta, Vagina

Tests for Down's syndrome These test several biochemical markers in the mother's blood stream; the usual ones are alpha fetoprotein, chorionic gonadotrophin and unconjugated oestradiol. They are a reliable indication of a number of foetal problems other than Down's syndrome (see page 337), including spina bifida, an undeveloped head (anencephaly) and, even rarer, an open abdominal wall (exomphalos). A firm diagnosis is not made on the blood tests alone; amniocentesis or chorionic villus sampling (see below) would also be offered.

Other tests

Amniocentesis It is possible to sample the amniotic fluid in which the baby floats, testing cells shed by the foetus into the fluid for abnormality. The test is done from about 14 weeks by passing a fine hollow needle through the mother's abdomen and drawing off fluid. The technique is used to confirm a diagnosis of spina bifida or Down's syndrome and for chromosome analysis. Amniocentesis carries a 0.5–1% chance of miscarriage, so it cannot be undertaken as a routine investigation. It takes about three weeks to get results.

Chorionic villus sampling This is another technique for deciding on the genetic make-up of the foetus. It can be performed from the tenth week of pregnancy. A needle is passed through the cervix or the mother's abdomen and guided, by ultrasound scanning, towards the placenta. The operator sucks up a small sample of the placenta, called chorionic villi, for analysis of the cells. The technique carries the similar 0.5–1% chance of causing a miscarriage. Results take just a few days but the technique does not detect spina bifida, anencephaly or exomphalos.

Ultrasound This can detect many cases of Down's syndrome by about 12 weeks but it is not yet accurate enough to replace other methods. In the second three months, ultrasound can detect spina bifida, abnormalities of the kidneys and heart and absence of a limb or fingers. Ultrasound is used to detect twins and to monitor the growth of the baby by measuring head size or length. It can establish the reason for bleeding in pregnancy, showing whether a foetus has survived a threatened miscarriage and whether there are abnormalities of the placenta, for example placenta praevia (see page 134). With newer techniques, such as scanning via the vagina, it is possible to detect foetal abnormalities by about 12 weeks. (See also page 349.)

Further investigations

Growth can be monitored by hormone blood tests and ultrasound of the baby's blood flow and heart rate. These tests help in deciding whether to let a high-risk pregnancy continue, for example if the mother has diabetes or high blood pressure (see page 135), or whether to induce labour or perform a Caesarean section (see page 139).

GENETIC ANALYSIS

The 'blueprint' of how to create life resides in the DNA (deoxyribonucleic acid) molecule (see page 132). DNA is organized into genes, sections of DNA which specify how to make each of the thousands of proteins on which life depends. The complete sequence of human DNA has recently been achieved. This fantastic achievement will probably transform genetic analysis within a decade.

Analysing DNA

From a blood sample, DNA is extracted using biochemical probes, which recognize particular sequences of DNA and break the molecule at those points. The fragments are separated by an electric current causing fragments to move at a rate dependent on their size.

Radioactive markers are then added which stick to known DNA sequences. By detecting the radioactivity on photographic plates, a picture of the DNA can be seen, showing whether particular fragments are present and thus whether the individual is susceptible to particular diseases or has abnormalities in his genetic make-up.

Polymerase chain reaction

This technique has opened up DNA analysis by 'amplifying' the minute amounts of DNA from just a single cell, for example as obtained from amniocentesis (see opposite). Biochemical probes targeted to the part of DNA of interest cause it to reproduce itself many times over, and after a few hours the technique produces millions of copies of a DNA sequence, enough for more detailed analysis.

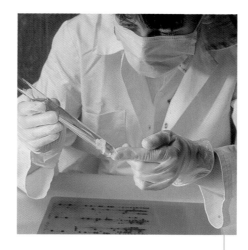

Above: A test tube of DNA over photographs of its genetic contents.

These are the techniques by which illnesses as diverse as breast cancer (see page 146) and schizophrenia (see page 84) are linked with particular DNA sequences.

Chromosomes

Humans have 23 pairs of chromosomes, including a pair of sex chromosomes that determine the individual's sex (see page 132). The chromosomes are revealed by staining cells and analysing chromosomes under the microscope.

The specialist looks for a full set of 23 pairs. Where there is a deficit or an excess of chromosomes, certain conditions can arise. For example, in Turner's syndrome, where there is a single female chromosome and no male chromosome, females are very short, have webbed neck skin and retarded sexual development. Extra chromosomes underlie conditions such as Down's syndrome (see page 337), where there is an extra chromosome 21, and Klinefelter's syndrome, where the presence of two female chromosomes plus a male one results in mental deficiency and abnormal male sexual development. Lack of a chromosome, apart from the sex chromosome, almost always causes gross physical abnormality and the death of the foetus. Apart from being absent or duplicated, chromosomes may be misformed in numerous ways.

Genetic family trees

If genetic disease is suspected, it is important to plot who else in a family is affected. This establishes whether a genetic condition has arisen spontaneously, for example most forms of Down's syndrome, or whether it is inherited, such as haemophilia or cystic fibrosis. The family pattern also shows whether the gene responsible is dominant (always causes the condition), or recessive (causes the condition only if no normal genes are present, as with sickle cell disease, see page 254).

The specialist can then calculate the risk of other members of a family or future children inheriting the condition. This is vital when counselling on the advisability of amniocentesis or chorionic villus sampling (see opposite), procedures which themselves carry risks.

Most important is knowing the risk of conceiving a child with an invariably fatal or disabling condition such as Huntingdon's chorea (leading to paralysis and dementia) or Tay-Sachs disease (causing blindness, mental retardation and early death). Parents may then decide not to have children or to abort on the basis of antenatal tests.

These heart-rending choices will probably become more common when further discoveries are made about the genetic contribution to disease. Already the latest technology allows rapid genetic analysis for a wide range of conditions not traditionally thought of as being genetically determined, such as high blood pressure (see page 38), but where research suggests some kind of genetic tendency. This is going to become one of the most controversial areas of medicine over the next few years.

COMPLEMENTARY DIAGNOSIS

Many complementary therapists arrive at a diagnosis in a similar way to conventional doctors, but with two major differences. First, such therapists concentrate on the whole person – the physical, emotional and psychological aspects, rather than only on the symptoms described and perhaps some personal factors. Secondly, each type of therapist will decide on a course of treatment based upon their individual speciality (see page 373).

Consultations with therapists often last longer than with conventional doctors, sometimes up to an hour, especially if you are seeing the therapist for the first time. Usually consultations fall into two parts.

Assessing the whole person

The therapist, like a conventional doctor, will ask about your physical symptoms – when they began, if they are intermittent or continuous and when they appear. Again, as with conventional doctors, the therapist will ask relevant questions regarding your personal, family, sexual and medical history, but will then broaden this to build up a complete picture of you as a person. This may entail finding out about your personality, behaviour, relationships, work, diet, lifestyle and current mental state in order to assess your overall physical and emotional health.

Physical examination

The type of examination will depend upon the therapist's speciality. For example, an acupuncturist will look at your appearance and posture, the colour of your skin, the lustre of your eyes and the condition of your tongue to assess

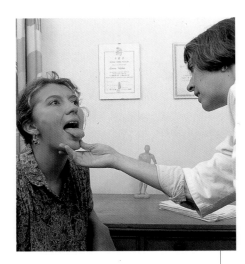

Above: A Chinese herbalist can determine a patient's health by checking the condition of the tongue.

whether there are energy blockages. A shiatsu-do practitioner will also look at these points but may feel parts of your body to see if there are underlying problems. Nutritional therapists may test hair, urine, sweat and muscles to see if there are deficiencies. A chiropractor will feel your spine and perhaps take some X-rays.

Diagnosis

The therapist will then discuss her findings with you, the treatment she proposes and the number of sessions needed.

HISTORY TAKING

During history taking, a doctor tries to obtain a precise description of your symptoms and form an overall picture of your state of health.

A doctor usually starts with open questions, such as 'What is troubling you?' or 'Tell me about this pain'. To complete a history he asks specific questions, such as 'Does coughing hurt?', 'Can you feel this?' or 'Do you feel depressed?'

Familiarity and fundamentals

In a long doctor–patient relationship a doctor already knows a great deal about you – problems you have had and your reactions to them. This helps decide on the significance of new symptoms and guides him through a physical examination (see opposite).

A doctor will want to know when the symptoms started, under what conditions they appear and what makes them better or worse. For pain, a doctor wants to ascertain its character, for example sharp or crushing, and whether it moves anywhere, for example from the chest into the neck. A doctor also wants to find out if there is anything else wrong, such as weight loss or fever.

Histories

Personal This concerns previous and current medical problems, your occupation, whether you smoke, drink or take drugs, and also whether you have done any recent foreign travelling.

Family Many illnesses run in the family, for example heart disease, so the health of parents, siblings and children is relevant.

Sexual It may be important to know whether you are at risk for AIDS or other sexually transmitted disease (see pages 122, 162 and 268).

Psychological This helps in assessing obscure symptoms or in deciding if depression or anxiety (see pages 70 and 72) may be causing physical symptoms, such as breathlessness or tiredness.

Diagnosis

At the end of history taking – which may take just a minute – a doctor should have a theory of what could be wrong and has probably decided upon the type of examination needed, the tests to be carried out and the likely diagnosis.

PHYSICAL EXAMINATION

Examining patients is one of the major skills doctors must master in order to arrive at a diagnosis.

A systematic approach

Doctors think in terms of body systems, for example the circulatory or cardiovascular system (see page 36) comprising the heart, arteries and veins, or the digestive system (see page 166) from the mouth to the anus. Examining each system follows procedures broadly the same worldwide.

Checking the circulatory system

These checks include:

♦ *Skin colour (blueness of fingers or tongue from lack of oxygen)*
♦ *Breathlessness*
♦ *Pulse rate (rapid, slow, irregular)*
♦ *Heart size (by feeling the chest wall)*
♦ *Heart sounds (regularity and any murmurs from abnormal blood flow)*
♦ *Blood pressure (see page 38)*
♦ *Veins in the neck (which distend in heart failure)*
♦ *Blood flow in arteries of the legs*
♦ *Ankle swelling (a feature of heart failure, among many other things)*

Detailed refinements are used if an abnormality is detected.

Physical examination in practice

Often patients complain of symptoms which span several systems. For example, breathlessness may result from heart, lung, hormone, kidney or psychological causes. It is inefficient and tedious to go through each of these systems in turn. Instead doctors make a general examination, probably starting at the head and working down, which they mentally analyse into the individual systems while they are thinking about possible causes.

With practice, a physical examination can be performed very rapidly – it takes just a few minutes to check the heart, lungs, abdomen and nervous system, although a very thorough total examination takes at least half an hour.

Looking and listening

Experienced doctors watch and listen to patients carefully and examine in a focused way, homing in on the likely problem area. While listening to your account of your symptoms and asking the questions posed during history taking (see opposite), the doctor is observing among many things:

♦ *Colour (the blueness from low oxygen, the pallor of anaemia or the yellow of jaundice)*
♦ *Gait, tremors and ability to use limbs*
♦ *Sweating or features of weight loss*
♦ *Features of pain (sweating, paleness or grimacing)*
♦ *Skin changes of eczema, psoriasis or acne*
♦ *Clubbed (highly curved) nails (typical of serious lung and heart disease)*
♦ *Mood, ability to speak, coherence and memory*

Basic tools

As well as the basic tools below, others are a sphygmomanometer to measure blood pressure and biochemically coated strips for testing blood for sugar (glucose) or urine for sugar, protein and blood. All of these help doctors reach reasonable conclusions about most symptoms.

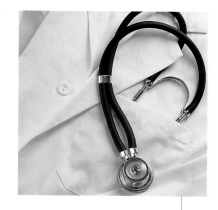

Above: Doctors rely heavily on their stethoscopes for diagnosis.

Stethoscope This is a device that amplifies sounds from the heart, lungs and intestines. Abnormal heart sounds or murmurs are found in heart disease and heart failure (see page 48). Taking blood pressure requires listening to sounds from the artery in the elbow as a pressure cuff is inflated and released. Lung sounds include the wheezing of asthma or bronchitis (see pages 57 and 58), the crackles of infection or fluid, or the absence of sound from a collapsed or fluid-filled lung. Listening to the abdomen may pick up a murmur from a diseased artery, the tinkling bowel sounds of obstruction, or the ominous absence of bowel sounds of peritonitis (infection within the abdomen).

Auroscope This bright light with ear pieces is used to inspect the ear, nose and throat.

Ophthalmoscope This is a bright light source with lenses to focus on the different parts of the eye. An opthalmoscope is used to check eye movements, reactions of the pupils and the health of the retina at the back of the eye.

Tendon hammer This is a stick with a weighted tip, which is used to test reflexes in the arms and legs. Variations in reflexes are an important sign of neurological disease, especially strokes (see page 80).

TYPES OF TREATMENT

HUMANS, IT HAS BEEN SAID, are a pill-taking animal. One hundred years ago, with modern surgery in its infancy, pills were almost the only choice of treatment. Today, people can be given treatments involving not just pills but electron beams, X-rays, sound waves, microscopic drills and transplantation of real and artificial organs. Even drug therapy has changed: now there are new ways of getting medication into the body, including implants, skin patches and hormone gels. And on the horizon there are smart drugs that will travel to targeted cells on specially designed molecules that latch on to tissues.

Behind these advances is an ever-more detailed knowledge of how the body works and increasingly sophisticated means of localizing the site of illness. This should allow doctors eventually to tailor treatments more exactly to the illness and deliver them more precisely to where things are going wrong.

This section reviews the major treatments possible. Many are exciting medical developments because they can reduce symptoms or cure serious illness as no other treatments in the past were able to do. This section also contains information about some complementary therapies.

'First, do no harm . . .'

Whatever the promise of a new treatment, doctors must bear in mind these words from Hippocrates 2500 years ago. The benefits should always outweigh the side effects. Treatments of all types are closely regulated by statutory authorities and need to prove their safety before they become accepted. The search for breakthroughs continues, but patient safety must always remain the number one priority. Patients are quite rightly now much more involved in choices of treatment.

Advances and breakthroughs

The development of techniques such as surgery and treatments for cancer is slower because it takes both courage for specialists to use untested procedures and time to use these new procedures on enough people to produce evidence of the benefits and drawbacks. Whereas drugs can be thoroughly tested in animals or in healthy volunteers, surgery and cancer therapies cannot be tested in the same way. The techniques can be trialled, but ultimately the only test is on ill people.

That said, certain medical advances are so clearly worthwhile that they become accepted rapidly. This has happened with laser and key-hole surgery and with surgical implants, all of which are revolutionary – the first two as less invasive treatments and the third as a means of prolonging or enhancing the quality of a person's life. True breakthroughs are unusual, however, despite the headlines. Behind such reports there is likely to be one of two things. The first is an advance in technology which can be applied to medicine, for example improved scanners. The second is a treatment which shows promise, but which is still years off full evaluation, such as a vaccine against cancer.

And yet true breakthroughs do occur and no more so than in the last 30 years. The most outstanding ones are transplantation of organs, ultrasound treatment for kidney problems and key-hole surgery as already mentioned. These will be described in detail in this section.

Other forms of treatment evolve through steady, careful research, achieving minor changes which, over time, together add up to big improvements. These include intensive care and drug therapy in general, both which are also covered here.

Treatment menus

For serious illnesses, medical care is now likely to involve a combination of treatments. For example, heart disease may begin with medication to reduce cholesterol, move to angioplasty to open up blocked coronary arteries, then end with a heart transplant and chemotherapy to keep rejection at bay. Cancers are often removed surgically, then treatment may continue with a combination of radiotherapy and chemotherapy. Treatment menus such as these appear to be the path of the future.

Right: We have begun the 21st century with treatments that were unimaginable at the beginning of the 20th century. The Surgeon by Jan Sanders van Hemessen (c.1504–66).

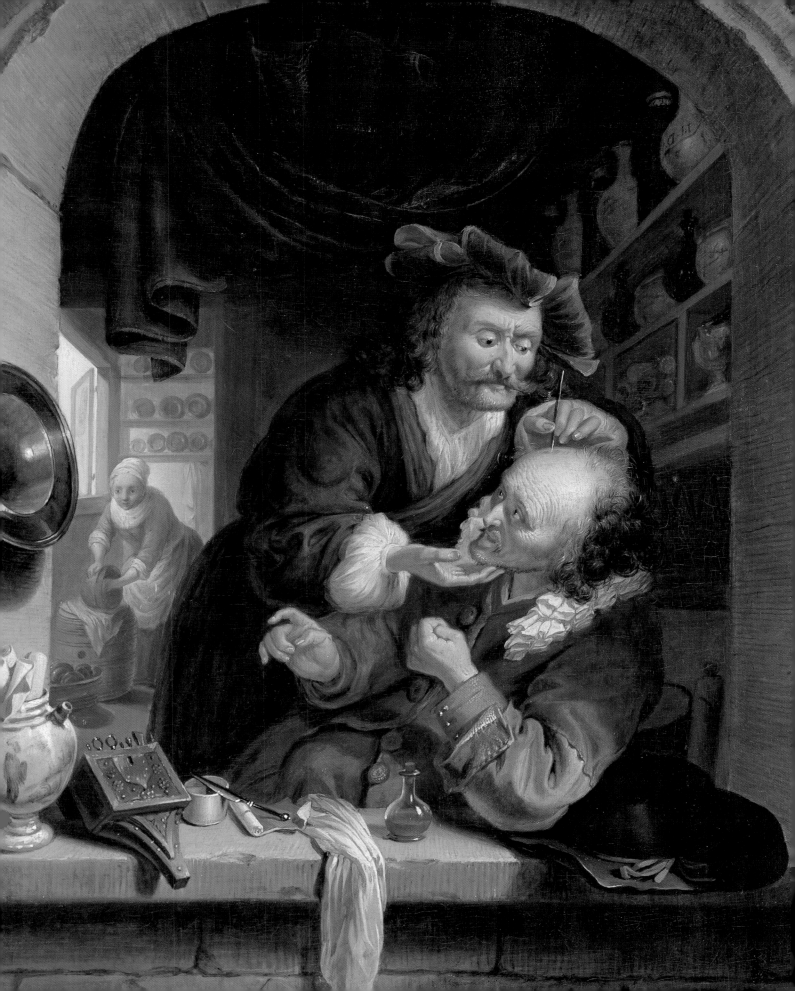

SURGICAL IMPLANTS

Living tissue is in some ways remarkably strong and resilient, but in other ways it is very delicate and easily damaged permanently. Over the centuries surgeons have used crude artificial replacements for damaged tissue, such as metal limbs, but the last century has seen particular advances in such techniques.

The great advantage of an artificial implant is that the body is unlikely to reject it, since rejection is what bedevils transplant surgery (see opposite). The following are the most common implants.

Artificial joints

Hips Hip replacement surgery started in the 1960s. Since then techniques have been refined to provide a wide choice of artificial hips.

There are two parts to the artificial hip: a plastic cup is set into the pelvic bone and the upper femur (thigh bone) is replaced by a metal tip, cemented into the rest of the femur.

Artificial hips last for ten to fifteen years. The main complications are infection, loosening and dislocation. Artificial hips can be replaced in an operation that is technically demanding.

Knees Implanting artificial knees is increasingly the treatment for severe pain. Part or all of the knee can be replaced with metal and plastic components, hinged to give a good range of back and front and side-to-side movement.

Other joints There are good results from the replacement of the whole shoulder joint and the small joints of the hand. These are likely to become more widely available operations in the future.

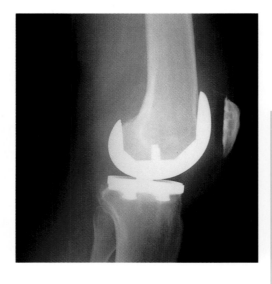

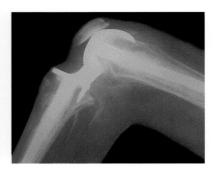

Above and left: Two of the many types of artificial knee joint available; different surgeons have their favourites.

Heart implants

Heart valves Valves damaged by atherosclerosis (see page 40), rheumatic fever or simply age cause breathlessness or heart failure. The Starr-Edwards valve, a ball within a cylinder, is still, after 35 years, the most widely used artificial valve. The flat Bjork-Shiley valve is another type. After implantation the patient must stay on an anticoagulant drug to prevent blood clots forming around the new valve.

Using valves from a pig's heart makes anticoagulation less of a necessity. The pig valves are treated so as not to provoke an immune reaction in the human recipient.

Artificial hearts Various pumping devices can assist the heart, using compressed carbon dioxide as a power source. Other devices support the heart while a patient is awaiting a heart transplant. The completely artificial, electrically driven heart has yet to be perfected. One major problem is getting power to the artificial heart without running wires through the chest wall by which infection can enter. This will probably be achieved using motors that generate electricity through magnetic induction across the chest wall.

Pacemakers These electronic devices are implanted under the skin of the upper chest (see page 49). Electrodes run from the pacemaker up veins into the heart, positioned under X-ray control. Pacemakers are sophisticated devices that deliver an electric shock to make the heart beat at a desired rate. They sense the natural beat of the heart and will therefore not 'fire' in competition with the heart. They can also vary the rate in reaction to exercise or stress. Pacemakers take about an hour to position, usually under a local anaesthetic, and their batteries last for five to ten years. There are very few hazards to wearing a pacemaker.

Other implants

A patient with cataracts (see page 195) can have the opaque part of the lens replaced with an artificial lens. Cochlear implants are artificial electronic sound detectors. Placed in the skull, they restore hearing reasonably well (see page 202).

The arteries to the legs and the great aortic artery within the abdomen commonly become blocked with atherosclerosis or are diseased in some other way. The affected part can be replaced with artificial fibre grafts.

The future

A challenging prospect is treating leg paralysis after spinal cord injuries. Experimental work is showing how electrodes in the spine could amplify natural nerve impulses to make the legs work again.

TRANSPLANTATION

Transplanting organs from a donor to another person (the host) is a relatively young science – the first successful heart transplant took place only in 1967. Transplantation raises important ethical as well as scientific issues. Transplants include the kidney, heart, liver, skin, bone and bone marrow. More ambitious transplants involve the lungs and heart combined or even a complete intestinal system. Timing is critical because donated organs survive just a few hours once detached from their blood supply.

The immune response and rejection

The body distinguishes its own cells from someone else's. By using special molecules called immunoglobulins and cells called lymphocytes, the host attacks transplanted tissues and can destroy the donor organ rapidly. The transplanted organ may itself react against its host. The great problem for transplant surgery has been to develop a means of reducing these immune rejection responses. Several drugs dampen the immune reaction, the best known of which is prednisolone. This is used with other drugs, the most effective being cyclosporin, which has relatively few side effects.

The ideal transplant tissue

This would be a duplicate of the damaged part of the body. Skin grafting, for example, transplants the patient's own skin on to the damaged area. It is beyond present capabilities to do this with more complex organs. It is easier to breed animals that provoke only a weak immune response in humans, for example pigs are bred for their hearts to be used as transplants.

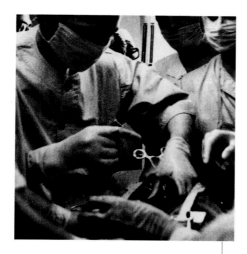

Above: Christian Barnard performing the first heart transplant. Risky and revolutionary in 1967, it is now an established treatment for serious heart disease.

The donor

A suitable transplant donor has a genetic make-up closely resembling that of the host so that less medication is needed to control rejection. Identical twins or close family are therefore often suitable donors.

Examples of transplantation

Kidney A kidney transplant has as good an outlook afterward as surviving on dialysis (see page 367) and is far more convenient for the patient.

Heart This is an option for people with diseased heart muscle, perhaps after infection or with congenital heart defects (see page 333). Four out of five people survive for a year after a heart transplant and many of these survive for more than five years. Most return to some kind of work and full activity.

Heart–lung Candidates for this surgery often have high blood pressure in the lung circulation. The results are almost as good as heart transplantation alone. It is impossible to transplant successfully lungs on their own without the heart.

Bone marrow This is used in forms of leukaemia (see page 252) and rare childhood diseases of the bone marrow. Without treatment these patients become severely anaemic, bleed profusely and succumb to trivial infections. This transplantation calls for the most careful matching of donor and host.

Liver, pancreas and intestine Liver transplants are used in treating liver cancer, chronic liver infection after hepatitis B and C or cirrhosis of the liver (see page 179) or, in children, congenital abnormalities of the liver. Liver transplants are quite successful, transplants of the pancreas and intestines less so.

Other Bone grafting has long been successfully performed. Close matching is not important because the transplant serves as a framework along which the host grows new replacement bone.

In the eye, corneal grafts are well known as a replacement for a cataract. Rejection is not a problem because there is no blood supply to that part of the eye and so no way for immunoglobulins and lymphocytes to destroy the graft.

Ethical issues

The donor of an organ loses it forever (except in the case of bone and bone marrow transplantation). The only organ a donor can survive giving is a kidney; otherwise for someone to have a new organ, someone else has to die. Tragically these potential donors are often young victims of accidents. Their families have only one or two hours in which to decide about donation while trying to cope with their tragedy. The increasing use of donor cards and 'advance directives' in wills may help reduce the trauma of what at present appears unseemly haste.

MICROSURGERY

Microsurgery is the general term for techniques that allow for surgery on very small or fragile parts of the body. The structures being operated can be a millimetre in diameter or less, and include nerves, arteries and veins. Microsurgery is particularly well established in operating on the eye.

The scope of the speciality has broadened with the development of operating microscopes and miniaturized equipment for cutting, probing and sewing. These are refinements of techniques first used in eye surgery. Microsurgery other than on the eyes took off from the 1960s, when it was first shown that it was possible to reimplant a thumb, and then other amputated limbs.

Equipment

The surgeon uses an operating microscope, which gives a magnified and full three-dimensional view of the operating field. The operating instruments include jewellers' forceps, electrodes to stop bleeding, fine probes and scissors. Of greatest importance was the development of ultrafine needles with nylon thread already attached to allow sewing of fragile structures without damaging them.

How microsurgery is performed

The surgeon works his way through each structure, cleaning, removing dead flesh where required, then repairing the site being operated on. After injury, such as an amputation, the first structures to be repaired are the blood vessels, because these are the most critical to the survival of the injured limb.

Each major vein and artery is identified, the ends brought together and painstak-

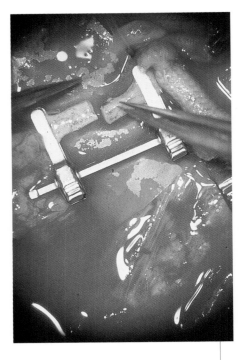

Above: Clamps holding the two ends of a cut blood vessel close enough for the surgeon to repair it.

ingly sewn. Then the surgeon finds the cut ends of nerves and carefully stitches them together. The tendons, muscles and bone are repaired similarly. The surgeon can see almost immediately whether the repair of blood vessels is successful, whereas it can take several months to know if repair of nerves has succeeded.

Uses of microsurgery

Nerve repair This is needed following accidental cuts, crushing or even amputation of a limb. After amputation of a hand or forearm, thumb and fingers, time is of the essence. The amputated part must be kept cooled, and it will then remain repairable for between six and twenty-four hours, depending on how much of the limb is injured.

Plastic surgery A common problem is the need to replace skin lost after trauma or surgery. This can now be done by transferring a whole segment of flesh with its skin from elsewhere in the body where

its loss is not so critical, for example transferring skin from the back to the face, or using a big toe to replace an amputated thumb. The procedure needs two teams of surgeons: one team removes the donor flesh, the other prepares the site where it is to go. The surgeon joins the various components – nerves, blood vessels and muscles – as detailed above. Often it is the scalp that requires reconstruction, but many structures around the face, including the cheeks, neck, floor of the mouth and jawline, also lend themselves to this type of surgery.

Gullet replacement This can be repaired using a section of intestine, joining the blood vessels by microsurgical techniques.

Brain tumours Certain rare tumours within the brain (see page 92) can be approached using miniature instruments. The tumour is cut out under microscopic control, reducing the chances of damage to surrounding brain material. Other uses are to repair aneurysms (arteries within the brain that bleed), abnormal blood vessels (haemangiomas) and spinal tumours.

Gynaecological surgery Microsurgery can unblock Fallopian tubes, the blockage of which is a cause of subfertility (see page 160). This blockage is often due to infection or tubes that have been tied previously or clipped for sterilization. Ovarian cysts are a common problem; their removal must be done delicately to preserve future fertility.

Safety

Bleeding is a problem in microsurgery, because just a small amount of blood may completely obscure the view. Although surgeons can use tiny scalpels, they also use lasers (see opposite) with very finely controlled beams that cut and stop bleeding at the same time.

LASER SURGERY

Since the 1970s, lasers have found a role in many parts of medicine. The thin, high-intensity beams of light offer a precise and bloodless operating tool.

Laser, which stands for light amplification by stimulated emission of radiation, is a beam of light with a high energy level. All the particles of the beam, called photons, move in precise step with each other and in a narrow beam that does not spread as an ordinary beam of light does. Different types of laser react on flesh in different ways, for example lasers of a certain type will pass through normal tissue yet burn tissue of a different colour because it absorbs the beam.

Laser beams can be fed through fibre-optic cables, and therefore can be manipulated into difficult positions in the throat, gullet, stomach and rectum.

Uses of laser surgery

Eye surgery Lasers are well established for operating for glaucoma and cataracts (see pages 194 and 195). They can deal with diseased blood vessels of the retina at the back of the eye which threaten vision, a common problem in diabetics. Ophthalmic surgeons use lasers to burn away blood vessels that look as if they may bleed, in a way that was impossible before lasers.

Gynaecological surgery Uses include unblocking Fallopian tubes (see page 160), cutting out cysts from the ovaries, removing the lining of the womb as a treatment for heavy periods (see page 152) and removing suspicious areas of the cervix (see page 148).

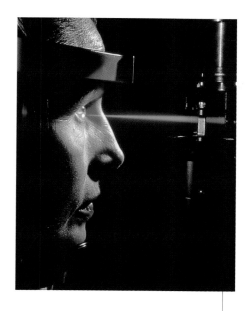

Above: A patient undergoing ophthalmic laser treatment. The laser is aimed using a retinal camera and its beam is delivered in a series of pulses.

Skin problems Lasers can remove small growths and coloured patches of skin. So-called tunable lasers are used for large patches of discoloured skin where scarring must be avoided, such as port-wine stains on the face. They emit light at wavelengths that are most absorbed by, and therefore destroy, coloured skin and cause little damage to less highly coloured normal skin nearby.

Tattoos, applied in haste and regretted at leisure, are another use for lasers. The laser emits very high energy for extremely short periods of time, enough to vaporize carbon, the black pigment in tattoos. However, the results are rarely as successful as would be desired.

Control of bleeding Bleeding from peptic ulcers is controlled by laser; small growths in the bowel or gullet can be removed by laser. These are not curative operations, but more to relieve symptoms, such as difficulty in swallowing, in otherwise inoperable illness. The laser can tunnel through the obstructing tumour in a way that could not be done by conventional cutting, because of all the bleeding that would be caused. Lasers can also cut out small cancers of the larynx and vocal cords.

Removal of prostate gland The laser burns away the prostate tissue, immediately relieving obstruction. This technique will probably become more widely used in future and may even make some prostate surgery (see page 118) an out-patient procedure.

Arterial and heart surgery Lasers initially appeared ideal for unblocking leg arteries obstructed by atherosclerosis (see page 40), but early enthusiasm has unfortunately not yet been matched by success. Using lasers to unblock coronary arteries is a more promising technique and will no doubt be improved over the next few years.

Safety

The main risk is from scarring nearby tissue. This is avoided by selecting the right lasers for the job, as mentioned above.

There is a risk of cutting through tissue, for example cutting through the stomach wall when operating on the stomach lining, but again this risk is reduced by selecting lasers which destroy only a millimetre or so of depth at a time.

The future

Photodynamic therapy is an exciting prospect, using the fact that lasers are absorbed differently by tissues of different colours. The patient swallows a photosensitizer that is taken up especially in cancerous tissues. When an appropriately coloured laser beam is shone on the affected area, it destroys only the cancerous cells, leaving the normal cells untouched. This remarkable advance is under intensive research.

DRUGS

Drugs are substances that affect the working of the body.

The modern drug industry began with aspirin, which is just a hundred years old. The first synthetic drug and one of the most successful ever, aspirin is a good example of how drugs are researched. A substance is found that appears to affect the body beneficially. For aspirin this was extracts from willow bark, which even the ancient Egyptians knew reduced pain and fever. The active ingredient is then identified, purified and tested to prove it works, and to check its dosage and side effects. Researchers can alter the ingredient biochemically to reduce side effects, and make the drug cheaper or more effective.

Dosage takes account of the patient's age and size, seriousness of the illness and function of the kidney and liver, the organs that usually get rid of drugs. Drugs rapidly eliminated by the body must be given frequently, hence penicillin is given every six hours whereas the antibiotic cefixime need be given only once a day.

How some common drugs work

Antibiotics These affect some unique part of the biochemistry of bacteria. For example, penicillin-type drugs destroy the cell wall of bacteria, making them burst.

Sedatives These alter brain chemistry, probably by interfering with neurotransmitters – biochemicals that pass from one nerve cell to another.

Painkillers Morphine-type painkillers attach to chemical receptors that normally respond to natural painkillers within the body (enkephalins and endorphins). Aspirin and other non-steroidal

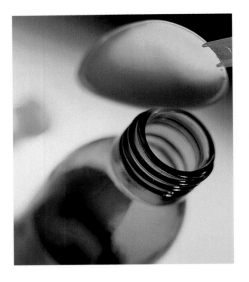
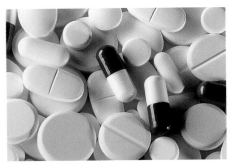

Above and right: It is difficult to imagine life now without drugs for pain relief and control of illness.

anti-inflammatory drugs (NSAIDs) such as ibuprofen affect biochemicals called prostaglandins, which regulate many body functions apart from pain.

Drugs for high blood pressure

Calcium-channel blockers (nifedipine and amlodipine) block calcium from entering muscle cells, letting blood vessels relax and reducing blood pressure (see page 38). ACE inhibitors (captopril and lisinopril) affect the uptake of potassium and sodium in the kidneys, thereby reducing blood volume and blood pressure. Betablockers (atenolol and metoprolol) have many not entirely understood actions on the blood vessels, kidneys and heart.

Taking drugs

By mouth (orally) These must taste acceptable and survive an attack by stomach acid. Drugs unable to resist this have to be given by other means. One of the best known is insulin, which has to be given by injection.

By injection Injected drugs work more rapidly than oral drugs, for example for rapid pain relief. Quickest of all is to inject drugs directly into the blood stream (intravenous therapy), which is used for intensive treatment of serious infections.

By patches, creams and ointments Drugs can be absorbed through the skin. This is a convenient method of administering them and allows the drug to bypass the liver at first, which would otherwise destroy much of the drug at the beginning of its journey in the blood stream. This route allows quantities lower than those taken by mouth to be used for hormone replacement therapy (HRT) or pain relief.

By suppository This method is very effective, working almost as fast as an injection. It is used to give painkillers and antiepileptic drugs rapidly, for example to someone having a prolonged epileptic fit.

Risks and benefits

Doctors are always weighing up possible side effects against possible benefits. This is why they advise against drug therapy for self-limiting problems or they select drugs with a low risk of side effects. However, for serious illness it is justifiable to use potent drugs such as gentamicin, despite there being a higher risk of side effects. Side effects vary from minor rashes and diarrhoea to the very serious – internal bleeding or liver damage. Always report possible side effects to your doctor.

Resistance

Over time germs become resistant to commonly used drugs. This is a serious problem with antibiotics and another reason why doctors try to limit drug use to essential circumstances only.

DIALYSIS

An estimated 500,000 people worldwide rely on dialysis to keep kidney failure (see page 112) under control. For some it is a temporary measure until a kidney transplant (see page 363) can be done, but for others it is a permanent way of life.

What dialysis is for

The kidneys perform many functions, one of the most important being the clearing of poisonous substances from the blood stream. These are accumulated waste products from metabolism which would otherwise cause kidney failure, with high blood pressure, anaemia, itching, general malaise and ultimately convulsions, heart disease and death.

Dialysis is a way of artificially filtering the blood stream to remove these substances. Additional medical treatment and careful diet can preserve many of the other functions of the kidneys.

The decision to begin dialysis is not straightforward and has to take into account social, personal and economic factors over and above purely medical considerations. It also depends on the local availability of kidney transplants, which varies greatly around the world. In the United Kingdom about half of the people with chronic kidney failure are maintained on dialysis.

How dialysis works

The kidney patient's blood is fed through a device that contains thousands of extremely thin-walled tubes of cellulose or plastic. The tubes rest in a liquid called the dialysate, which contains water with precisely calculated quantities of sodium, potassium, salt, sugar and other chemi-

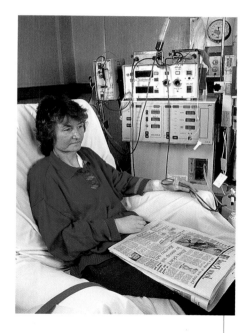

Above: While never routine, kidney dialysis can be fitted around everyday activities.

cals. With the blood flowing in one direction and the dialysing fluid flowing in the other, chemical forces called diffusion make waste products move from the blood stream across the membrane of the tubes and into the fluid, which is then pumped to waste.

How dialysis is performed

Once someone is judged as needing regular kidney dialysis, a surgeon fashions a permanent shunt called a fistula, usually in the patient's arm. This links a large artery to a large vein; the vein grows so it can be easily accessed by a needle. This allows a large blood flow to be taken rapidly every two to three days, the filtered blood being returned via another needle further down the shunt.

Blood at about 300–500 ml/approx 10–17 fl oz per minute flows through the dialysing machine, the whole sequence taking about five hours for an adult. The technology is largely automated, allowing many patients to have a dialysing machine at home and to deal with their dialysis themselves. However it is a complex technology and often patients prefer to be treated in a hospital setting.

This dialysing method is suitable for people with long-established kidney failure (chronic renal failure). Other dialysing techniques are suitable for people who go into sudden kidney failure (acute renal failure) as a result of serious blood loss or extensive burns.

Peritoneal dialysis

Conventional dialysis takes up a major part of a kidney patient's time and ability to work. Peritoneal dialysis is an attempt to reduce this burden. Instead of using an artificial membrane and machine, peritoneal dialysis uses the natural filtering properties of the lining of the abdomen, called the peritoneum.

Access is secured by fitting a permanent catheter tube, through which 2–3 litres/ 3½–5 pints of dialysing fluid is poured into the patient's abdomen, and let out again after an hour or two. In between changes the patient can be mobile. Again, there are refinements and some automated delivery systems.

Problems

The main potential problem in peritoneal dialysis is infection via the access sites; this can be extremely serious and difficult to manage. Despite this, death from peritonitis is rare as long as it is treated aggressively. In machine dialysis there is a risk of removing too much fluid, leading to low blood pressure with light-headedness and weakness. Some people understandably cannot cope with the technology or with the associated anxiety. Otherwise the outlook with dialysis is good, with patients managing on it for 20 years or more.

INTENSIVE CARE

Intensive care units are wards that are equipped to deliver intensive medical and nursing care to the seriously ill.

Those patients who require intensive care treatment include victims of serious accidents or illness, such as burns, head injury, heart attack, lung infections or major trauma with multiple injuries; those who are recovering from heart or abdominal surgery; and people who have taken drug overdoses. These patients all share the risks of collapse of blood pressure, infection, poor lung function and biochemical disturbances leading to heart irregularities and epileptic fits. They will be in pain and often unconscious, and will be disorientated when they regain consciousness. It is a carefully considered decision to put someone on intensive care; sometimes medically there is no point because of brain death or irreversible physical damage.

Intensive care is delivered by specialized doctors and nurses, skilled in relieving pain and dealing with infection and who know when to call in experts in kidney or heart diseases. They are also experienced at keeping relatives informed of progress and breaking bad news.

The first priority in intensive care is to keep the patient's circulation going with blood plentiful in oxygen.

Equipment used in intensive care
Central venous pressure (cvp) line A tube is inserted into a large chest or neck vein and is connected to a display unit. This measures the pressure of blood returning to the heart, indicating how well the heart is working and whether there is enough blood and fluid to keep the patient's circulation going.

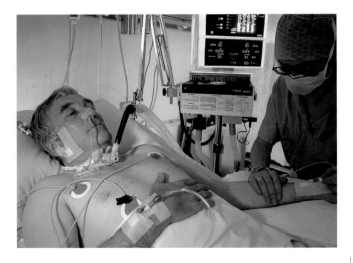

Left: A patient with a nasogastric feeding tube, a drip attached to one hand, a tracheostomy for breathing, a CVP line and ECG electrodes.

Pulmonary artery pressure line This is a catheter in the pulmonary artery, which supplies blood to the lungs. It is inserted from a vein in the groin and guided up to the chest.

Drips These feed fluids and drugs directly into the blood stream, enabling rapid therapy for sudden bleeding or collapse of blood pressure. A hollow needle in an arm vein is connected by tubing to a fluid-filled bag and the fluid is delivered at the desired rate. There may be two drips, one for blood and one for other fluids and medication.

Ventilators (artificial respiration) These machines push air and oxygen into the lungs. A tube is guided down the throat into the trachea (main airway), then connected to the ventilator. The type of ventilator varies greatly: some do all the work for a patient who cannot breathe at all, while others work in between the patient's own breaths. Once someone can breathe by themselves, they can have oxygen via a face mask.

Tests
Blood oxygen The simplest technique is called pulse oximetry. This is a device placed on the finger or ear lobe that shines bright light through the skin; the redness of the transmitted light is related to the amount of oxygen in the blood.

In addition, blood samples are taken from arteries in the wrist or groin.

Blood tests These monitor such critical things as potassium, sodium, sugar (glucose), kidney function, levels of medication and signs of infection.

Kidney function This is critical after a collapse of blood pressure. It requires frequent blood samples and accurate measurement of urinary output from a urinary catheter, a tube passed into the bladder that drains urine continuously into a bag.

Brain function It is a constant worry whether a serious illness has critically damaged the brain. There are scoring systems that rate responsiveness to stimuli, such as touch or commands, pupil dilation in response to pain, choking reflexes and the ability to breathe.

Leaving intensive care
Guided by tests, specialists gradually wean people off the various devices, starting with the respirator then abandoning drips and catheters. Some people remain deeply unconscious, unable to exist without artificial input. The management of such cases involves difficult ethical issues; a decision to switch off support will be made jointly by doctors, nurses, relatives and if possible, the patient, in what is called an advance directive.

LITHOTRIPSY

Developed in Germany in the 1970s, this technique has revolutionized the treatment of stones in the urinary system.

Kidney stones, which are very common, cause excruciating pain and possible damage to the kidney (see page 111). The preferred treatment is to allow the stone to pass spontaneously down the ureter, which happens in 50% of cases. However, many stones are too large or irregular to pass through the ureter to the bladder and out. Such cases formerly required surgery to expose the kidney and to remove the stone, or else to pass a tube up from the bladder to encircle the stone and pull it out. Both methods were unpleasant and traumatic.

How lithotripsy works

The term means wearing away of stones. The idea is to create a shock wave of energy which is focused on to the stone. The energy is created by a spark plug device, a piezo electric effect (compressing a ceramic plate) or something like a very powerful loudspeaker. The energy source rests within a specially shaped container which focuses the energy where it is needed. For technical reasons, the earlier lithotripsy devices required the energy source to be in water, so the patient had to sit in a water-bath. Newer devices still require water around the energy source, but are portable and the patient no longer has to sit in water.

Each shock wave causes tiny bubbles to form on the surface of the stone. When those bubbles collapse they release an enormous amount of energy and heat that crumbles the stone. A course of treatment may involve as many as two thousand rapid shocks.

How lithotripsy is performed

The apparatus is positioned very close to the affected kidney and precisely focused under X-ray guidance. The shocks are given automatically, in rapid succession. As originally designed, the shocks were powerful enough to be painful, and therefore lithotripsy was performed under general anaesthetic. Second-generation machines are deliberately less powerful, avoiding the need for a general anaesthetic. On the other hand, this means that it can take several treatments to shatter the stone.

Success and safety

Lithotripsy works very well for stones within the kidney, upper ureter and bladder, and less well if the stone is in the lower ureter. It may cause bleeding around the kidney, although this is rarely of any significance. People feel as if they have been bruised around the kidney, but again, rarely to any great degree. Occasionally the fragments of stone fail to pass so that further surgery is needed.

Other applications

Ultrasound lithotripsy This is a refinement using an ultrasound generator. Under anaesthetic the surgeon guides this tube device to the bladder and up the ureter to the stone, or he can insert it directly into the kidney through a cut in the loin. The probe vibrates vigorously and shatters the stone, as if it were being hammered. The instrument includes a suction device to suck up the fragments of stone. Ultrasound lithotripsy is used to shatter very hard stones resistant to the usual form of lithotripsy.

Laser lithotripsy The laser is guided in a tube up the ureter then focused against the stone. The high energy from the laser shatters the stone and the fragments pass out in the urine.

Gallstones It was natural to try to apply the same lithotripsy technology to destroying gallstones (see page 180), which are even more common than kidney stones. Surgeons have used ultrasound lithotripters guided to the gall bladder from the small intestine, with the patient under light sedation. However, the shattered fragments do not pass out as reliably as do the fragments from kidney stones. With the advent of key-hole gall bladder surgery (see page 372), gallstone lithotripsy is rarely used.

RADIOTHERAPY

In the 1920s scientists showed that radiation could affect cancerous cells more than normal cells. With that realization a search began for ever-more selective forms of radiation. The goal is still to find treatments that affect cancerous cells as much as possible but have the minimum effect on normal cells.

The selection includes X-rays (see page 348), which are the most common, and gamma rays, electron beams and neutron beams, which are the least used. Radiotherapy may be given by implanting radioactive material within the tumour, a technique especially used in treating cancer of the cervix and womb (see pages 148 and 149).

How radiotherapy works

Radiotherapy uses high-energy atomic radiation. X-rays and gamma rays interfere with the electrons orbiting around atoms, whereas proton and neutron beams destroy the nucleus of atoms and tend to have more devastating effects. Radiotherapy interferes with the normal working of the cell, stopping the cell reproducing, destroying vital proteins and altering DNA structure (see page 132).

Each type of cancer responds differently to radiotherapy. This depends upon many factors, including how quickly the tumour grows, how good its blood supply is and how quickly the tumour cells can repair damage from radiotherapy.

Uses of radiotherapy

Destroying cancers Radiotherapy is most effective for cancer of the cervix, the bladder (see page 113), the head and neck (the larynx and tongue), the prostate (see page 118), Hodgkin's disease (see

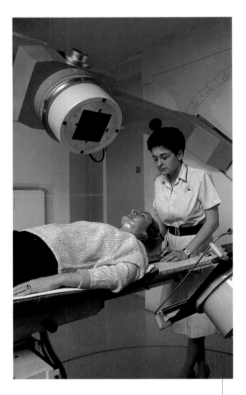

Above: Rotating radiotherapy equipment maximizes radiation on the target, minimizing damage elsewhere.

page 250) and cancer of the testicles (see page 120). It may be curative for these cancers. Radiotherapy alone does not cure leukaemia (see page 252), but it is often used before giving chemotherapy (see opposite) to destroy deposits of leukaemia at sites chemotherapy may not reach, such as the brain and spinal cord. Radiotherapy is also used with surgery for breast cancer (see page 146).

Radiotherapy is unlikely to cure cancers of the brain, lung (see page 66) and gastrointestinal system, including the bowel and stomach (see pages 174 and 175), but it may still help to relieve symptoms.

Relieving symptoms Even though a cancer is incurable, relief of symptoms may be valuable, especially if a tumour is causing pain or pressing on nerves in the spine. Radiotherapy shrinks the tumour enough to give relief, making it an extremely important application of the treatment.

Other uses An overactive thyroid gland (see page 105) is treatable using radioactive iodine. The thyroid gland takes up iodine and the concentrated radioactivity slowly destroys just those cells.

Planning treatment and the amount necessary

The tumour must be precisely localized. This is straightforward if it is visible on the surface, but often the tumour is deep within the body. Modern scanners have greatly improved localization, for example, CT and MRI scans (see pages 350 and 351). The radiotherapist needs to know the type of the tumour, the position and its volume in order to aim the radiotherapy and calculate a total dose.

Often radiotherapists use a plastic shell, which the patient wears and which allows rapid realignment for each treatment. The point to be aimed at may be marked by a tattoo or a light beam.

It is normal to have several sessions of radiotherapy, each lasting for just a few minutes. Treatment may be given every day for a couple of weeks or weekly sessions for a couple of months. The schedule is calculated so as to reduce the risk of damage to normal tissue, while hitting the cancerous tissue at its most vulnerable time as it recovers from the previous session. This varies greatly from tumour to tumour.

Side effects

Common side effects include nausea, tiredness and burns where radiation beams pass through the skin. These occur immediately or within a week or two of treatment. Long-term effects include damage to the organ where the cancer lies, such as inflammation of the lung. It is always difficult to weigh side effects against the benefit of therapy. This is best done by complete honesty and discussion with patients.

CHEMOTHERAPY

This type of cancer treatment uses medication taken by mouth or by injection. Researchers believe that chemotherapy ultimately offers more hope for curing some forms of cancer than either surgery or radiotherapy (see opposite).

How chemotherapy works

The drugs used in chemotherapy are, for all practical purposes, poisons because they interfere with normal cell function. Among the first chemotherapy agents and still very important are those drugs that work by destroying the structure of DNA. Examples of these are cyclophosphamide and melphalan. Such drugs were originally developed for chemical warfare. Other drugs work by blocking normal metabolic pathways in cancerous cells. Examples are methotrexate, 5-fluorouracil and doxorubicin. Platinum is a metal which, in certain forms, can disrupt DNA, so it is put in some drugs. Finally, there are several drugs derived from plants which disrupt DNA or the internal structure of cells. Examples are vincristine, from the periwinkle, and taxol, from the bark of the Western yew.

Suitable cancers

The most responsive cancers are those that are fast-growing. This is because fast-growing cells take up the poisonous agents much more than normal cells, which means that side effects can be limited. Such cancers include leukaemia (see page 252), Hodgkin's disease (see page 250) and childhood cancers.

Then there is a group of less rapidly growing tumours where chemotherapy is still effective. Examples are breast cancer (see page 146) and cancers of the ovary (see page 150), bladder (see page 113), head and neck.

Certain cancers do not respond particularly well to current chemotherapy, such as cancer of the pancreas, lung, bowel and stomach (see pages 66, 174 and 175).

Deciding on the suitability of chemotherapy very much depends on the appearance of the tumour's cells under the microscope, the age and general health of the patient and whether the kidneys and liver are healthy enough to excrete the chemotherapy.

How chemotherapy is given

Usually the medication is given intravenously into the blood stream to avoid the patient immediately vomiting up the dose. Typically, treatment is given every three to four weeks to cause the maximum damage to the tumour while at the same time as little upset to the patient as possible. It has been found that chemotherapy is most effective if several types of drug are given at the same time, even at the risk of more side effects. This is called a 'cocktail' of drugs, and many cocktails are standardized for particular forms of cancer.

Side effects

While it is true that side effects are to be expected, modern chemotherapy is much less likely to cause these than was the case even as recently as the 1980s. Nausea can be controlled by the latest drugs such as ondansetron, with the result that therapy that entailed an overnight stay in hospital can now be given on an outpatient basis.

Hair loss is a feared side effect of chemotherapy. It is sometimes avoidable by the selection of drugs but often it is not. Cancer centres will advise on a temporary wig, but the hair always regrows after therapy.

The major side effects from a medical viewpoint are destruction of the bone marrow, leading to risk of infection, anaemia (see page 251) and bleeding, and damage to the liver and kidneys from the medication. Regular blood tests should detect these problems to allow for an adjustment of dosage or more intensive care in hospital.

Combinations of treatment

Often chemotherapy is one of several types of treatment given for cancer. This is the case in both breast cancer and cancer of the bowel. Surgery removes the obvious tumour and radiotherapy destroys cancers not visible at operation; then chemotherapy destroys deposits of cancer spread elsewhere in the body (metastases).

The future

Many experts believe that future developments in chemotherapy will make it much more specifically targeted to the cancer cells and less toxic elsewhere. This will be achieved by drugs using antibodies to cancerous cells that carry chemotherapeutic drugs with them, or with new forms of chemotherapy that directly target the growth of cancer cells.

KEY-HOLE SURGERY

Surgeons have long been able to look inside the body with a variety of tubes, such as cystoscopes for the bladder and bronchoscopes for the lungs (see page 355). A technique called laparoscopy, which uses a single rigid tube as opposed to flexible tubes, is well established for operations on the prostate gland (see page 118) and in gynaecological surgery for sterilization and inspection of the womb.

The breakthrough leading to key-hole surgery came with the availability of small television cameras that pick up the images from fibreoptic probes guided inside the body. This means that the electronic image could be magnified on to a television screen in full colour and detail, displayed for the surgeon and his assistants. Coupled with miniature instruments and bright illumination, key-hole surgery has rapidly become the method of choice for several common operations and is especially suitable for abdominal ones. The technical term is endoscopic surgery or minimally invasive surgery.

How key-hole surgery is performed

Most key-hole operations require three tubes inserted into the body. One tube carries the lighting and the optical equipment. At present these use fibreoptics, but soon they will have miniature cameras at the tip. The other two are access tubes. These are pushed through the surface and positioned close to the operation site. Once these are in place the surgeon passes the actual operating instruments through the access tubes to probe, cut, sample and staple. These operating instruments have long handles for manipulation; often they are disposable.

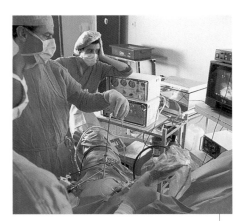

Above: In key-hole surgery the surgeon manipulates the instruments, watching the results on a television monitor.

In abdominal operations, in order to create room to operate, gas (usually carbon dioxide) is pumped inside the abdomen during the operation. Afterwards the gas dissolves harmlessly within the tissues. Some parts of the body are natural cavities, such as the sinuses of the face, so inflation is unnecessary.

Key-hole *versus* conventional surgery

Key-hole surgery is totally different from conventional open surgery, posing a considerable challenge to surgeons. Some traditional procedures do not work well – for example a conventional cut produces so much blood that it obscures vision. Therefore new instruments and methods have been devised to allow cutting with electrical currents (diathermy) or lasers that seal blood vessels as they cut. Conventional stitching with needle and thread is virtually impossible; instead surgeons use stapling instruments, clips or specially designed needles.

Patients benefit from smaller surgical cuts and scars, quicker healing and less time spent in hospital or recovery. This also has economic benefits for hospitals. On the other hand, there are the high costs of training surgeons and of expensive instruments.

Training for key-hole surgery is rigorous: surgeons have to learn to look in one direction (the television monitor) while moving the instruments elsewhere. There are sophisticated training workshops to teach the skills. The next generation of surgeons are learning the techniques more easily, having grown up with computer games.

Uses of key-hole surgery

The first and still most accepted operation is cholecystectomy, the removal of the gall bladder (see page 180). It is remarkable that this now universal use was first achieved in just 1987. Other abdominal operations are removal of the appendix, removal of part of the bowel and surgery around the stomach. Key-hole techniques are used to repair hernias in the groin (see page 170), operate on the sinuses and even pass small endoscopes into the skull. The benefits of all of these procedures are accurate surgery, minimal cutting and a rapid recovery for the patient.

The future

The fast-developing field of key-hole surgery is being carried along on a wave of enthusiasm. However, it may be that some operations are simply not worth doing through a key hole. For example, a key-hole hernia repair turns a simple, highly effective procedure into a difficult and more hazardous one. As with any new technique, it will take time to reach agreement about situations where key-hole surgery is suitable.

COMPLEMENTARY TREATMENTS

The type and length of treatment depends on the therapy used; the severity of symptoms and whether the condition is acute or chronic; whether the practitioner is performing the therapy or teaching you how to do it yourself; and whether follow-ups are required. Note that some therapies can be used to treat a variety of different conditions. Below are some typical complementary treatments. See page 404 onwards for more detailed information.

Circulatory and respiratory disorders

High blood pressure (see page 38) can in part be controlled by stress reduction methods (see below). Naturopaths can also devise a low-fat, low-sodium, high-fibre diet. Autogenic training is particularly good for dealing with negative emotions that raise blood pressure.

For respiratory disorders homeopaths recommend herbal dilutions like phosphorus to relieve the coughing and breathlessness of bronchitis (see page 57). Acupressure can help the wheezing of asthma (see page 58) if you press on a specific pressure point. Autogenic training can show you how to prevent attacks. Reflexology can relieve symptoms and yoga reduces stress that starts an attack.

Mind, brain and nerve problems

Therapies to reduce stress (see page 74) include using acupuncture to release energy; putting aromatherapy oils in a bath or inhaling them from a bowl of hot water; taking Bach flower remedies such as rock rose to reduce anxiety; using bio-dynamics to release tension; chakra

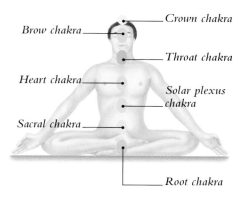

Above: Chakras are energy centres in the body and are linked to the nervous and endocrine systems.

balancing for relieving energy blocks; and trying Hellerwork to realign the body. Other stress-relievers include massage with oils and creams to help relax the muscles, hypnotherapy, shiatsu-do for tension relief and yoga. Relaxation techniques such as meditation, deep abdominal breathing and progressive muscle relaxation have also proved beneficial.

Other mental and emotional problems can be helped by arts therapies, bio-dynamics, Chinese herbalism, healing, play therapy, tai chi and yoga.

Urinary and digestive problems

For cystitis (see page 109), nutritional therapists will recommend dietary changes. Herbalists will prescribe infusions to soothe the bladder.

Some stomach problems result from stress, others may be symptomatic of other conditions. For heartburn and indigestion (see pages 172 and 173), Ayurvedics prescribe alterations to lifestyle and diet; naturopaths recommend changes to the diet; both Chinese and Western herbalists offer stomach-calming infusions made with herbs; and nutritional therapists will investigate your diet

and recommend changes to your eating habits. Autogenic training may help with irritable bowel syndrome. For food allergies and intolerances (see page 181), naturopaths can recommend food-elimination diets to ascertain the cause.

Musculo-skeletal problems

Back, joint and muscle pain can be stress related or symptomatic of other conditions. Therapies for pain relief include the Alexander technique, which teaches you to move smoothly so that your body is put under less stress, chiropractic to manipulate joints and vertebrae and massage to relax muscles. Osteopathy, which releases strain in tissues, muscles and joints, is especially good for RSD (see page 242). Rolfing is beneficial for body realignment, shiatsu-do for easing joint pain and yoga for improving muscle tone. Acupuncture, acupressure and auricular therapy can also help to control pain.

Skin disorders

Dry or chapped skin, on its own or as a result of eczema or allergic reactions, can be soothed by creams, ointments and infusions recommended by a Western herbalist. Naturopaths will suggest dietary changes.

Infections

Aromatherapists suggest soothing a sore throat by inhaling steam from a bowl of hot water which contains eucalyptus and sweet thyme oil. For colds and flu, acupressure may alleviate symptoms generally. Chinese herbalists suggest specific infusions to reduce fever and encourage sweating, relieve mucus and ease sore throats, while homeopaths offer remedies that deal with these symptoms or boost the immune system, reducing the chances of future infection. For sinusitis, both Chinese herbalists and homeopaths prescribe remedies to relieve pain and eliminate the underlying infection.

ALTHOUGH ILLNESS IS NEVER ROUTINE, there are circumstances when it is particularly worrying – in the cases of children and the elderly and when someone requires hospital care. The following section contains information about dealing with illness in these circumstances.

The old wisdom

The fundamentals of caring for the sick have not really changed much over the centuries, although the technology and range of medication available have expanded enormously. Sick people still need reassurance during their illness and rest while recovering. Comfort, fluids, light food and amusement are still the cornerstones of care. These are best delivered by carers familiar with the individual who combine compassion with competence, who recognize when the sick person wants company and when not, and when to intervene and when to let nature heal. Most doctors believe that it helps to involve patients in choosing treatment and in discussing illness and progress.

Children

We worry about our children at the best of times, but especially when they are unwell. Children are more likely than adults to fall ill repeatedly, so some familiarity with how to nurse them back to health is desirable. The basic principles are not difficult and may even seem common sense, but they are no less important for that. You can expect your children to experience many fevers, pains, episodes of diarrhoea and vomiting and minor injuries and accidents during their childhood. It might be tempting to have a medical opinion each time, but this is not a realistic option nor is it in your child's best interests. The more you can become experienced in dealing with 'routine' illness, the better you will recognize episodes of illness that may be out of the ordinary.

It goes almost without saying that all caring parents naturally fear for their children's health even when logically they realize that serious illness is uncommon. It is hoped that the information about childhood illness here and elsewhere in this book will help you to assess the severity of your child's illness with more confidence.

The elderly

On the whole, most elderly people are able to cope for themselves and remain reasonably active, both physically and mentally. But, like an old car, when one thing goes wrong everything else may go wrong at once. The reason is that the elderly do not have large reserves of stamina and strength to

CARING FOR THE SICK

deal with illness. Even though the underlying illness may be relatively mild, such as a urinary infection or a chest infection, they may very quickly neglect themselves, or they may fall, become confused or be unable to walk. The burden of seeing them through illness then falls on to their carers. Dealing with an elderly person who is ill can be especially draining, but by following basic guidelines you can make a potential crisis less likely and minimize the strain on yourself.

Hospital treatment

Although as a society we are healthier, large numbers of us go into hospital each year following accidents, for investigation or for planned surgery. Increasingly treatment is done on a day case basis, as evolving technology has reduced the need for in-patient care. But no matter how brave people say they are, few really are immune to the anxieties generated by the unfamiliar hospital setting and the sense of vulnerability that comes with being in someone else's hands.

Hospitals run on routines; it is easy for staff to forget that what is familiar for them is an exceptional experience for a patient. This section explains what being a patient entails on a practical and psychological level and describes the basics of care in order to better prepare you for hospital treatment.

Right: A comforting and caring attitude
is as important as ever, whatever the
wonders of modern medicine.
Sweet Dreams by Thomas Brooks
(1818–91).

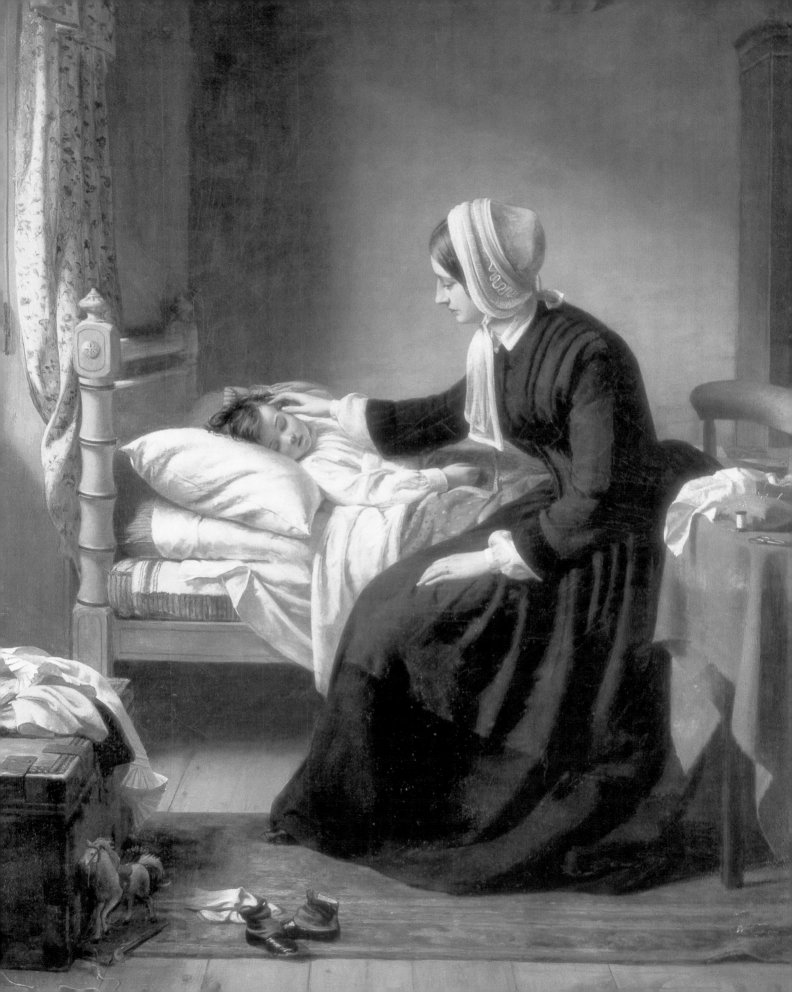

HOSPITALIZATION

Going into hospital is an important life event, regardless of whether it is for the removal of a benign lump or for further investigation of worrying, puzzling symptoms. Doctors and nurses are all now trained to be aware of the psychological effects on patients of hospitalization, but the following should be borne in mind.

Psychological factors

Entering hospital requires a considerable degree of trust. It is normal to have mixed feelings: apprehension, uncertainty and relief that things are going to happen. People can rapidly adopt what has been called the 'sick role' – acting the invalid, becoming passive and focusing on feelings of ill health. Enjoy this while you can. Modern speedy medical procedures mean you are likely to be back in your own home more rapidly than you expected.

Practicalities

The hospital staff will tell you what you need by way of clothing, washing equipment and so on. Bring a list of your medication and allergies. It may be comforting to have a relative escort you and remain there to listen to what the doctor or surgeon says. It is easy to forget things when you are in a state of anxiety.

Tell the hospital staff if you are on the contraceptive Pill or if you have had a problem with blood clots, for example, a deep vein thrombosis or a pulmonary embolism (see pages 51 and 67). The contraceptive Pill increases very slightly the risk of thrombosis, so you should stop taking it four weeks before major (abdominal, chest, heart or hip) surgery. Discuss this further with your doctor.

Being admitted

This is a formal procedure. The hospital staff have to know that you are who they think you are. They will check your age and address and make a note of your next of kin. A nurse will take a nursing history. This is a thorough document which includes social information, food preferences, nursing preferences, how you like to be addressed and an exploration of your feelings about your stay in hospital.

You will be medically admitted by a junior doctor. This involves reviewing the problems that have led to your admission, double-checking medication and asking about things that may affect treatment, such as previous thrombosis or allergies. You will be examined and this will possibly be very thorough, especially if you are being admitted for tests. You will probably be re-examined by other members of the medical team and at some point by the consultant.

Teaching hospitals

These are where both nursing and medical students learn their jobs, so students will be involved in some of your care. It is often a precondition of admission to such hospitals that you agree to this arrangement. If you have objections you should make this clear beforehand.

Tests

For procedures involving a general anaesthetic, some patients will require an ECG of their heart (see page 46), tests to check for anaemia, liver and kidney function to exclude diabetes and possibly a chest X-ray (see page 348). More detailed tests will be performed depending on the reason for the admission, for example scans or special blood tests (see page 354).

If you have been admitted because of a serious medical problem such as a suspected heart attack (see page 43) or a severe chest infection, it is normal to have an intravenous drip. This involves passing a hollow needle into a vein, normally in the arm, securing it in place, then running in fluid or blood. The reason for this is that you may require sudden urgent treatment with drugs directly into the blood stream via the drip, or there may be a risk of sudden bleeding or a drop in blood pressure requiring rapid administration of blood and other fluids.

Consent for procedures

All medical procedures require your informed consent. This means you agree that the procedures or surgery have been explained to you, including risks and side effects, and that you accept these. Doctors want to ensure you understand treatment, so ask questions until you are satisfied. Simply entering hospital implies consent to many routine procedures. Before surgery a doctor, usually the junior doctor, will explain the procedure and ask for your written agreement.

Below: The inevitable anxieties of being in hospital can be reduced by discussion and explanation.

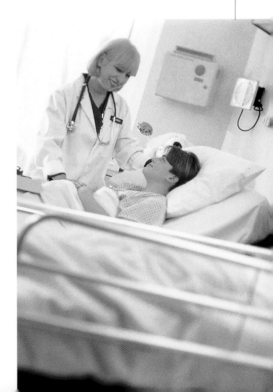

Preparation for surgery

You must not eat or drink for at least six hours before a planned operation under general anaesthetic. This is a very strict rule because eating increases the chance of vomiting during surgery and breathing stomach contents into the lungs, which is a very serious event.

The anaesthetist will visit you to satisfy himself that you are fit for surgery. The area to be operated on will be marked and possibly shaved. You will probably be given premedication – mild sedatives – by injection or tablet. These also reduce saliva flow during the operation.

Day surgery is increasingly the norm. You will be advised about whether you need to fast and any other preparations you should make, for example having a laxative to clear the bowel for bowel operations, and whether you need an escort to see you home.

Recovery from surgery

After surgery, you will come round in a recovery room where staff will monitor your blood pressure and breathing and check for any bleeding. Once you are stable they will transfer you to a ward unless you have had major surgery, in which case you will go into intensive care (see page 368) for a while.

Even after undergoing just a minor operation it is normal to keep a drip in place until you can swallow – usually just a few hours. After major surgery doctors will keep a drip going until you are out of the danger period.

Very often after major surgery you will have a urinary catheter, which drains urine directly from the bladder, and probably other tubes draining fluid from the operation site. Most tubes can be removed within a few days.

Preventing thrombosis

Blood clots in the legs and lungs are an important hazard after major surgery,

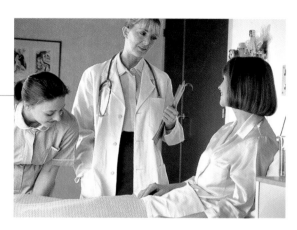

Right: Reassurance and explanation are aids to a patient's recovery; it is important that medical staff do not overlook this fact.

especially orthopaedic (for example for a hip replacement) and abdominal surgery. Therefore you may find that you are given compression stockings to wear to stop blood pooling in the leg veins, and injections of heparin to reduce the tendency of the blood to clot.

Pain relief

The many techniques include nerve blocks to provide long-lasting anaesthesia after the operation, epidural anaesthetics, painkillers in drips and syringes and of course painkillers by mouth. Be sure to let the staff know if you are in pain – pain relief is an important component of your care and enhances recovery.

The routine of the ward

You will be reviewed frequently by the nursing staff, so that they can check if you are comfortable and deal with medication, feeding, special diets, wound care and any problems you are having. Once or twice a day a junior doctor will review you, examining you and, in consultation with senior colleagues, adjusting medication, removing tubes and so on. You will probably see the consultant only once or twice; he will review the technicalities of your case, check the surgery and consider the results of tests. Ward life tends to start early in the day

and finish early and it can be extremely wearing as a result of constant interruptions, emergencies and noises. For this reason many patients, once mobile and comfortable, actually look forward to leaving hospital.

Leaving hospital

You should have a clear idea of what has been done to you, what medication you need, when stitches need to be removed, what follow-up visits are required and any special instructions during recovery with respect to activity, diet and resuming sex. Many hospitals provide leaflets covering these topics.

Being a patient

Patients can expect to be treated with dignity and to be given clear and detailed explanations. All authorities believe that keeping patients informed improves cooperation and reduces stress. Sharing the often inevitable uncertainties of medical treatment also improves patient satisfaction and incidentally reduces complaints if things go wrong or do not go as you would have wished. However everyone is an individual: some people want to be told everything, others nothing. Hospital staff are not mind-readers, so you should tell them if there is something causing you concern.

THE CHILD IN HOSPITAL

◆

Every year an estimated three million children in England and Wales go to Accident and Emergency, and over one-third of all children under the age of five have day surgery or stay in hospital for at least one night. Staff make every effort to welcome children and their families, and all wards provide facilities for parents to stay overnight. Yet going into hospital is still daunting for a child; studies have shown that children are afraid of going in and feel lonely and frightened when they get there. Procedures such as blood tests that seem quite routine to hospital staff, and even some parents, can be very traumatic, especially for young children. In an unfamiliar environment children cannot predict what will happen to them and this increases their anxiety.

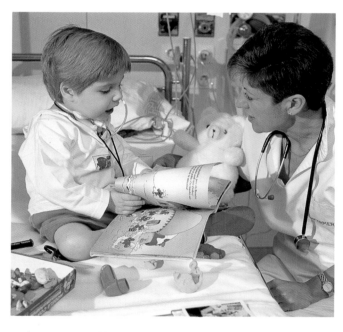

Above: Young children can find their dependence on support systems extremely tiresome. Babies tend to loosen or pull out catheters unless they are restrained, and even older children need constant distraction. This child is suffering from a rare respiratory disease in which the normal breathing reflex does not work overnight.

Preparing for admission Find out everything you can about your local hospital before your child is admitted.

If you are visiting someone else who is in hospital before your child is due to be admitted, take your child with you to get him or her used to the idea.

Ask whether the hospital has open days. A few children's wards hold open sessions in their playroom for children who

are booked in for surgery the following week. Your child may be able to join in. When explaining to the child about going into hospital, tell a young child only a day or two in advance and always include information about getting better and coming home. Children worry that they won't recover. Don't, however, promise a precise day for returning home if you don't know one.

Going to Accident and Emergency Many hospitals have a separate area in Accident and Emergency that is set aside especially for children, with a separate waiting room and staff who have been trained to look after children. Within a few minutes of arrival children are assessed by a triage nurse, but they may then face a long wait or series of waits to have further investigations or treatment.

If you have time, before you set off for hospital pack a bag containing cash and overnight essentials in case you need to stay until the following day. However reassure the child that this is 'just in case'. Most children who go to Accident and Emergency come home the same day.

A common reasons for children's admission to Accident and Emergency is broken bones. Diagnosis involves at least two periods of waiting – first for X-rays, and then for the X-ray films to be sent to the attending staff. The child will be given pain relief before a plaster cast is applied to the fracture. If the bones need re-aligning before the plaster is applied, an anaesthetist will give your child a general anaesthetic. The plaster cast will be removed later with an electric saw. Many children find this frightening; ask if a fine hand saw or cutters can be used for the layers nearest the skin.

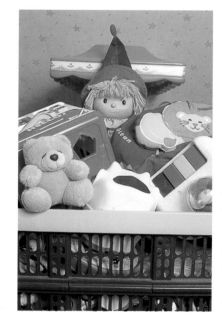

Left: Toys and puppets help in therapeutic role-play in hospital, with puppets entrusted with important messages, while treatments can be role-played on toys, allowing child to come to terms with feelings of anxiety or anger.

Hospital essentials bag

- The child's health record, including information about any illnesses, such as asthma. Any drugs the child takes
- Your child's favourite comforter, teddy or bottle. It doesn't matter if it is scruffy – most are
- Light day and night clothes, socks, trainers, slippers or shoes
- Money, including coins or cards for public phones. (You can't use mobile telephones in all hospitals)
- Telephone numbers of family and friends
- Small rewards for bravery
- Washing bag with toothbrush and toothpaste, soap, face cloth, hairbrush, towel
- Your child's favourite drink
- Toys and books and a walkman for an older child. However limit valuable possessions as hospitals are public places

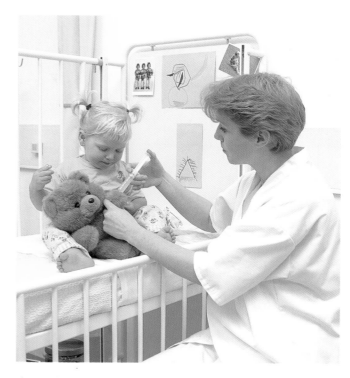

Above: Play specialists are central to children's preparation for many hospital experiences. They can explain and act out procedures, and use diversionary tactics even when the anaesthetic is administered. Integrating play with therapy relaxes children and makes their hospital admission a more positive experience.

Going to a clinic In many hospitals outpatient clinics are designed with children in mind and may be connected to the children's department. There should be a play area but toys may be limited, and as waiting periods between different investigations are almost inevitable, it is worth bringing a supply of activities, toys or games that do not require too much concentration. You should be seen within 30 minutes of arrival, and if you are not you should be told why. It is very helpful if you bring your child's health record with you as well as any drugs your child is taking. Most children in outpatients departments are likely to be examined, so dress your child in clothes that are easy to remove. If you think your child may be upset by tests or treatment take a small reward with you to give for bravery.

Planned admissions Some hospitals have a member of staff who is in charge of establishing links with children's families and who will contact you before your child's admission. If not, ask them if you can visit the hospital before your child is admitted.

It is important, if at all possible, to stay in hospital with your child. Sick children are known to get better much faster when they have the confidence and security of having their parents near them. Hospitals make overnight accommodation provision for parents, which may be free of charge. In a regional centre or in special circumstances there may be accommodation for the rest of the family.

On arrival at the hospital the ward clerk will take down basic details, and the nurse who will be looking after your child will draw up a care plan. After basic checks – temperature, pulse, weight – have been carried out the nurse will give your child a hospital wristband. The doctor who admits the child will carry out an examination, reviewing the reason for which admission is necessary and, if the child is to have surgery, examine the child's chest. The anaesthetist may visit the child as well.

Boredom and restlessness are major problems both for children and parents. There may be a play specialist who can help prepare the child for medical procedures such as blood tests or an anaesthetic and provide alternative activities during the day. A store of undemanding games and activities from home is helpful, and it may be necessary for the child to keep up with school work. Primary schools are particularly good at building a class member's stay into the learning process.

Access to a telephone as well as a walkman makes all the difference to an older child confined to bed. Older children also like to keep up with their friends by watching their favourite television programmes.

Parent partnerships While you are with your child you can look after them as you would at home – washing and feeding, playing and settling the child for sleep. If your child is to be hospitalized for more than a very short while, nursing staff may show you how to help with some of the caring procedures, such as taking and recording temperatures. The longer the stay, the more you will do. Staff should also observe and learn from you.

Stay with the child when they most need you – when they are having investigations or treatments, or when they are in the anaesthetic room or the recovery room following surgery. Observe your child's responses sensitively. Children often don't feel brave enough to speak up for themselves in hospital, in which case the parents need to speak up for them.

One disadvantage of staying in hospital with a child is that you can feel trapped. Living in hospital is tiring and often boring. Bring plenty of activities that are not too demanding for yourself, and take a break at least once a day, if possible while your child has a visitor.

Surgery Surgery may be elective or an emergency. Sometimes you have time to prepare your child briefly – for example, if surgery is needed to re-set a fractured bone. An elective operation is one that is planned, so there is ample time to prepare the child. Children and parents are told what is likely to happen, either during a session with the play therapist or during discussions with the surgeon.

Preparation for day surgery may take place at a weekend session before admission; otherwise it usually takes place on the day of the operation. Individual hospital practices vary, but you can usually expect the following sequence of events. Children may have to fast overnight, or at the least have no milk or solid food for four hours prior to surgery and no clear drinks such as apple juice or water for two hours before. They will have a bath and dress in suitable clothing. If your child's nightwear or T-shirt is cotton or mainly cotton, they may be able to wear their own clothes if that is how they feel most comfortable. However hospital gowns are easier to remove and may be preferable if clothes are likely to get stained during surgery. Jewellery or nail varnish will have to be removed.

Just before surgery staff will put an anaesthetic cream on the back of the child's hand and may give a sedative drink, although this is often not needed for a day surgery procedure. Children are usually allowed to take a favourite object to the anaesthetic room and choose how they go – in their parent's arms, on foot, on a trolley or on a hospital bed. The anaesthetic may be given as gas from a mask or as an injection. For young children gas is often preferred. If the anaesthetic is given into a vein, simply asking the child to cough can be sufficiently distracting so that they do not notice the needle

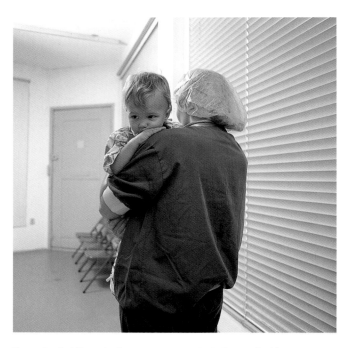

Above: In deciding whether or not to remain in hospital with your child, you should consider whether he is used to group play and whether he is old enough to go on holiday without you. If the answer to either of these is no, you should stay with him if you can. Hospitals can be frightening places even for adults, more so for a child.

entering the vein. Parents are asked to leave the anaesthetic room once the child is unconscious.

Following surgery you will be able to sit with your child in the recovery room. If the child is asleep it is better not to wake them. When the child does wake, offer a drink. After day surgery, once the child is able to walk again, go to the toilet, drink, eat and is comfortable, you can help them get ready to leave. This is usually two to four hours following surgery. Before you leave you should be given an information leaflet, a follow-up appointment and instructions explaining how to give any prescribed drugs. You should also be given the name and telephone number of a staff member whom you can contact if you are worried. Try not to use public transport to get back from the hospital and do not let your child play outside for the rest of the day, as it can take 24 hours for the full effect of an anaesthetic to wear off.

Pain and pain relief
Procedures that are painful for most children include anything involving needles – blood tests, immunizations or injections; recovery from surgery; fractures; and having dressings changed. Such pain can usually be prevented, but fear and anxiety make pain worse, so no child should ever have to wait

for pain relief. Parents can help by asking about analgesics when they see their child is in pain. Signs include a change in behaviour – the child may be noisier or quieter than usual or look flushed or pale.

Pain relief without drugs Pain relief without administering drugs may be appropriate while waiting for the next scheduled drug dose, or in circumstances when drugs are not available or are contraindicated.

Warmth eases pain, and a child who is generally in pain may be helped by sitting in a warm bath if this is practical. A well-wrapped hot water bottle can temporarily ease toothache or earache. If a procedure is going to be painful, children should be told and given an explanation. For a mild, brief pain such as an injection, numbing the skin with ice cubes for a second or two may be all that is needed.

You can prepare a child for a painful procedure by keeping them calm and relaxed. Deep breathing, stroking and massage help some children. Blowing bubbles helps to control breathing; alternatively count four slow breaths in and four slow breaths out. Distraction with a story tape, video or hand-held computer game is helpful, particularly if the child is in charge of the controls. A simple appeal to the child's imagination (a technique known as imaging) can also have powerful results.

Control is an important part of pain. If children know that they can stop the pain with a pre-arranged signal, then they will feel better about allowing a certain amount of it.

Pain relief with drugs For mild pain, paracetamol works quickly, building up to maximum effect within 30-45 minutes. Alternatives for moderate pain include the anti-inflammatory drugs diclofenac and ibuprofen (but these should be given only when directed by hospital staff). For a local procedure such as a blood test, an anaesthetic gel or cream numbs the skin. For a short but painful procedure such as having a dressing changed, the pain can be lessened if the child takes a warm bath. A child who is old enough to cooperate may be able to breathe in nitrous oxide (Entonox). For severe pain, such as that experienced from a fracture, morphine works quickly and, taken as part of treatment, is not addictive. It can be given as an injection, intravenously (when it works in 10 minutes) or by use of a device that allows the child to control their own pain relief. This is known as patient controlled analgesia (PCA). It can be used by some children over five years of age who are in severe pain. When the child experiences the onset of pain they press a button, which activates the device to release a dose of the pain-killing drug.

Children should not wake up in pain following surgery. Immediately after surgery they may be given an injection of local anaesthetic into the wound or into a nerve to a specific area. A caudal block is one type of nerve block, in which anaesthetic is injected around the nerves at the base of the spinal cord, numbing the genital and buttock areas. The effect lasts for four to six hours.

Hospital tests

Some tests carried out in hospital are completely painless, while others are uncomfortable. For any which are painful a child will be offered pain relief. The parent's presence is, however, often the best form of pain relief and the best form of reassurance child can have.

Blood tests Blood tests can provide important information about the state of a child's health. Children who are hospitalized may need to give blood samples to help doctors diagnose illness such as anaemia or evaluate the efficacy of treatment. If only a small amount of blood is needed it can be taken from a capillary just under the skin. In babies it is usually taken from the side of the heel, while in older children it can be taken from a finger or thumb. Taking blood like this does cause a pricking sensation, and if a child needs repeated blood tests their fingers can become tender. Keeping the child warm taking blood helps children to relax, and it also helps to keep their blood vessels dilated.

A larger blood sample is usually taken from a vein, often on the inside of the elbow. A few ice cubes held against the area prior to inserting the needle provide instant numbness. Otherwise a child can have a local anaesthetic cream or gel applied to the site half an hour to an hour in advance. This is almost always done before an injection into a vein, or when a cannula (a very fine tube) is to be inserted into a vein, in which case the wriggling of the tube can feel uncomfortable. A cuff similar to a blood pressure cuff may be put around the child's arm to help the veins stand out so they are more visible which makes the procedure easier. Children deserve a reward afterwards – even if it is just a cuddle.

X-rays X-rays do not hurt, but children can feel frightened by the size of the machine, particularly if it has to come very close to them. They also have to lie or stand quite still and may have to adopt an uncomfortable position so that the technician can obtain a clear picture. Parents can normally stay with their child during the procedure, but they must wear a lead apron to protect their reproductive organs. Any mothers who might be pregnant will not be allowed into the X-ray room with the child but can watch through a glass screen. To reassure them, you can tell them that the X-ray machine is large and will come close to them, but never comes very close, and that it never hurts.

Radio isotope tests These tests are used specifically to find out whether the kidneys are functioning normally. The child lies on a table which has a large isotope camera underneath it. Anaesthetic cream is rubbed on to the back of the child's hand and a fine tube is inserted into a vein. The child is then given an injection of liquid containing a tiny amount of radioactive substance; this is tracked by the X-ray camera under the bed. While the X-ray pictures are being taken staff will usually ask the child to take up different positions. To help them lie quite still the nurse or technician may tie light straps around the child's body.

MCUG The MCUG (a micturating cysto-urethrogram) shows how well the bladder and its outlet are functioning. It specifically checks whether any urine is flowing back from the bladder towards the kidneys instead of draining out normally. The test does not hurt, but it is uncomfortable and takes about 30 minutes. The child lies on a table in the X-ray room. After cleaning the genital area, the doctor inserts a catheter into the child's urethra and bladder. Fluid is then passed into the bladder until the bladder distends. X-rays are taken when the child urinates. Urinating after the catheter has been removed may cause a stinging sensation, but drinking quantities of fluid will help to relieve this.

Barium swallow or meal These tests are carried out to investigate structures in the digestive tract. The child swallows a white, chalky liquid containing barium; X-rays are taken as the barium travels through the digestive tract. For a barium swallow, the baby or child is X-rayed in an upright position, but when taking a barium meal they lie down. The test can cause constipation, which you can help to prevent by giving the child plenty to drink for the next 24 hours. When the child does pass stools, you may notice tiny white pieces or streaks in them, which are the remains of the barium. They will soon disappear.

EEG (electroencephalogram) An EEG measures the patterns produced by tiny electrical impulses in the brain. It is useful for diagnosing epilepsy. The child usually wears between 16 and 20 small electrodes attached to their head. The electrodes pick up the impulses, which are enlarged in the computer and then either viewed on a monitor or printed on to paper. There is no pain involved – the electricity goes from the brain to the machine, not vice versa. It takes 30-90 minutes, depending on how still the child can lie.

During the recording staff may ask the child to open and close their eyes and breathe deeply in and out; a light may be flashed in their eyes. As the electrodes are sometimes fixed in place with a special glue, the child will need to have their hair washed after the test. Some children have the test at night to examine their brain waves while they are asleep. Many hospitals can offer children a portable EEG, which allows recordings to continue at home.

CT scan (computed tomography) A CT or CAT scanner records images of the brain or other soft parts of the body. The child lies on a table that slides into a tubular disc – scanner – that rotates around the patient, building up a scan of the brain by means of X-rays. A computer then integrates the images to build up slices or cross-sections of the part of the body X-rayed. The test is painless but as the X-rays are taken the machine sometimes produces sounds, which the child may find disturbing. As the child has to lie very still for the test they may be given a sedative, or possibly even a brief general anaesthetic.

MRI (magnetic resonance imaging) As far as the child is concerned, this is very like a CT scan, because the child has to lie quite still on a table in a tubular structure rather like a tunnel while images are recorded. However the images show far more detail than X-rays and more than a CT scan.

The scan takes about 30 minutes. The MR scanner looks frightening and is noisy, and as the child has to lie alone and perfectly still inside, they are usually given a sedative or general anaesthetic. An older child or teenager who is not sedated can communicate through an intercom with the staff operating the machine.

ECG (electrocardiograph) The child undresses to the waist and lies down while patches are stuck to their arms, legs and chest. These are attached to a machine that picks up the heart's electrical impulses and records them as a printout or on a monitor, showing the rhythm and rate of the heartbeat. The test is completely painless and normally takes about five minutes to perform.

Echocardiogram This is like the ultrasound used in pregnancy. A picture of the heart, its structure and blood flow is produced on a screen. The procedure takes between 15 and 60 minutes.

The care of premature babies

About one baby in ten in the United Kingdom needs extra medical care immediately after birth. Of the 70,000 babies a year who spend time in special care units in British hospitals, some 52,500 are premature. Most have a low birth weight; more than 1% of babies born in England and Wales in 1995 weighed less than 1500 g/3 lb 5 oz. Yet in recent years the prognosis for very premature babies has steadily improved. A few babies survive at 23 weeks and from 24 weeks survival rates start to climb steeply.

The cause of some premature births is still not understood, but it is possible that some otherwise inexplicable premature births are triggered by a common vaginal infection, bacterial vaginosis. In some pregnant women the membranes break before term, or the foetus begins to grow too slowly or stops growing altogether, and the doctor decides that they would thrive better outside the uterus.

Predicting prematurity is the subject of much current research. A range of tests is now being investigated, including swabbing the vagina to detect infection, screening for fibronectin (a foetal protein that usually disappears by the fifth month) and scanning the cervix for early signs of changes that herald labour. If delivery can be delayed long enough to give the mother a steroid drug to protect the baby's lungs, the chances of any breathing problems developing later on can be halved.

Special care baby units All babies are different, but a baby born after 36 weeks can usually be treated like a normal term baby and will not need special care. A baby born between 33 and 36 weeks should have few difficulties, but may find coordinating sucking and swallowing too difficult for normal breast- or bottle feeding. Babies born between 28 and 32 weeks have immature lungs, and those born before 27 weeks need support for many of their body systems.

Until the baby is 32–34 weeks old the lungs are physically very small. They do not produce surfactant, the substance that allows expansion when the lungs fill with air. In some babies the breathing control in the brain is still immature. Ventilators take over the breathing by gently inflating the lungs.

Some premature babies receive negative pressure ventilation, which reduces the air pressure around the baby and makes breathing easier. Others receive oxygen-enriched air through nasal prongs (rubber tubes, which are inserted into the baby's nostrils, while others lie with their head in a transparent headbox containing oxygen-enriched air. Babies are often given artificial or animal-derived surfactant at birth. Research is under way into liquid ventilation, in which the lungs are not filled with air or oxygen but with a fluid in which oxygen is dissolved.

Paediatricians balance the amount of ventilation the baby needs with the knowledge that ventilation over a long period, especially at a high pressure, can damage the internal surfaces of the lungs, giving rise to a condition called chronic lung disease (also called bronchopulmonary dysplasia or BPD). Babies who do develop this condition have a tendency to catch respiratory infections and to wheeze in their first few years; however they outgrow their difficulties by late childhood.

Premature babies lose heat very quickly, so they need to be kept extremely warm, either in an incubator or, if they need constant medical attention, under an open radiant heater.

Until coordinated sucking and swallowing develop around 34 weeks, babies can be fed essential nutrients by intravenous drip directly into the bloodstream, or given milk through a tube that passes through the nose and down the oesophagus into the stomach.

The major impact on parents who have a baby in special care is emotional. At first parents often feel shocked (at not having produced a healthy, full-term baby), anxious (about the baby's immediate health and long-term development) and perhaps either alienated or fiercely protective of a baby who depends on high-technology medicine to survive. Staff in neonatal units are acutely aware of parents' difficulties. When it is appropriate, parents are encouraged to become involved in the baby's care and to talk to, possibly touch or even hold them. Some units foster kangaroo care, in which the baby is placed on the parent's chest in an upright position, warm inside their clothing, for up to an hour a day.

Outcome The development of babies born prematurely depends on many factors but most grow up with no long-term difficulties. Because development may initially be delayed or follow an unusual pattern, in the first two years of life allowances are usually made for the child's prematurity. Beyond the age of two years the effects of having been premature are less noticeable, although a minority of children are left needing long-term support. It is impossible to predict the outcome for any individual baby, but generally speaking, the closer the baby was to term the more unlikely they are to have long-term disability. Babies born after 32 weeks have a 98% chance of developing in a perfectly normal way.

CARING FOR CHILDREN AT HOME

Illness is a normal part of childhood, and parents should get to know how to deal with the child who has a minor illness and when to call for help. The following guidelines apply to children with illness in the developed world where, thanks to immunization, good nutrition and good hygiene, serious illness is relatively uncommon.

Give comfort . . .

Ill children, even more than ill adults, want comfort, help and the knowledge that someone is at hand. Simply being there for your sick child is a major factor in relieving her discomfort.

You are the one best placed to know your child and how she responds to illness. Perhaps your child makes a fuss about being ill, groans, moans and demands attention. Or perhaps you have a child who curls up in a ball on the sofa and tries to make the best of things. As well as providing revealing insights into your child's character, it is important to know your child's normal reaction to illness as a means of judging when she is 'unusually' ill. When doctors talk about a parent's instincts, this is what they have in mind, and a wise doctor will take seriously a parent's instinct about illness.

. . . but do not make a drama out of illness

You would not be a responsible parent if you did not worry about your child being ill. However, children pick up parental panic and soon learn if illness gets them treats and extra attention. It is not in your child's long-term interest for her to learn that minor illness has compensations. Childhood illness in the developed world is usually no more than a nuisance and an inconvenience, to be handled with care and concern, but without going overboard on sympathy. Of course you will comfort, hug and reassure your sick child, but it is a mistake to let her see you worry over every trivial symptom.

Reduce fever

A high temperature is not an illness in itself, although parents often believe it is. Fever is no more than a symptom of illness, probably an infection, but on its own it does not allow a doctor to make a diagnosis. Parents must develop confidence to cope with a feverish child and to allow time for other symptoms of illness to appear.

In the meantime, give paracetamol syrup or ibuprofen syrup (but not to asthmatics) in a dose appropriate to the child's age. These help regardless of the cause and can be given without masking other symptoms. Bear in mind that fever often persists despite medication and that fevers tend to rise at night.

Keep your child cool by removing layers of clothing. In summer leave her in a tee shirt in the shade; in winter put her in just enough clothes so she feels comfortable. The younger the child the more important it is not to let her get overheated, otherwise there is the risk of a fit. If an infant remains very hot, cool her with a fan or sponge over her brow with tepid water.

Give fluids

Give increased fluids, such as fruit cordials, low-sugar fizzy drinks allowed to go flat or water. A sick child should drink 1–2 litres/1¾–3½ pints a day depending on her size, and she should take small, frequent sips rather than large quantities all at once. Avoid milk and very sweet

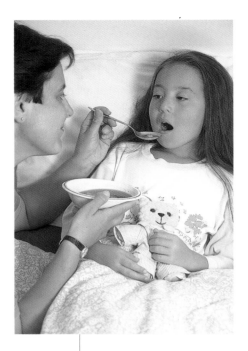

Above: Starting to eat again is a reliable sign that your sick child is recovering.

fizzy drinks, which distend the stomach and which the child is more likely to vomit. For babies there are specially formulated salt and sugar drinks, available from your pharmacist. Encourage your child to drink even if she is reluctant and especially if she has a fever or diarrhoea.

Do not worry about eating

Going off food is a basic symptom of illness. Save yourself frustration by recognizing this and not even bothering to serve up a tempting morsel. If your child is hungry, offer her a light snack such as bread, pasta, a biscuit or some soft fruit. If she can cope with that, you can give her something more substantial, but take it slowly and be prepared if a child who manages one bite of biscuit vomits up a rice pudding. Children will not starve through missing meals for a few days.

Let your child rest

Being ill takes energy: the child's body pours resources into fighting an infection and has less energy left over for the usual childhood mayhem. Brothers and sisters should leave their sick sibling alone, and if the child simply wants to sleep just let her. On the other hand, encourage a sick child to get up, to wash and to go to the toilet, perhaps with your help.

There will be times when an unwell child suddenly appears full of energy and begins to rush around; do not be fooled. Let her get it out of her system then encourage her to calm down again. It is especially common for a child to appear well again first thing in the morning only to wilt as the day goes on. So do not abandon your care on the basis of a single good hour.

Bed is not necessarily best

There is no reason for a sick child to stay in bed if she feels comfortable elsewhere.

Beds get hot, sheets get twisted; she may find it difficult to get out in a hurry to be sick or to go to the toilet. And it gets boring. Lying on a sofa is often more comfortable and convenient, and a carer can keep an eye on the child while going about other tasks.

Deal with boredom

For the first couple of days an unwell child will not need amusing, but she is likely to get bored as she starts to feel better. Some children will happily amuse themselves with books, magazines and games. Others prefer to watch television or a video or play computer games. The healing powers of Disney are an under-researched area of medicine; half an hour giggling at cartoons can work wonders.

Giving medicine

If a doctor has decided that your child needs medication, you should give it to her. Drug manufacturers make their medicines palatable for children with sweeteners and flavourings – banana or strawberry are apparently guaranteed winners. Some children reject certain antibiotics but will accept others. Tell your doctor about this because often the exact choice of antibiotic does not matter and it makes sense to prescribe an alternative that the child prefers. You can disguise flavours by diluting medicines, mixing them in a cold drink or hiding a tablet in jam, but check the drug information leaflet first to be sure this is allowed.

What should you do with the child who refuses medication? You must try again and then again. Bribery? Offering a treat? Why not? But medication is not a game and illness is not a diversion, so you may have to insist she takes her medicine. If it all keeps ending in tears and tantrums, discuss it with your doctor. There may be another option or your doctor may judge that the child has had enough of a course and can stop.

Babies

Babies are different: they cannot tell you how they feel, they become ill more quickly and with fewer symptoms and they recover faster. It is entirely reasonable to seek advice about a sick baby, even if the only feature is vomiting, a rash, fever or constant crying. Your doctor can examine and reassure, prescribing medication only if it is really necessary. Your baby is bound to have several minor illnesses during her first year of life, each of which is an opportunity to learn how your baby reacts during 'normal' illness so you become confident in recognizing when your baby is more than usually unwell and needs help.

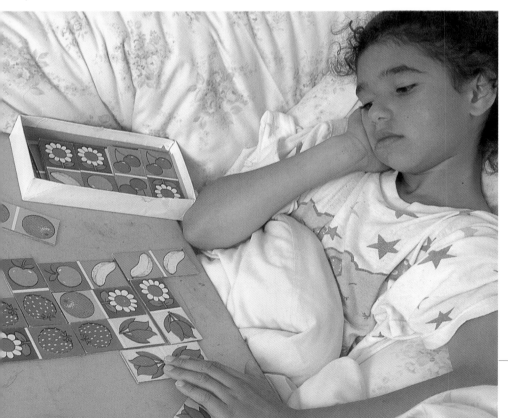

Left: Illness can be boring as well as unpleasant. Your child will welcome amusements while she recovers.

CARING FOR THE ELDERLY

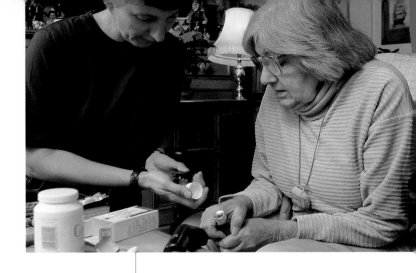

Above: In the elderly, 'a pill for every ill' can end up as a confusing array of drugs, calling for close supervision.

Unprecedented numbers of people in the developed world are now surviving into their 80s and beyond. Despite all you read about illness and dementia in the elderly, the majority do cope, with support from family, friends and care agencies.

This is the time of life when things can go seriously wrong and may do so very suddenly, the most common problems being chest pains, bleeding, strokes and immobility. While many illnesses show obvious symptoms, elderly people may have significant illness without any dramatic signs, although they may experience breathlessness, dizziness, falls or confusion or go off their food.

However, minor illness is still more likely than a serious one. Carers become familiar with an elderly person's normal health and mobility, allowing them to judge whether the person is significantly off colour. In this respect care of the elderly is similar to that of sick children.

Factors contributing to illness

The following may directly or indirectly cause illness in the elderly.

Accidents These are common. Elderly people become giddy, tripping and falling for no apparent reason. If, after a fall, an elderly person cannot walk or appears in pain, have him checked over for fractures. As a preventive measure, reduce the chances of accidents by making the elderly person's home safer.

Medication The elderly often take several medications, increasing the possibility of reactions to medication and accidental overdose. If an elderly person appears confused or falls, medication is one of the first things to consider.

Poor diet There is a temptation as one gets older to eat less and more simply, with a diet low in iron, protein, vitamins and fibre from fresh fruit and vegetables. Combined with lack of mobility, this can lead to malnutrition.

Lifestyle Although many elderly people keep active and interested, others allow themselves to become reclusive and take little exercise. This can degenerate into an isolated existence cut off from social activities, leading to and worsening the inevitable stiffness of old age. Such people may occupy only one room in a house which, through habit or lack of money, they keep inadequately heated.

Remaining at home: decisions and guidelines

A decision has to be made about whether a sick elderly person can stay at home. A few questions need answering before a decision is made. If he can cope, some guidelines must be followed to ensure that he is given the best care possible.

Is he safe? Critical factors are whether he can get to a toilet, prepare food, keep warm and not fall. Many communities and families can provide temporary home care for a week or two during recovery. Otherwise hospital admission is unavoidable (a so-called 'social admission'), even though the underlying medical problem may not be serious.

Will he take his medication? Another factor to consider is whether he can cope with medication at home – remembering, for example, to take tablets every eight hours. This can be made easier by drawing up a list or using a medication holder that holds the day's medication. The person should also be able to recognize if he is becoming more unwell and be capable of summoning help if this were the case.

Taking fluid Just as with children, it is important for the elderly to drink more fluids when unwell. They should have at least 3 litres/5 pints a day – more if they have a fever or diarrhoea. Dehydration in the elderly is difficult to be certain about, but you should suspect it if the person becomes more confused, passes little and concentrated urine, and has a dry tongue and sunken eyes.

Taking food Loss of appetite is inevitable during illness, so high-carbohydrate drinks that will provide a lot of energy in a small quantity are advisable. There are also many liquid feeds that can completely supply necessary nutrition during a prolonged illness.

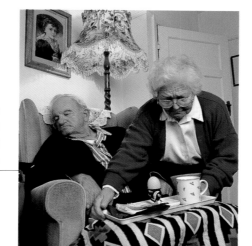

Right: The sick elderly person needs warmth and light, and nourishing food with plenty of fluids.

Rest A sick elderly person will naturally want to doze and will not feel inclined to do anything. Simply going to the toilet can be a major effort. It also takes longer for an elderly person to recover from even a minor illness. A cold or chest infection that a younger person recovers from within a week may leave an elderly person feeling debilitated for a month, without signifying any serious complication.

Warmth Body temperature control becomes poor in the elderly. Keep the house warm – 18–21°C/65–70°F is reasonable but be guided by the individual's preferences. It is vital to keep a good temperature in the evening by leaving heating on, because if an elderly person falls in a cold room during the night and is unable to move it could lead to hypothermia.

Amusement Illness is as boring at 90 as it is at 9. Television, radio, magazines and computers can pass long uncomfortable hours. Buy a daily newspaper as time disorientation can occur quickly during illness.

Bed rest It takes only a few hours of resting heavily in bed for the skin to break down, so encourage the elderly person to sit in a chair. This is better both for the skin and for draining the lungs if there is a heart or chest problem. Resting in bed also leads to constipation (see page 169), a common problem anyway in the elderly.

Some elderly people find it more comfortable to sleep in a chair covered with blankets rather than in a bed, but they must keep warm during the night.

Aids Temporary aids can make all the difference in allowing someone to stay at home. Some of the aids available include a commode, soft bedding and air mattresses to reduce the chance of bedsores, raises placed under chair legs to make it easier to rise from a sitting position, meals on wheels, syringe drivers which supply medication continuously through the skin (especially useful for controlling severe pain) and incontinence devices such as pads and catheters.

Skilled help for the patient

It can be difficult to care for an elderly person who appears demanding and critical of the help they are given. While professional helpers are used to this, it can be extremely difficult for relatives. Try to accept that it is the illness causing this and discuss how you feel with other helpers you meet.

However devoted a helper you may be, you might need assistance from a district nurse to deal with dressings and bedsores. Call a doctor if you are in any way concerned about the condition of an elderly person in your care, because his symptoms may be minimal despite serious illness. It is also reasonable to ask for reassessment if the patient fails to improve within a few days, always remembering that full recovery can take a number of weeks.

Long-term care

Advances in medical care mean that large numbers of the elderly now survive with chronic disabling conditions. Examples are following strokes (see page 80), chronic bronchitis (see page 57) and severe arthritis (see page 234). This puts a great physical and psychological burden on their carers.

In coping with this you need to:

- *Have a routine – daily, weekly, monthly*
- *Get home aid assessment for showers seats, grab handles and stair lifts*
- *Investigate other services available, e.g. meals on wheels, district nurses and physiotherapists*
- *See what government benefits apply, both for the individual and for you as a carer*
- *Let professionals know if the elderly person's condition changes*
- *Arrange respite care to give yourself a break*

In the United Kingdom these facilities are accessed via social services and the patient's doctor. Hospitals often provide a day centre to give both you and your elderly person a rest.

Guilt

This is normal for a thoughtful carer to experience. It may arise through your own feelings of inadequacy at the level of care you can provide, resentment at the demands made by the elderly person and how responsibilities encroach on your own life. Coping with a demented but otherwise perfectly healthy elderly person is draining. You should explore all means of having a break yourself and consider long-term institutional care if the burdens are affecting your own physical and emotional health.

ALTHOUGH FIRST AID cannot be entirely learnt from books, you can learn certain basic techniques to deal with minor injuries and health problems. Anyone should be capable of dealing with minor cuts, wounds and burns, for example.

When it comes to skills such as artificial respiration, there is no substitute for proper training but there may be circumstances where it is better to have a go than not to do anything. Even a little knowledge of first aid will give you a confidence which will communicate itself to the casualty. That comfort alone is very worthwhile.

This section will give you some practical guidance for more common problems. It is not a complete first aid manual. For that, and especially to learn the physical techniques of resuscitation, enrol on a first aid course.

The principles of first aid

The important principles in administering first aid in any situation are as follows:

- *Do not endanger yourself*
- *Assess the situation*
- *Protect a casualty from further harm*
- *Attend to the most serious problem first*
- *Support life where possible*
- *Get help if necessary*

Do not endanger yourself Do not go into hazardous situations without thinking or without proper equipment. At fires, stay away; similarly, beware of exposure to chemical spillages and fumes. At a road traffic accident, put up hazard signs to keep other vehicles clear. If someone is drowning, be sure that you can stand the cold and swim strongly enough before attempting to help the victim.

Assess the situation Can you deal with the situation alone, or is your most useful action to call for help? Are there any people around who can assist? You could organize them to comfort the casualty, make dressings or go for help.

Protect a casualty from further harm Help those people who can move by themselves into a comfortable position, away from fire or fumes and so on. Otherwise do not move anyone unless it is essential for their further safety. If someone is unconscious, place them in the recovery position (see page 390), unless there is a possibility that they have a neck or spinal injury.

FIRST AID

Attend to the most serious problem first Check each casualty for breathing and pulse – if absent, the person will need resuscitation (see page 391) (unless obviously dead). Then deal with people who are unconscious, bleeding heavily, choking, breathless or who have fractures and so on. Finally, deal with the minor cuts and bruises and those who are emotionally shocked.

Support life where possible Give resuscitation (see page 391) until help arrives; it is for healthcare professionals to decide when efforts are hopeless. You may have to balance the risk of moving someone with a possible neck injury against the need to resuscitate.

Get help Many minor injuries can be dealt with perfectly well by first aid. You may need help for a fuller assessment, more intensive treatment or transfer to hospital. Call for help if in any doubt; do not attempt first aid beyond your capabilities or confidence unless the situation is absolutely desperate, in which case it is better to have a go rather than leave someone to their fate.

Right: It is reassuring, and potentially life saving, to learn a few basic first aid techniques. A painting by Issac Koedyck (Koedijck) depicting a barber surgeon tending a peasant's foot, c. 1650.

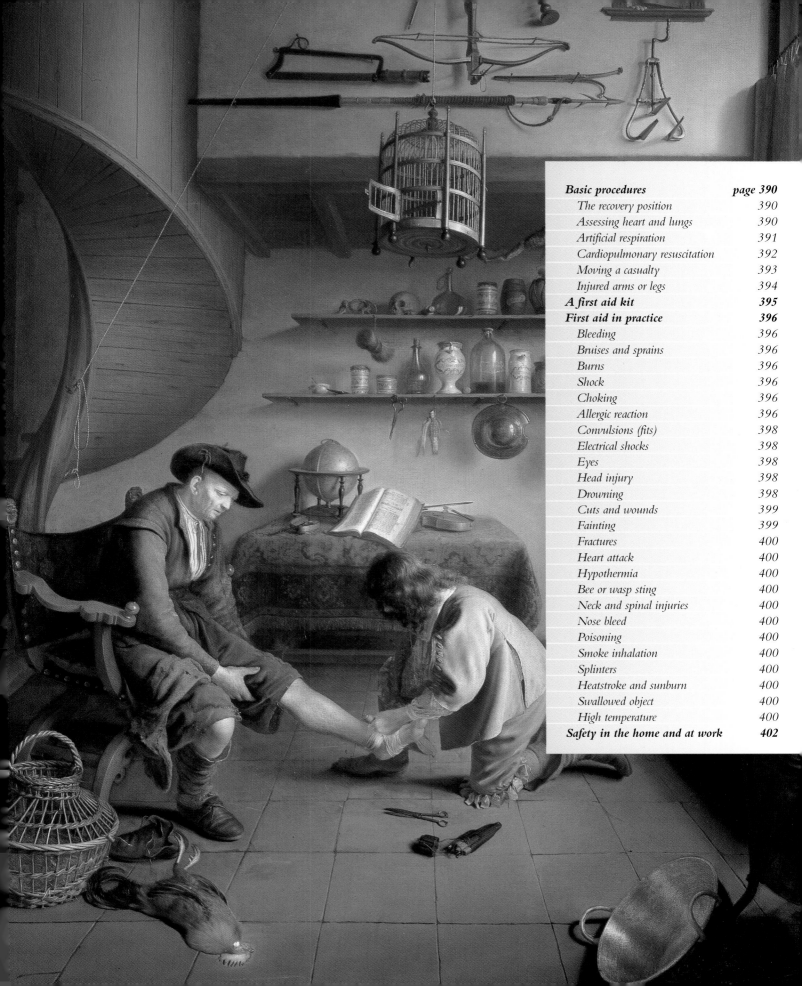

BASIC PROCEDURES

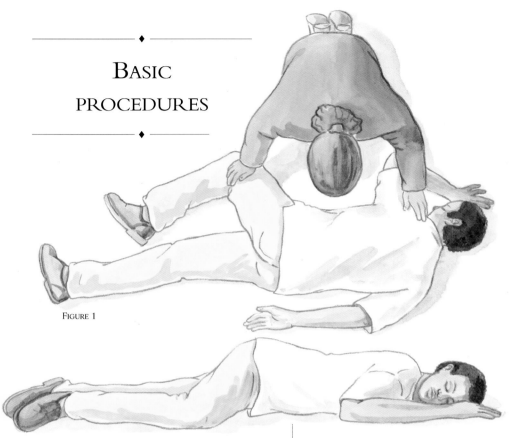

FIGURE 1

FIGURE 2

THE RECOVERY POSITION

Purpose: To prevent an unconscious or drowsy person from inhaling vomit; to allow drainage of material from the mouth. It is not necessary for someone who is conscious and who can move into a comfortable position.

WARNING: Do not use if there is the possibility of a neck or spinal injury.

To place someone in the recovery position, first roll the person on to his front (Figure 1). Turn his face to one side, resting against that hand. Place the other arm down his side (Figure 2).

To assess heart and lungs,
check **ABC:**
    AIRWAY
    BREATHING
    CIRCULATION

ASSESSING HEART AND LUNGS

Purpose: To make sure the casualty's heart and lungs are working. Check 'ABC': airway, breathing, circulation.

Airway (throat, windpipe)
Look for and clear away vomit, fluid, food, foreign body or a swallowed tongue. Tilt the chin upward.

Breathing
Check if the casualty's chest is moving and feel for breath. If he is not breathing start artificial respiration (see right).

Circulation
See if the heart is beating by feeling with two fingers for a pulse in the carotid artery in the neck (or in the inner arm above the elbow in a baby – the brachial pulse).

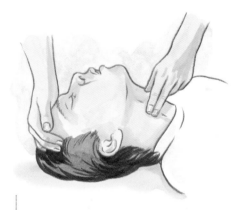

FIGURE 3

To check for a pulse in an adult or child, first feel for the Adam's apple. Move your fingers to one side and press gently over the artery (Figure 3). If no pulse is felt after ten seconds, assume the heart has stopped and start cardio-pulmonary resuscitation (see page 392).

ARTIFICIAL RESPIRATION (MOUTH-TO-MOUTH RESUSCITATION)

Purpose: To breathe for the casualty.

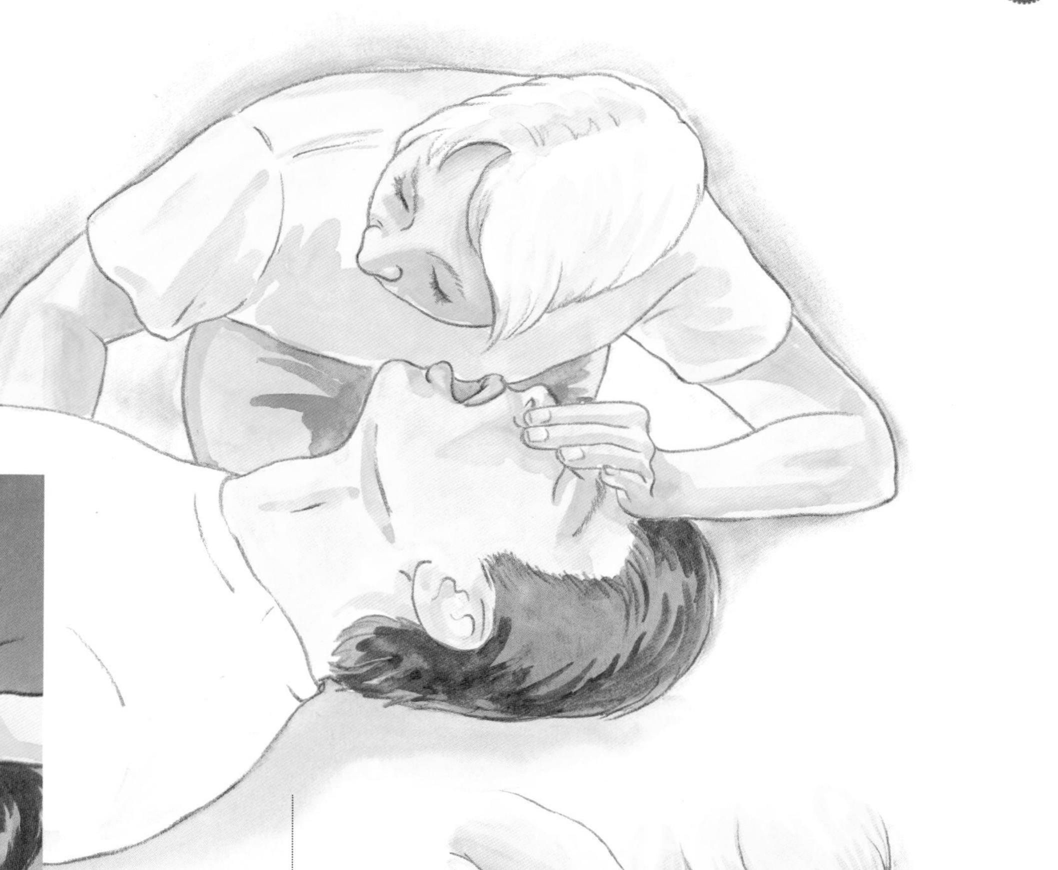

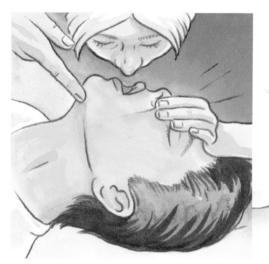

FIGURE 4

FIGURE 5

To give artificial respiration to an adult or child over the age of one year, keep the casualty on his back. Clear the airway, tilt back the chin and pinch his nostrils shut. Place your mouth over his and blow in for two seconds at a time (Figure 4). His chest should rise; if it does not, look again for an obstruction. Remove your mouth; the chest should fall (Figure 5). Repeat. Keep checking the pulse; if absent start cardiopulmonary resuscitation (see page 392).

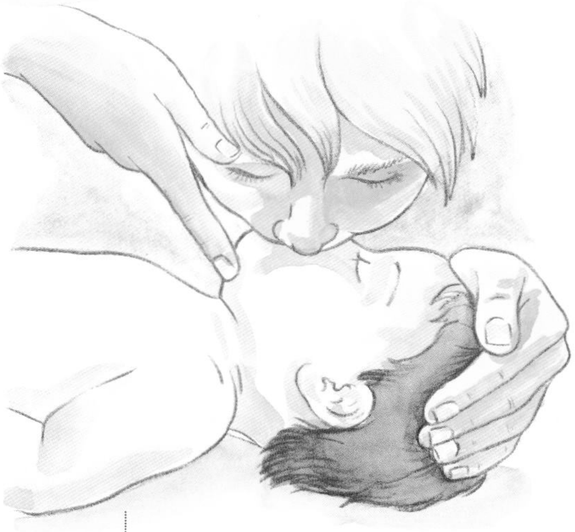

FIGURE 6

To give artificial respiration to a baby less than one year old, keep the baby on her back. Clear the airway and tilt back the chin, as for an adult. Place your mouth over the baby's nose and mouth. Breathe into her nose and mouth (Figure 6) then let the baby's chest fall, allowing three seconds for this process of breathing into the baby and letting her chest fall. Keep checking for circulation, or else begin cardiopulmonary resuscitation (see page 393), giving one breath every five heart compressions.

CARDIOPULMONARY RESUSCITATION (CPR)

◆

Purpose: To keep the blood pumping if the heart has stopped. It always has to be combined with artificial respiration (see page 391), hence the name cardiopulmonary resuscitation (CPR).

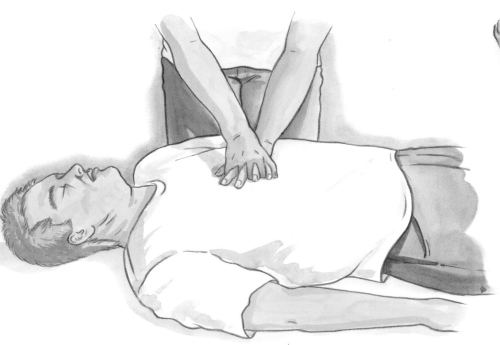

FIGURE 7

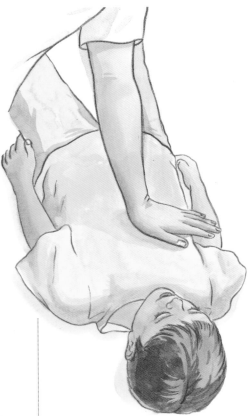

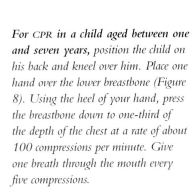

FIGURE 8

To administer CPR to an adult or an older child, keep the casualty on his back. Kneel over him, place the heel of one hand over the lower breastbone, place your other hand on top (Figure 7). With your arms straight, press down 4–5 cm / 1½–2 in firmly at a rate of about 100 compressions per minute. Give 15 compressions, then 2 breaths and keep repeating. Check for a pulse after the first minute (see page 390) then every few minutes, until help arrives or the heart restarts.

For CPR in a child aged between one and seven years, position the child on his back and kneel over him. Place one hand over the lower breastbone (Figure 8). Using the heel of your hand, press the breastbone down to one-third of the depth of the chest at a rate of about 100 compressions per minute. Give one breath through the mouth every five compressions.

MOVING A CASUALTY

◆

Purpose: Move a casualty only if it is necessary to get the person out of danger and not at all if there is a possibility of fracture to the person's neck or spine. Take care not to strain your own back – if in doubt wait for help and equipment.

If the casualty has been electrocuted, do not touch her until the electricity has been turned off at the mains (see Electrical shocks, page 398).

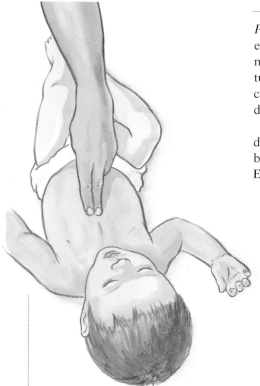

FIGURE 9

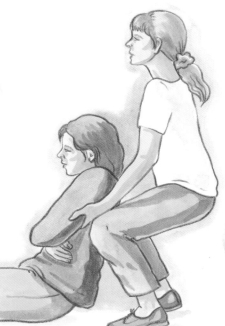

FIGURE 10

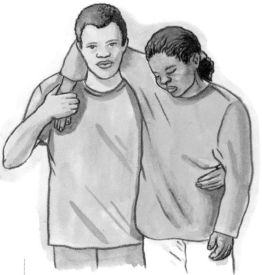

FIGURE 11

For CPR in a baby less than one year old, *place two fingers over the lower breastbone (Figure 9). Press the breastbone down to one-third of the depth of the chest at a rate of about 100 compressions per minute. Give one breath (through the nose and mouth) every five compressions.*

To drag a casualty, *fold the person's arms over her chest. Squat, then place your hands under her armpits (Figure 10). Move smoothly, without jerking.*

To support a casualty to walk, *stand on her injured side – but if the arm is injured, stand on the opposite side. Place her arm across your shoulder and hold her hand. Place your other arm across her back at waist level, holding her clothing (Figure 11). Walk with small steps, starting off with your inner foot.*

INJURED ARMS OR LEGS

Keep the limb comfortable and supported until help arrives. Move it as little as possible, but check for bleeding from cuts. The injured limb will swell so do not hesitate to cut away anything that might constrict the swelling.

An injured arm

Purpose: To keep an injured arm or shoulder immobile and supported. Gently place the injured arm across the person's chest and improvise a support using bandages, clothing or a towel, tied behind the neck. In the case of an injured elbow do not use a sling if it is too sore to bend; instead keep it in the position of the least pain, tied against the body if possible.

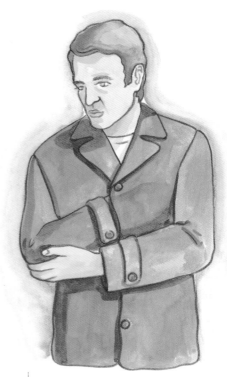

FIGURE 14

A sling can usually be improvised if a triangular bandage is not available. One method is to tuck the hand of the injured arm into a buttoned shirt or jacket at chest height (Figure 14).

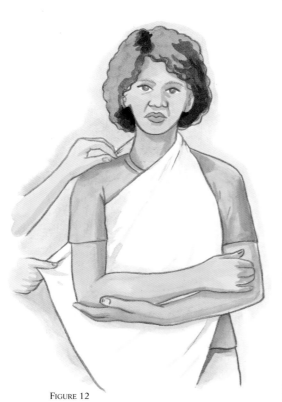

FIGURE 12

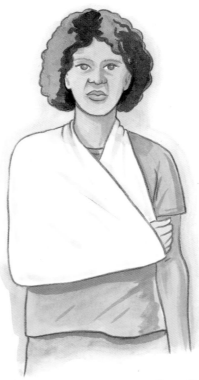

FIGURE 13

To make a sling using a triangular bandage, run one point of the triangle over the shoulder and around the neck (Figure 12).
Lift the lowest point of the bandage up over the forearm to meet the end at the shoulder. Knot these ends together just below the level of the shoulder. Tuck in the third point at the end of the elbow (Figure 13) and secure with a safety pin.

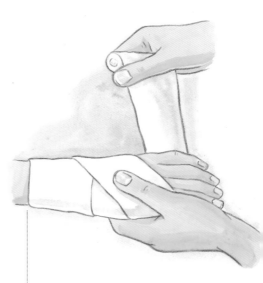

FIGURE 15

To bandage a hand, for holding pads to control bleeding or for support after a sprain, begin at the wrist (Figure 15).

An injured leg

Purpose: To keep the leg immobile in the position of the least pain and slightly elevated to reduce swelling.

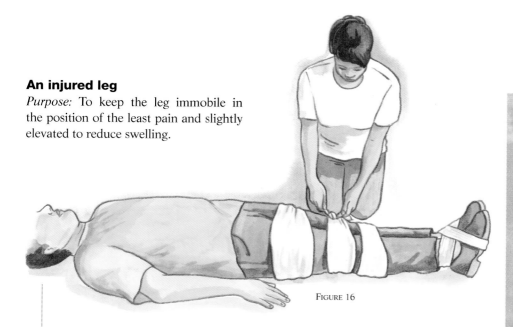

FIGURE 16

To immobilize a leg, lay the casualty down. Move the limb only if it is essential for comfort. Place a support under the injured part, for example rolled-up clothing or a towel. Bandage the injured leg against the good one (Figure 16) if the ambulance is going to be delayed.

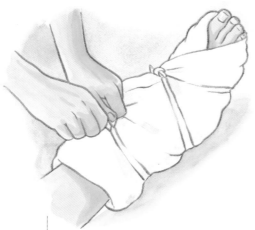

FIGURE 17

For an injured foot and ankle, use a piece of cloth or a flat cushion secured with narrow bandages for support (Figure 17), until you can get professional help.

A FIRST AID KIT

Keep a well-labelled kit where it is most likely to be used, for example the kitchen, the garage, the car or at work. Select items according to common sense. If you live in town, you probably need enough only for minor injuries; if you live, work or drive somewhere remote, keep a more comprehensive kit. Kits for public places such as offices and factories must meet approved standards – discuss with your health and safety representative or supplier. Replace things you use immediately, and discard anything that is out of date.

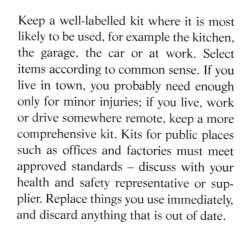

DRESSINGS

◆

Sticking plaster of various sizes
Sterile dressings of various sizes (non-stick if possible) – to cover wounds
Gauze pads – for absorbency over cuts and burns
Adhesive tape – to fix pads and bandages
Rolls of bandage of various widths to hold dressings in place and support limbs
Tubular bandages plus applicator for injured fingers
Triangular bandage – to support an injured limb, bandage the head or pad large wounds
Eye pad
Swabs – for cleaning wounds
Cotton wool – for padding and washing, but not to be used directly on wounds

MEDICATION

◆

Antiseptic cream – for cuts
Antiseptic liquid – to clean wounds and skin
Antihistamine cream – for insect bites and stings
Paracetamol tablets (liquid for children), or ibuprofen – for fever or pain relief

EQUIPMENT

◆

Tweezers – for splinters
Thermometer
Eye bath
Disposable gloves
Safety scissors
Safety pins

FIRST AID IN PRACTICE — WHAT TO DO WHEN

BLEEDING

Assuming this is from a minor injury, raise the bleeding limb or lay the patient down if the wound is on the body. Apply firm pressure over the bleeding point for two to four minutes. Once the bleeding has stopped, do not disturb the clot. Cover with a clean dressing.

Beware of the following: bleeding from a deep wound; arterial bleeding (spurts, bright red); heavy bleeding; the victim becoming pale and faint with rapid pulse. In such cases apply pressure or a pad to the bleeding point. Get the casualty to hospital immediately.

BRUISES AND SPRAINS

The swelling that accompanies these injuries is from bleeding under the skin and fluid in the tissues.

For bruises cool the area with an ice pack – a pack of frozen peas is ideal. Keep it there for ten to twenty minutes to reduce further bleeding under the skin. No other treatment is necessary.

A sprain is a pulled ligament – usually of the ankle or knee. The area is tender and you may not be able to walk properly. Carry out 'RICE': rest, ice, compression, elevation (see box, above right).

See a doctor for severe bruising, or if you cannot put weight on a sprain, since you may have torn the ligament.

Carry out **RICE**:

- ♦ **REST:** *Stop walking or playing sport as soon as possible*
- ♦ **ICE:** *Put the injured part in ice-cold water for ten to twenty minutes, or apply an ice pack – a pack of frozen vegetables is perfect*
- ♦ **COMPRESSION:** *After cooling, apply a compression bandage to reduce further swelling*
- ♦ **ELEVATION:** *Keep the injured part slightly raised for several hours after the injury*

BURNS

Remove the source of heat, i.e. fire or hot liquids. Remove hot clothing from the skin carefully – but do not attempt to remove anything that appears stuck to the skin. Cool the burn with cold water for 15 minutes to reduce tissue damage. Cover with a dry, non-stick dressing. Do not burst any blisters. If the burns are extensive, give the person drinks and keep him lying down and warm until help arrives.

Seek medical advice for any burn that is larger than 5 cm²/2 sq in, for severe blistering, charred skin and burns from chemicals or electricity.

SHOCK

Medical shock is a collapse of blood pressure caused by bleeding, heart attack, poisoning, burns or dehydration. Symptoms include cold clammy skin, weak pulse, feeling faint, going unconscious, blue lips and difficulty breathing. Lay the casualty down with her legs raised and keep warm. Do not give food or fluids. Be prepared to resuscitate until help arrives.

CHOKING

Food or foreign objects may stick in the throat, obstructing breathing. The victim may be coughing or clutching his throat, or has collapsed and looks blue.

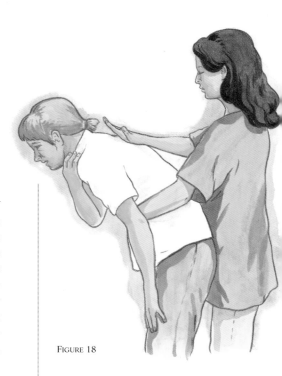

FIGURE 18

For choking adults and older children, first try to pull out the obstruction if it can be done. Get the person to bend forwards and try to cough. Slap firmly between the shoulders five times to move the obstruction (Figure 18). If it does not work, perform the Heimlich manoeuvre.

ALLERGIC REACTION

Suspect if someone's mouth and lips swell, they cannot breathe or swallow. If mild give an antihistamine. See if they have an adrenalin injection pen – many allergy sufferers carry them. If so, give the injection, otherwise get urgent medical help.

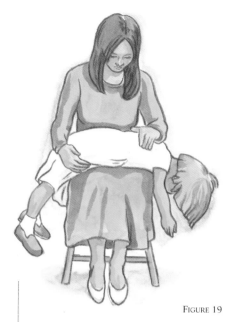

FIGURE 19

Lay a choking toddler face down over your lap (Figure 19) and give five quick slaps between the shoulders. If this fails, try the Heimlich manoeuvre (see right), then more back slaps if still choking. Keep checking if the obstruction has been dislodged and can be easily removed.

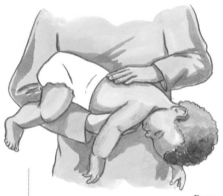

FIGURE 20

For a choking baby less than one year old, lay the baby face down across your knees or arm, head well down (Figure 20). Give five firm slaps to her back; see if the obstruction can be removed. Otherwise, turn the baby on her back, head down. With two fingers, push firmly and sharply several times over the lower breastbone. Repeat as necessary.

For victims of any age, give resuscitation if required until help arrives.

Performing the Heimlich manoeuvre (abdominal thrusts)

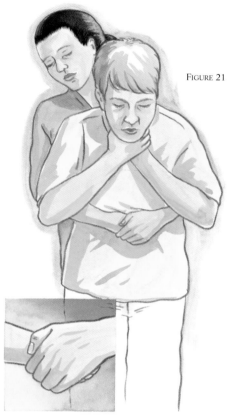

FIGURE 21

FIGURE 22

For the Heimlich manoeuvre in an adult, stand behind the person who is choking. Place your hands over her upper abdomen, just below the bottom of the breastbone (Figure 21). Link your hands and have one thumb pushing against her abdomen (Figure 22). Pull sharply in and upwards five times, then slap her back five times. Repeat if necessary if the obstruction has not been dislodged.

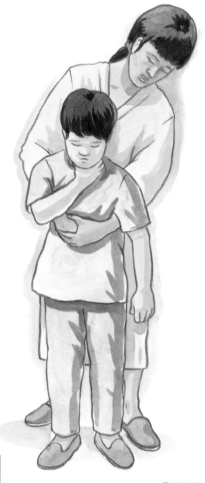

FIGURE 23

For the Heimlich manoeuvre in a child aged one to seven years, stand or kneel behind the child. Place your fist over the lower breastbone, your other hand over it. Thrust firmly in and upward five times, then slap her back five times. If there is no success, place your hands lower, over the upper abdomen (Figure 23). Give five thrusts upwards, then slap her back. Repeat if necessary.

WARNING: Do not use the Heimlich manoeuvre on a child less than one year old.

CONVULSIONS (FITS)

Recognize a fit by the following symptoms:

- *Collapse*
- *A few seconds of clenched teeth and muscles, followed by jerking movements for several minutes*
- *Finally, drowsiness and a gradual return to consciousness*
- *Children may be very hot*

Lay the individual down; put him into the recovery position. Do not otherwise interfere. Do not put anything in his mouth, even though he might bite his tongue. Cool a hot child (see High temperature, page 401). Take the person to hospital if it is a first fit, if it lasts longer than ten minutes or if it keeps repeating.

ELECTRICAL SHOCKS

Turn the electricity off at the mains before attempting anything else. Do not endanger yourself by directly touching the appliance or the victim.

FIGURE 24

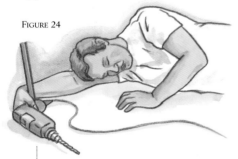

If you cannot turn off the electricity, you need to separate the casualty and the live electrical appliance: push away the appliance or the victim's limb with a broom or a wooden chair since dry wood does not conduct electricity well (Figure 24). Stand on a dry chair or paper while doing this – a telephone directory is a good insulator. Resuscitate the person if necessary, and treat any burns.

EYES

Foreign bodies or splashes in the eye cause irritation, watering and redness. Get medical help if the problem cannot be immediately sorted out or if vision remains blurred.

Foreign body in the eye

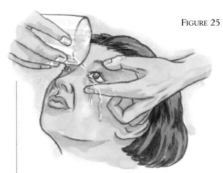

FIGURE 25

To remove the irritant, first locate it by pulling up the eyelid. Gently wipe away the object with a clean tissue or hand kerchief. Otherwise pour cool water over the eye (Figure 25) or get the person to blink under water. Do not attempt to remove an object which appears embedded in the eye.

Chemical splashes in the eye

Wash out the eye immediately using running water or cups of water; continue for ten minutes. Apply an eye pad and have the patient checked at hospital.

FIGURE 26

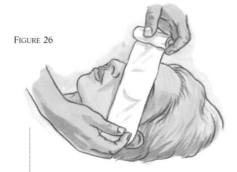

Protect the eye with a pad, held in place with a bandage (Figure 26), while transferring the casualty to hospital.

HEAD INJURY

Blows to the head can be serious, although minor knocks are unlikely to cause a problem.

If someone is knocked unconscious, put them in the recovery position (see page 390) and arrange for transfer to hospital. If someone is conscious, treat any cuts. Transfer them to hospital if any of the following occurs:

- *They cannot move all of their limbs normally*
- *They have a fit*
- *Their pupils are irregular in size*
- *They begin vomiting*
- *They become drowsy or unconscious*
- *They were knocked out*
- *They have amnesia (loss of memory)*

If the casualty seems all right otherwise, reassure her but she should seek professional help if any of the above features appear during the next few days.

DROWNING

The risks of drowning are from inhaled water and from chilling (hypothermia, see page 400) while in the water or once rescued. Rescuers also risk hypothermia and exhaustion, so attempt a rescue only if confident about your own safety – it may be better to manoeuvre a boat or raft, or wade out attached to a rope, for example.

Lay the victim in a sheltered area on his back, his head lower than his feet to allow water to drain out. Clear debris from his mouth, check 'ABC' (see page 390) and resuscitate if necessary. Once he is conscious, put him in the recovery position (see page 390) and keep him warm until help arrives – further assessment in hospital is always essential.

CUTS AND WOUNDS

Most minor cuts can be dealt with by first aid alone. Check the casualty's tetanus coverage – a booster may be required for a dirty or penetrating wound.

Wash dirt away from the injury with water or antiseptic solution. Put pressure on the injury until bleeding stops – two to four minutes. Then clean it more thoroughly, without dislodging the blood clot. Apply a plaster or a non-stick dressing.

Hand wounds

Wounds to the hand often bleed heavily, requiring padding.

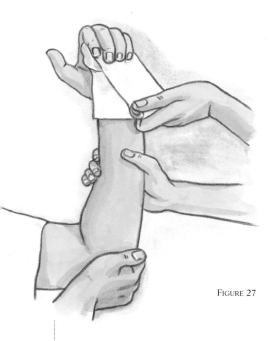

FIGURE 27

To treat a cut palm, put a clean gauze or handkerchief in the person's palm. Get the person to squeeze it and wrap the hand with a bandage (Figure 27). Get the person to hospital.

Embedded objects

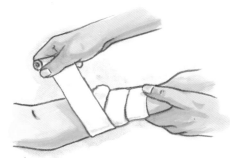

FIGURE 28

Bandaging around an object may be necessary in the case of deeply embedded objects such as glass (Figure 28). Do not pull out embedded objects since you may set off heavy bleeding. Get the patient to hospital.

Fish hooks

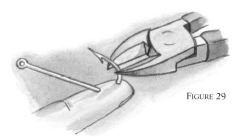

FIGURE 29

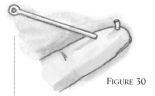

FIGURE 30

Removing a fish hook often requires hospital attention. Only attempt the following if it is unavoidable: if the barb has come completely through, cut it off (Figure 29) then withdraw the rest of the hook (Figure 30). If the barb is still buried, do not withdraw it. Attempt to push it quickly through and out of the flesh; cut off and withdraw as above.

FAINTING

Faints are common in people having to stand for long periods, especially in the heat, during pregnancy or after missing meals, and often even for no obvious cause. Blood pressure falls, the person feels light-headed and dizzy, then slowly collapses. She looks pale, sweaty and has a slow pulse.

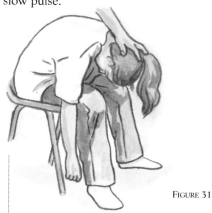

FIGURE 31

If someone feels faint, help them to lie down or to sit with their head between their knees (Figure 31).

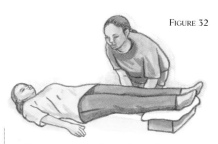

FIGURE 32

If someone has fainted, check that they have a pulse and are breathing – if neither, begin resuscitation (see page 390) and call for help. Lay the person down and raise her legs to a level above her head (Figure 32). She should recover within a few seconds but do not let her sit up or stand until she feels back to normal – ten to fifteen minutes. Give her a drink of water and a light snack if she has not eaten for some while. Get help if the victim is bleeding, has a fit or remains unconscious.

FRACTURES

◆

Suspect a fracture if, after an accident, someone has pain over a bone, difficulty using that part of the body or deformity of a limb. Deal with any bleeding and cover any protruding bone or open wound. Do not let the victim put weight on a fracture. If an arm or shoulder is involved, support the limb with a sling (see page 394), then get the casualty to hospital.

HEART ATTACK

◆

Suspect a heart attack if someone complains of chest pain and then has difficulty breathing, looks blue around the lips or collapses. Lay the person down; check for pulse and breathing – if absent begin resuscitation (see page 390). Arrange for immediate medical help.

HYPOTHERMIA

◆

This is most likely to occur in the elderly, in outdoor enthusiasts, or in someone who has fallen into cold water.

The person feels cold, is confused or unconscious. Remove any wet clothing, and place the person in a warm or sheltered place. Warm him gradually with blankets or your own body heat. If conscious give him warm drinks – but do not give him alcohol. A mildly affected person can have a warm bath; someone severely affected must not – continue warming them gradually until help arrives.

BEE OR WASP STING

◆

Brush the sting off; do not squeeze it. Use tweezers if available. Apply a cold dressing to reduce swelling. If stung in the mouth, suck ice cubes. Get help if there is severe swelling or difficulty in breathing.

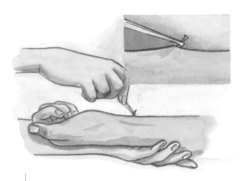

FIGURE 33

To remove the sting, place tweezers below the poison sac, as close to the skin as possible, then pull it out (Figure 33).

NECK AND SPINAL INJURIES

◆

Such injuries happen after accidents and falls – often through sporting activities. Beware of paralysis, severe pain or tingling down the limbs. If these symptoms are present, do not allow any movement of the back; get urgent help. Keep the patient's neck well supported.

To improvise a neck support, use towels, rolled newspapers or clothing to keep the casualty's neck still but comfortable (Figure 24).

NOSE BLEED

◆

Most nose bleeds are a result of inflammation of the lining of the nose through colds or the heat.

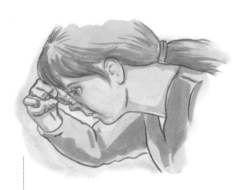

FIGURE 35

To deal with a nose bleed, lean forward. Firmly pinch the soft part of the nose just above the nostrils for ten minutes (Figure 35); breathe through the mouth. Do not wipe or blow your nose for several hours afterwards. If bleeding persists, seek hospital treatment.

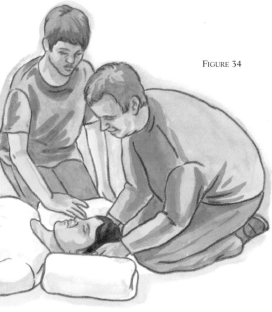

FIGURE 34

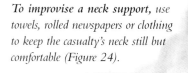

POISONING

Suspect poisoning if a child or adult becomes suddenly drowsy or unconscious; if there are chemical burns around the mouth or hands; or if someone has been drinking heavily or using drugs.

Give resuscitation if required. If someone has swallowed a caustic substance give artificial respiration (see page 391) only via a face mask. Do not make them vomit. Wash mouth burns with water. Wash chemical contaminants off the skin. Identify the poison or keep a sample of it and try to establish how long ago it was taken. Get medical help urgently. Keep the casualty safe until the antidote can be given. Remember alcohol is a poison, too; treat drunkenness as poisoning.

SMOKE INHALATION

Smoke causes damage by suffocation and by irritation of the lungs. Do not risk your own safety by entering smoke- or fume-filled areas without proper equipment.

Escape from smoke or fumes if possible. Otherwise find a room with a window; put towels or clothing at the base of doors to prevent smoke entering. Keep yourself low because smoke rises. Open the window to help you breathe.

Avoid opening doors or windows in a

SPLINTERS

Remove splinters as soon as possible, before the skin swells. Clean the area around the splinter. Use tweezers to grip the splinter where it meets the skin. Pull it out in the direction in which it entered. After removal, clean the wound more thoroughly with antiseptic solution.

HEATSTROKE AND SUNBURN

Heatstroke can appear within minutes in someone exposed to heat through exertion, illness or a hot atmosphere. Symptoms include nausea, a bad headache, confusion, a fast pulse and very hot skin. This is an emergency – call for help. Move the heatstroke victim into the shade, remove his clothing and fan him. Put wet clothing or towels on him to reduce temperature quickly. Resuscitate if necessary.

Sunburnt skin is red, hot and tender. Get the person out of the sun. Cool the skin with cool water or a cooling cream such as calamine. Give fluids. Seek help if the burns are extensive or blister.

Keep yourself low down in a smoke-filled area. Cover your nose and mouth with a wet cloth to keep out fumes

SWALLOWED OBJECT

It is unusual for swallowed coins or similar objects to cause problems unless they are sharp, for example fragments of glass or bones.

Give plenty of fluids. Seek hospital treatment if the object was sharp or large, i.e. more than 1 cm/½ in in diameter, or if the person was coughing and may have breathed it in. (An X-ray at hospital may be used to locate a swallowed object which fails to pass within 48 hours, is large or may have been inhaled.)

HIGH TEMPERATURE

A fever is almost always due to infection; it may be 48 hours or more before the cause is apparent. The younger the person, the more important it is to reduce temperature to avoid a fit.

Children

To take a child's temperature place a thermometer under the arm for one minute – never in the mouth – or use an ear thermometer. Normal underarm temperature is 36.5°C/97.5°F. An alternative is a fever strip which is placed across the forehead to measure skin temperature. Although a useful guide, this is not nearly as reliable as using a standard thermometer.

Give paracetamol or ibuprofen syrup. Never give aspirin to children below 12 years of age. Remove clothing apart from a light vest. Use a fan if necessary or sponge the child's brow with tepid water. Give the child plenty of drinks.

Adults

Place a thermometer in the mouth, under the tongue, for one minute. Normal temperature is 37°C/ 98.4°F. Take paracetamol or aspirin. Wrap up or undress, whichever is more comfortable for you. Drink plenty of fluids.

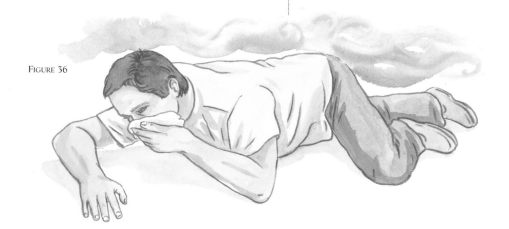

FIGURE 36

SAFETY IN THE HOME AND AT WORK

Many accidents happen in the home through falls, cuts, burns, domestic chemicals and so on. Make your home a safer place by identifying and eliminating hazards before harm comes. Similarly, you can make your workplace safer, too, by reporting unsafe working practices and making suggestions for improvements.

In the bathroom

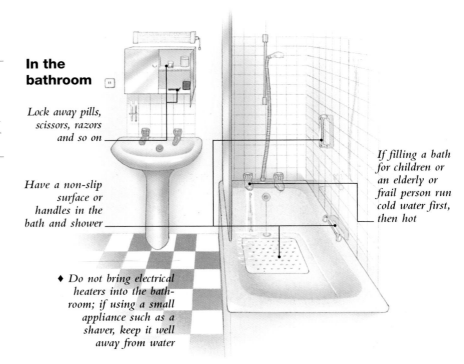

Lock away pills, scissors, razors and so on

Have a non-slip surface or handles in the bath and shower

If filling a bath for children or an elderly or frail person run cold water first, then hot

♦ *Do not bring electrical heaters into the bathroom; if using a small appliance such as a shaver, keep it well away from water*

In the kitchen

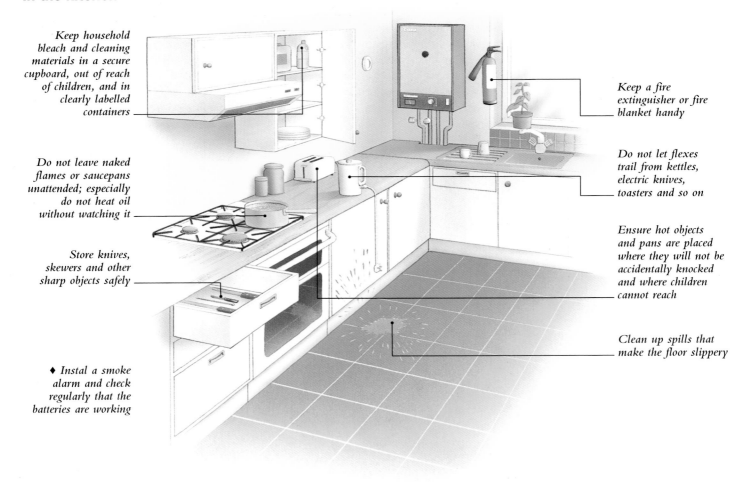

Keep household bleach and cleaning materials in a secure cupboard, out of reach of children, and in clearly labelled containers

Do not leave naked flames or saucepans unattended; especially do not heat oil without watching it

Store knives, skewers and other sharp objects safely

♦ *Instal a smoke alarm and check regularly that the batteries are working*

Keep a fire extinguisher or fire blanket handy

Do not let flexes trail from kettles, electric knives, toasters and so on

Ensure hot objects and pans are placed where they will not be accidentally knocked and where children cannot reach

Clean up spills that make the floor slippery

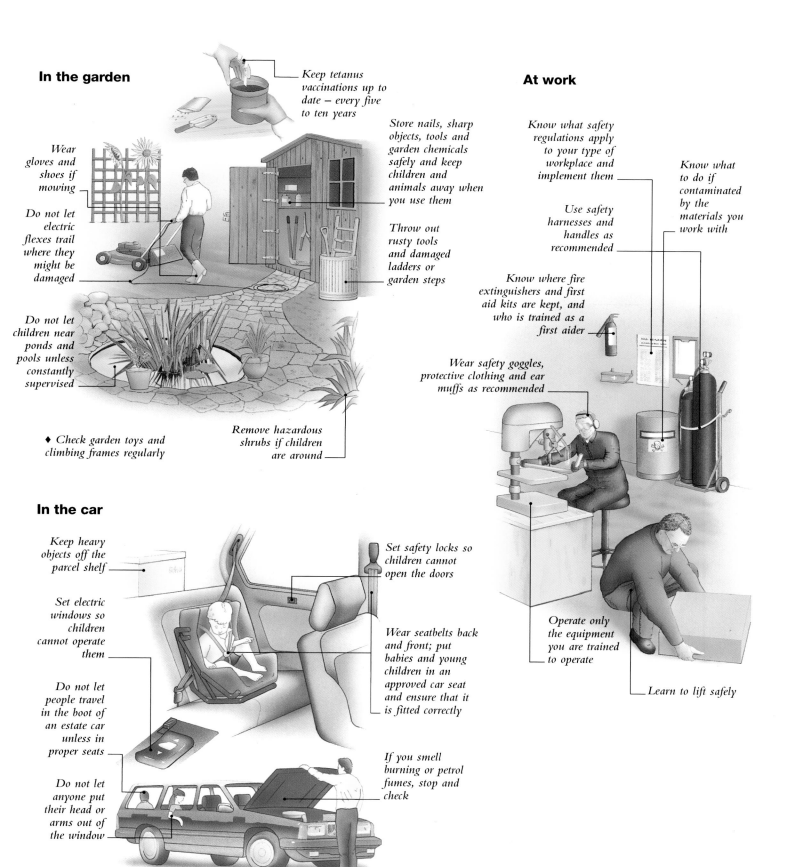

In the garden

Keep tetanus vaccinations up to date – every five to ten years

Wear gloves and shoes if mowing

Do not let electric flexes trail where they might be damaged

Do not let children near ponds and pools unless constantly supervised

Store nails, sharp objects, tools and garden chemicals safely and keep children and animals away when you use them

Throw out rusty tools and damaged ladders or garden steps

♦ Check garden toys and climbing frames regularly

Remove hazardous shrubs if children are around

At work

Know what safety regulations apply to your type of workplace and implement them

Use safety harnesses and handles as recommended

Know where fire extinguishers and first aid kits are kept, and who is trained as a first aider

Wear safety goggles, protective clothing and ear muffs as recommended

Know what to do if contaminated by the materials you work with

Operate only the equipment you are trained to operate

Learn to lift safely

In the car

Keep heavy objects off the parcel shelf

Set electric windows so children cannot operate them

Do not let people travel in the boot of an estate car unless in proper seats

Do not let anyone put their head or arms out of the window

Set safety locks so children cannot open the doors

Wear seatbelts back and front; put babies and young children in an approved car seat and ensure that it is fitted correctly

If you smell burning or petrol fumes, stop and check

COMPLEMENTARY THERAPIES

I N THE FAST PACE of today's world where everyone is under constant pressure, people are now taking more interest in maintaining good health and wellbeing. There is general concern about disease and the environment, in particular about the way pollutants are affecting our health and the way in which pesticides or contaminated animal feeds are affecting the vegetables and meat that we eat in our daily diets.

Today, adults and children also seem to be developing more allergic reactions to food and general pollutants in the environment, and diseases such as asthma are now particularly affecting children. One theory is that childhood asthma is on the increase because of increased traffic fumes, and also dust mites that are present in everybody's homes.

Resistance to antibodies

People are developing an increasing resistance to antibiotics given to treat different infections and are starting to investigate complementary treatments which will help build up their immune systems. There are also new diseases, such as ME, which can start after a viral infection, that have arisen over the last 10–15 years. There is no cure at present for ME. However, complementary treatments such as aromatherapy, Western herbalism and nutritional therapy have been found to help sufferers by improving and balancing their general diet and boosting their immune systems, which are often at a very low ebb.

A new attitude

There has also been an overall rejection of the materialistic values of the hedonistic Eighties. Since the more caring Nineties, people have had to work harder, often juggling careers and children, and have suffered more stress because of it. But today they are more willing to undertake holistic therapies such as yoga, tai chi and massage to help them cope with tension and overwork by relaxing both their bodies and their minds.

The way forward

Complementary therapies are definitely becoming more popular. In fact, recent research in Britain showed that eight out of ten people had tried a complementary treatment and three-quarters of them reported that it had either helped or cured them. Doctors are also becoming more aware of the benefits of complementary health therapies in cases when orthodox treatment alone does not seem to help. In fact, they will now often refer a patient to an osteopath or chiropractor, for example, for manipulation of a nagging back problem that is proving difficult to resolve. Some doctors are also trained in a complementary therapy, such as homeopathy, and this treatment is now becoming more widely available in Britain under the National Health system.

Emphasis on 'complementary'

Complementary health treatment can do so much to improve a person's mental attitude and to help or cure ailments, but in cases of serious or terminal illness only certain therapies will be suitable and should never be taken instead of orthodox treatment, but rather alongside it. Acupuncture, for example, can greatly boost the immune systems of cancer or HIV patients while also improving their overall mental attitude and their perspective on their disease.

Right: Complementary treatments come from many parts of the world but they all have the well-being of the patient at heart. Pierre Quthe, apothecary by François Clouet (c. 1510–72).

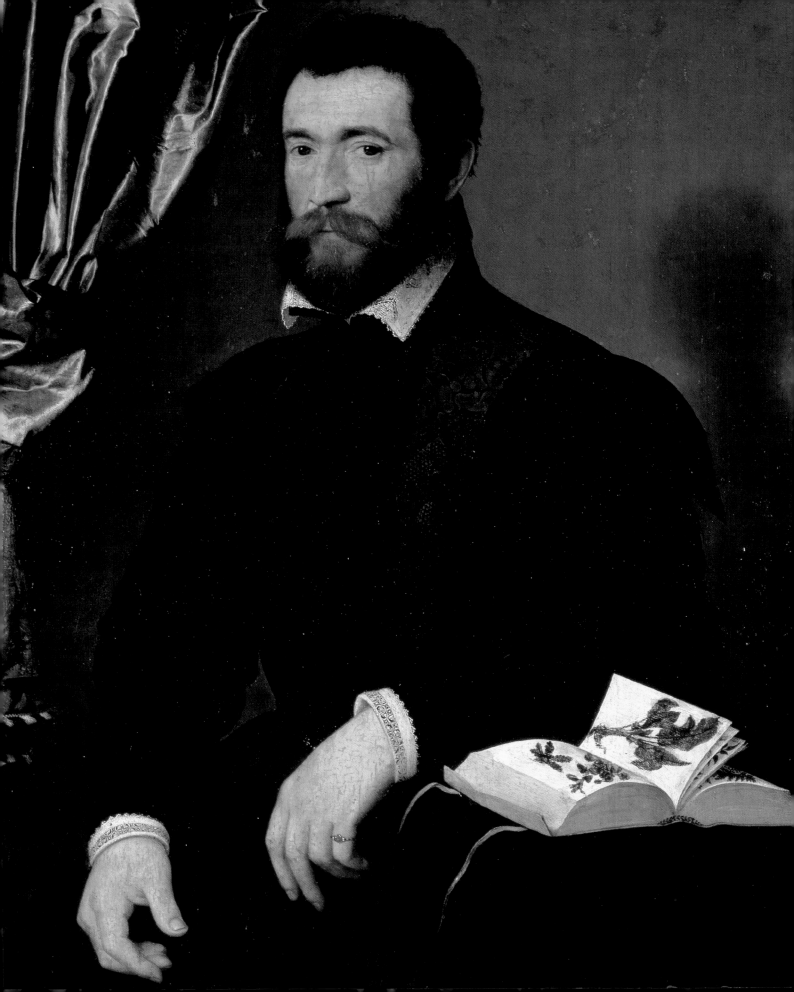

NATURAL THERAPIES

AROMATHERAPY

Aromatherapy is the fastest growing complementary therapy in Britain. It is used in homes, therapy rooms, clinics and beauty salons all over the country.

The Greeks, Romans and ancient Egyptians all made use of aromatherapy oils. However, it was not until the 1930s that French chemist René-Maurice Gattefossé developed the use of aromatherapy as we know it today. He originated the term aromatherapy to define the therapeutic use of essential oils as a discipline in its own right.

Aromatherapists believe that the therapy works on the mind and body at the same time, making it a perfect, gentle, mind and body medicine.

Aromatherapy means 'treatment using scents'. It refers to the use of essential oils to improve health and emotional wellbeing and restore balance to the body. Essential oils are aromatic essences extracted from plants. They have therapeutic, psychological and physiological properties, which improve and prevent illness. Around 150 have been extracted, each with its own unique scent and antiseptic and healing property.

In fact, all the properties, and none of the side effects, of tailor-made drugs occur naturally in plants and their benefits are extracted through essential oils. These pure oils are usually extracted by steam distillation, but other methods, such as solvent extraction, enfleurage, and expression can be used.

How does it work?
Leading aromatherapist Valerie Worwood describes essential oils as 'the little keys that can unlock our physical and mental mechanisms'. Some oils, such as lemon and lavender, adapt to what the body requires of them at the time. Nobody really understands how plant essences can do this. It may be because chemically we are much closer to plants than we care to think. However it happens, we know that essential oils are absorbed into the body and exert an influence on it. They also affect our minds. They enter the body in two ways: by inhalation or absorption.

Inhalation Essential oils have a direct effect on our emotions through our sense of smell. No one knows how smells affect the brain, but the theory is that a smell enters the nose and connects with cilia (the fine hairs lining the nose). The receptors in the cilia are linked to the olfactory bulb (the end of the smelling tract) which, in turn, is linked to the brain. Smells are converted into electrical impulses which, through the olfactory system, are transmitted to the limbic system of the brain, associated with our moods, emotions, memory and learning. So a smell that reaches the limbic system has a chemical effect on our emotions, and improves mental alertness and concentration.

Absorption through the skin Essential oil molecules are so small that they can be absorbed through the pores of the skin, affecting the skin itself, the bloodstream and the whole body including the brain. Absorption is considered to be more effective than inhalation, and massage is believed to be the best method. It can take anything from 20 minutes to several hours for essential oils to be absorbed into the body, but the average time is about 90 minutes. Heat also helps their absorption, so warm hands and a warm room work best. Hot water also helps them to be absorbed from bath water. Applying oils to the body is more powerful than inhalation because they begin to work on the fabric of the body as soon as they touch the skin.

How the oils are used
Essential oils are used in a variety of ways, most of which you can do at home.

Inhalations These can be direct or by steam. Place one or two drops of your chosen oil on a handkerchief and you can inhale while at work or travelling. Two drops of a relaxing oil on a tissue inside your pillow helps you sleep. Steam inhalations with three or four drops in a large bowl of hot water helps clear congestion or catarrh. Eucalyptus, pine, lavender, black pepper, lemon or peppermint oils are helpful for coughs, colds, bronchitis, sinus problems and headaches.

Diffusers and vaporizers These release the scent of essential oils into the air, providing an attractive natural fragrance and distributing their therapeutic benefits at the same time. Diffusers can be electrical devices, burners which use candles, or simple ceramic rings that are warmed by a light bulb. Choose a stimulating oil such as lemon or rosemary for the office or a relaxing oil such as lavender or camomile for the bedroom.

Massage This is the most common form of treatment used by aromatherapists, simply because it is so effective (see Massage pages 428–9). The combination of touch and the therapeutic benefits of the oils improves circulation and releases trapped energy from tense muscles. The fragrance also promotes a feeling of wellbeing. The essential oil is diluted in a vegetable carrier oil such as grapeseed or sweet almond oil. Aromatherapists usually recommend a dilution rate of five drops of essential oil to 5ml (1tsp) of the carrier oil for adults, half that strength for children under seven, and a quarter of the strength for children under three. For newborn babies it is best to avoid essential oils altogether.

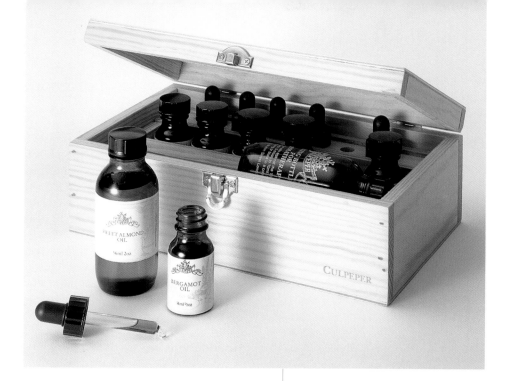

Above: There are over 150 different essential oils from which to choose.

Baths Scent with your chosen oil(s). Any oil can be used in the bath. Add up to eight drops for adults, four for children over two, and stir though the warm water with your hand. Five or six drops of grapefruit essential oil on a sponge will invigorate during your morning shower.

Neat Lavender oil has an amazing healing effect when used undiluted on burns. It soothes pain, eases the shock, promotes healing and reduces scarring. Tea tree is particularly effective on cuts, grazes, spots, bites and stings. Other essential oils, however, should not be used neat as they can cause irritation.

What happens in a consultation?

Your first appointment with the aromatherapist will last between 60 and 90 minutes. The room should be warm, comfortable and clean with soft lighting and relaxing music. There will, of course, be a massage table, towels, probably a sink and the therapist's stock of oils. As with all forms of holistic therapy, the therapist will begin by interviewing you. She will want to know about you and your medical history and why you have come.

She will need to decide which oils to use, but also which ones to avoid. If you are pregnant, have sensitive skin, blood pressure problems, epilepsy, or have had a recent operation there are some oils that are not safe to use. If you are pregnant she will avoid basil, rosemary, sage, thyme, clary sage, juniper oils and others, because they are toxic or may harm the foetus or even induce a miscarriage.

The therapist will ask about your stress levels, as many people use aromatherapy for stress relief. She will ask if you are taking any medicines or homoeopathic remedies as strong smells can negate the effects of homoeopathic remedies. She will also want to know how you feel, what mood you are in and what kind of day you have had. This consultation will take about 20 minutes and you may be asked to sign a consent form at the end of it.

Then you will be asked to undress and lie down on a massage table with a towel over you. You need not undress completely if it makes you uncomfortable. If you lie on the table with a towel over you the therapist will move the towel as she works around your body.

She will decide on a blend of oils that she thinks will suit you, or ask if there are any oils that you like. As a rule of thumb, those you like best often work best for you. Then with a blend of oils, mixed in a carrier oil, the therapist will begin, using traditional Swedish massage techniques, perhaps incorporating shiatsu, a type of massage that works on pressure points of the body (see Shiatsu and Acupressure, pages 446–7). Most people prefer to relax rather than talk. A full body massage lasts 30–45 minutes. When it is over, you have a few minutes to relax before dressing. The therapist may conclude by giving you oils to use in the bath at home.

How many sessions do I need?

For relaxation or reducing stress, you can have a treatment whenever you like. But for a specific health problem you will need several visits depending on the problem, the length of time you have had it, and your body's healing abilities. A condition like PMS may need three or four treatments before improvement is noticed, and up to 10 weekly treatments to relieve the symptoms.

Which problems can it help?

Like all forms of holistic medicine, aromatherapy works on the whole body to make you feel better. It is particularly effective for stress and anxiety-related problems, muscular and rheumatic pains, digestive disorders and women's problems, such as PMS, menopausal complaints and postnatal depression.

Is it safe?

Essential oils are safe for all, but can be strong. Always follow instructions and do not exceed dosages. Be careful if you are pregnant, have an allergy or a medical condition such as eczema, high blood pressure or epilepsy. In such cases consult a qualified practitioner for treatment. Take care when using essential oils on young children. If neat oils splash on your skin or in your eyes, wash them off with water. If you swallow an essential oil, drink plenty of milk, eat soft bread and consult your doctor immediately.

HOMEOPATHY

Millions of people worldwide use a safe, reliable, natural form of medicine called homeopathy. Homeopathy, which uses neither drugs nor surgery, is based on the belief that everyone is an individual and should be treated accordingly. It first gained prominence in the 19th century after extensive pioneering work by the German physician and chemist Samuel Hahnemann, but its origins date from the 5th century BC, when the Greek physician Hippocrates – known as the father of medicine – introduced homeopathic remedies to his medicine chest.

Homeopathy is a form of medicine that treats the body as a whole and helps it to heal itself. The treatment works for short-term and chronic ailments and the aim is to prevent illness as well as treat it. The name comes from the Greek word *homios* meaning like and *pathos* meaning suffering. So homeopathy simply means treating like with like.

In practice, this means a substance that causes symptoms in a well person can cure similar symptoms when they result from illness. This view is the opposite of conventional medicine which treats illness with an antidote rather than a similar substance. For example, a doctor would treat diarrhoea with a substance that causes constipation, while a homeopath would treat it with a minute dose of a substance that would cause diarrhoea if given in a larger dose.

The minute substances used in treatment are called homeopathic remedies. These remedies are prescribed for the person and how they are reacting to the ailment, not just the disease. In addition to homeopathic remedies, homeopaths (and other therapists such as medical herbal-

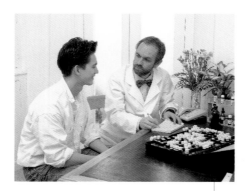

Above: A homeopath will ask questions so he can treat you, not just your illness.

ists), also prescribe tissue salts. These are homeopathically prepared ingredients which were introduced at the end of the 19th century by a German doctor, Wilhelm Schussler. He believed that many diseases are caused by a deficiency of one or more of 12 vital minerals, and that a deficiency in each salt would manifest itself in specific symptoms. Lack of *Calcerea phosphorica* (Calc phos), for example, would show up as a problem with the teeth or an inability to absorb nutrients properly. He replaced the missing mineral with a minute dose of the tissue salt to correct the problem.

Tissue salts are prepared from mineral sources, but homeopathic remedies are made from animal, vegetable and mineral sources, which are all diluted to such an extent that there can be no possible side-effects from even the most toxic substances. Extracts of the natural ingredient are dissolved in alcohol and water and left to stand for 2–4 weeks. They are shaken occasionally and then strained. The strained solution is known as the mother tincture. The mother tincture is then diluted to make the different potencies.

Between every dilution the remedy is 'succussed' (shaken vigorously). To make a 1c dilution, one drop of the mother tincture is added to 99 drops of an alcohol and water mix and succussed. To produce a 6c potency, this happens six times, each time the one drop is taken from the previous succussed solution. By the time it is diluted to the 12c potency, it is unlikely that any of the original ingredient remains. This is often the reason why sceptics are so reluctant to believe that homeopathic remedies can work. Finally, these drops are added to tiny lactose tablets, pillules, granules or powder and stored in a dark bottle.

How does it work?

Conventional doctors treat the symptoms of disease because they see the symptoms as a manifestation of the illness. They prescribe pharmaceutical drugs in a dose great enough to dampen the symptoms of the condition or kill the bacteria causing it.

Homeopaths, however, see symptoms as an expression of the body's attempts to heal itself, a positive sign that the body is fighting illness. Homeopathic remedies are aimed at supporting the body's healing mechanism. For this reason they can sometimes provoke what homeopaths call an 'aggravation', whereby symptoms may get worse before they improve.

The law of similars This states that a substance, which in large doses can produce symptoms of illness in a well person, can, in minute doses, cure similar symptoms in a sick person. According to Hahnemann, this is because nature does not allow two similar diseases to exist in the body at the same time. To rid the body of a disease, homeopaths introduce a similar artificial disease that pushes the original one out, but is too fleeting to cause any long-term suffering.

The minimum dose This states that extreme dilution enhances the curative properties of a substance, while eliminating any side-effects. You only need a minute dose of the active ingredient to stimulate a health improvement.

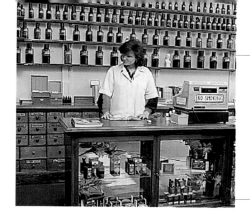

Left: Homeopathic remedies come in pills, granules, powders or liquid form.

Whole person prescribing This is the third and vital principle of homeopathy. A homeopath studies the whole person: their temperament, personality, emotional and physical responses. Therefore a homeopath will not treat flu, but a person who has flu-like symptoms. So, although a conventional doctor could see 10 people with flu and prescribe the same treatment for all of them, a homeopath may give each a different remedy.

Most people have difficulty in understanding how homeopathic remedies work when they contain such minute traces of the remedy. Homeopaths believe it is the energy or 'vibrational pattern' of the remedy, rather than its chemical content, that stimulates healing by activating what Hahnemann called the Vital Force. The vital force is simply the healing power or energy that exists within all of us. It is what the Chinese call chi and the Indians call prana. It fuels the body, mind and emotions, keeping us healthy and balanced. But when the balance is disturbed by stress, pollution, inadequate diet and lack of exercise, it becomes weakened and illness can result. The symptoms of illness are the body's way of attracting attention to the fact that the vital force is struggling to fight off disease.

Hahnemann could not prove how minute doses of homeopathic remedies could restore health, but he could prove that they did. His own belief that they somehow strengthened the embattled vital force, enabling it to restore the body to health, remains the predominant belief among homeopaths today.

What happens in a consultation?
The consultation will begin with the homoeopath asking numerous questions about yourself and your lifestyle and making copious notes. This will build up a picture of your mental, physical and emotional health so that the practitioner can prescribe the best remedy for you.

Typically, the questions asked focus on five different aspects of your life concerning the physical, mental, emotional, spiritual and general aspects. The first four include such information as:

♦ *Details about your past illnesses and any inherited family health problems*
♦ *How you feel about taking on new challenges*
♦ *If you are afraid of the dark and any other relevant details*
♦ *General information includes such details as how you tend to react to hot and cold, whether you are at your best in the morning or evening, your favourite season, and whether you prefer to eat sweet, salty or spicy food*

When your homeopath feels he has all the information he needs he will prescribe a remedy. He will normally only prescribe one at a time, although the prescription can change as your symptoms change.

For example, you may need to take one remedy four times a day for three days and another remedy once a day for the next week. The remedy will be small pills, tablets, granules, powder or a tasteless, colourless liquid. You will be advised not to touch it but to take it on a spoon or tip a pill under your tongue, and to keep it away from strong-smelling substances as these can negate the remedy.

You may also be asked to abstain from eating peppermints and drinking coffee during your treatment. Your practitioner may advise taking the remedy in a 'clean mouth', that is not to eat, drink or smoke for half an hour before. When you take the remedy let it dissolve under your tongue.

The homeopath may also advise on diet and lifestyle changes. Your first visit will probably end with you making a follow-up appointment, usually for a month later so that the practitioner can assess your progress.

How many sessions do I need?
Some people recover more quickly than others, depending on the ailment and their response to the remedy. Treatment may take only one or two visits, but it can take more. Sometimes a homeopath will change your remedy if the first one proved unsuitable and this can take some weeks. The length of treatment also depends on the severity of your illness and how long you have had it. However, if there is no improvement after four or five visits, see another homeopath or try an alternative therapy.

Which problems can it help?
It is probably fair to say that homeopathy works well for everything, but doesn't work for everyone. Minor ailments such as colds, constipation, vomiting and diarrhoea respond well. In the way of more serious conditions, it can help rheumatoid arthritis, fibrositis and psoriasis. Because a homeopathic remedy stimulates your body to heal itself it will help rectify emotional, mental or physical complaints, but some people respond better than others.

Is it safe?
Homeopathic remedies are so diluted that they are safe for everyone to take, from babies to pregnant women and the elderly. However, as with all medicines, take the remedies only as long as you need to. You can happily take homeopathic medicine while receiving conventional treatment, although some chemical drugs may affect its action.

NUTRITIONAL THERAPY

Nutritional therapy is the use of a special diet to balance the body and prevent illness. A macrobiotic diet is based on the Chinese philosophy of yin and yang. Yin and yang foods can be adjusted by the therapist to restore the body to health.

For years nutrition has formed the backbone of healthcare. Food and herbs were our first medicines, which were used to treat a large number of conditions ranging from wounds and insect bites, to infection and broken limbs.

From the earliest days, it became clear that food had a medicinal effect, and that a varied diet, rich in natural ingredients, was a prerequisite for good health. So diet became a fundamental part of most early health therapies, and an integral element in almost all later medical systems. In the 18th century English sailors were given lime or lemon juice in order to prevent scurvy, a disease caused by lack of vitamin C, which occurred due to long periods at sea without fresh fruits or vegetables.

In the late 19th century naturopaths drew attention to the use of food and how nutritional elements could be used as medicine, a concept which was not new, but which had not been acknowledged as a therapy in its own right until that time. Naturopaths used a nutritional diet and fasting to cleanse the body and encourage it to heal itself. As knowledge about food, its make-up and its effects on the body became greater, the first nutritional specialists treated specific ailments and symptoms with the food components.

By the mid 20th century, scientists had put together a profile of proteins, carbohydrates, fats, vitamins and minerals, which were essential to life and to health. More than 40 nutrients were discovered. It was found that minerals were needed for healthy body functions, and a new understanding of the body fed the growing interest in the subject.

In the 1960s, Stanford chemistry professor Linus Pauling published a paper in the journal *Science*. He talked about creating the best molecular environment in the mind by supplying the right levels of biochemicals such as vitamins. He used the term 'orthomolecular'. The now controversial fields of orthomolecular psychiatry and orthomolecular medicine were then defined, and doctors began to treat patients with special diets and supplements, which were prescribed according to symptoms, health problems and special needs. While conventional doctors still discussed nutrition in terms of basic food groups (it is only studied briefly in medical school), orthomolecular nutritionists were regularly prescribing high levels of vitamin supplements.

Nutrition then spread from being a mainly doctor-led dietary therapy, also called clinical nutrition, into a more profound theory of health based on treating the patient as a whole (holistic health), and looking for specific deficiencies that could be causing illness in an individual.

The term 'macrobiotics' comes from the Greek words *makros* which means large and *biokos* which means life, and macrobiotics is based on the fundamental belief that everyone should be healthy enough to enjoy life to the full.

Macrobiotics has a rich heritage which originated in Tibet and China, where the early philosophy was largely inspired by three books – *The Nei Ching, The I Ching*, and *The Tao Te Ching*. The emphasis of these books was the idea that humanity is part of the environment and the cosmos, and that health is a reflection of our appreciation, connection and intake from the world around us.

In the 1880s, a Japanese doctor, Sagen Ishizuka, discovered that many health problems could be treated with dietary changes, often involving wholegrains and vegetables. Refined carbohydrates and white rice were removed from the diet. His work was published in two volumes, and was later used for reference by George Ohsawa, who, by 1945, had synthesized all the beliefs and adopted the term 'macrobiotics'. Ohsawa wrote over 300 books which dwelt on the importance of a healthy, balanced, diet, seasonally and individually adjusted. Remedies and first aid were drawn from Japanese folk medicine, and practical guidelines for a healthy lifestyle were drawn from the *Nei Ching*, – a comprehensive study of anatomy, physiology and diagnosis. This book also held a cosmological view of human beings, derived from the major world religions.

In the 1960s, Michio Kushi, one of Ohsawa's students, began teaching the philosophy in the US and Europe, and he broadened the dietary guidelines and further developed Ohsawa's ideas. The result is modern-day macrobiotics, which has evolved from being a fairly strict regime to include all of the essential elements of basic nutrition. The idea is that you can live life to its full potential, assisted by a diet promoting physical, mental, emotional and spiritual health.

What is nutritional therapy?

Nutritional therapy is using diet to treat and prevent illness, and to restore the body to a natural, healthy equilibrium. It is believed that sub-clinical deficiencies are responsible for much of the disease and weakness in the body. These are in fact vitamin and mineral deficiencies which are too slight to produce obvious deficiency diseases, such as scurvy or anaemia, but which are enough to reduce the body's ability to function efficiently. These minor deficiencies can often start with niggling and annoying symptoms which may not, on their own, be enough for most people to seek medical attention.

Indeed, we have today come to accept many of these symptoms as just part of our day-to-day stressful living. Problems like fatigue, susceptibility to colds and other viruses, skin ailments and lethargy are common symptoms of nutritional sub-clinical deficiency.

One of the problems is that the diet of the modern Western world fails to provide adequate nutrition. In fact it contributes not only to ill-health but to obesity, heart disease, cancer, digestive disorders, premature ageing, and in many cases death. The Western world is overfed but undernourished and, although food is plentiful, it is often devoid of any nutritional value. Over the past few years research has indicated that many health conditions are caused by allergies or intolerance to foods, but that certain foods have therapeutic properties. For example, some are known to aid digestion, reduce inflammation or mucus production, and many conditions such as asthma or eczema can be treated almost entirely by changing the diet. Similarly, rheumatism and arthritis can be greatly improved by diet.

The modern world has also placed new stresses on our bodies, exposing them to environmental and psychological demands which did not exist even two decades ago. This means that our bodies are often depleted of protective and important nutrients, which results in ill-health plus a variety of other common ailments.

In an ideal world it should be possible to get all of the nutritional elements that we need from a balanced diet, but with intensive farming methods, pesticides, preservatives, additives and hormones, our diets are often far less nutritious than they appear. The soil is no longer as rich with minerals as it used to be, and vegetables and fruit are therefore less nutritious. Cattle grazing on the land reap much less

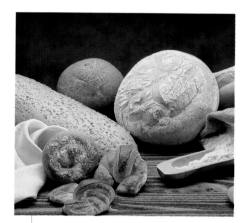

Above: Bread is an important source of carbohydrate. Choose wholegrain types.

nutritional goodness from the grass because it grows in depleted soil. Also alcohol, tobacco, drugs, stress, environmental pollution and additives all rob the body of nutrients, so even a healthy individual can suffer from living in the modern world. Today as manufacturers and food producers strive to make food last longer they now contain a mixture of:

♦ *Colourants, preservatives, flavourings, emulsifiers and polyphosphates*
♦ *Contaminants from agriculture, antibiotics and growth promoters, industrial contaminants and also radioactive contamination*

Nutritional therapy is a sophisticated system of healthcare, which depends on an increasing knowledge of biochemistry, physiology and nutrition to address the health needs of the individual. There are three basic diagnoses made by the nutritional therapist: allergy (or intolerance) to food, nutritional deficiencies (often subclinical) and toxic overload.

Food allergies

Many practitioners believe that 20% of people have an allergy, although this is controversial. A food allergy can be caused by almost any kind of food, and common symptoms include nausea, vomiting and diarrhoea. The most common allergens are dairy produce, nuts, eggs, yeast, shellfish, wheat, flour, citrus fruit and artificial colourings. Many children are affected by food additives, especially tartrazine and benzoate, which cause hyperactivity and behavioural problems.

If you suspect an allergy, your therapist might suggest an elimination diet, which will allow her to pinpoint which foods are causing your symptoms. Elimination programmes should never be undertaken without professional supervision. Some common allergy-causing foods are:

♦ *Gluten, tea, seafood, tomatoes, coffee, bananas, dairy produce and animal fats*
♦ *Yeast, oranges, peppers, eggs, rye, cheese and potatoes*
♦ *Alcohol, onions, strawberries, pineapple, tap water, condiments and garlic*
♦ *Corn, wine, nuts, oats, chocolate and mushrooms*
♦ *Rice, pork and soya*

Nutritional deficiencies

Few people show signs of a serious vitamin or mineral deficiency, such as scurvy, but many people suffer slight shortages. These can be tested by symptom analysis, hair mineral analysis, muscle testing, and perhaps blood or sweat analysis.

Toxic overload

Toxic overload is identified by the combination of the symptoms experienced and the normal lifestyle of the sufferer. Toxins are effectively poisons which can be in our food, or are created within our bodies by intestinal bacteria or as waste products.

How does it work?

Nutritional therapy is based on the knowledge that each part of the body is made up of elements that were once the nutritional elements of food. The idea is that functions deteriorate when some of these elements are in short supply or the body is being mildly poisoned. The nutritional therapist will decide how to improve these functions, using a good nutritional diet and body knowledge.

Dozens of laboratory tests measuring everything in a patient's body from sugar intolerance and blood levels of vitamins and minerals, to thyroid function and levels of insulin, can help the nutritional therapist to find out what may be causing illness. Hair analysis can be used to evaluate levels of trace minerals.

A healthy body is strong and resistant to illness, so while the nutritional therapist will treat the symptoms of one illness by meeting the body's needs, very often other unrelated conditions will be cured.

A nutritional therapist believes that many of the ailments common to Western people are provoked by a toxic overload, food allergies or nutritional deficiencies in their diet. She may recommend vitamin and mineral supplements and other substances to restore the body's natural balance, along with a diet that includes plenty of vegetables, fruit and whole grains. Nutritional therapists believe that the recommended level of intake of vitamins, minerals, and other elements, do not take into account the very wide range of individual requirements. Certainly any difficulty in absorbing one particular vitamin, or even a slight deficiency in another can set the whole system awry, because they are all necessary to complete the chain of nutrition. After a consultation, and perhaps some tests, a nutritional therapist will diagnose possible nutritional deficiencies and ensure that your diet is better balanced to incorporate these elements. She might also prescribe supplements or some herbs to speed up the healing process. Possible food allergies and intolerance may be identified, and some extra foods suggested to give the body a therapeutic effect.

Some controlled use of supplements may be recommended as research suggests they can treat certain conditions. For example, there is increasing evidence that some PMS sufferers are deficient in gamma-linolenic acid (GLA), found in evening primrose oil, and a course of this supplement may be recommended. Some types of neuralgia or carpal tunnel syndrome may indicate a deficiency of B vitamins; tyrosine, an amino acid, has been successfully used to treat depression and anxiety. A deficiency in vitamin A may aggravate skin conditions.

These are only some of the treatments offered by a nutritional therapist, and treatment will always be tailored to the individual. The consistent use of supplements or mega-doses should, however, always be supervised by a registered therapist because many supplements can be toxic in high doses.

A healthy diet

The Western diet is generally high in cholesterol and fats, especially saturated fats, low in fibre, and high in refined sugars and animal products. Diets which are low in fat and cholesterol, but high in dietary fibre, fruits and vegetables, are healthier

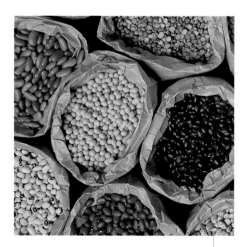

Above: A balanced, healthy diet relies on whole, unrefined foods such as pulses.

and provide much more energy. Ailments such as aches and pains, headaches, some types of diabetes, immune deficiencies, skin problems and digestive disorders all disappear when the right diet is followed.

A healthy diet is one in which the food you eat contains all the nutrients needed by the body for it to grow, heal and to function normally on a day-to-day basis. A balanced diet provides energy, and allows you to function at your optimum level, free from disease and malaise.

There are three essential nutrient food groups: proteins, carbohydrates and fats plus minerals and vitamins. You also need water, which is found in most foods and which makes up a large proportion of our body. Roughly speaking, proteins should make up about 15% of the diet, carbohydrates 60% or more, and fats a maximum of 25–30%. Vitamins and minerals are found within each of these groups, and a balanced diet should have all or most represented in adequate levels. Dietary fibre is also important for your health.

Choosing wholesome foods

Fresh fruits, vegetables and salads should form part of your daily diet, and ideally fresh meat and fish should be used instead of packaged or frozen foods. Many of the processes used to preserve food, such as freezing and canning, can result in a loss of nutrients. Wherever possible, try to choose local and fresh produce, as long storage or transportation can cause nutrients to be lost. It is essential that you read food labels carefully. Products which contain flavourings, preservatives and colourings have been linked with health problems.

A balanced diet is based on eating whole foods, which means unrefined foods. With refined foods, certain parts are removed during the refining process and in this way vital nutrients and natural fibre are lost. The result is a product with a reduced nutritional value, and one which is less easily digested, since natural fibre aids the process of elimination and digestion. Generally speaking whatever your age, you should have two servings a day of protein, preferably meat, fish, poultry, nuts, beans, peas or lentils; one serving of milk, cheese or another dairy product; four servings of complex carbohydrates such as bread, brown rice, pasta, potatoes or muesli and finally five servings of fresh fruit, vegetables or salads, and as little fat as possible. Children and pregnant or breastfeeding women may need more dairy produce and they may need more fat than other groups.

Ideally, organically produced foods should be eaten when possible as they are more healthy and nutritious. However, they are usually more expensive than their non-organic equivalents and fruit and vegetables can appear less attractive because pesticides have not been used.

There are a number of diets which are based around special needs: for example, sufferers of heart disease should eat a low-fat and low-salt diet. There are also a wide range of diets to treat different illnesses, for example, fasting or eating raw food diets to cleanse the system. Unless strictly short-term, all diets should be varied, with as few restrictions as possible.

The benefits of fibre

Doctors increasingly believe that fibre-rich diets contribute to good health. Fibre swells the bulk of the food residue in the intestine, and then helps to soften it by increasing the amount of water retained within it. This lessens the strain on the bowel and decreases the amount of time that toxins being eliminated remain in the body. Many practitioners believe that this reduces the likelihood of cancer, since cancer-causing substances are eliminated from the body quickly.

Fibre also reduces the number of calories that are absorbed from food, while ensuring that the remaining calories are absorbed into the body more slowly. It also helps to increase the content of friendly bacteria which work to protect the body against infection and yeast conditions such as thrush. Rich sources of fibre include wholemeal bread, brown rice and other cereals, vegetables (both leafy and root), fruits (fresh and dried), salads, beans, peas and other pulses.

What happens in a consultation?

Nutritional therapists are often medical doctors who are interested in nutrition. The practitioners of other complementary therapies may also offer healthy eating advice as part of their treatment. A consultation normally takes up to an hour; the therapist will take a full case history

♦ *She will look at your current diet and habits, including drinking or smoking*
♦ *She will discuss your exercise patterns and your emotional and physical history*
♦ *She will ask whether you take medication or drugs, such as the pill, and note any physical symptoms that you experience*

Many practitioners suggest testing hair, urine, sweat and muscles and use a questionnaire to pinpoint specific deficiencies. Therapy will also be based on physical symptoms. The practitioner will take into account any nutritional deficiencies, food intolerances and also the possibility of a toxic overload. A special diet plan will be produced for you and any vitamin or mineral supplements will be prescribed. An exercise programme and some herbal treatments may also be incorporated. You may also be referred to another complementary therapist. Nutritional therapists will always advise you to consult a doctor as well if you have not already done so.

How many sessions do I need?

The number of sessions required depends on how quickly you respond to treatment, how long you have suffered from your symptoms or illness, and how carefully and thoroughly you incorporate the lifestyle and dietary changes suggested.

Which problems can it help?

Nutritional therapy can help with almost anything, since food is the basis and the fuel of all the chemical processes which take place in the body. Therefore, almost all types of ill-health can stem from missing or insufficient nutritional elements within the diet.

Nutritional therapists have had great success treating conditions such as rheumatism and arthritis, high blood pressure, fatigue, constipation and other digestive disorders, the healing and recuperation processes following injury or surgery, skin problems and many psychological and behavioural problems. Neuralgia, osteoporosis, PMS, post-natal illness, pregnancy problems, reduced immunity, stress and viruses may also respond to dietary treatment. In effect, however, all the body systems will be improved by a healthy diet. In a fit state you are much more likely to fight off infection and deal efficiently with any health problems or injury.

The benefits of a healthy, balanced diet are profound. A large proportion of today's ailments are caused by food allergies, and these can be pinpointed by your therapist. If the relevant foods are avoided many illnesses can be prevented.

Is it safe?

In the hands of a trained practitioner, nutritional therapy is one of the safest complementary therapies. Reputable practitioners will always be wary of promoting extreme or highly restrictive diets administered for lengthy periods of time. Nutritional therapy should always be undertaken on the advice of a registered practitioner and he or she should always be informed of every other aspect of your current physical and mental condition.

There are many ailments which contraindicate the use of certain supplements, as they would be dangerous, and it is essential that your therapist is aware of everything which may affect your health.

People of any age can benefit from the prudent use of nutritional therapy, and there are always different regimes for babies, pregnant women, young children, the elderly, and those suffering from chronic (long-term) health conditions.

MACROBIOTICS

Macrobiotics is based on the Chinese philosophy of yin and yang, which are two qualities that balance one another, and which exist in every natural object and cycle. Yin is the flexible, fluid and cool side of nature, while yang is the strong, dynamic and hot side. There are yin and yang elements in everything, including people, and macrobiotics is a philosophy aimed at balancing them to promote good health.

Yin qualities are peacefulness, calm, creativity, sociability and a relaxed attitude and behaviour. Yang qualities include activity, alertness, energy and precision. Most people have a combination of both of these qualities. However, when one becomes stronger than the other, a state of imbalance can occur, which can result in illness. Too much yin can lead to depression, fatigue and sleeping problems; whereas too much yang can cause tension, irritability, hyperactivity and also possibly insomnia.

The macrobiotic therapist would attempt to right that balance by suggesting an increased intake of yin foods for someone who is suffering from too much yang, and an increased intake of yang foods for someone with too much yin. There are various other factors involved in this theory, among them exercise, which is broken into yin and yang (yoga is yin while aerobics is yang), temperature and climate.

The macrobiotic diet

The macrobiotic diet is similar to that of the traditional Japanese peasant, which consists of:

♦ *50% cooked whole cereal grains, pasta, bread, porridge, stir-fried rice or noodles*
♦ *25% local seasonal vegetables, cooked in a variety of ways (for example, raw, pickled, steamed, sautéed, or boiled)*
♦ *10% protein, to be drawn from local fish, beans and soybean products such as tofu or tempeh*
♦ *5% sea vegetables, used in soups or stews*
♦ *5% soups, including miso soup, fish soup, bean soup and vegetable soup*
♦ *5% desserts and teas, including simple teas and grain coffees, and desserts using fruits and fermented rice (amaskae), agar agar (sea vegetable), seeds and nuts*

In fact, surveys show that most macrobiotic practitioners use the diet as a basis for healthy living but include a 5–10% intake of other foods either socially, or to give a dietary balance. Emphasis is placed on the art of cooking, and on the variety of cooking styles and ingredients.

Foods which are excluded from the diet include sugar, spices and alcohol (which are said to be too much yin), and meat, eggs and cheese (which are said to be too much yang). These foods are believed to be too strong for human consumption, unbalancing the system and causing illness. The best balanced foods containing yin or yang are:

♦ *Yin – fruit, leafy green vegetables, nuts and seeds, tofu and tempeh, fruit and vegetable juices, jams (made without refined sugar), barley malt*
♦ *Yang – wholegrain cereals, such as brown rice, bread, flour, whole oats, root vegetables such as potatoes, parsnips and turnips, fish and shellfish, cottage cheese, beans, peas and lentils, salt, miso and shoyu soya sauce*

The macrobiotic lifestyle

Macrobiotics is believed to be the natural cycle of life, an example of the universal rhythms of yin and yang which occur everywhere and in everything. During your more difficult periods, it is suggested that you read case histories and accounts of others whose lives have been radically improved by macrobiotics.

Macrobiotic practitioners urge you to live each day happily, without being preoccupied with your condition, or dwelling on negative thoughts, ideas or emotions.

It is a fundamental belief that nature is essential to life, and that regular contact with nature is necessary to enjoy optimum health and wellbeing. There are five daily practices which create a more stable and harmonious lifestyle:

♦ *Greet everyone happily and with appreciation*
♦ *Initiate and maintain a regular correspondence with all family members, expressing thanks for their part in your life*
♦ *Enlarge your circle of friends and acquaintances, including people from different lifestyles*
♦ *Share your food more often by having people around; food prepared in larger quantities is more satisfying and the act of sharing food is a universal gesture of human kindness and brotherhood*
♦ *Put aside some time each day for peace and quiet, and thank your forebears and teachers for their help. Repeat your dedication to aid and support those who look to you for guidance*

Macrobiotic philosophy

The macrobiotic philosophy is essentially one of being responsible for your health, aspirations and actions. This comes through clearly in the works of Ohsawa, and he and the early Chinese doctors made it clear that their job was to prevent illness rather than 'fixing things' later, when they were not working properly.

As the Yellow Emperor said thousands of years ago in the *Nei Ching*: 'it is hardest to treat someone who has become rebellious [sick] – a wise doctor helps those who are well and have not become rebellious'.

How does it work?

Macrobiotic practitioners believe that macrobiotics changes the condition of your blood, which is made of three main components – plasma, red blood cells and white blood cells. Plasma amounts to 50% of the cells, and this changes every 10 days. Therefore, the changes to your health will be noticeable in 10-day cycles.

When you begin a macrobiotic programme, you will notice some large changes during the first 10 days, mainly as a reaction or a 'discharge process'. Tiredness, irritability, sweating, insomnia and cravings are common. After 10–30 days, reports vary, but generally people tend to feel brighter, and more alert, with an increased appetite, and a calmer, more focused and flexible outlook.

When people continue for 6–8 months on a macrobiotic programme, their blood will show a great improvement and have perfectly balanced yin and yang. If regular physical activity is kept up, and there is plenty of variety in the diet and lifestyle, then long-term or chronic ailments should start to show a noticeable improvement.

Changing your diet is a big step to take; approaching it in the right way and getting support and feedback are essential to minimize mistakes. It takes commitment and patience, but macrobiotic practitioners say that when it becomes easy and you are enjoying all the food you eat, then you have become macrobiotic.

What happens in a consultation?

Practitioners are skilled in Oriental diagnosis, with the same background as an acupuncturist or Chinese herbalist. There are four methods of diagnosis:

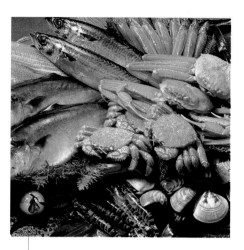

Above: Fish and seafood and sources of vegetable protein should make up 10% of a macrobiotic diet. They should be locally caught to cut down on travelling time.

♦ *Seeing – visual diagnosis of the face, tongue, fingers and nails*
♦ *Listening – studying your voice during the interview to ascertain whether the condition is yin or yang*
♦ *Touching – feeling the pulses on the inside of the wrist*
♦ *Questioning – about lifestyle, habits, diet, symptoms and medical history*

The practitioners will then give advice, generally aimed at the three branches of macrobiotics. The first type of advice is dietary advice which suggests which foods to avoid for 30 days, and which foods to incorporate in your diet. It will possibly include other extras such as special herbal teas. This advice is based on Michio Kushi's Standard Macrobiotic Diet, with any necessary adjustments, deletions, or extra dishes.

The next type of advice will be lifestyle and exercise suggestions to improve your general health and wellbeing. There may also be suggested referrals to other practitioners working within the Chinese medical field. The third type of advice is philosophical advice. On the philosophy side, suggestions for a more harmonious lifestyle will be offered by your macrobiotic practitioner.

How many sessions do I need?

Normally two sessions, 30 days apart, are needed with the macrobiotic therapist to sort out your diet. Each session will take about an hour.

Which problems can it help?

Macrobiotics helps to strengthen the immune system and enables the person to maintain good health. It is also good for preventing or reducing digestive complaints, obesity, fatigue, poor concentration, physical inflexibility or lack of stamina. Some practitioners claim to have had success even in treating and curing arthritis and some forms of cancer.

The macrobiotic diet is considered to be excellent for healthy individuals as it can help prevent disease forming.

Is it safe?

In the 1970s and 1980s there was a dangerous version of macrobiotics being practised. This system involved eating little other than brown rice. Many men, women and children developed severe malnutrition, which instantly gave the therapy a bad reputation. Since that time, the diets have been modified to reflect current thinking on balanced nutrition within the diet. Under the supervision of a registered practitioner, macrobiotics is normally very safe.

Many children adopt a liberal macrobiotic diet without any problems, however, it should only be undertaken under the guidance of a doctor. Similarly, breast-feeding mothers, pregnant women, and those wishing to conceive should discuss the possibility of adopting macrobiotics with their doctor before attempting to start the diet. Most registered practitioners will be quite happy to modify the diet to suit your individual needs.

WESTERN HERBALISM

The tradition of using herbs for healing dates from ancient times. Herbalism forms part of our Western heritage, but it has proved equally important in Africa, India and China (see Chinese Herbalism pages 448–9).

Medical herbalism is the use of plants as medicines to restore and maintain health by keeping the body balanced. It relies on the curative qualities of plants, flowers, trees and herbs to stimulate our healing system when the body is ill. Like most holistic practitioners, herbalists believe that we all possess healing energy within us, which they call the 'vital force'. This vital force works constantly to maintain our whole health, physically, mentally and emotionally. Sometimes, however, the vital force is weakened by factors such as stress, poor diet and pollution and we get ill. Herbalists see the symptoms of disease as the result of the vital force's attempts to maintain harmony in the body when it is under threat from illness. Herbal remedies are prescribed to support the affected body systems in their fight against disease.

Medical herbalists combine traditional knowledge of herbs and healing with modern scientific developments. They are trained in the same examination techniques as a doctor and have a thorough medical knowledge of the body.

How does it work?

Despite extensive research and analysis, scientists are still unable to identify every chemical component of which herbs are composed and so far have not been able to reproduce them synthetically. They have discovered, however, that herbs contain

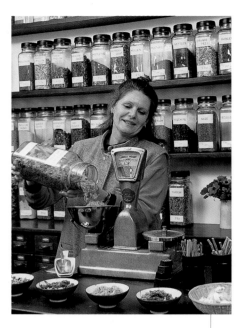

Above: Herbal remedies can be taken as decoctions, tablets, compresses or creams.

vitamins, minerals, carbohydrates and trace elements and healing agents such as tannins, bitters, volatile oils, mucilage, glycosides, saponins and alkaloids. These help herbs to aid the body's fight against infection, to sedate overactive organs, relax tense muscles and nerves, improve circulation, and reduce any inflammation.

Herbs are classified in a similar way to drugs, but are often prescribed to support body systems rather than relieve symptoms. The skill lies in prescribing the most suitable herb for an individual.

The remedies

Herbal remedies are prescribed to be taken internally or applied to the skin. They come as tinctures, creams, compresses, poultices, infusions, decoctions, oils to use in the bath or as tablets and capsules. You may even be given fresh herbs to incorporate into your diet.

Tinctures These are the most common type of internal remedy prescribed. They are made by soaking the flowers, leaves or roots of the chosen herbs in alcohol to extract and preserve their useful properties. Tinctures keep and store well, and you only need take a small amount at a time.

Infusions Always less concentrated, these are an easy way to take herbs at home. The herbalist prescribes fresh or dried flowers, leaves or green stems of the herbs that you make into a not very pleasant tasting 'tea'. To make an infusion use one teaspoon of dried herbs to one cup of boiling water, leave to infuse for 10–15 minutes, strain and drink hot. Sweeten with honey if preferred. Herbs such as comfrey, marshmallow and valerian root are destroyed by heat so they should be 'macerated' in cold water for up to 12 hours.

Decoctions are similar to infusions but these are made from materials such as roots, barks, nuts and seeds. Using the same proportions as for an infusion, place the herb mixture and water in a saucepan and bring to the boil. Simmer for about 10 minutes. Strain and drink hot.

Tablets and capsules All are taken in the same way as a prescription drug (often with water after food) and are useful for people who would rather not taste the remedy.

Creams and ointments These are applied externally to soothe irritated or inflamed skin conditions or to ease sprains or bruises. When applied, the herb's active ingredients pass through the pores of the skin into the bloodstream to encourage healing.

Hot or cold compresses Both can help with aches, pains and swollen joints. Fold a clean piece of cotton into an infusion of the prescribed herb and apply to the painful area. Repeat as the hot compress cools or, with the cold compress, hold there until the pain eases.

Poultices These are made from bruised fresh herbs or dried herbs moistened into a paste with hot water. They are good for painful joints or drawing out infection from boils, spots or wounds. Place the herb paste on a clean piece of cotton and place it on the affected area with a bandage. Leave for a couple of hours or until symptoms ease.

Herbal baths These are the ultimate in pleasant herbal treatments, and are a useful supplement to other treatments. Lemon balm, lavender or elderflowers make a fragrant, relaxing bath and can help you sleep or calm your nerves. Tie a handful of herbs in a muslin bag and hang from the bath tap so that the water runs through it to activate the herbs' properties. Alternatively, use essential oils (see Aromatherapy, pages 406–7). In both cases they pass into the bloodstream and when inhaled they pass through the nervous system, to the brain, healing both the mind and the body.

What happens in a consultation?

Visiting a medical herbalist is rather different from seeing your doctor. Your first consultation will last for about an hour. The herbalist will begin by taking down details such as:

♦ *Your name, address, age and occupation*
♦ *Your personality and what things are important to you, for example whether you worry about the state of your children's health or if you get concerned about the state of the environment*
♦ *She will also ask if you are you a perfectionist, a rebel, money-conscious, or fashion-conscious*
♦ *She will ask about your childhood, your appetite and sleeping patterns, family, job, previous illnesses and any medicines you have been prescribed in the past*

She will also want to know how you feel and will note the condition of your hair and skin, your facial expression, posture and how you move. These all provide important clues to help diagnosis.

While you explain why you have come and your main symptoms, the herbalist will write down your case details in her notes. When the herbalist has collated all this information, she will aim to establish how your problem started, what conditions caused it or are making it worse, how it relates to previous illnesses and how you feel at this moment.

During the consultation the herbalist will also ask you about the health of your body's systems – the respiratory, circulatory, digestive, reproductive and so on.

Medical herbalists are qualified to carry out a physical examination. This will be similar to a check-up from your doctor and may include checking your pulse, taking your blood pressure, testing your reflexes and probably listening to your heart and chest.

Only after a full consultation and examination will the herbalist be able to make a diagnosis and choose a suitable remedy. She will also advise on how you can help your healing by improving your diet and exercise regime and relaxing more.

The remedies can be prescribed in any of the forms listed above, but most are given as creams or ointments for skin conditions and tinctures to be taken internally. The herbalist may mix several tinctures in one bottle to make your remedy and you will be told how and when to take the medicine.

The remedies you will receive are prescribed for you, not for your ulcer, hay fever or eczema. As with many forms of alternative treatment, herbal remedies can occasionally make you feel worse before you feel better. This is because they are not prescribed to alleviate your symptoms, but to eliminate the problem from your system.

Your appointment may end with you being asked to return for a follow-up appointment in a few days, a week or even two weeks' time, depending on the nature and severity of your problem.

How many sessions do I need?

Acute (short-term) conditions can be resolved within a few days and you may need one or two appointments. Chronic (long-term) conditions, such as arthritis or eczema, need several appointments. Repeated appointments may be necessary so that the herbalist can check on your progress and possibly change your prescription as your condition improves.

Which problems can it help?

Herbalism can help with most illness and disorders, but it does seem particularly effective with skin conditions such as eczema, urinary problems such as cystitis and digestive problems such as irritable bowel syndrome.

A herbalist cannot reverse damage caused by very serious or life-threatening diseases such as cancer, diabetes or Aids, but she can relieve the symptoms, support your immune system and improve your overall wellbeing.

Is it safe?

Herbal medicines have proved their efficacy over centuries of use and have a much better safety record for everyone from babies to pregnant women and the elderly than that of pharmaceutical drugs. But it is a mistake to think that natural means harmless as any substance can be abused if overused.

Some herbs are toxic when taken in large doses. A herbalist will not usually prescribe these herbs even in small doses and the dosage of certain herbs is controlled by law. Safe herbal preparations for minor or acute ailments are also available over the counter, but if unsure ask your herbalist for guidance, especially if you are taking the herbs during pregnancy or giving them to babies or children. When taking herbal medicines with conventional medicine, let your doctor know about the herbs and your herbalist about your medical treatments.

NATUROPATHY

Only nature heals is the philosophy of naturopathy, a system of holistic medicine that has been around since ancient times. Hippocrates, the Greek father of medicine, could more specifically be called the father of naturopathic medicine since, like modern naturopaths, he incorporated diet, fasting, hydrotherapy, exercise and manipulative techniques into his healthcare.

Naturopathy as a scientific discipline did not make an impact until the 19th century, and it remained a fringe therapy. The 1970s and 1980s saw a shift in health consciousness from the pharmaceutical to the natural and holistic, and the message of early 20th-century naturopaths such as Dr Henry Lindlahr, Stanley Lief and Alfred Vogel started to receive wider recognition. They maintained that living in harmony with nature was the only way to achieve lasting good health.

Naturopathy actually means a treatment system that uses natural resources to help the body heal itself. It is founded on the following basic principles.

The body can fight disease and recover from illness because it possesses a vital curative force that enables the body systems to return to a state of harmony known as homoeostasis. This state tends towards perfect health, both physically and emotionally, and the naturopath's aim is to restore and preserve it.

Naturopaths see disease as a natural phenomenon. Disease occurs in plants, animals and people when any part of the whole organism is not working well. The aim of the naturopath is to identify the cause of the illness, help the vital force eliminate it, and restore the body to a state of balance.

The symptoms of disease are often evidence of the healing process in action. They are the signs that the vital force is striving to balance the body and they ought not to be suppressed in healthy individuals. Going through acute (short-term) illnesses such as measles or flu is seen as normal in a healthy body to develop a strong adult immune system.

Treatment should be holistic and natural. This is prescribed to activate and strengthen the body's innate healing ability and to bring the diseased body part into balance with the rest of the body. The treatment is based on naturally occurring substances such as water, wholefoods, sunlight, relaxation, fresh air and exercise and the emphasis is not only on natural treatment, but on a natural lifestyle.

Naturopaths believe in the triad of health. This in simple terms means that good health depends on maintaining a balance between three things: the body's structure, its biochemistry and the emotions. The health of the body's structure, good posture, the bones, muscles, tendons and ligaments are vital to the body as a whole as any structural problems can have an effect on the nervous system and organs. Biochemical health refers to the effects of food and drink on the body. Good nutrition is essential for growth and repair and immunity to disease.

Like many other natural therapists, naturopaths also believe in the law of cure. This states that in healing, all disease moves from within out, from the top to the bottom, and symptoms disappear in reverse order of their appearance.

How does it work?
Naturopathy is a philosophy for life. Naturopaths aim to prevent and treat disease by detailed diagnosis and a wide range of treatments, many of which must be integrated into a person's lifestyle for lasting health.

Diagnosis
The main purpose of diagnosis is to find out how well the vital force is working. Practitioners carry out normal medical investigations such as taking the pulse and blood pressure, listening to heart and lungs, and assessing breathing capacity, if necessary. Naturopaths are usually trained osteopaths, so observing the body structure also provides information about vitality and how well the body's systems and organs are functioning.

Practitioners also make use of biotypology to assess health trends in the individual. Everyone is classified according to biotype or constitution.

Iridology Iris diagnosis also gives insights into a patient's general constitution and has been shown to be effective in pinpointing areas of weakness.

Mineral analysis Hair and sweat can be tested for mineral levels, trace elements and also for any heavy metal poisoning. A spectroscope can measure the energy frequencies of minerals in a hair shaft.

Bioelectronic diagnosis This form of dowsing is also used to take a reading from a hair sample, toe nail clipping, drop of blood or saliva. The hair or other body material is used as a 'witness', from which the naturopath can read the patient's energy using special equipment.

Treatment
Treatment is diverse and flexible. Different practitioners incorporate or emphasize different aspects of treatment. Below are the most widely used.

Diet This is the most important factor in naturopathy. It can be broken down into good diet and the more specific form of nutritional medicine. Wholefoods form the core of the naturopathic diet. Food should be close to its original state. The diet should tend towards vegetarianism and be organic, with as many raw foods as possible. Some protein (preferably plant) and unrefined carbohydrates and grains should be included.

Nutritional medicine involves special diets to alleviate specific ailments. Food allergies or intolerances may contribute to ill health. Elimination diets which avoid certain suspect substances, often wheat and dairy produce, can be important in naturopathic treatment.

Fasting This means abstaining from food for a specified time, usually one, three, five or seven days. Fasting gives the digestive system a rest, it detoxifies the system and stimulates the metabolism so that healing and renewal can take place.

Naturopaths recommend that most of us should fast one day a month, even when healthy. Most common fasts are short fasts on juice or water.

Hydrotherapy This improves circulation and increases vitality so that the vital force can work more efficiently. It can also ease pain. Hot, cold and alternate hot and cold water is used to achieve specific effects. Hot water is initially stimulating but has a secondary relaxing effect; cold water has an invigorating and tonic effect.

Osteopathy Most naturopaths will work on posture, joints and muscles, not just to correct structural problems, but because structural integrity also affects the organs and body tissue. Naturopaths work on the body's soft tissues using neuro-muscular techniques. This particularly gentle technique is suitable for the elderly, for freeing adhesions that occur after an operation and for relieving abdominal pain.

Psychotherapy The mind and emotions are an integral and vitally important part of total health. Naturopaths approach

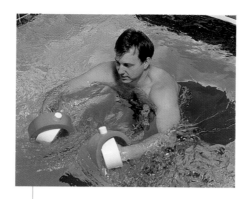

Above: Hydrotherapy is used to improve circulation and general vitality.

mental health from the perspective of removing destructive emotions and pinpoint and eliminate the origins of psychosomatic illnesses, mostly through counselling and relaxation techniques.

Naturopaths are often trained in herbalism or homeopathy, which they may include in the treatment.

What happens in a consultation?
The consultation will take about an hour. The naturopath will ask you questions, such as:

♦ *What and how much you eat and drink*
♦ *Details about your bowel movements*
♦ *How you sleep*
♦ *Details of your job*
♦ *Your relationships with family, friends and colleagues*

He will then give you a routine medical check-up, and use some or all of the diagnostic techniques described.

For the osteopathic examination you will be asked to undress to your underwear. If further medical tests such as blood or urine analysis or scans are needed, the naturopath will arrange for these to be carried out at your nearest hospital. If he discovers a serious problem he will recommend you see your doctor.

The treatment is gradual and can be adapted as your health improves. Early recommendations often include dietary changes, perhaps a detoxifying fast, or a diet to build up strength and immunity and perhaps some relaxation exercises.

Hydrotherapy can either be carried out in the clinic or you will be advised on how to use it at home. Any diet and exercise changes need to be implemented at home. It is normal to make a follow-up appointment as you leave for a week or two later, depending on how acute your condition is and the treatments you are receiving. If any problems occur during treatment, ring your practitioner.

How many sessions do I need?
The length of treatment depends on your illness, how long you have had it, how long it has been suppressed, your age and how healthy you are. Established disorders could take six months or more of advice and treatment for self-sufficiency.

Which problems can it help?
Naturopathy can help with many problems such as anaemia, allergies, arthritis, bronchitis, candida, circulation disorders, constipation, cystitis, eczema and other skin diseases, hangovers, irritable bowel syndrome, migraine, PMS, sinusitis and ulcers. In the case of serious disease, it can improve your resistance to infection so there is less risk of complications.

Is it safe?
As with all medicine, naturopathy is safe when practised by a qualified practitioner.

Responsibly practised, naturopathy is good for young children because their vital force is more easily brought into balance. It can also be used with most elderly patients who can benefit from nutritional and dietary improvements.

Pregnant women who are suffering with morning sickness can also safely benefit from naturopathy.

BACH FLOWER REMEDIES

There are few therapies as simple and gentle as the Bach Flower Remedies. These 38 little bottles of tincture are on sale in most chemists and healthfood stores and are being used by everyone from students to company executives. Rescue Remedy, in particular, has become as popular as the mobile phone, establishing itself as an indispensable ingredient of modern living. No doubt the creator, Dr Edward Bach (pronounced 'batch') who gave up a thriving practice in the 1930s to develop the simple natural remedies, would have been delighted to see them embraced with such fervour.

Dr Bach was a trained homeopath, and was unusual among doctors of this time because he believed in treating people, not their illnesses. He believed that a person's nature had a direct impact on their physical health. After considerable study, he concluded that disease is a manifestation of negative thoughts such as fear, anxiety, grief or despair. The way to heal people, he believed, was to cure the negative thoughts that made them ill.

There are 38 Bach Flower Remedies developed to support every conceivable personality, attitude and negative state of mind. They were developed as a complete system and, before his death, Bach gave instructions that no more remedies were to be added. His aim was to keep the system simple, and although some therapists may find the system restrictive, the remedies were devised for self-help and most users value their simplicity. Bach classified all emotional problems into seven major groups: fear, uncertainty and indecision, insufficient interest in the present circumstances, loneliness, oversensitivity, despondency or despair, and overcare for the welfare of others. Through their subtle vibrational energy the remedies work to heal every negative aspect of all seven types of emotional illness, thereby restoring mental harmony and preventing any physical illness from taking hold. Flower remedies can complement other therapies such as herbalism, homeopathy or aromatherapy or can be used alone.

The remedies were produced by Bach when he was looking for pure natural remedies that could work in a similar way to his homeopathic remedies. Every morning he went out walking and noticed the dew on flowers. He thought that while dew rested on the plant it must absorb some of the plant's properties. He collected and tested the dew from certain flowers and noticed that it could have a positive effect on the mind. He tested several flowers and plants, apparently by instinct, and arrived at 38 remedies.

Bach tested the remedies on himself. For several days before he found each flower, he would experience a particular negative state of mind and the resulting physical symptoms which needed a remedy. Then he would go in search of the flower that would restore his peace of mind and body. He tested each flower by placing a petal on his tongue or in his hand and immediately felt the benefits of the one that worked. He would first feel the mental benefits and then the physical symptoms would disappear.

He discovered that the dew from the flowers exposed to sunlight was more potent and the plant's energy was most concentrated when the flower was in full bloom. Having satisfied himself that the flowers could yield their energy to sun-warmed dew, he decided to devise a more practical method of extraction. In fact, he developed two methods: the sun method and the boiling method. Both of these methods are still used.

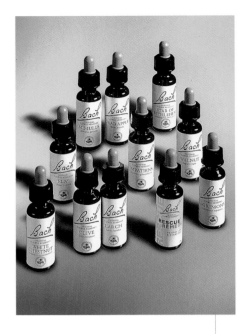

Above: There are 38 Bach Flower Remedies to suit different emotions.

The sun method The best flowers are picked and put in a glass bowl of spring water. The bowl is left in strong sunlight for several hours to allow the plant to energize the water. The blooms are removed with a twig or part of the parent plant to avoid human contact with the essence, and it is poured into bottles half filled with brandy. The brandy preserves the essence which becomes known as the mother tincture. This is further diluted in brandy to make the stock remedies, sold in small brown bottles.

The boiling method This is reserved for essences which qualify for a stronger extraction process. In this process the buds, cones or flowers of the plant are simmered for 30 minutes in a pan of spring water. When cooled, the liquid is filtered, mixed with brandy and bottled.

How do the remedies work?

Bach Flower Remedies are so simple that they are often dismissed as placebos. They do not work in any biochemical way and because no physical part of the plant remains in the remedy, its properties and actions cannot be detected or analysed like a drug or herbal preparation can.

Therapists believe the remedies contain the energy or imprint of the plant from which it was made and work in a similar way to homeopathic remedies – that they provide the stimulus needed to kick-start your own healing mechanism. Some of the remedies are known as 'type remedies'. Your type remedy is effectively the remedy that is most compatible to your personality or basic character, and you take it when the negative side of your character threatens the positive.

The difficulty with the type remedy lies in analysing your character and deciding which remedy matches it best. You may not be the best person to decide on this as it is easy to read through the list of remedies and think that most of them could apply to you to a degree, or be appropriate at a different times in your life. However, usually only one truly complements your basic nature, although some people do seem to be a mixture of two types. To find your type remedy, sift through the events in your life and make a note of how you reacted to them:

♦ *Think of how you were as a child*
♦ *What did you feel like when you started school?*
♦ *How easy or difficult was it to make new friends?*
♦ *Think of how you are in your present relationships*
♦ *How do you respond to criticism?*
♦ *How do you cope with crises, illness or pain?*

These are all tests to find out about your true nature. This memory dredging may suggest several similar remedies. For example, if you think that you are an outspoken extrovert and natural leader, remedies such as Vine, Impatiens, and Vervain are possibilities. But, by a process of elimination, you must try to narrow it down to one that is most like you. Alternatively, ask a friend to tell you, or consult a therapist who uses the remedies.

You should also consult a therapist if you have serious or long-term emotional problems that need resolving. You can use any number of remedies for mental and emotional balancing, but most people take only one or two at a time, keeping Rescue Remedy on hand for emergencies.

There are no rules about taking the remedies. Four drops at least four times a day is suggested, but not the rule. Let your instinct guide you. All remedies are available in ready-to-use preparations that you drop on your tongue or mix in water.

What happens in a consultation?

Bach remedies were created to be so simple to use that people could treat themselves. However, many practitioners of other disciplines such as herbalism, homeopathy and aromatherapy use Bach remedies to complement their own remedies. A few Bach Flower therapists use the remedies exclusively.

Most therapists have their own ways of working, but every consultation should begin with an interview between you and the therapist. This can last for 15 minutes or go on for over an hour. The therapist will explain the Bach system to you if you do not already know how it works. She will ask why you have come to see her and will listen while you talk about yourself and your worries. She will observe your posture and appearance and will listen to the tone of your voice and the way you say things as these can be as revealing as what you actually say.

While you talk, she may take notes and ask questions to work out, by a process of elimination, which remedies would be best for you. She might ask questions about your fears, how you feel about your children, or how easily you give up when something you attempt does not work out. It is not enough for her to know that you have a problem at home or at work. She needs to know how you feel about it and how you react to it.

For example, if your boss does not appreciate how hard you work in the office, you could respond in any number of ways. You might hate him, or the situation may make you even more desperate to please him, or you could pretend you simply do not care. Each of these reactions points to a different remedy. At the end of the consultation the therapist will prescribe the remedies she has chosen. The number of remedies prescribed depends on the individual, but it is unlikely to be more than six, usually fewer. Most people feel better at the end of the consultation because they have been able to talk through their problems.

How many sessions do I need?

The number of sessions you need depends on the individual. If you have quite complex problems you may want to visit a therapist several times. When you are self-prescribing you can take the remedies as and when needed. The length of time it takes to notice an improvement also depends on the person and the problem. Many people notice an immediate benefit, but it can take some time to get back in balance. It is possible to have an emotional or physical reaction while taking the remedies. Therapists would say 'you cannot stir a muddy pool without bringing silt to the surface'.

Which problems can it help?

The Bach remedies help with mental problems and emotions rather than physical ailments. Problems such as fear, anxiety, loneliness and depression can all be relieved by using the right remedy.

Is it safe?

The remedies are not addictive, dangerous, nor do they interfere with any other treatment. They are suitable for all ages. They are safe for pregnant women, babies and children and can also be given to animals and plants.

MANIPULATIVE THERAPIES

◆

OSTEOPATHY

◆

Osteopathy was devised in 1874 by an American doctor called Andrew Taylor Still who worked on the belief that muscle tension and misaligned bones place unnecessary strain on the whole body. Osteopathy is a manipulative therapy which works on the body's structure (the skeleton, muscles, ligaments and connective tissue) to relieve pain, improve mobility and restore all-round health.

Much of osteopathic practice focuses on easing muscular tension, which does more than simply alleviate pain and stiffness. The osteopathic belief that a relaxed muscle is a well-functioning muscle is based on the fact that muscles use up enormous energy when they contract.

Stress, either mental or physical, can cause muscles to contract, wasting energy and making the muscles less elastic so that they are more prone to damage. Tense muscles can also impede the circulation of blood and lymph fluids which flow through them. By relaxing tight muscles these important fluids can flow freely, allowing blood to carry nutrients and oxygen to where they are needed and enabling the waste-carrying lymph to drain away. The ribs and diaphragm are also surrounded by muscles. Treatment in this area can improve respiratory conditions such as asthma and chronic bronchitis.

The nervous system is the most complex system in the body. It comprises the brain, spinal cord and millions of nerve cells, involved in both voluntary and involuntary movement, which reach into every nook and cranny of the body. They register pain, taste, temperature, sight, sound, in fact every sensation it is possible for humans to experience. They affect secretions from glands such as the endocrine glands (thyroid, parathyroid, thymus, suprarenals, pituitary, pancreas, ovaries and testicles), which make hormones.

The nerve cells also regulate blood and lymph circulation and breathing. The whole-person benefits of osteopathy are achieved through the effects that manipulation has on the nervous system.

How does it work?
Through a series of established manipulative techniques, an osteopath can diagnose and treat people with many physical and emotional problems. Osteopaths use many techniques depending on the muscles that are being treated. Most of the techniques are not violent nor usually painful. Admittedly some, such as the high-velocity thrust, are more forceful than others, but even this is not painful.

Cranial techniques (see Cranial Osteopathy pages 424–5) employ the lightest touch to achieve astonishing results. The techniques below are some of the most commonly used today.

Soft tissue manipulation This is used on the soft tissue of the body: skin, connective tissue and muscles. Soft tissue techniques are similar to massage, but are aimed at effecting specific changes in the tissue and are only applied to areas that need treating. Light or heavy pressure is used on the skin or deep in the muscle with fast or slow movements.

Articulatory techniques These are gentle and rhythmic and are also known as refined passive movements. The osteopath might use your arm or leg to apply a leverage through the affected area. He does this to use less force and to cause less pain. Articulatory techniques are used mainly on ligaments and muscles. They also free adhesions, which are thick fibrous bands of tissue that weld muscles together, often in older people.

Articulatory techniques stretch the muscle or ligament and the gentle pull gradually allows the tight tissue to relax and lengthen. Ligaments will resist a short sharp movement such as a high-velocity thrust, and in degeneration and osteoarthritis, shortened ligaments restrict movement as much as damage to the joints themselves. Articulation techniques can restore normal function by lengthening this tight tissue. Patients with osteoarthritis in the hip can get some relief from this treatment.

Traction (pulling) is another type of articulation technique applied to ligaments, capsules and muscles over a joint. Traction can treat back pain or a frozen shoulder. The osteopath will use pressure along the arm to separate the halves of the shoulder joint and relieve pain and stiffness. He will use his hands rather than a traction table so that he can feel the effect of the manoeuvres and once he has achieved the desired effect he will stop.

The high-velocity thrust This technique is common to both osteopaths and chiropractors and is used mainly on the spinal area. High-velocity thrusts can trigger dramatic improvements with muscle relaxation and pain relief. The thrust is a swift, painless movement and only takes three seconds to achieve.

The osteopath puts his hand on the joint parts he wants to adjust. The part of the hand used varies according to the part of the spine being adjusted. The practitioner then takes the joint to its extreme range of movement and applies a direct high-velocity thrust into the joint to make the adjustment. This is characterized by a cracking or popping noise as the joint moves. The noise is caused by gas bubbles in the fluid between the joints bursting under the force of the movement. What is in fact a small pop resounds through the joint as a crack.

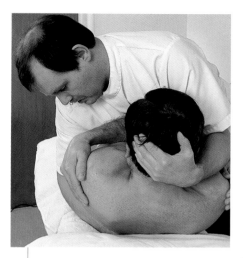

Above: The osteopath may place the patient in rather awkward positions to make the necessary adjustments.

The dramatic therapeutic effect occurs as the thrust separates the joints. The nerves on the covering of each joint send a message to the spinal cord to say that the joint has been stretched. The spinal cord responds by relaxing the tight muscles which had caused the pain.

Muscle energy techniques These are quite new techniques that originated in the United States. Again they are used on tight contracting muscles and are effective on sports injuries to encourage muscles to heal while forming little scar tissue. The techniques involve the patient contracting his muscle against a specific resistance in a particular direction. The osteopath provides a gentle, but definite counterforce to try to encourage the muscles to let go. These techniques require skill and experience to be effective.

Indirect techniques These are so gentle that many patients fall asleep during treatment. They relieve tension in stressed tissue, but aren't used by all osteopaths. They rely on gentle palpation to reduce tension and find a point of balance, where the tissues are subjected to minimal stress. Cranial osteopathy (see pages 424–5) and functional techniques are forms of indirect techniques. They rely on subtle positioning of joints rather than noticeable force.

What happens in a consultation?

Your problem and the type of osteopathic treatment you require will be discussed at your first appointment. This will usually last about an hour and will concentrate mostly on asking questions, examining your body structure and diagnosis. The osteopath will ask you:

♦ *Why you have come to see him*
♦ *When and how your problem started*
♦ *What the problem feels like*

If it is painful, he will want to know what type of pain and where, and how often you feel it. Crushing, burning, stabbing pain or a dull ache and stiffness all stem from different origins. A spot of pain indicates a different problem to pain that runs the length of your upper leg or covers your whole hip. He will also ask about:

♦ *Your current physical and emotional health*
♦ *Your medical history to date*
♦ *What your home life is like*
♦ *What type of work you do*
♦ *Your general lifestyle*
♦ *Whether you have a regular exercise routine*
♦ *The names of any medicines or remedies you are taking*

The practitioner will want to assess your body framework and posture. He will ask you to undress to your underwear so that he can make an accurate assessment. As previously mentioned, many factors can affect your body structure and the associated functions. So, before he can treat you, the osteopath will want to establish the cause of your problem. By observing your body he can get an idea of whether your problems are related to misuse, injury or other causes.

He will evaluate the way your body functions before checking parts such as your spine, hips and legs. He will ask you to stand while he looks at your spinal curves, then ask you to walk across the room, lean forwards, backwards and to each side, lie down and sit as you would sit at your desk or at home. He will study your posture and movements. His intention is not to make you suffer, so if any movements cause you too much pain you will not have to do them.

The osteopath will observe you from the front, back and both sides, he will note the shape of your chest and your muscle tone, especially in the abdominal area as this can relate to lower back problems, as well as your posture and spine.

He will ask you to repeat the movements, while he tests your joints to find how well you can move them. This time he will also palpate the tissue as it moves. He will carry out passive movement testing, which means that he will move your body through the motions of sitting, lying down and walking while feeling your body's response to the movement. The way in which movement is restricted can reveal the cause of your problem.

By feeling the whole body he can detect tissue changes that may be affecting or are being affected by the function of the tissue. He will run his hands over your spine, feet and hands to feel the temperature and muscle tone. Sometimes the tissue can feel boggy or spongy, cold or hot depending on good circulation, or even inflammation, or reveal any number of other problems.

What happens in an examination depends very much on you and the problem you have. The extensive testing will also focus on your reflexes, muscle strength and flexibility. Sometimes you may need further tests or X-rays at a hospital. If this is necessary, the practitioner will explain why and taking your consent, he will make the necessary arrangements with your doctor. Otherwise, he will probably end his diagnosis by telling you, as simply as he can, what he believes to be the cause of your problem and what he can do to help you.

If he believes that osteopathy could help with your particular problem he may begin treatment immediately, especially if you urgently need pain relief. However, it is more usual for treatment to start at your second appointment.

For a treatment, you will be asked to lie down on the therapist's table. Practically every treatment begins with the soft tissue massage to relax the muscles, before moving on to any other techniques. The amount of pressure is also adapted to suit individual needs. Not everyone, for example, is treated with the high-velocity thrust. Children and elderly or frail patients are always treated with more gentle release techniques.

Your first appointment will usually end with the osteopath advising you on useful ways to help yourself and how to avoid any further damage. He may give you diet and lifestyle advice and remedial exercises for you to do while at home. After treatment with gentle techniques you may feel relaxed, while joint manipulation can cause slight aching and tenderness for up to a couple of days afterwards.

How many sessions do I need?

As with any form of treatment this varies according to your individual symptoms. Most people need at least three treatments to see any improvement. If after five treatments you still feel no better, the osteopath will reassess you and may advise you to consider another form of treatment instead of osteopathy.

Which problems can it help?

Osteopathy can help muscular and joint pain, backache, neck problems, sciatica, sports injuries, migraine and dizziness. It can also help to relieve PMS, constipation, arthritis, many respiratory conditions, abdominal pain and problems, and rheumatism. Pregnancy conditions such as backache and other discomforts can also be treated.

Is it safe?

All treatment is safe if you visit a qualified practitioner. Osteopathic techniques can be adapted to treat almost anyone. However, there are some conditions that are not suitable for osteopathic treatment. People with very weak or fragile bones, such as those with severe osteoporosis cannot be treated. Neither can people with inflamed joints from rheumatoid arthritis, although the unaffected parts of the body can. Broken bones and diseases such as bone cancer are also not suitable for treatment.

◆

CRANIAL OSTEOPATHY

◆

In the 1930s American osteopath William Garner Sutherland, a disciple of Andrew Still, developed cranial osteopathy. His interest in the potential for cranial treatment began some years earlier while still a student. His training taught him that the bones of the skull, which are separate at birth, grow together into a fixed structure, but he noticed they retained some potential for movement even in adulthood. If they could move, he surmised, they could also be prey to dysfunction.

Dr Still had taught his students that cerebrospinal fluid (the clear watery fluid surrounding the brain and spinal cord) was 'the highest known element in the human body'. Sutherland discovered that the fluid had detectable rhythms which he called 'the breath of life', as the rhythms appeared to be influenced by the rate and depth of breathing.

By gently manipulating the skull he found he could alter the rhythm of this fluid flow and postulated that it might stimulate the body's self-healing ability

and help cure conditions which appeared unrelated to the cranium. Modern cranial osteopaths call the pulse the cranial rhythmic impulse (CRI).

Cranial osteopathy is a specialist technique used to manipulate the bones of the skull with a touch so light that many people claim they can barely feel it. Sceptics doubt that so light a touch could have any therapeutic benefits and claim that the often amazing results may be due to some sort of spiritual healing. Advocates claim it is based on sound anatomical and physiological knowledge combined with finely tuned palpatory skills and extremely sensitive qualities of touch.

Another therapy called cranio-sacral therapy also grew out of Sutherland's treatment. It is similar in technique and philosophy, but without the detailed examination. The most notable difference, however, is in practitioner training. An osteopath who practises with cranial techniques will have had full osteopathic training and should also be a member of the General Council and Register of Osteopaths. A cranio-sacral therapist may have a background in osteopathy, but this is not always the case.

How does it work?

The human skull is made up of 28 bones which are not fixed but can move slightly, thanks to a complicated system of flanges and bevelled joints. Inside the skull the brain is surrounded by cerebrospinal fluid. The fluid is secreted in the brain and from there flows out of the skull and down the spine, enveloping the spinal cord and the base of the spinal nerves. The brain is held between membranes and sheets of connective tissue, which pass down through the base of the skull to form the lining of the spinal canal and are attached at the end of the spine to the sacrum which forms part of the pelvis (hence the term cranio-sacral in the therapy of the same name).

Practitioners believe that cerebrospinal fluid is pumped through the spinal canal by means of a rhythmic pulsation called the cranial rhythmic impulse, which is distinct from the cardiovascular pulse or the breathing rhythm. As the bones of the skull are moving normally the cranial rhythm remains balanced, but any disturbance to the skull bones can affect the normal motion and consequently alter the cranial rhythm which, in turn, affects other functions in the body. Typical examples of disturbance can occur at birth, when the bones of a baby's skull compress to allow her to pass through the birth canal, or can be caused by a head injury later in life.

A trained osteopath can feel the rhythm of the cranial pulse anywhere in the body, but principally at the skull and the sacrum. In a healthy adult it is supposed to beat at 6–12 beats a minute, but this alters in the case of ill health. By holding and exerting very gentle pressure on the skull the practitioner can feel the rhythm of the cranial pulse and detect irregularities. He can then manipulate the bones of the skull to restore rhythmic balance.

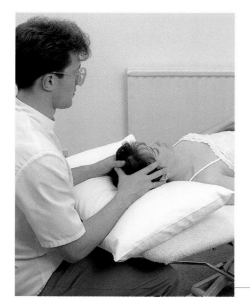

Left: A cranial osteopath balances the flow of cerebrospinal fluid to help problems of the nervous system.

What happens in a consultation?

Your first appointment will last about an hour, although subsequent treatments usually last for 30–40 minutes. As with any osteopathic consultation, the practitioner will begin by taking a detailed case history:

♦ *He will ask about aspects of your life in general*
♦ *Your medical history will be discussed*
♦ *He will need details of any falls, or head injuries, although it is often difficult to remember these*

Most practitioners will also ask you to undress to your underwear for a full physical examination (see Osteopathy page 423). This sort of examination is important in all osteopathic diagnosis, regardless of the practitioner's area of expertise.

You will normally lie on a couch for treatment, although you can occasionally be treated while sitting or standing. The osteopath then places his hands on your body, concentrating on the head and sacral areas to feel for the rhythm quality. He may ask you some questions about your physical and emotional health, based on the information he can pick up from the rhythm. Many people are surprised at the accuracy of this diagnosis. He may carry out some manipulative techniques on your body, using gentle pressure to release tension from specific areas and to rebalance the rhythm.

The amount of body work carried out depends on the practitioner and how he feels it would benefit your condition. He will also work on your head, holding or cradling it and manipulating the bones with a touch so light that you will barely feel it. Most people find this a very pleasant relaxing sensation. However, do not be surprised if your symptoms seem to become slightly worse over the next day or two. This is a normal reaction as treatment stimulates your body's own healing system to bring more problems to the surface. However, if you are at all worried about your reactions, contact your osteopath. Treatments are usually weekly, although the frequency of appointments can vary depending on the severity of your problem.

How many sessions do I need?

It depends on the person and the problem. If there is no noticeable improvement after three or four treatments ask the osteopath if it is worthwhile continuing with your treatment.

Which problems can it help?

It is particularly beneficial for children, easing the effects of a traumatic delivery. It can also help to relieve the discomfort of colic, constant crying, fretfulness, feeding problems and spinal curvature. Childhood problems such as glue ear, breathing problems, learning disabilities, and hyperactivity can also benefit.

Cranial techniques are also suitable for nervous adults who prefer the gentle techniques to the vigorous manipulations of full body osteopathy. It also proves beneficial with cases of migraine and dizziness, sinus problems and head, neck and spine injuries.

Is it safe?

Treatment is extremely gentle and when given by a fully qualified osteopath, it is safe for everyone from babies to the elderly. It is not, however, suitable for severe psychological disturbance.

The aim of the treatment is to balance the cerebrospinal fluid and stimulate the body to heal itself.

CHIROPRACTIC

In the world of alternative therapies, chiropractic is a relative newcomer, although numerous versions of the therapy have been practised for centuries. The name itself derives from the Greek *cheir* meaning hand and *praktikos* meaning done by. In 1895 Canadian magnetic healer Daniel David Palmer founded chiropractic as it is practised today.

Chiropractic is a therapy that works on the musculo-skeletal system of the body, focusing mainly on the spine and its effects on the nervous system. The term musculo-skeletal refers to the body's structure: the bones, joints, muscles, ligaments and tendons that give the body its form. Through a series of special examination and manipulative techniques, chiropractors can diagnose and treat numerous disorders associated with the musculo-skeletal system. The emphasis chiropractors put on the spine has led many people to believe that the therapy is useful only for treating back pain. This is a gross underestimation of the power and range of chiropractic. In fact skilled therapists can treat every structural problem from headaches caused by misalignment through to ankle pain.

The spine itself plays more than a purely structural role in the body. It is the bony structure that surrounds the spinal cord. The brain and spinal cord make up the central nervous system and give rise to nerves which spread to all parts of the body. Part of the central nervous system is called the autonomic nervous system, which controls involuntary body functions. The bony structures of the spine protect the central nervous system and the autonomic nervous system which, in turn, is linked to most body functions.

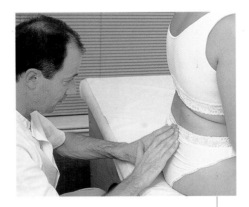

Above: A McTimoney practitioner looks at the alignment of a patient's sacrum before starting corrective treatment.

Consequently any damage, disease or structural change of the spine can affect the health of the rest of the body. Through spine manipulation, chiropractors can improve bone structural problems such as sciatica or ones relating to sports injuries, but can also help with other conditions which you may not think of as being related to the body's structure. For example, asthma can be helped by easing tension in the chest muscles.

How does it work?
Chiropractic is a complicated and highly specialized therapy that may be best understood in terms of its principal aim, systems of analysis and techniques. It is similar in theory and practice to osteopathy and can help with similar problems. But it differs from osteopathic treatment in several ways: chiropractic concentrates on specific adjustment, manipulating one joint at a time, while osteopaths can stretch several joints at a time using 'long lever' techniques. Chiropractors may also use X-rays as part of the diagnosis, while osteopaths rarely do.

The aim is to restore a person's spine to its natural, perfectly functioning form. Chiropractic treatment can benefit both structural and non-structural illnesses because manipulating the spine and musculo-skeletal system not only restores mobility to the body structure but also takes the pressure off the nervous system which connects the spine with all the major organs of the body.

Chiropractors diagnose problems through observation and palpation (hands-on examination). X-rays are used to pinpoint the area of damage, assess the injury, and decide if chiropractic treatment is suitable. They aim to restore the spine and musculo-skeletal system to normal function by using different manipulative techniques. Whereas mobilization involves moving a joint as far as it will comfortably go within its normal range of movement, manipulation involves shifting it even further. There are around 150 different chiropractic techniques, the most common of which are:

Direct thrust techniques These are rapid, forceful movements, also known as high-velocity thrusts, which are central to chiropractic treatment. The chiropractor will make contact with different parts of the hand on the specific joint he wishes to adjust. There may be a cracking noise when the joint moves, due to gas bubbles in the fluid between the joint surfaces.

Indirect thrust techniques These are used where the previous technique is too uncomfortable. With this method it takes a few minutes to gently stretch the joint over a pad, towel or wedge-shaped block.

Soft tissue techniques These manipulations are often used just before an adjustment to reduce the muscle spasm and to relax the joints to allow easier adjustments. They are also commonly used to release 'trigger points', which frequently become tender with musculo-skeletal conditions and can feel like having a trapped nerve.

What happens in a consultation?

Your initial appointment will last 30–45 minutes. That time will be divided between discussion, examination, diagnosis and possibly treatment, although that may not begin until your second visit. Like any other holistic treatment it is important for the chiropractor to know as much as possible about you and your particular problem, so that he can diagnose and treat you as effectively as possible.

Consequently, the chiropractor will take a detailed case history. He will ask why you have come, where you feel pain, when it started, how long you have had it and if you have had similar pain before.

The chiropractor will then examine you. For this you may need to strip down to your underwear. The chiropractor will also carry out routine medical tests, such as taking your pulse, testing blood pressure and checking reflexes. Such tests can help the chiropractor with his diagnosis.

He will then examine your spine while you sit, stand and lie on his treatment couch. While you are lying down, he may ask you to raise your leg, then ask you to stand up and bend your spine forwards and backwards as far as you comfortably can and then bend from left to right.

To find out exactly where the spine is malfunctioning he will ask you to sit on a stool while he palpates or touches the spine, first using 'motion palpation' to move each part of the spine through its normal range of movements until he can locate where the joints are either not moving freely enough or are moving more than they ought. Then he will check the spine and surrounding muscles and tissues; this is called 'static palpation'. The chiropractor may then complete the examination by taking X-rays. X-rays form a very important part of the diagnostic process as they can help to pinpoint the problem and reveal the extent of damage, and most chiropractors have facilities on the premises.

Treatment may involve soft tissue work and then manipulation. It can sometimes feel uncomfortable, but the treatment and the amount of pressure used is done to suit you. Often very little force is necessary. Ice treatments may also be used to reduce pain and any swelling.

The type and frequency of treatment depends on whether your problem is short-term or long-term. Short-term problems can vary. For example, a sports injury can be treated quickly and easily. The practitioner may see you two or three times in one week and then do a check-up a week later. A prolapsed disc in the back may take much longer to sort out. You might find you need 10–12 treatments over a period of 6–8 weeks. It is likely that long-term problems would be treated at your second visit, after the chiropractor has studied your X-rays.

After treatment your body may need a couple of days to settle down. Reactions vary – some people find they are buzzing with energy, others just want to go home and sleep. The effectiveness of the treatment depends on your age and health: if you are young and fit with no other illness you will recover faster than an elderly person with other health problems.

How many sessions do I need?

You can often feel an improvement after just one treatment, but recovery time depends on your problem. You may need two or three visits in the first 7–10 days and then weekly or bi-weekly visits until the condition clears. After that you may need a check-up every few months. The average number of visits is about seven.

Which problems can it help?

Any kind of pain or disability relating to the musculo-skeletal system, and the associated nervous system. It can help neck, shoulder and lower-back pain and give relief to indigestion, constipation, menstrual pain, headaches and asthma.

Is it safe?

Chiropractic is not suitable for damaged bones or for people with bone disease such as bone cancer. Otherwise, it is safe for everyone, from newborn colicky babies to very elderly people suffering from osteoporosis.

Pregnant women can also be treated. Chiropractors do not use X-rays to diagnose pregnant women as this can pose a risk to the unborn child. The practitioner will adapt treatment to ensure it is safe and suitable for pregnancy; different techniques can particularly help back pain.

McTIMONEY CHIROPRACTIC

◆

This particular branch of chiropractic follows the teachings of John McTimoney (1914–80). He trained originally in Palmer's method and then developed the technique to treat the joints of the whole body rather than just the spine.

The McTimoney philosophy and method is similar to straight chiropractic. It works on the structure of the body with the emphasis on the spine and the nervous system, but it also works on other areas, such as arms, legs, hands and feet, thorax and skull, where joints can go out of alignment. Practitioners take a thorough case history, observe posture and check your spine and the angle of your pelvis.

McTimoney chiropractic is a very gentle form of chiropractic treatment that involves manipulation by the practitioner's hands only. Choose a McTimoney chiropractor if you prefer a practitioner who studies your whole body, rather than just your spine.

MASSAGE

Massage as a therapy has evolved out of one of our most instinctive desires – the desire to touch and be touched. We touch each other for many reasons: to show love, offer security, but also to make us feel better. As a species we can exist without many things, but physical contact is not one of them.

The father of therapeutic massage was the Swedish gymnast-turned-therapist Professor Per Henrik Ling (1776–1839). Ling gave us an updated form of therapeutic massage, known as Swedish massage, which still forms the basis for modern massage. Massage is the manipulation of the soft tissues with specific techniques to promote or restore health. Massage therapists use their hands to detect and treat problems in the muscles, ligaments and tendons in the soft tissue.

Most therapists, and certainly those who work holistically, believe that regular body massage can release emotional tension and gradually restore the whole person to balanced health. Massage also forms the basis of other therapies such as aromatherapy, shiatsu and physiotherapy, and plays an important part in Chinese and Ayurvedic medicine. Massage is primarily about touch, and touch in itself has healing qualities for reasons that are beyond our understanding.

How does it work?

There are many different types of massage, some which work on pressure or reflex points such as shiatsu, reflexology and Chinese massage, while others concentrate on relieving specific conditions, for example, remedial massage used to treat sports injuries and muscle strains, and manual lymphatic drainage used to

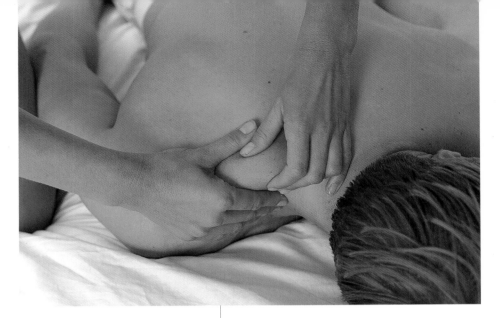

Above: A massage is a very relaxing experience that eases muscle tension, particularly in the neck, back and shoulders.

stimulate the lymphatic system. But basic massage techniques such as stroking, kneading, wringing, pummelling and knuckling have been shown to stimulate physical and emotional healing in two ways: by a mechanical and a reflex action.

The mechanical effects of massage are the physical results of pressing, squeezing and moving the soft tissues. Depending on the techniques used, this can be relaxing or stimulating. Tense muscles cause sluggish circulation because they force the blood vessels to constrict. Massaging the muscles relaxes them and stimulates the circulation so that blood flows freely, carrying oxygen and nutrients to where they are needed. By working on the circulation regular massage can help normalize blood pressure, easing pressure on overburdened arteries and veins. Massage also stimulates the lymphatic system, which is responsible for nourishing cells, carrying waste products out of the body and defending the body against infection.

The reflex action is the involuntary reaction of one part of your body to the stimulation of another part. Because the body, mind and emotions form one intricate organism, stimulus in one part of the body can effect several other parts. So a relaxing back massage can also help to ease leg pain.

Massage is a physical therapy, but one with a strong emotional content. Austrian psychoanalyst, Wilhelm Reich (1897–1957) was the first modern therapist to understand the effects of massage on emotions. He introduced the concept of 'body armouring', the belief that unexpressed emotions, such as anger or grief, are held in the body. Tense, rigid muscles are not healthy and suppressed emotions are not good for the mind. Reich's philosophy paved the way for massage as a holistic therapy. It was developed by the Esalen Institute in California into a therapy for releasing and promoting personal growth.

Massaging the skin releases peptides which affect the mind, stimulate the immune system and improve health.

The four stages of healing

It helps to understand how healing takes place. Massage can have immediate benefits but, if you are ill, recovery takes time. Massage therapists have identified four stages in the healing process:

Relief The first few treatment sessions relieve pain, reduce tension and sedate stressed nerves. They do not necessarily solve the problem, but ease the symptoms.

Correction When the pain has lifted the therapist works on the underlying cause to prevent the return of the problem. Correctional work involves retuning muscles, decongesting a sluggish lymph system, or freeing knotted or scarred fibres.

Strengthening This is important in a badly damaged area. Weaknesses at the injury site can mean recurring problems. For example, sports injuries can cause problems long after they have healed if the tissues around them is weakened by the injury and slow recuperation. Massage can strengthen the surrounding tissues enabling them to provide adequate support when the injury has healed.

Maintenance This is both the final stage of healing and the first step in preventative care. Therapists recommend occasional massage treatments to keep problems at bay and prevent annoying problems from becoming major health issues.

What happens in a consultation?
The type of treatment you receive will depend on your problem, your personal preferences and the therapist's skills. You should not eat or drink heavily before your appointment or attend with an inflamed or infectious skin condition. There are no hard and fast rules, but your appointment should normally begin with the obligatory interview about:

- *Why you have come*
- *Your current state of health*
- *Your medical history*
- *Details of any medication that you take*
- *General lifestyle enquiries*

The therapist will usually then not talk unless she needs to ask you something or you want to discuss something. She may play relaxing music and dim the lights.

For the massage you will need to undress, normally in privacy, and lie on the massage table. You can keep on your briefs, if you wish, but even if you strip completely the therapist will cover you with a towel and only uncover the part of your body on which she needs to work. It is important that you like the massage and feel comfortable, warm and happy with it.

The therapist may use some essential oils. She may choose a blend she thinks appropriate or ask you if there is anything that you like. She might massage your back, work down your body, then turn you over and work down the front, paying particular attention to knotty or tense areas. The massage should be relaxing, although you may feel pain in tense areas. You should not feel severe pain, however, so speak out if an area hurts badly.

A full body massage can last 60–90 minutes. Afterwards you may be left alone for a few minutes. This is important as massage can leave you feeling a little spaced out. Everybody reacts differently to a massage. You may feel relaxed, energized, slightly tired or ache a little the next day. You might cry – this is not unusual if you've been bottling up feelings.

How many sessions do I need?
You can enjoy a massage as often as you like. If you are receiving massage therapy for a specific condition, the number of appointments depends on how serious the problem is and your powers of recovery. Be prepared for extensive treatment.

Which problems can it help?
Massage can treat many complaints. It is particularly good for stress and stress-related conditions, insomnia, depression and circulation problems. It is also good for helping aching and strained muscles, arthritis, rheumatism and sciatica. People with digestive disorders such as irritable bowel syndrome and constipation also benefit, as do women with PMS.

Is it safe?
Massage is a proven, gentle and effective therapy suitable for everyone from premature babies to pregnant women. It can be given to the weak and terminally ill, but only by a qualified therapist. Basic massage for healthy adults can be performed by anyone with essential skills.

MASSAGE GUIDELINES

Before you start to massage at home, take note of these tips:

- *Choose a firm massage surface. A bed is not suitable as it tends to 'give' under pressure. Instead spread several thick towels on the floor. Position a duvet under the towels if it is too uncomfortable*
- *Make sure your partner is warm and comfortable*
- *Relax and concentrate on the massage. If you are unsure about what to do just start by stroking, then concentrate on tense areas*
- *If you use aromatherapy oils, mix five drops to one teaspoon of a carrier oil, such as grapeseed or almond for adults. Use half the strength for children under seven and a quarter strength for children under three. Do not use essential oils on babies*
- *Never pour oil directly onto your partner's skin. Warm it in your hands. If you add oil during the massage, pour it over the back of your hand to warm it before rubbing it into your partner's skin*
- *Vary the pressure and the length of the strokes you use – take your lead from the person you are massaging*
- *Make your massage strokes flowing and rhythmic, keeping one hand in contact with the body at all times*
- *Work in a comfortable way, but always stroke towards the heart and finish by holding your partner's feet for a few seconds to 'ground' him*
- *Do not massage anyone who has an infectious skin disease, an inflammatory condition such as thrombosis, is pregnant, chronically ill, in severe pain, or who has just eaten*

REFLEXOLOGY

People often take some convincing to try reflexology for the first time and for many it is the last resort after many failed treatments. It is difficult to understand how pressing a point on your foot could relieve toothache or eczema, but results can be so impressive that many people have regular treatments to overcome illness, to stay healthy or simply to relax.

Like most complementary therapies reflexology is not a new therapy. It has its roots in the ancient civilizations of Egypt, India and China as well as among African tribes and Native Americans.

But the therapy did not make any real impact in the West until the early 20th century when Dr William Fitzgerald, an ear, nose and throat specialist at Boston General Hospital, became interested in zone therapy, which provided the foundations for reflexology. In zone therapy the body is divided into ten vertical zones, running from the tips of the toes to the top of the head and back down to the finger tips, and all the parts of the body within one zone are linked. By applying pressure to one part of the body, Fitzgerald was delighted to discover that it was possible to relieve pain in other areas within the same zone.

It is not clear where or how Fitzgerald found out about zone therapy, but it is assumed that it was while he was in Europe, because on his return to the United States he began to introduce his patients to zone therapy. He applied pressure to their feet and hands to relieve pain in other parts of the body. He shared his knowledge with a colleague Dr Joe Riley.

Through Riley, a physiotherapist named Eunice Ingham got to know about zone therapy and began to use it on her patients. To her satisfaction, Ingham noticed a marked speeding up of her patients' healing abilities. It was Ingham who developed and renamed zone therapy as reflexology. Ingham also made the important discovery that applying pressure to reflex points could have a much wider therapeutic effect than just pain relief. Reflexology was brought to Britain in 1966 by Ingham's pupil, Doreen Bayly.

The technique involves applying pressure to points on the feet and hands, usually the feet, to stimulate the body's own healing system. A reflex action occurs in a muscle or organ when it is activated by energy from a point of stimulus on the body. In reflexology the point of stimulus is on the hand or foot.

Reflexologists believe that applying pressure to these reflex points can improve physical and mental health. Depending on the points chosen, therapists can use the therapy to ease tension, reduce inflammation, improve circulation and eliminate body toxins. Reflexology is a safe, effective form of treatment, which works by acting the physical body to stimulate the healing at physical, mental and emotional levels.

How does it work?

No one knows exactly how reflexology or zone therapy works beyond the physical act of stimulating nerve endings in the

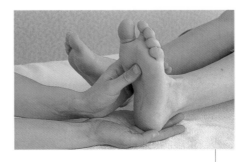

Above: Reflexologists apply pressure to reflex points on the feet which stimulate other body parts linked by nerve pathways.

foot. It has been explained in terms of electrical or electro-chemical energy which operates along the pathways of an autonomic reflex system, working with the autonomic nervous system.

In a healthy body the brain is constantly sending out and receiving messages along the pathways of the nervous system. Good communication is necessary for good health. But sometimes the pathways get blocked and messages cannot get through. Reflexology may operate by stimulating the autonomic reflex system to clear blockages, so that the communication lines stay open and the body, mind and emotions stay healthy.

We know that there are over 70,000 nerve endings on the sole of each foot which, when stimulated, send messages along the pathways of the autonomic nervous system to all areas of the body and brain. Pressure applied to nerve endings can influence the body systems, including the circulation and lymphatic systems. Improvements in circulation and the lymphatic system result in improved body functioning because nutrients and oxygen are transported more efficiently round the body and toxins are eliminated more easily. Through this physical reflex action, reflexology stimulates the body's energy to improve general wellbeing and effectively clear out congestion.

The body is divided into ten vertical zones or channels, five on the left and five on the right. Each zone runs from the head down to the reflex areas on the hands and feet and from the front through to the back of the body. All body parts within any zone are linked by nerve pathways and are mirrored in the corresponding reflex zone on the hands and feet.

By applying pressure to a particular point, known as a reflex point or area, the therapist can stimulate or rebalance the energy in the related zone. For example, the left kidney, which is in zone two of the left-hand side of the body, is reflected at

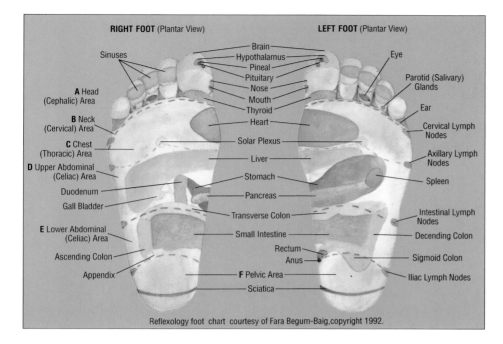

RIGHT FOOT (Plantar View)   **LEFT FOOT** (Plantar View)

Sinuses

Brain
Hypothalamus
Pineal
Pituitary
Nose
Mouth
Thyroid
Heart

A Head
(Cephalic) Area

B Neck
(Cervical) Area

C Chest
(Thoracic) Area

D Upper Abdominal
(Celiac) Area

Duodenum

Gall Bladder

E Lower Abdominal
(Celiac) Area

Ascending Colon

Appendix

Solar Plexus
Liver
Stomach
Pancreas
Transverse Colon
Small Intestine
Rectum
Anus
F Pelvic Area
Sciatica

Eye

Parotid (Salivary)
Glands

Ear

Cervical Lymph
Nodes

Axillary Lymph
Nodes

Spleen

Intestinal Lymph
Nodes

Decending Colon

Sigmoid Colon

Iliac Lymph Nodes

Reflexology foot chart courtesy of Fara Begum-Baig, copyright 1992.

the same point in zone two of the left foot. If an energy blockage occurs in a zone, it can affect several body parts within that zone, causing more than one symptom of ill health. For example, someone with a problem in the left kidney can sometimes develop problems in the left eye because the eyes and kidneys are both linked by the energy in zone two.

What happens in a consultation?

The reflexologist's therapy rooms should be warm and comfortable and may have pleasant music playing. Treatment varies from one practitioner to another. Your first appointment will probably last for about 90 minutes to allow for consultation time, but subsequent appointments are 30–60 minutes. The reflexologist will ask you questions about yourself:

◆ *She will ask details about your medical history, including childhood illnesses, accidents or operations*
◆ *You will need to tell her if you are under the care of a doctor at present or receiving drug treatment for an illness or any chronic (long-term) condition*

The reflexologist will also want to know how you feel about yourself and your life. She will ask about your work and leisure activities, your diet, drinking and lifestyle.

Throughout the treatment the therapist will ask you to sit in a reclining chair or to lie on a treatment couch. She will ask you to remove your shoes and socks and may wipe your feet with cotton wool soaked in witch hazel. She may then apply talcum powder or cream to make treatment easier. Reflexologists often say that feet tell your body's history, so do not be surprised if she picks up on past health problems.

The therapist usually begins and ends with some relaxation techniques to relax the diaphragm, free the ankle and loosen the joints. She will work over all the foot, before giving specific attention to any problem areas. If you feel pain or tenderness, it is an indication of a blockage or imbalance in the corresponding organ or body part. The reflexologist will then pay extra attention to these tender areas.

The intention is not to cause you pain, but pain is a sign of blocked energy, and she will want to free the blockage to stimulate the healing process. Blocked energy is often indicated by crystalline deposits under the skin, which can feel like grains of sugar, or the reflexes can be taut or spongy. The reflexologist will spend time working on these areas.

For most people, treatment is relaxing rather than painful, although you can experience various sensations. It is normal, for example, to feel a tingling in your

arms and hands, a good sign as it points to increased circulation. After treatment you may feel tired or revitalized, it depends on you. You will usually make a follow-up appointment for a week later. Some people's symptoms get worse before they get better. This can sometimes happen if you are fighting an infection or overcoming a painful condition.

How many sessions do I need?

The number of treatments depends on your problems, how long you have had them, and whether or not they have been suppressed by drugs. The effect is usually accumulative: you may feel more relaxed, or sleep better after your first treatment and this will encourage you to continue.

Which problems can it help?

Reflexology is a good all-round 'whole system' therapy for people of all ages. However, it works well for any conditions that need to be cleared or regulated, for example: digestive and menstrual irregularities, stress and fatigue, aches and pains and inflammatory skin conditions such as eczema. Studies have shown impressive results when reflexology has been used to aid pregnancy, and to help childhood problems such as glue ear.

Is it safe?

Reflexology by a qualified therapist is safe for everyone. It can be a wonderfully relaxing treatment during pregnancy as it relieves back pain, nausea and heartburn. If you are in the early stages of pregnancy, tell the therapist so she can tailor the treatment to your needs. Children also benefit from short reflexology sessions; infants' feet just need gentle stroking.

Self-treatment is safe for minor ailments, but is not recommended if you are pregnant, diabetic, epileptic or receiving medical treatment for a serious illness. If you are under a doctor's care let him know before treatment begins.

ACTIVE THERAPIES

ALEXANDER TECHNIQUE

The Alexander Technique is a special method that re-educates us to regain our natural posture and use our bodies more efficiently. It can help relieve stress-related conditions, breathing disorders and neck and joint pain. It was developed by Frederick Matthias Alexander who believed that, 'Every man, woman and child holds the possibility of physical perfection; it rests with each of us to attain it by personal understanding and effort'.

Alexander, an Australian actor born in 1869, was giving recitals of 'dramatic and humorous pieces' when he started to lose his voice for no apparent reason. His doctor diagnosed inflamed vocal cords and prescribed various treatments and rest, but his condition worsened. When faced with an operation or giving up his career Alexander resolved to find the cause himself.

He noted that his voice was all right when he was not working so he began to analyse what he did differently when he spoke on stage. He arranged mirrors all around the room to watch himself and noticed that as he recited he sucked in air and pulled his head down, depressing his larynx. This reaction shortened his spine and narrowed his back, affecting his breathing. He noticed that when he spoke normally, he adopted a similar stance but in a less exaggerated way. He realized that this posture represented a pattern of misuse that affected his voice, and that this related to general body tension.

Over the years he tried many new ways of using his body to prevent his old habits affecting his voice. He finally discovered that the relationship between his head and neck and how the head and neck

related to the rest of his body were crucial to correct body use. He called this 'the Primary Control' because this relationship determines the poise and quality of the whole body. He believed that when the head, neck and back worked in harmony it balanced the whole person.

The Alexander Technique is not a therapy as such, but a process of re-education, which aims to teach us to rediscover our natural poise, grace and freedom, and use our bodies more efficiently. It is often referred to as posture training, which is not strictly correct, although improved postural balance is a benefit. It is taught in lessons by a teacher, not a therapist, and the individual taking the lessons is known as a pupil, not a patient or client.

The Alexander Technique works on the principle that mind and body form a complex and integrated whole. Today, with advances in psychosomatic medicine, this principle does not seem so radical. Most of us now accept that mental, emotional and physical health are linked. But when Alexander was writing at the turn of the century, his holistic theories were considered revolutionary. As a holistic system, the technique is not taught in order to alleviate specific ailments, such as a stiff neck or aching back, but to address the source of problems. However, it has been found that in restoring harmony to the whole person, the specific problems will often disappear.

The Alexander Technique does not emphasize correcting poor posture but aims to get people to move with ease and grace and walk with increased balance and poise. Alexander claimed that we began to misuse ourselves when we became more involved in occupations that restricted our natural movements.

Alexander also believed that our stressful modern lifestyle takes its toll on our mental, physical and emotional health and that we develop poor postural habits.

Today we also lead sedentary lifestyles hunched over office desks, computers, counters, and production lines. We force our bodies into unnatural postures which cause aches and pains. Alexander believed that his technique could help people to undo and prevent the bad habits that so often lead to aches and pains and poor functioning.

How does it work?

The Alexander Technique has to be experienced to be properly understood. It is difficult and confusing to understand the principles from reading about them in a book. However, the people who have taken the lessons are amazed at how simple it all seems.

It may best be understood in terms of the Primary Control. This refers to the dynamic relationship between the head, neck and back. The aim is to direct the head away from the spine without tensing and narrowing the back. The Primary Control can be thought of as a barometer for our general state of psycho-physical health. When the head, neck and back is working well, we tend to feel good. But when the neck is unnecessarily tense it pulls the head back and down towards the spine. This causes the spine to shorten and the back to narrow, a sign of misuse that corresponds to the 'startle pattern' which we instinctively adopt when we brace ourselves for a shock. Through education, the Alexander Technique aims to change this startle pattern so that it only happens in appropriate situations.

This system of changing the startle pattern can be achieved through the Alexander practice of inhibition. Inhibition refers to the potential not to react immediately to stimulus. Alexander claimed that success with his technique could only be achieved if we stopped being dominated by unconscious impulses and made reasoned choices about every movement that we made. In his opinion the way to lasting health was to develop conscious use of ourselves in our daily activities. Through inhibition we gradually sustain good primary control of our head, neck and back and achieve a postural homeostasis (balance) that corresponds to mental balance.

It is difficult to explain exactly how this can be achieved, but it can be allied to the osteopathic concept of spinal health and postural alignment, to emotional health in psychotherapy, to the enhancement of skills of the performing artist and to improved self management. Ultimately the technique can only be understood through practice.

What happens in a lesson?

Lessons take place on a one-to-one basis. The lesson will begin with a discussion between you and your teacher about why you have come and what you hope to get from the course. If you have a particular problem that needs resolving, ask her if she thinks Alexander can help and how many lessons she thinks you need. Wear loose, comfortable, casual clothes for the lesson. You do not need to remove any clothes, although some teachers may suggest taking off your shoes so that you can feel more 'centred' by keeping contact with the floor.

Each teacher will have her own system, but every lesson will involve guidance and verbal instructions to help pinpoint and unravel patterns of misuse and restore your natural reflexes.

For example, the teacher may ask you to get up from a chair or sit down on a chair, while she guides and instructs you. You may have to carry out several movements such as walking, bending, sitting, talking and lifting. The teacher will guide and direct you in all of these activities so that you can feel how effortless and smooth the movements can be compared to your usual patterns of misuse.

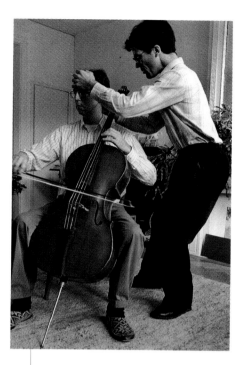

Above: During a lesson, the teacher will point out your bad postural habits and show how to replace them with good ones.

Throughout the lesson the teacher will talk to you about what she is doing, pointing out your bad habits and teaching you to replace them with good ones. This is when your inhibiting skills come into play; you must make a conscious decision to refuse to contract into each movement and think about new ways of using your body to keep your spine free of tension. The lesson may involve some table work. The teacher will ask you to lie on your back on a therapy couch with your knees bent and a small stack of books under your head so that your neck is roughly parallel with the table top. This is what is known as the semi-supine position and it is believed to be the most restful posture for the spine. The teacher will gently coax you to let go of muscle tension, release your joints and lengthen your spine.

At the end of a lesson most people say they feel taller and lighter. You may also feel any number of other sensations: rejuvenated, energized, relaxed and 'centred'. After several lessons you will start to react and move without tension and eventually without the guidance of the teacher.

Before you leave each lesson the teacher may give you some 'homework' to practise regularly. This may be a suggestion to observe how you hold your breath when you are tense or how you brace yourself before performing a simple activity. You may also be asked to adopt the semi-supine position for 10–15 minutes every day to reinforce the learnt techniques and to relax and lengthen your spine.

How many sessions do I need?

Alexander recommended a minimum of 30 lessons, but most teachers believe it depends on the individual. However, about 25–40 lessons is normal. Lessons usually last 30–45 minutes and it is best to begin with two or three a week.

Which problems can it help?

The Alexander Technique is not a cure for any condition or illness, although many symptoms improve during practice. There is not much scientific evidence for the benefits of the technique, but students and teachers report an improvement with numerous problems. Stress-related conditions, fatigue and lethargy, anxiety, breathing disorders, back, neck and joint pain can all benefit from the technique. It can help recovery from illness or injury, and is believed to improve both personal and professional relationships.

Is it safe?

When taught by a qualified teacher, the Alexander Technique is safe for everyone. Young children do not usually need the technique as they have natural balance, but they can be taught it as a preventative technique. Children with physical handicaps such as polio and scoliosis of the spine can also benefit. The technique is safe to learn in pregnancy. Pregnant women may find that it helps them to cope with their changing shape and spinal pressure and it is believed to encourage easier labour.

HYPNOTHERAPY

There is no single accepted definition of hypnotherapy, but it can be described as a form of psychotherapy that works on the subconscious to change thought and behaviour. Hypnosis refers to the trance-like state, somewhere between waking and sleeping, which you enter when you are hypnotized, and hypnotherapy is the practice of bringing about healing or facilitating change while under hypnosis.

Modern therapists build up a rapport with their clients which enables them to 'suggest' changes. Modern hypnotherapists use simple techniques to induce a light trance which can have the most amazing results. While in a trance you are much more suggestible and compliant than you would be normally and your mind is more willing to accept new information, but only what you want to hear.

Consequently, the therapist can make suggestions that you·will store in your mind, effectively reprogramming it to accept or reject certain beliefs or patterns of behaviour. If you have a fear of spiders, for example, she can suggest that you are no longer afraid of spiders. If you want to overcome your phobia, your eager mind will absorb the suggestion and replace the old fear with the new lack of fear. The same can happen with pain. If, under hypnosis, your mind accepts that you do not feel pain, then you will not feel it.

The mind is incredibly powerful and is inextricably linked to the body. This is demonstrated during a hypnotic trance when breathing, heart-rate and metabolism can be slowed, allergic reactions stopped and pain reduced.

Hypnotherapy can be used alongside other therapies such as osteopathy or acupuncture to reinforce their benefits.

How does it work?

There is not complete agreement about how hypnosis works, but the commonly accepted theory is that the mind has two parts: the conscious and the subconscious. We are aware of the conscious mind because we use it to make everyday decisions. But the conscious mind is ruled by the larger subconscious, as are all mental and physical functions from regulating blood pressure to storing memories. A subconscious desire is so strong it will triumph over a conscious desire.

Hypnotherapists believe the subconscious mind is the source of human energy and power and the home of the real you. If you do not learn to understand your subconscious, you will never understand yourself and if you do not use it you will never realize your true potential. One other important point about the subconscious is that it will believe anything you tell it. Hypnotism exploits this mental submission by putting the conscious mind to sleep temporarily to reach the subconscious where you can replace negative beliefs or emotions with positive ones. This reprogramming is done by the therapist suggesting targets or beliefs to counteract your problem. Hypnotherapists reach the subconscious by inducing a trance.

Therapists begin hypnosis by encouraging you to relax. There are several ways of doing this, the most common is through the use of your imagination. Alternative methods include the heavy arms and semaphore techniques.

Imagination The therapist talks to you in a relaxing, controlled way, which encourages you to concentrate on her voice. She asks you to focus on a point such as a real or imagined spot on the ceiling or an object in front of you. She may ask you to take several deep breaths, suggesting that with every breath you feel more relaxed and sleepy. On the final breath you are told to close your eyes. The

therapist then asks you to imagine a particular scene such as a beautiful sunlit garden and talks you through what you will see there, encouraging you to use all of your senses to make sure that you hear the birds, smell the flowers and see the beautiful colours around you.

She may count you down imaginary steps, counting them back from ten to one. At this point she might test the depth of your trance by instructing you to perform a simple action such as raising your right arm. Throughout, the therapist encourages you to let go of the conscious world by enticing you into this imaginary one. In unaccustomed subjects it can take up to 20 minutes, sometimes more, to get to a level where you are open to suggestions. After several sessions, a trance can be induced in seconds.

Direct/autosuggestion therapy When you are in a trance the therapist gives you direct suggestions, which are always specific, positive and in the present tense. Your mind accepts these suggestions because the trance state causes the critical factor of your mind to shut down. This therapy is excellent for calming exam nerves, and stopping nervous habits.

The first session is usually the most difficult. Some therapists record the session and give you a tape to play at home to reinforce the treatment. Several sessions of autosuggestion may be needed, during which the therapist will change the suggestions as changes start to take place.

Age regression The therapist uses this technique to take you back to discover how your present problems may result from past incidents. She enables you to see childhood events in context from an adult perspective. In most cases the event itself was meaningless, but as a child, you may have attached some significance to it. Interpretation of events is what retains such a hold on the mind and exerts con-

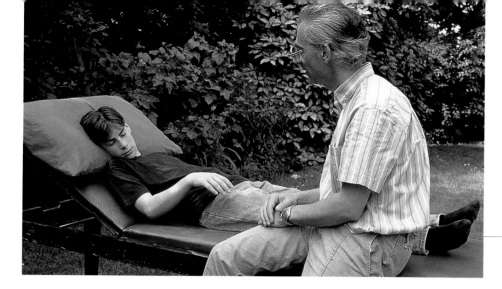

Left: A hypnotic trance is a state between waking and sleeping, during which you will still be in complete control.

trol over our behaviour. Many people are afraid to be regressed, but returning to review a painful situation does not mean going through it again.

Hypnohealing is aimed at healing pathological disease. The therapist helps you uncover the cause of your illness and through visualization encourages you to release it. The therapy is based on the belief that every thought has a physical response in the body and that nothing is more positive than thought. The therapist shows you how to think, imagine and feel diseases such as asthma, angina or cancer being eradicated from your body. She encourages you to see your healthy cells as a powerful force, regenerating and growing in strength to defeat the diseased cells and clearing the way for new, healthy cells. The technique is so successful that some of Britain's leading hospitals are encouraging patients to use it.

What happens in a consultation?

The initial consultation can last for 60–90 minutes, although subsequent sessions rarely last for longer than one hour. The first session is principally an assessment and conversation with the therapist:

♦ *She will ask you why you have come to see her, explain how hypnosis works and advise you on what you can hope to get from treatment*
♦ *She will hopefully put your mind at rest about the safety of the therapy and encourage you to voice any fears that you may have and win your trust*

Trust is important in any therapy, but especially in hypnosis as your cooperation is essential. Different therapists can use different techniques, so it is best to know what will happen from the outset.

If there is time, the therapist may induce hypnosis in the first session, but often it will start at the second session.

The treatment itself is often much less dramatic than many people expect. You lie on a couch or sit in a comfortable chair while the therapist induces a trance-like state. This can be done in many different ways depending on what is best for you. She then uses suggestions to deepen the relaxation into a trance. When in the trance you may look like you are asleep but it will not feel like it. Most people feel relaxed, others feel dreamy, or as if they are floating or watching themselves sleep. You will, however, be aware of what is happening throughout.

It is important to remember that while in a trance you are in complete control and the therapist cannot make you do or say something that you do not want to or that goes against your principles. If there is any part of the treatment with which you feel uncomfortable, you can leave.

While you are in the trance, the therapist will address the problem with which you consulted her, possibly in one of the ways mentioned above.

At the end of the session, she will encourage you to work your way slowly back to consciousness. For example, she may say, 'You will awake on the count of three, and when you do, you will be feeling relaxed and refreshed'.

During treatment the therapist will probably encourage you to learn self hypnosis to use at home to back up the work you have done with her and to equip you to overcome any future problems.

How many sessions do I need?

It is difficult to say. It depends on the person, the problem, and the treatment method. For a straightforward problem such as stopping smoking or losing weight, you may need four or five weekly sessions, sometimes less. For chronic health problems or deep emotional problems, about 12–15 weekly sessions are more likely. Some people can be taught self hypnosis in one or two sessions.

Which problems can it help?

Hypnosis can help with many physical, psychosomatic and mental problems. It has been successful with habit problems and addictions; problems which originate from past traumas; phobias, and stress-related problems such as irritable bowel syndrome, eczema, anxiety and insomnia.

Is it safe?

There is understandably concern about the safety of hypnotherapy. Horror stories abound about people not being counted out properly or of women being taken advantage of. You are safe in the hands of a qualified practitioner, so check their credentials with their association. It also pays to see someone that you like. Children under the age of four cannot be hypnotized as they are too young to cooperate with the therapist.

YOGA

Yoga is an ancient exercise system that uses stretching movements and meditation techniques to relax body, mind and spirit. With regular practice it can help relieve such conditions as anxiety, backache, arthritis and depression.

Yoga is often portrayed as a mystical Eastern relaxation system that involves intricate postures that only the most supple and double-jointed people would dare to attempt. But the movements can be so simple that even the very stiff, elderly, ill and disabled can benefit from yoga.

Certainly, the discipline appears to be Eastern in origin. Ancient Indian statues illustrate that it was practised in northern India at least 4,000 years ago, but the details of its origins are indistinct. We do know, however, that it was originally practised by Indian philosophers or yogis who lived hermetic lives of meditation. But today the benefits of yoga have spread internationally and it is now practised in non-religious, non-cultural-based classes all over the Western world.

What is yoga?

Yoga is a gentle exercise system that benefits both the body and the spirit. The word yoga comes from the Sanskrit (Indian) word for union of mind and body. Practising the discipline of yoga is believed to encourage a better union of mind, body and spirit and restore the whole person to balance. Yoga benefits the body by relaxing muscles and improving suppleness, fitness and physical function. It also relaxes the mind, and teaches us how to control stress, destructive emotions and unhealthy habits. A relaxed mind encourages the concentration and serenity that make life easier and allow spiritual development.

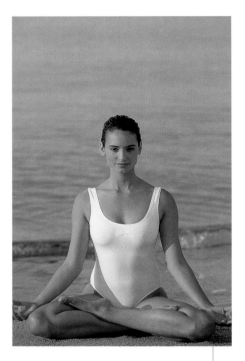

Above: Meditation in yoga is usually done in the famous Lotus position, but many other moves require less flexibility.

There are many different forms of yoga, including four mental yogas called *Bhakti yoga* (emotions), *Gyana yoga* (wisdom), *Raja yoga* (meditation) and *Karma yoga* (actions) but most Western forms are based on the physical yoga called *Hatha yoga*. The principles of hatha yoga were laid down by the 8th-century Indian sage, Patanjali.

Patanjali's yoga code advocates developing healthy attitudes and values such as honesty, non-acquisitiveness and moderation in preparation for the more serious business of spiritual enlightenment. The three aspects of the code on which yoga concentrates most are: Pranayama (breathing), Asanas (postures) and Dhyana (meditation). Through rigorous practice of these principles the yoga practitioner aims to achieve the ultimate goal of self-enlightenment.

How does it work?

Harmony between body, mind and spirit is achieved through correct breathing, postural exercises and meditation. To yoga practitioners, breathing correctly is a way of controlling all mental and bodily functions and is essential for relaxation and meditation. Most of us tend to breathe incorrectly: anxiety and tension cause us to take short breaths that are centred in the upper chest, while lack of energy can cause weak breathing lower down in the diaphragm.

Yoga breathing, on the other hand, encourages us to make full use of our lungs, so we strengthen them, increase our energy and vitality, and improve our circulation.

The yoga postures exercise the body muscles and encourage relaxation and meditation. They are easier to demonstrate than describe and they must be practised regularly to be really appreciated and to make a difference. The famous Lotus position represents self-awareness and is the pose most often adopted by people who are experienced in meditation. Other postures with names such as Cheetah, Cobra, Ostrich, Butterfly and Praying mantis are based on the naturally relaxed and graceful movements of animals. These movements stretch the muscles to release pent-up tension and encourage strength and flexibility in the limbs and spine.

Asanas are performed in a particular sequence, designed to exercise all the major muscle groups in the correct order, to encourage good circulation and to flush toxins out of the body. They build muscle tone, and eliminate fat that has accumulated in the body cells. They can also help to reduce cellulite and regulate the metabolism to maintain a regular weight. By practising asanas regularly as you get older you can keep your metabolism stable and avoid unnecessary weight gain. Yoga is also believed to help to strengthen the immune system so that you can become less likely to suffer from colds and other viruses.

Meditation is a form of deep relaxation used to calm or focus the mind. It is an important, but not essential part of yoga, and most beginners start with the postures only. Yoga practitioners often see meditation as a natural progression from becoming competent at performing the postures and breathing exercises.

What happens in a class?

Yoga is taught in classes of about 15–20 people and each one lasts from one to two hours. You do not have to complete a questionnaire or be interviewed before the class, but you ought to tell the teacher if you suffer from any physical disabilities or illness so that she can advise you on which movements you should avoid or possibly adapt. Some specially trained practitioners give one-to-one sessions or teach small groups of people with specific medical problems.

To carry out the postures with ease and comfort, you should go barefoot and wear clothes which allow movement – a leotard or T-shirt and leggings or shorts is best. You will also need a rubber mat on which to work. The teacher often provides these, but many people buy their own so that they can carry on practising at home. Classes vary in structure, but in a 90-minute class you would usually begin by focusing on breath control for about 10 minutes, followed by 15–20 minutes of gentle warm-up exercises.

It takes time to master the postures, so be realistic about what you can achieve and do not push yourself too hard. Perform them slowly and smoothly and hold each posture only for as long as is comfortable, concentrating on your breathing throughout. Postures are usually performed for about 25 minutes, followed by 20 minutes of relaxation exercises. The class may end with 5–10 minutes of reflection and the advice to practise at home in a warm, quiet, well-ventilated room.

Early morning sessions are recommended, but you can practise yoga at any time of the day, providing you do so at least two hours after eating.

POSTURE AND BREATHING

◆

To sit or stand in perfect posture is an important part of yoga, and many of the asanas have been developed to help strengthen the back muscles so that you can hold your spine in alignment. When you are sitting, kneeling or standing, keep your head up, and open out your chest by pushing down your shoulders.

Learning how to breathe correctly is an important part of the yoga practice. Babies always breathe naturally from the diaphragm, but as adults we get into bad habits and tend to breathe shallowly from the chest. Shallow breathing is increased when we are under stress. By breathing correctly you will improve your lung capacity, which will in turn send more oxygen into your bloodstream to revitalize and cleanse your internal organs. Deep breathing also helps to calm the nervous system and still the mind.

Good posture

1) When standing, keep your feet firmly on the ground with your weight evenly balanced between your toes and heels. Keep your arms by your side, your shoulders down, and your stomach and bottom tucked in.
2) When sitting cross-legged, place your hands on your knees, keep your head held high and your spine straight, but your shoulders relaxed.
3) When sitting on your heels, keep your head up, put your hands on your knees, lift up your spine and keep your elbows straight.

Good breathing

1) Stand or sit in good posture as above. Inhale deeply from your diaphragm, pushing out your stomach, but don't let your chest move and keep your shoulders down.
2) Now exhale deeply. Keep up a steady breathing rhythm for at least 10–12 breaths. Always do this before you start a yoga session to calm and relax your mind.

How many sessions do I need?

Like any other exercise or relaxation system, yoga needs to be practised regularly to have lasting effect on you. It should become part of your everyday lifestyle and routine. However, even after one session most people feel more relaxed and many will start to sleep better immediately.

Which problems can it help?

Regular yoga can help any type of problem related to stress. Ones that particularly benefit are anxiety, high blood pressure, circulation and heart problems, backache, asthma, digestive problems such as irritable bowel syndrome, fatigue and depression. It can also help to relieve rheumatism and arthritis.

Is it safe?

Yoga is safe for everyone. It is suitable for people of all ages and levels of fitness. Children, pregnant women, the elderly and people with chronic health problems can all practise yoga under the guidance of a qualified instructor. You may want to talk to your doctor if you are suffering from an ongoing ailment and remember that yoga is complementary rather than an alternative to conventional treatment.

TAI CHI

Tai chi is a gentle martial art that involves a combination of meditation and flowing exercises to help improve the health of the body and mind. With regular practice it can relieve stress and improve the functioning of the metabolism and the immune system.

Like many ancient skills there are numerous theories about the origins of tai chi. One of the most popular is that it was founded by Taoist monk and martial arts expert, Chang San Feng, who lived in the Sung dynasty (AD 960–1279). Legend has it that Chang San Feng watched a battle between a crane and a snake, in which the snake outwitted the much bigger stronger bird by dodging and weaving each attack and retaliating with lightning speed. The monk is believed to have been so impressed by the flexibility and natural grace of the snake's movements that he decided to integrate them into his own special system of martial arts.

The new postures were combined with ancient Taoist breathing exercises, which were used to stimulate chi (inner energy), and this formed the basis of tai chi. From this beginning the present exercises are believed to have been further developed.

Research has shown that regular practice of tai chi relaxes and destresses the muscles and the nervous system. Through the nervous system the benefits then filter through to the glandular system, improving metabolism and enhancing the overall working of the immune system. The body also benefits from improved posture and joint flexibility, and blood circulation and breathing also get a positive boost.

If you combine these benefits with the mental and spiritual aspects of a system steeped in meditation, it is easy to see why

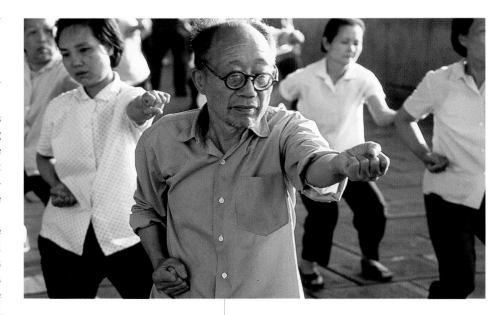

Above: In China, the gentle and relaxing movements of tai chi are regularly practised outside by all age groups.

so many people today who are leading busy, stressful lives have been convinced to include tai chi in their current programme of preventative healthcare.

What is tai chi?
Tai chi is more accurately known as tai chi chuan, which means 'the supreme way of the fist'. It is a non-combative martial art system that includes meditation and exercises to promote and enhance total body health. It can be used to heal and rejuvenate the body, and to encourage spiritual growth.

Tai chi is part of the complex system of Oriental medicine which also includes acupuncture, acupressure, herbal medicine and massage. Together with these other areas, tai chi is used to promote a long, healthy life.

The system itself has in time developed and divided into many different styles such as the Yang style, Chen style, Lee style and Wu style. The Yang style, for

example, is slow, strong, rhythmic and flowing, while the Chen style is varied, and constantly changes pace from slow to fast. These various styles illustrate that there is no one correct way to perform tai chi. Ultimately, it is a very personal endeavour. And, although an instructor can show you a particular style and how to perform the different movements, it is basically up to you to make tai chi your very own.

How does it work?
The basis of every style of tai chi is the practise of 'the form'. A form is a set of slow-moving, graceful exercises performed in a definite pattern. There are short forms and long forms, which vary from one style to another. Traditionally, a long form involves 108 movements and can take anything from 20 minutes up to one hour to perform. A short form can involve 48 or sometimes only 37 movements, and rarely takes more than 5–10 minutes to perform.

The movements of the form are essentially self-defence movements; they have names such as, 'Kick with right heel' and 'Punch with concealed fist'. They are practised in a slow flowing sequence in order to encourage general relaxation and harmony between the mind, body and spirit. The movements achieve this harmony because they are designed to rebalance the flow of chi or energy that flows through channels in the body that are called meridians (see Acupuncture, pages 444–5). It also helps to regulate the circulation of body fluids, such as blood and lymph.

To perform tai chi you need to relax and focus your mind. It can help to develop balance, a good posture and control. It also aims to build up a strong 'inner' power in a body that is responsive and supple. Although not outwardly aggressive, tai chi masters in the past have been known to defeat many younger martial arts experts who have trained in the more combative 'outer' forms of karate and kung fu.

Ideally, tai chi should be practised outdoors. In China it is traditional to practise the form near trees so that the performers can absorb the positive energy that is given off by these natural living forms.

Wherever you practise tai chi it is important to relax and focus your mind and concentrate on how you breathe, so that you can coordinate breathing with all the movements of your body. This special attention to breathing has earned tai chi the special title of 'meditation in motion'.

What happens in a class?

Tai chi can be learnt on a one-to-one basis from a tai chi master, but is usually taught in a class of about 15–30 people. When deciding on a class it is important to feel happy with the instructor's qualifications and experience, so often recommendation from a contact or friend can be the best way of finding the right one. The class usually lasts for about 90 minutes and although no special clothes are necessary, it is customary to wear loose comfortable clothes, such as T-shirt and leggings and shorts, and socks or soft flat-soled shoes

to perform the movements. Tai chi classes in the West usually take place indoors in a well-ventilated, quiet space. There is no consultation, nor does the instructor take down a case history, but you should tell him if you are suffering from any health problems that might affect your ability to do the movements or possibly render some of them to be unsuitable. The instructor may explain the purpose of tai chi and advise you to take the exercises at your own pace.

The class will usually begin with 10–30 minutes of basic warm-up exercises before you move on to learning the components of a form. Learning a form is not as easy as it sounds. It can take up to a year to learn a short form and possibly two years to learn the long form, as continual practice is needed in order to perfect the execution of each movement.

The tai chi exercises are meant to encourage you to feel more balanced and relaxed. So early lessons may focus on encouraging you simply to feel rooted or 'centred'. You are taught to stand and move in ways that allow your 'awareness' to move down into your abdomen and legs, making you release tension and feel strong and balanced. A tai chi class should not make you feel sore or tired as you are advised from the outset not to overstretch or overreach yourself. At the end of the class you will be advised to practise the movements you have learnt often at home.

How many sessions do I need?

You need to practise tai chi on a regular basis to gain any noticeable benefits. A weekly class is believed to be the minimum to consider, especially when you first start as a beginner.

Which problems can it help?

Tai chi can help stress-related problems. Anxiety, muscular tension, depression, insomnia, high and low blood pressure

and circulation are all problems that have been alleviated by the exercises. Tai chi has been shown to benefit people suffering from arthritis, to aid recovery from injury, and even to assist in the rehabilitation of heart attack or stroke patients. Those people who practise the art long-term have been shown to be more flexible and less susceptible to spinal problems and some debilitating bone conditions such as osteoporosis. It is also used by the Chinese for the treatment of people suffering from chronic disease.

Is it safe?

As with any therapy when it is taught by an experienced and knowledgeable instructor and practised correctly, tai chi is a gentle art and a perfectly safe system of exercise for people of any age and all levels of fitness. However, if you are at all worried about joining a new class, consult your doctor before you go along.

CHI KUNG

♦

This is a similar exercise movement to tai chi. Slow, fluid, elegant movements are performed which help regulate the body, while deep breathing and some visualization techniques help to still the mind. The movements tone and make the abdominal muscles more flexible. The aim again is to improve the flow of chi in the body.

It is an ideal preventative exercise, and it is good for people who find it hard to meditate as it produces the same relaxing benefits. It is believed to help conditions such as anxiety, depression, insomnia, asthma, arthritis, stomach disorders and even heart disease.

AUTOGENIC TRAINING

Autogenic training involves teaching people a series of special mental exercises to help them relax mentally and physically from day-to-day stress. This calming process can help relieve conditions such as asthma, high blood pressure and colitis.

For thousands of years Indian yogis have known that the mind can be trained to influence our body systems. Breathing, blood circulation and the autonomic nervous system, which controls muscle and gland responses to stress, can all be regulated by a well-trained mind. Mental training, however, was neglected in Western medicine until Autogenic Training took the principles of Eastern meditation and made them more acceptable for Westerners.

Autogenic Training was developed in Berlin in the 1920s by a German psychiatrist and neurologist, Dr Johannes H Schultz. He had been a student of neuropathologist Oskar Vogt, who was involved in research into sleep and hypnosis. From Vogt he learnt that people who had been hypnotized quickly learnt how to hypnotize themselves and while in a hypnotic state were deeply relaxed and free from the psychosomatic disorders that plagued them in everyday life. Schultz pinpointed two effects of this type of self-hypnosis: a heavy sensation in the body brought about by deeply relaxed muscles, and a feeling of warmth associated with the increased dilation of the blood vessels.

He believed that we could all be taught to bring about these sensations by suggesting to ourselves that they were happening in our bodies. By doing so we could go into a state of 'passive concentration' and effectively switch off the body's alarm system long enough to let our bodies and minds really relax and get some rest, especially after a stressful, debilitating day.

The technique was first introduced into Britain in the 1970s by Dr Malcolm Carruthers. It has since become one of the most consistently researched stress-relief methods that is available. If it is practised daily, the mental and emotional effects felt are similar to those associated with meditation. Physically it produces the same chemical and physiological changes in the body that come after a bout of vigorous athletic training.

The beauty of the technique is that it can be practised anywhere – you can do the exercises travelling on a train or plane, in a doctor or dentist's waiting room or even do some of them while out walking or driving. They could even be done just because you are feeling bored. They can also be performed when you are in a business meeting to keep your stress levels under control. There is no limitation to when and where they can be practised, it is just down to the individual and their imagination.

What is autogenic training?

Autogenic training is a form of deep relaxation, using mental exercises to relieve the effects of stress and illness on the mind and body.

It has been compared to self hypnosis, but it is actually closer to meditation. The term 'autogenic' means 'produced by the self' or 'generated from within'. And this is the key to how Autogenic Training differs from the hypnosis technique. In hypnosis you or the therapist plants suggestions into your subconscious to make you change your beliefs and behaviour. In Autogenic Training you focus your attention on certain words or phrases which will then trigger your relaxation response.

Mastering the technique consists of learning a series of easy mental exercises that switch off the body's stress response. Research into the therapy has shown that over 80 physiological changes actually take place in the body during a single autogenic exercise.

How does it work?

Autogenic training works by achieving a shift in consciousness that enables you to control your autonomic nervous system, switching it from the sympathetic (which reacts to stress) to the parasympathetic (which instills rest and relaxation) at will. Research shows that it helps to rebalance the left and right hemispheres of the brain, to enable a person to move towards a balanced state in which the conditions are right for self-healing.

Once the technique has been learnt individuals will also be able to get in touch with, and express, any latent artistic or creative talents that have previously been hidden or undiscovered.

Learning the technique involves mastering two groups of exercises that are introduced progressively. The first group consists of six standard autogenic exercises which use key phrases such as, 'My arms are warm and heavy' to focus your attention on the physiological changes occurring when you start to relax. These changes are:

♦ *Heaviness and warmth in limbs*
♦ *A calm and regular heart beat*
♦ *Regular breathing*
♦ *Warmth in the abdomen*
♦ *A feeling of coolness on the forehead*

The second group are called 'intentional exercises'. These are taught with the autogenic exercises and should be practised at home. They focus on releasing emotional and physical tension in direct ways such as crying, shouting and punching pillows. Over the weeks you build up several techniques to equip you to deal effectively with your body's reaction to general stress.

In primeval days when we encountered trouble we would just run away or get into a fight and our bodies produced physical reactions to deal with these situations. Today, however, this physical tension is kept inside which can bring about high blood pressure or conditions such as irritable bowel syndrome.

What happens in a consultation?

Training is taught by a practitioner, individually or in small groups. When you first go along, you will need to complete a form about your health and medical history and attend a preliminary session for a general assessment. Then begins the first in a series of about eight weekly sessions during which you will be taught the simple exercises. There is no need to wear special clothes, to remove them or to get into any unusual or difficult positions. The exercises are purely mental ones. You just sit in a chair or lie comfortably on the floor and relax. All sessions last an hour. You must also practise the exercises for no more than 15 minutes, three times a day, every day.

Early on in the training it is not uncommon to experience 'autogenic discharges'. These are temporary symptoms which may mimic past illnesses or emotional problems, and their coming out is all part of the overall healing process. You also may experience some muscular strain or have the odd dizzy spell as your body lets go of all its pent-up stress.

Generally when the techniques have been mastered most people report experiencing wonderful physical and mental relaxation, plus feelings of calm and tranquillity that are generated from within. These feelings are not dependent on any external philosophies or values, religious beliefs, or on a therapist's help. The physical benefits of these exercises are that

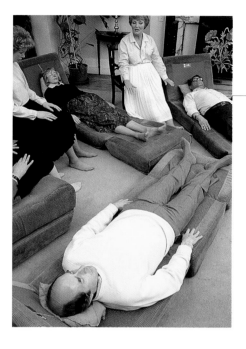

Left: In an autogenic session, you will be asked to sit or lie comfortably as you are talked through the relaxing mental exercises.

heart and breathing rates decrease and muscle tension is released, allowing blood to flow much more easily through the circulatory system.

About six weeks after your last session you will have a follow-up one to assess how you are progressing. Tapes can also be purchased which detail the autogenic technique. These can help to remind you of all the exercises that you have learnt.

How many sessions do I need?

A course of autogenic training is eight to ten weeks, except in exceptional circumstances such as in the case of chronic depression where more will be needed. You must practise the techniques regularly to reap the benefits fully.

Which problems can it help?

As a holistic therapy, autogenic training focuses on the physical, mental and emotional health of the whole person rather than on individual ailments. However, numerous conditions seem to respond well to the exercises. These include: irritable bowel syndrome, asthma, diabetes, eczema, tension headaches, migraines, the menopause, insomnia, high blood pressure, anxiety, PMS, bladder problems, epilepsy, arthritis, colitis and infertility. Sufferers of the circulatory illness, Raynaud's disease, seem to experience relief from their symptoms when they practise the technique.

Is it safe?

People of all ages can safely practise autogenic training provided they are taught by a qualified teacher. Pregnant women in particular can benefit from the calmness that is induced by the exercises. Sometimes, it is necessary to inform your doctor of any plans to have training, especially if you suffer from a medical condition such as diabetes, as the exercises can affect blood sugar levels and your medication may need to be adjusted. If you experience persistent 'autogenic reactions' during the course, see your doctor.

Certain people are not suitable for autogenic training. These include those who are suffering from personality disorders or acute psychoses.

♦

PILATES

♦

This modern system of maintaining the body was named after Joseph H Pilates, who invented it. He originally called it Contrology but it is commonly known as Pilates. The system has a holistic approach as although it involves physical exercise the aim is to balance the mind, body and spirit.

Joseph Pilates was born in 1880 in Germany. He was a sickly child and suffered from asthma, rickets and rheumatic fever. Striving to overcome these illnesses he built up strength by taking up sports such as skiing and boxing. He developed a strong interest in studying human physiology, while at the same time he learnt Eastern exercise forms such as yoga. Contrology was devised out of these combined interests.

In 1912 Joseph Pilates came to England where among other things he worked as a boxer and a self-defence instructor. The outbreak of war with Germany 1914 brought a period of internment in a prisoner of war camp. And it was during his confinement here that he devised a system of exercises to keep himself and the other internees fit. The beds and pieces of furniture he used have now been developed into the equipment that is seen in Pilates studios today.

When he was released he returned to Germany where he worked on his new technique. It was back in Germany that he met Rudolf von Laban, who had invented a method of dance notation called Labanotation. Von Laban was impressed with Joseph Pilates' exercises and incorporated some into his teachings. He even taught his techniques to the Hamburg police force, but declined to teach the German army and decided to

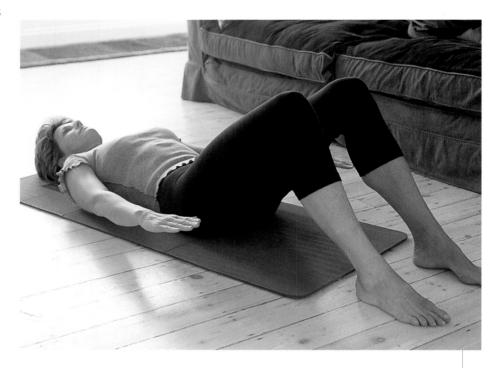

Above: Pilates movements are aimed at improving postural problems, and also the mind.

emigrate to America. During the voyage he met a nurse called Clara, and they spent the rest of the journey together discussing health and how to keep the body fit and well. By the time they reached America they had decided to open a physical fitness studio together, which they did in the same building as the New York City Ballet. The relationship between them flourished and they were later married.

What is Pilates?

It is a combined training of mind and body to achieve correct postural alignment. Pilates works on the whole body, rather than just targeting areas with problems. The aim when practising Pilates is to achieve a body that is naturally aligned, rather than one that is governed by the fashion of the day.

The main aims of Pilates are:

♦ *To lengthen short muscles and to strengthen any weak muscles*
♦ *To improve how you move*
♦ *To focus on core postural muscles to stabilize the body*
♦ *Working to breathe correctly*
♦ *To control even small movements*
♦ *To understand and improve good body mechanics*
♦ *To induce mental relaxation*

How does it work?

When Pilates worked out his muscle theory, his aim was to develop the body in a uniform fashion. He acknowledged that people often wanted to work on certain sets of muscles; they often wanted to achieve a flat stomach, for example, and so would only exercise these muscles. He wanted to emphasize that this would not promote good muscle health, or overall good health as good muscle tone of all the muscles is necessary to keep the body organs in place and working well.

The aim of Pilates is to gain control of your whole body. Repeating the exercises and performing them in a mindful way will in time allow you to acquire a natural muscle coordination, which is normally associated with subconscious activities.

This natural coordination and control is always seen with animals. A cat when it wakes up first stretches all its muscles before it moves. Pilates may have taken this element of his theory from Eastern practices such as yoga, chi kung or tai chi (see pages 436–9) where many of the postures are named after the animals that they emulate. The reason behind imitating animal movements is that the person doing them will acquire the balance, suppleness and strength that these animals have, as well as increased health and vitality that accompany them.

As children, we have a natural, relaxed posture, but as we get older our bodies reflect the strains and pressure of life. We acquire incorrect posture without even noticing it, and this then affects our physical functions and drains our energy.

Some posture problems arise because of repetitive work patterns – this can be sitting badly for hours on end, or for working in a job such as hairdressing where it is necessary to stand for long periods. Others have an emotional basis – your shoulders can literally seem to bend under the strain, and finally you can inherit postural problems.

The Pilates exercises can help to correct the postural problems and also improve your mind. Joseph Pilates was convinced that a lack of regular, conscious exercise also caused the functioning of the brain to deteriorate. So when Pilates developed his theory he surmised that the ideal condition is for our muscles to obey our will, and that our will should not be dominated by our reflex actions. With this theory Pilates was influenced by the views of German philosopher Schopenhauer.

Simplistically, Joseph Pilates believed that we do physical movements without conscious thought and that this is not good for either the mind or body. However, conscious movement uses brain cells, preventing them from dying, which in turn increases brain activity. This was what Pilates believed accounted for the 'feelgood' factor that people experienced after regularly practising his exercises.

Muscle memory

One part of the relationship between mind and muscles is muscle memory. This plays a part in learning any new exercise, but is particularly important in understanding Pilates as the main aim of the exercises is to re-educate the body and its muscle memory.

For example, if you sit working at a desk you will sit in a particular way. If you try to change it you feel some discomfort because your muscles will want to return to the position to which they have become accustomed. This is why Pilates places so much emphasis on mindfulness or conscious exercise, because it is when you lose focus on what your body and muscles are doing that your body does what it feels like, not what you want it to do.

What happens in a class?

Pilates is taught on a one-to-one basis, in small groups or larger classes. As with other therapies you need to find a teacher with whom you feel comfortable and who has a good understanding of you and your physical condition.

When he or she first sees you they will assess your individual problem and work out an exercise programme accordingly. This will be based on musculo-skeletal harmonization, where they do not just look at the injured area but will also assess the functioning of the supporting muscles and joints.

Always make sure that you find a teacher who has had the correct training and accreditation. It takes two years to do the full Pilates training.

Loose, comfortable clothing can be worn for the classes which, in a studio, normally last for about 90 minutes.

When your first learn Pilates you listen to the teacher and follow their instructions and practise what you have been taught. At the second stage when you believe that you have learned your lessons well, you can then start to improve on them and incorporate your own ideas into the movements. Your teacher may well advise you to carry on practising the exercises at home.

Core stabilization is the focal point of Pilates. It is a set of 17 exercises that is taught to students to provide the basis of the Pilates technique. The exercises work the key muscles necessary for good posture, which in turn affect the rest of the body and the mind. Pieces of equipment are also used to add resistance to the exercises.

For example, the reformer uses tension springs to add resistance. It works the whole body by strengthening and lengthening the muscles.

The cadillac has special attachments for working on spinal articulation and muscle strength.

The chair is a bit like a step machine. It supports and works the whole body.

Correct breathing technique will also be taught, where you will learn to breathe deeply from the diaphragm. This can help with stress control and also with how you perform the exercises.

How many sessions do I need?

You need to practise Pilates regularly to notice the benefits. Teachers advise that you attend a class twice a week on a regular basis, but are aware that only once is more likely.

Which problems can it help?

Pilates can help to prevent muscle injury, it corrects imbalances that have occurred through injury and it can heal backache and back problems.

Is it safe?

When taught by an experienced teacher Pilates is safe for all age groups and levels of fitness. It can be beneficial to pregnant women provided they receive qualified instruction.

However, it is not advisable to exercise after a heavy meal or after drinking alcohol. If you are undergoing medical treatment, always consult your doctor before taking up Pilates.

EASTERN THERAPIES

◆

ACUPUNCTURE

◆

Acupuncture literally means 'needle piercing', where very fine needles are inserted into the skin to stimulate specific points called acupoints. The acupoints are stimulated to balance the movement of energy in the body; the process can cause slight discomfort rather than the pain that its name suggests. Acupuncture is a major part of traditional Chinese medicine, a sophisticated and complex system of healthcare that also includes the use of moxibustion, herbalism, massage, dietary therapy and also exercise such as tai chi.

Acupuncture has become very popular in recent years among conventional doctors in the West, some of whom now use it to treat symptoms of disease as if it were just another part of Western medicine. But it has been shown to work best when it is kept within the context of the Chinese tradition.

How does it work?
There are a variety of scientific theories about how acupuncture works. These range from the belief that acupuncture works on the nervous system to the fact that it helps release endorphins – the body's natural pain relievers. But, although scientific theories can in part explain the immediate pain-relieving effects of acupuncture, they cannot explain acupuncture's ability to relieve chronic health problems, conditions which are not pain-related, and the effect of the therapy on the whole person.

The acupuncture system is based on the Chinese belief that our health is controlled by two types of energy that exist in the body called yin and yang. Yin is dark, passive, feminine and cold, yang is light, warm and male. To keep healthy, the right

balance of yin and yang is needed. So to correct any imbalances in energy flow, needles are inserted at certain points to release 'blockages' or to adapt the energy flow. There are 365 main points that are situated on 12 invisible energy channels – meridians – six of which are yin, six yang. These channels are thought to be connected to the body's organs.

The Chinese believe that disease affects us on every level – a physical illness upsets the mind and emotions and mental anxiety registers in a related organ. So a worrier could have a stomach ulcer, because excessive mental activity affects the functioning of the stomach, while an imbalance in the liver can express itself as inappropriate anger. For this reason illness is never treated as a set of isolated symptoms or diseased organs, but as an expression of disharmony within the mind, body and spirit.

What happens in a consultation?
On your first visit to an acupuncturist he or she will ask you about yourself as a person, your current lifestyle, diet, sleep patterns as well as taking a thorough medical and family history. The practitioner will also ask about the functioning of your digestive and circulatory system and ask about your emotional wellbeing.

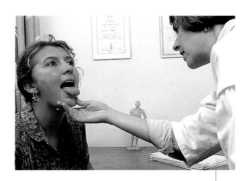

Above: Acupuncturists always examine a person's tongue. A healthy tongue is pale red with a thin white coating.

When he examines you, he will study your tongue's structure, its colour and coating – a healthy tongue should be light red with a thin whitish coating. Pulse readings will also be taken from your wrists. There are three on the inside of each wrist from which the practitioner can check for up to 28 pulse qualities relating to an organ or function. Isolated symptoms are not being looked for, but a pattern to work out your problem.

When a diagnosis has been made he will decide on a course of treatment to restore your energy and get your body back in balance. For the treatment you will have to lie on a couch and undress sufficiently to allow the practitioner to reach the relevant points of your body. The parts not being worked on can be covered by a sheet or blanket. Needling or moxibustion are the most common treatments given. Very fine, sterile stainless steel needles are inserted into the skin at the site of the relevant points. Moxibustion is sometimes used to warm and stimulate energy in a patient with cold, damp conditions or to reinforce a treatment. Moxa is the herb used, and often a small cone of it is burnt on the skin over the acupuncture point. When the patient feels the heat it is removed.

When needles are used, they may cause a pinprick sensation when they first go in followed by tingling or numbness, or a slight ache. It depends on the point being treated and the depth to which the needle is inserted, but it is not a big ordeal. The acupuncturist can use just one or two needles, but usually between four and eight and will manipulate them to stimulate or calm the point. The needles can either be in and out of the body in a second or left in for up to half an hour.

You may feel no different after treatment, but some people feel sleepy, revitalized or sometimes a little 'spaced out'. You can feel an immediate improvement

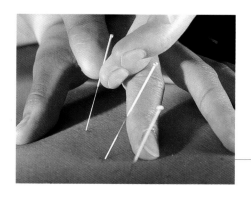

Left: The needles used are sterile, very fine and about 12–24mm (¹/₂ –1 inch) long.

after acupuncture, especially if you have gone specifically for pain relief, but it usually takes a couple of days to feel any other benefits. It is common to feel a little worse before you feel better as acupuncture brings physical, mental and emotional problems to the surface. This is a positive sign. As with any treatment, complete recovery takes time and patience.

How many sessions do I need?

The length of treatment depends on the type of illness that is involved, its duration, your age, and your healing abilities. Normally you should see some improvement after three or four treatments.

Which problems can it help?

The acupuncturist would not make a distinction between you and your illness and would aim to improve your overall health. However, in Western medicine, acupuncture has benefited all types of aches and pains from arthritis to back pain and sports injuries, stress, depression, fatigue, circulation and digestive problems. It can also help menstrual, gynaecological and sexual problems, hay fever, asthma and unspecified ailments such as ME and fatigue.

In general, it works best as a preventative treatment, helps acute (short-term) conditions or relieves the early stages of an illness. As with any other form of medicine, acupuncture cannot reverse tissue damage, so although it can reduce pain, stiffness and swelling and improve mobility in rheumatoid arthritis, for example, it cannot reverse muscle wasting or bone deformities that have already occurred in the body.

Acupuncture treatment is also particularly good to use for the following:

Pain relief Pain in muscles and joints is the most common problem that acupuncturists are asked to treat. This may be for two reasons. Acupuncture has a strong analgesic effect, which has been scientifically explained by theories such as the endorphin theory and 'the gate' theory. The endorphin theory states that stimulating points releases pain-relieving endorphins. The 'gate theory' states that the spine is made up of 'gates' which can open to let pain in or close to shut it out. The gates open or shut in response to messages from the nervous system.

Supporters of this theory believe that acupuncture works on the nervous system to instruct the gates of the spine to shut out pain. But acupuncture's high success rate with pain relief in particular may simply be because many types of pain, especially back pain, are so responsive to treatment that more cases get referred.

Addictions Ear acupuncture – auricular therapy – in particular has proved very successful with treating drug addictions, because it lessens the withdrawal symptoms. Ear acupuncture points are stimulated by fine needles, light therapy, electro therapy or magnetically-charged ball bearings. This treatment is beneficial in weaning people off hard drugs such as cocaine and heroin as well as more common substances such as cigarettes and alcohol. Successful withdrawal usually involves intensive specialized treatment.

Childbirth Acupuncture is proving effective for pain relief in labour and the back pain before and after birth. It is particularly beneficial because it does not harm the baby and eliminates the need for drugs which could affect the child. Acupuncture can calm an anxious mother-to-be and is believed to reduce labour pain by up to one-third. A well-known point on the little toe can help turn the foetus if it is in breech position.

Surgery Acupuncture has been used as a form of anaesthetic in China and is suitable for some patients, especially those at risk of anaemia, but it is not widely used in the West. One of the main problems is that not everyone responds to the treatment and it is more time consuming than giving a conventional anaesthetic.

Lack of energy Acupuncture can have a dramatic impact on people who feel generally unwell or constantly tired. This may be due to its ability to restore harmony to the body and normalize body systems. It also has a psychological effect. Studies show changes in brain activity, which can result in a relaxing or 'energizing effect'.

Acupuncture for animals The remarkable success of acupuncture in treating animals appears to disprove that acupuncture works simply because you believe in it.

Is it safe?

When it is practised by a qualified practitioner acupuncture is perfectly safe for everyone. In fact young children often respond very well because their imbalances can be treated before they become a health problem. If you think acupuncture could help your baby or child, it is advisable to see an experienced practitioner and preferably one who specializes in child acupuncture. Acupuncture can be used during pregnancy, and it can also give pain relief and stimulate contractions during labour. However, as with all responsible forms of healthcare, acupuncturists avoid unnecessary intervention during pregnancy.

SHIATSU AND ACUPRESSURE

Shiatsu originated in Japan as a holistic therapy for treating the mind, body and spirit. It is very much a 20th-century therapy, but one which is closely related to its oriental ancestor called 'amma'. This ancient massage therapy involved rubbing and pressing on different parts of the body to treat common ailments.

It evolved alongside acupuncture and Chinese herbalism, but became much more established in Japan around the 16th century. Early this century, practitioners of amma started borrowing knowledge and techniques from osteopathy and chiropractic and combined these with the traditional oriental body work to develop what we now know as shiatsu.

Today in the West shiatsu is becoming popular as people recognize that it helps them to release stress and maintain a healthy, balanced lifestyle.

What is shiatsu?

Shiatsu is a Japanese word which means 'finger pressure'. The term is slightly misleading as practitioners use their fingers, palms, elbows, arms, knees and feet to apply pressure to points called 'tsubo', which are dotted along the body's 12 main energy channels called meridians. The treatment has been described as similar to acupuncture but without the needles. This is a reasonably accurate assessment as both therapies share similar philosophy, principles, diagnostic methods and treatment points. Again in the same way as acupuncture, shiatsu aims to bring about a balanced energy flow through the meridians and to increase the vitality of the person being treated.

However, shiatsu practitioners may argue that a shiatsu treatment is more nurturing than acupuncture as it also incorporates therapeutic touch.

How does it work?

Shiatsu works on the body's energy system. Practitioners apply pressure to points or tsubo on the meridians to stimulate 'ki', the Japanese word for chi or energy. Diagnosis is similar to the Chinese method. There are several strands in the diagnostic process: looking (Bo-shin), touching (Setsu-shin), asking (Mon-shin) and sense diagnosis (Bun-shin), which also involves intuition.

Treatment involves techniques to relieve pain and release energy blockages that may be causing your problem. The therapist treats your whole body using various methods for different areas. For example, he may rotate and manipulate your leg to relieve associated back pain, or use his elbow to stimulate points on the spine that relate to the chest, digestion or circulation problems. He will often rub and apply finger pressure to specific points to open up a blocked meridian and may even walk on the soles of your feet to stimulate the kidney meridian. The pressure used depends on what the practitioner feels, but areas such as the face will be given less pressure, for example.

Sometimes parts of the body may feel sensitive or possibly painful as they are touched and manipulated by the practitioner, but this does not normally last long and passes as the treatment continues.

Body stretches will help to release any tension held in the muscles and promote a feeling of calm and relaxation. Gentle manipulative techniques are often also used to give better mobility in the joints.

What happens in a consultation?

You do not have to undress for treatment, although some parts of your body may be briefly exposed during examination, so wear loose, comfortable clothes. For your treatment practitioners recommend that you refrain from drinking any alcohol and eating food for two hours beforehand. If you have a particular medical condition, bring any medication details with you. The session usually lasts an hour, with at least 40 minutes devoted to the actual treatment. The first appointment starts with the practitioner taking a case history. Practitioners ask questions about:

♦ *Your current health and medical history*
♦ *What type of work you do*
♦ *What sort of diet you eat*
♦ *Your relationships with friends and family and your lifestyle*

These facts are needed to discover what is causing your problem. The look and feel of certain parts of the body can also give an indication of underlying problems. A red face, for example, points to problems with circulation and the shoulders give information about the digestive system, the chest and upper back reflect heart and lung energy and your emotional health. In fact, the back and the abdomen are the most important areas of all. The abdomen or 'hara' is called 'the ocean of ki', and is used to diagnose and treat problems in all 12 meridians. Touching the hara and other parts of the body helps to give the practitioner the most detailed information about your body.

Some therapists take readings from the same pulse points on the wrist used by acupuncturists and all feel the muscle and skin tone for signs of excess or deficient ki. They also listen to your breathing and the sound of your voice .

To arrive at a final diagnosis the practitioner will piece together these different diagnostic strands and then back them up with his basic gut feeling about what he believes to be your health problem.

Most treatment takes place with you lying down on your back on a mat on the floor. It is important that the therapist feels as comfortable as you do. Sometimes you will need to lie on your front or possibly on your side if you are pregnant or have neck problems. The therapist will work at superficial and deep levels, producing a relaxing sensation described as 'pleasurable pain'.

Some people feel good after a treatment, often saying they are revitalized and refreshed, but others can feel unwell for about 24 hours. This is because shiatsu can trigger a sort of 'healing crisis' as toxins are released and ki is unblocked. Common symptoms include fatigue, headaches, flu-like symptoms or changes in bowel movement. Try to relax until the symptoms pass, but call your therapist if they end up persisting for several days.

How many sessions do I need?

On average it takes four to eight treatments to get rid of common problems, but this varies depending on the problem. Chronic (long-term) conditions can require extensive treatment to bring noticeable relief.

Which problems can it help?

Shiatsu improves health generally by relieving stress, calming the nervous system and stimulating the circulation and immune systems.

It is particularly effective for stress-related tension and illnesses, insomnia, headaches, menstrual problems and digestive upsets. It can encourage a better posture and will relieve pain being experienced in the back and neck. Better con-

centration and an improved mental state is often felt after a treatment, and many clients go away with an increased feeling of wellbeing.

Is it safe?

Shiatsu given by a qualified therapist is safe for everyone and is particularly beneficial for women during pregnancy. Some therapists also treat small children and the elderly. It is not suitable, however, for people with cancer of the blood or lymphatic systems, an infectious disease or a high fever. People with heart disease or who are weak should always be treated cautiously using the more gentle techniques. Techniques should also not be applied to areas where there are open wounds, inflamed areas or scar tissue.

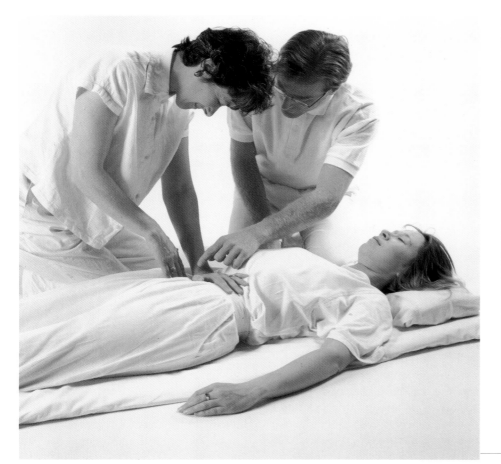

WHAT IS ACUPRESSURE ?

◆

Acupressure is similar to shiatsu in that it involves using finger pressure on acupuncture points throughout the body to stimulate the flow of chi through the body's energy channels (see Acupuncture pages 444–5). Unlike shiatsu, acupressure involves mostly thumb and fingertip pressure, although it can also incorporate massage along the meridian lines. In the West the use of acupressure has been largely overshadowed by shiatsu. It is usually incorporated into other therapies such as shiatsu or Chinese massage, or used simply for self-help. There is no central body of acupressure practitioners in Britain.

Left: For shiatsu treatment, you lie on the floor and finger pressure is applied to points on your body.

CHINESE
HERBALISM

Chinese herbal medicine is part of the ancient system of traditional Chinese medicine, which after 5,000 years of practice in its homeland, has taken the West by storm. Many people, disillusioned with quick-fix Western medicine, are taking advantage of this more sympathetic system.

Chinese herbalism uses herbs to treat and prevent mental, physical and emotional ill health. Together with acupuncture, it forms the bulk of Chinese medical treatment. Although in the West acupuncture is often seen as being more important than herbalism, the number of Chinese doctors who use herbs exclusively is greater than those who use only acupuncture. However, most practitioners combine both to complement each other.

In the Chinese philosophy of the complementary opposites yin and yang, acupuncture is considered yang, because it moves from the outside in, while herbalism is yin because it works from the inside out. Herbalism can support acupuncture treatment, or be used on its own for conditions such as viral infections and blood disorders like anaemia or menstrual problems, which can sometimes be better suited to herbal treatment.

Herbs also strengthen people who are too weak for acupuncture or who dislike needles. Acupuncture works with the body's own energy, but weak patients have little energy. Herbal treatment, however, adds nourishment to the body. Traditional Chinese diagnostic techniques determine the cause of ill health and 'patterns of disharmony' in the body, and herbs are prescribed to restore harmony to the mind, body and emotions.

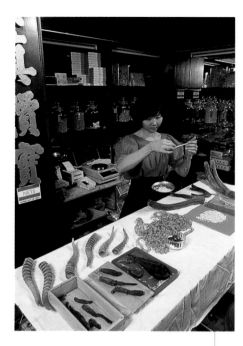

Above: In a Chinese dispensary, a girl is precisely weighing out a special herbal preparation.

How does it work?

To understand Chinese medicine you need a basic understanding of the concepts of yin and yang, the eight principles, chi or energy, and the five elements and their role in maintaining health.

The Chinese believe that each one of us is governed by the opposing, but complementary forces of yin and yang. Yin and yang are the opposites that make the whole, they cannot exist without each other and nothing is solely one or the other, there are elements of each within everybody.

The tai chi symbol illustrates how yin and yang move into each other with a little yin always within yang and vice versa. When the two forces are in balance you feel good, but if one force dominates the other, the imbalance can lead to ill health.

This concept of balance affects us through the eight principles, which include yin and yang and more detailed subdivisions of these two, namely cold and heat, internal and external, deficiency and excess. As aspects of yin and yang, the principles apply to every part of us. While they work in harmony you stay healthy, but any imbalance can cause illness.

Chi is also important to health because it is the energy that binds yin and yang. Together with blood and moisture it flows around the body keeping us healthy. When chi flows freely, yin, yang and the whole person are in balance. But when it is blocked, stagnant or unbalanced it can lead to illness. Chi flows through meridians. There are 12 major meridians, and numerous other meridians including tiny ones called collaterals which intersect these. Six of the 12 major channels are yin and six are yang. They all relate to and are named after major organs. These are the Lungs, Large intestine, Stomach, Spleen, Heart, Small intestine, Bladder, Kidney, Pericardium (heart protector), San jiao (triple warmer), Gall bladder and Liver. If there is disharmony in a meridian it can affect the corresponding organs. Likewise disharmony in the organ can also disrupt the meridian. Herbalism works directly on the meridians and their associated organs to rebalance yin and yang by helping chi flow smoothly along the meridian pathways, thereby restoring harmony to the whole person.

Through detailed diagnosis the Chinese herbalist can identify energy imbalances. For example, a diagnosis such as 'kidney yang deficiency with exterior heat in the stomach meridian' involves details about yang, deficiency, heat and exterior, which are four of the eight principles; kidney and stomach, which refer to organs and meridians and also to the five elements, where kidney is water and the stomach is earth. A combination of herbs would be prescribed to rectify these disharmonies.

What happens in a consultation?

The consultation and diagnosis is similar to that given by an acupuncturist:

Looking This examination is the first of the four procedures. The practitioner will note your general appearance, your size and shape and general demeanour. He will check the colour of your face and examine your tongue – its colour, coating and condition. Close examination of your face and posture are important in revealing the state of the Shen or spirit. Shen is the power behind your personality, it guides the emotions and rules over all the organs. The eyes reveal the state of Shen so the practitioner will take a look at your eyes. If they are bright and shiny it is a sign that the Shen is in harmony, but blank lustreless eyes show disharmony of spirit. The colour of your face is also significant: a white face indicates a cold disharmony and is linked to an imbalance in the metal element, a yellowish complexion is related to dampness and the earth element, while a red face is a sign of too much heat and points to an imbalance in the fire element.

The practitioner will then look at your tongue. Tongue diagnosis and pulse taking form the most important part of the examination. Chinese herbalists treat the tongue and its coating as two separate elements in the diagnosis.

A normal tongue should be pale red and moist, which is a sign that chi and blood are flowing smoothly. If you are sick, a healthy-looking tongue is a sign that your illness has caused no long-term damage and that you should recover well. The tongue coating should always be white, moist and thin enough to be transparent.

Listening and smelling The herbalist will listen to your breathing patterns, your speech and your cough if you have one. Shortness of breath usually suggests deficiency and loss of voice would point to pernicious influences. Your voice can help the practitioner diagnose an element imbalance. For example, a shouting voice is a sign of a wood imbalance which can point to liver or gall bladder problems and can also show itself emotionally as inappropriate anger.

Asking Like all therapists the Chinese herbalist will ask you questions about yourself, your lifestyle and your health. He will want to know about your home, work and relationships. He will also want to know your medical history, your symptoms, any pain you have had, sleep patterns, sensations of hot and cold, dizziness, eating habits and toilet habits.

Touching This is the last examination. The herbalist may palpate your body where there is pain such as your back or abdomen, and will touch your skin if you have a rash, but more importantly, he will take your pulses. He will test three pulse positions in each wrist with the index, middle and third finger of one hand. Using a combination of light, moderate and heavy pressure he will look for 28 different pulse qualities.

This incredibly detailed diagnostic procedure will take about an hour and maybe longer. Some Chinese herbalists will prescribe herbs at the end of your first consultation, give you patent (ready-made) remedies as pills or they may prescribe a mixture of concentrated herbal powders. You may, however, leave your first consultation empty-handed and return a week later for a mini check-up and to receive your herbs. Your herbal prescription will be aimed at balancing your mind and body, although you may also be given something else to alleviate any particularly distressing symptoms that you are experiencing. You will probably be asked to return a week later. Each time you return the herbalist will carry out a mini check-up.

How many sessions do I need?
It is difficult to say. Serious or chronic (long-term) illnesses, especially those that have been suppressed by years of drug treatment will need several weeks of treatment to show any improvement, and

maybe months for significant changes. However, it is possible to notice improvements after a week's treatment, especially with related symptoms such as insomnia.

Which problems can it help?
The World Health Organization (WHO) has published a list of ailments which can benefit from Chinese herbalism. Many health problems from arthritis to depression, eczema, hay fever, infertility, sciatica, herpes, insomnia, PMS and vaginitis appear on that extensive list, with some surprising entries such as cerebral palsy, impotence, diabetes and strokes.

Is it safe?
Chinese herbs are available over the counter, but apart from patent remedies for minor ailments, you should not buy them without a prescription from a qualified practitioner who has made a full diagnosis. Some herbs are not safe for public use, or are safe only in specific doses. When prescribed by a qualified Chinese herbalist, the remedies are usually suitable for everyone.

However, there have been a few rare problems with Chinese herbs. Often these have been because the herbs have been prescribed by non-qualified practitioners, in non-traditional ways, or can be linked to poor quality control. These problems can be avoided by consulting a fully trained and qualified practitioner. Very rarely someone, perhaps one person in 10,000, experiences an allergic reaction to the herbs (particularly those used for skin diseases). If you feel unwell or have flu-like symptoms, nausea or diarrhoea while taking the herbs, stop taking them immediately and contact your practitioner. Because this rare allergic-type reaction affects the liver, you should tell your practitioner if you have ever suffered from a liver disease such as jaundice or hepatitis. A good practitioner will always be available if you need to contact him.

AYURVEDIC MEDICINE

Ayurvedic medicine is the traditional system of medicine practised in India and Sri Lanka. Like traditional Chinese medicine, or Western medical practices, Ayurveda ('the science of life') is a complete and complex system of healthcare. As such, its many components – detoxification, diet, exercise, herbs, and techniques to improve mental and emotional health – work together to contribute to a way of life rather than an occasional treatment.

The fundamental belief in Ayurveda is that everything within the universe, including ourselves, is composed of energy or 'prana'. We may look like solid structures of bone, muscles and tissues, but this appearance belies the fact that we are simply bundles of vibrating energy. Consequently, we are forever changing in ways that are either positive or negative. To ensure that most of the changes are positive, we must live in a way that encourages energy balance. Ayurvedic practitioners recognize that there is no one prescription for health that caters for everyone. The balance of energies that contribute to good health in your body may lead to sickness in someone else. In Ayurvedic medicine every person must be treated individually. The practitioner's skill lies in identifying each person's constitution, diagnosing imbalances and treating them accordingly.

How does it work?

Your individual constitution and how it relates to your energies is the key to understanding Ayurvedic medicine. A good constitution is your best defence against illness. If you are functioning well, disease cannot take hold, but when your constitution is weakened you can get ill. Ayurveda aims to prevent disease by working with your body. Each of us has a unique constitution, determined by the balance of three vital energies in the body, known as the three doshas or 'tridosha'. The three doshas are known by their Sanskrit names of *vátha*, *pitha* and *kapha*. Everyone's constitution is governed by these doshas in varying degrees, but each of us is also controlled by one or possibly two dominant doshas, so that you are classed as either a *vátha*, *pitha* type or *kapha* type, or a *vátha/pitha*, *pitha/kapha* and so on.

Your dosha not only determines your constitution, and the illnesses to which you might succumb, but it also determines your temperament, the colour of your hair, your tendency to put on weight, and which type of foods you should eat.

You keep healthy when all three doshas work in balance. Each one has its role to play in the body. For example, *vátha* is the driving force; it relates mainly to the nervous system and the body's energy. *Pitha* is fire; it relates to the metabolism, digestion, enzymes, acid and bile. *Kapha* is linked to water in the mucous membranes, phlegm, moisture, fat, and lymphatics. The balance of the three depends on many factors, principally good diet and exercise, maintaining good digestion, and balanced emotional and spiritual health.

Your constitution is determined by your parents' doshas at the time of your conception and each individual is born with levels of the three doshas that are right for them. But, as we go through life, diet, environment, stress, trauma and injury cause the doshas to become imbalanced. When this imbalance becomes excessively high or low it can lead to ill health. Ayurvedic practitioners prescribe treatment to restore the balance.

In Ayurveda all ill health is related to disturbances in the three doshas. The doshic imbalances affect other body factors, culminating in imbalances that cause disease. These other factors include the five elements (*panchabhuta*), the ten pairs of qualities (*gunas*), agni, the three malas, and the sekaphaen tissues (*sapha dhathu*).

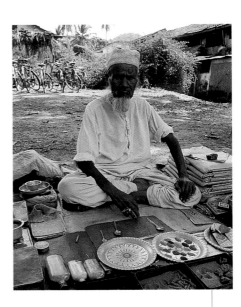

Above: Much of Ayurvedic medicine relies on herbal remedies, or samana, to correct imbalances in the three doshas.

The five elements

The elements are ether (space), air, fire, water and earth. All five elements exist in all things, including ourselves. Ether corresponds to the spaces in the body: the mouth, nostrils, thorax, abdomen, respiratory tract and cells. Air represents muscular movement, pulsation, the expansion and contraction of the lungs, and intestines, even cell movement. Fire controls enzyme functioning. It shows itself as intelligence, fuels the digestive system and regulates metabolism. Water is in plasma, blood, saliva, digestive juices, the mucous membranes and cytoplasm, the liquid inside cells. Earth manifests in the body structures: the bones, nails, teeth, muscles, cartilage, tendons, skin and hair.

All five elements are also related to the five senses and the sense organs. In a healthy body all five work in harmony, but an imbalance in any one stimulates changes in the others. Imbalance can occur through changes in the 20 fundamental qualities or *gunas*.

Digestion

In Ayurveda good digestion is considered the key to good health; poor digestion produces *ama*, a toxic substance believed to cause illness, seen as a white coating on the tongue. *Ama* occurs when the metabolism is impaired due to an imbalance of *agni*. *Agni* is the fire which, when working, maintains all functions. Imbalanced *agni* is caused by irregularities in the doshas, eating and drinking too much of the wrong foods and repressing emotions.

Agni also ensures that the three *malas* are working effectively. These are sweat, urine and faeces. For example, acid urine is a sign of too much *pitha*.

What happens in a consultation?

Your first consultation is mainly diagnostic and can last an hour. The practitioner will ask you detailed questions:

♦ *He will want to know about yourself, your health and your parents' health*
♦ *He will want to know how you were as a child and a teenager in order to determine your dominant dosha. Asking you relevant questions about yourself, lifestyle, job, diet, likes and dislikes can also help*
♦ *He will also inquire about your appetite, bowel movements and digestive system*

The physical examination begins with the practitioner noting the way you look: your colouring, size, shape, speech, the way you move and your behaviour. He will study your face, its lines and colourings, eyes, tongue, lips and nails to find out about your doshic imbalance and any particular problems that you might have.

Each finger and thumb indicates the state of the five elements in the body and the organs to which they relate. The practitioner will take your pulse to check the state of each organ, the quality of the blood, and the doshas relating to the five elements. An experienced practitioner can detect up to 32 pulse qualities.

Treatment

Traditionally there are two main types of treatment that are generally used in Ayurvedic medicine:

Shodana In Ayurvedic medicine it is essential to detoxify the body before prescribing restorative treatment. *Shodana* is used to eliminate disease, blockages in the digestive system, or any imbalance in the doshas. Where *shodana* is required the practitioner can use *panchakarma* therapy and sometimes a preparatory therapy called *purwakarma*. Not all practitioners carry out this detoxification as it is a two-day treatment, which is best carried out in a residential clinic. But it is becoming more common.

Samana (herbal remedies) After detoxification the practitioner may prescribe herbal or mineral remedies to correct imbalances in the doshas. These have the necessary medicinal qualities to stimulate *agni* and restore balance in the doshas. They are not prescribed to eradicate disease because the disease is just a symptom of doshic imbalance.

Herbal remedies are usually prescribed in liquid form or as dried herbs, although they can also come as powder or tablets.

During your consultation, the practitioner will also advise on lifestyle, a suitable diet (the practitioner may prepare a special diet sheet for you) and exercise.

Exercise, such as yoga, is important for physical and emotional health and the practitioner will advise on the exercise best suited to you. Follow-up appointments can be weekly, fortnightly, or monthly depending on your problem. A condition such as serious asthma may need two or three treatments a week.

How many sessions do I need?

The number of sessions needed depends on several factors such as your age, your doshic imbalance and the severity and length of time you have had it. But a condition such as irritable bowel syndrome could improve in two to six visits.

Which problems can it help?

Because it is a complete system of medicine, practitioners say that Ayurvedic medicine can help with any ailment – mental, physical or emotional. It has been found to be particularly beneficial for digestive complaints such as irritable bowel syndrome, constipation, indigestion and associated conditions that can arise from eating inappropriate foods, for example, eczema, water retention and circulation problems. Certain conditions such as cancer and some hernias are not suitable for Ayurvedic treatment.

Is it safe?

With a qualified practitioner, Ayurvedic medicine is safe for everyone. A competent practitioner would never ask you to give up your conventional medicine and would adapt treatments to suit you. *Panchakarma* treatments are mostly for adults and not suitable for pregnant women or very frail patients.

CHAKRA BALANCING

This is another Indian therapy that promotes healing by allowing energy blocks to be relieved in the chakras – the spiritual energy centres of the body. There are seven main chakras to which treatment is given, starting at the top of the head with the crown chakra, third eye chakra, throat chakra, heart chakra, solar plexus chakra, sacral chakra and the root chakra. Deep relaxation is felt after treatment which aids both mental and physical recovery.

THERAPIES INVOLVING EXTERNAL POWERS

SPIRITUAL HEALING

Spiritual healing is when energy is transmitted through a healer's hands to the person who needs it. The treatment works on the body, mind and spirit, which are seen as one unit that must balance and be in harmony for a person's wellbeing and to be in good health. This healing can help mental and emotional problems as well as physical conditions such as a frozen shoulder.

Many people are benefiting today from spiritual healing, which is now an established therapy in its own right. In 1995 there were 7,000 spiritual healers registered in Britain and the therapy has also won the respect of the medical establishment; doctors can now refer patients for spiritual healing, if they wish. Many doctors are so impressed with healing that they are now undertaking training to develop their own healing powers.

What is spiritual healing?
The channelling of healing energy from its spiritual source to someone who needs it is called spiritual healing. Christians say it is the work of God; while some spiritualists claim that the spirits of physicians are healing through them, other healers say that they receive help from angels. Some healers believe they are channelling 'cosmic' or 'universal energy'. The channel is usually a person, whom we call a healer, and the healing energy is usually transferred to the patient through the healer's hands. The healing, however, does not actually come from the healer, but transfers through him, through his hands to where its needed, otherwise the healer would be constantly drained. The word

'spiritual' refers to the divine nature of the energy, which healers agree comes from one external, invisible intelligent source. The healing energy from this source is available to all.

Healers see the body, mind and spirit as one interdependent unit and believe all three must work in harmony for a person to maintain positive health at all times. Any problem – be it physical, such as a broken leg, or mental, such as depression – needs the power of healing to restore the balance of the whole person. It is felt that sickness often starts in the mind, or at the deeper level of the spirit, and it is often here that healing begins first.

How does it work?
The theory is that everyone has a healing mechanism that flows as an energy force around the body and through the mind and spirit to keep them in perfect order.

Unfortunately, stress, an inadequate diet, a negative attitude and other adverse factors can block our healing mechanism so that it cannot function correctly and this is when we tend to get run down or ill. Spiritual healing provides the energy needed to crank our own healing mechanism back into action. When a healer lays his hands on you, he acts as a conductor or channel for the healing energy which he believes has the 'intelligence' to go where it is needed in the body.

Healers say that all of us have the power to heal, if we choose to develop it. However, some people do seem to be born with a special healing gift.

Many physicians and scientists, however, still remain sceptical about the effectiveness of treatment, despite the fact that controlled studies have shown the power of healing. Babies and animals seem to respond well to treatment, and in experiments with plants and seeds a definite growth response has been noted. Experiments with distant healing, which

can either be sent as a prayer or thought to people in another place, has also been found to have good effects.

Healing does not always work at a physical level; the illness may remain but the ability to cope with it improves. Sometimes it does not work at all. This may be because the sick person chooses to 'block' the healing forces – this is because it is believed that some people subconsciously prefer to be ill because of all the fuss and attention they are getting. It may also be because we 'need' to remain ill. Healing is not just about living well, but also about dying well. People who are healed when they are dying can feel more at ease with the world and the life they have led and die more peacefully.

What happens in a consultation?
Healing sessions can take place in groups or on an individual basis. They are generally held in informal, warm and comfortable rooms. Try to find a healer that you like and feel relaxed with if you are going to have several treatments as you can resist or block the healing energy if you feel unhappy or stressed.

Avoid using any healers who demand a large fee upfront or who insist that you stop taking prescribed medication or abandon specific religious beliefs that you have.

When you have a treatment there will often be soft music playing in the background in order to create a relaxed atmosphere. You do not have to undress, you just need to take off your shoes and coat. You will then be invited to sit on a chair while the healer sits opposite and asks questions such as:

♦ *The problems you are experiencing, and previous treatments*
♦ *He will want to know about any emotional or spiritual problems*
♦ *He will also want to be told about any physical complaints*

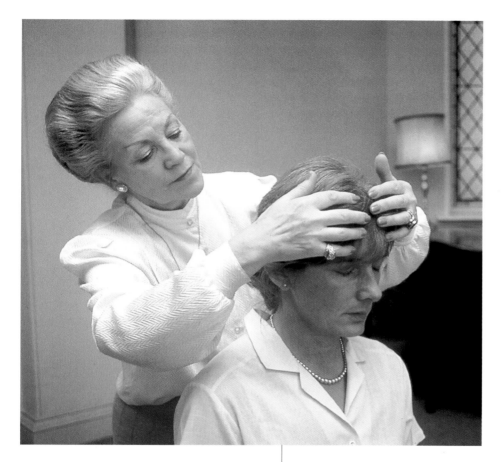

Above: A healer will place his or her hands on or over the part of your body that needs healing. How long the healer spends on each location depends on your needs.

This discussion usually takes about 20 minutes and the healer may take confidential notes. He will then stand up to begin the healing. He may ask you to remain seated or to lie down on a treatment couch. He will put his hands on or over the part of your body that needs healing and hold them there for a few minutes. If the healing is to be concentrated on the breasts or genitals, his hands will not touch you. And if you prefer not to be touched at all he will work in your energy field 'aura' with his hands hovering above you.

To begin the treatment the healer will first attune with the healing energy. Then he may scan your body with his hands hovering just above you. This scanning is to take a reading of your body's energy levels and to locate the areas of low or blocked energy where healing is particularly needed. How long the healer spends on each area is determined by your body's needs. Generally, the session lasts for about an hour. All healers work in this way, but some employ additional healing tools such as visualization, past lives therapy, aura healing or they may concentrate on using the 'chakras' – the seven main spiritual energy centres of the body.

If they decide to use these methods, they will discuss them further with you. During the treatment you may feel heat coming from the healer's hands, although some people feel a cold draught, a tingling sensation or pins and needles. You may also experience a general feeling of lightheadedness. Some healers will combine healing with other treatments such as massage or crystal or colour therapy.

After treatment, most people say they feel relaxed and peaceful, although you may also feel thirsty or sleepy. You will be advised by the spiritual healer to leave a few days or a week between sessions to give the healing time to work right through your system.

How many sessions do I need?

According to most spiritual healers you should feel an improvement in your condition after experiencing six healing sessions.

Which problems can it help?

Healing can help with any problem, mental, physical or emotional, although it does seem to be especially effective for musculo-skeletal problems, such as frozen shoulders, stiff necks and bad knees. 'Miracle' cures for illness are unusual, but most of the people who seek treatment get some benefit from it, getting relief from stressful conditions, depression, pain and other ailments. It has also been found that many chronic and potentially terminal illnesses have been alleviated with healing treatment.

Is it safe?

Healing cannot harm anyone – if a person does not want to be healed they just subconsciously reject the energy. A respectable healer will not promise to cure you or ask you to give up any conventional treatment that you are receiving. Healers are not allowed to attend women in childbirth or for ten days afterwards and are not to give healing to children under 18 years old, unless the child's parents or guardian has sought medical help and have given their permission for healing.

CYMATICS

Cymatics is a therapy using sound waves that operate on the same level as healthy cells to heal a body that has become unbalanced or which is suffering from disease. The treatment that is given is completely painless and can help to relieve conditions such as rheumatism, arthritis and back pain.

Cymatics was developed in the 1960s by British medical doctor and osteopath, Dr Peter Manners. The therapy grew out of early research into electromagnetic energy and the concept that every living thing – person, animal, plant or organism – is surrounded by an energy field that resonates at its own particular frequency.

Professor Gauvou of the Sorbonne in Paris, Dr Brauna from Germany, Dr Harold Burr from Yale University and Swiss scientist Dr Hans Jenny were all individually involved in research into the sound wave phenomenon back in the 1950s.

The results of their work was collated by Dr Manners and he further developed into it the therapy of cymatics.

Unlike many other types of complementary therapy, cymatics exploits the scientific possibilities of 20th century medicine and according to Dr Peter Manners, is 'founded on a true knowledge of man'. Consequently, the conventional medical profession is mostly appreciative of what it has to offer. In fact, the treatment has proved to be so successful, painless and easy to perform that it is rapidly growing in popularity. There are now cymatic clinics available in Britain, other parts of Europe, America, Canada, Japan, Australia, and others are soon to open up in countries further afield such as Brazil and Mexico.

What is cymatics?

Cymatics comes from the Greek word *kyma* meaning 'a great wave'. Cymatic therapy is a form of sound therapy, based on the principle that every cell in the body, of which there are believed to be millions, is controlled by an electromagnetic field that resonates at its own particular sound frequency. When we are well this frequency is steady and constant, but any dysfunction or disease upsets the harmony of the body and the area that is affected then generates a different, increased resonance.

The practitioner uses the cymatic machinery to generate a frequency identical to that of healthy cells which he then pulses to the ailing area. His aim is to support what the cells are trying to do naturally, therefore aiding the healing process and restoring the body back to its normal good health and overall harmony.

How does it work?

Cymatics practitioners use special equipment to generate the required frequencies of harmonics to stimulate the affected cells in all areas of the body. Originally, the equipment was very large, cumbersome and expensive, but today it is much smaller in size, in fact the machine is now normally about the size of a small briefcase.

Treatment is applied either by means of a large hand-held applicator, is directed through electrodes which attach onto the body, or is applied via cymatic probes which are small pencil-like applicators that are used to treat small dysfunctional areas. The practitioner chooses the treatment from around 850 frequencies, all of which have been calculated over a period of years.

The treatment is then directed at the area of the body that is causing the problem. This may be at the point of the pain, but often it is not and is situated elsewhere in the body.

Treatment works in the same way for all problems. If you have muscular pain, for example, the energy of that muscle and the frequency of its field will have been changed by the injury or condition affecting it. Transmitting a corrective frequency into the muscle can rebalance its energy and almost immediately relieve the pain that is being experienced by the patient.

When someone is suffering from an asthmatic condition, for example, the asthmatic tension is released by the cymatic treatment so that the patient feels less congested and is able to breathe more freely and easily. Viral conditions on the other hand can be cured because the sound waves set up a condition in the body which makes it intolerable for the virus to remain or survive there.

What happens in a consultation?

The first treatment lasts for an hour or more and begins with a normal medical check-up. If necessary the practitioner will take your pulse, blood pressure, listen to your chest and carry out any other relevant conventional medical diagnostic tests to check the condition of your body organs. But in the case of a specific injury where the nature of the condition is obvious these tests are not usually necessary or required. The practitioner will then go on to ask you for further details about:

♦ *Your general health and any conditions that you might be currently suffering from*
♦ *What sort of food you eat in your normal daily diet*
♦ *He will also require details of your occupation and will want to know about any aspects of your lifestyle that may also be contributing to your condition*

Practitioners trained in other forms of complementary therapy, such as acupuncture or osteopathy, may also use elements of those systems in the diagnosis. When

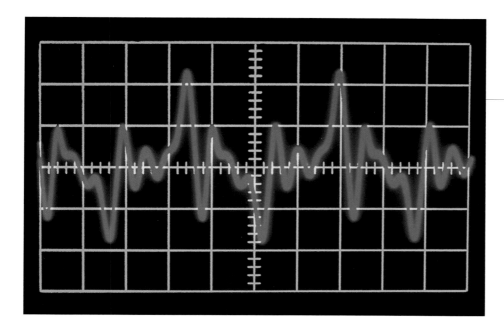

Left: Cymatic treatment works by generating corrective sound waves to the part of the body that is injured, thus rebalancing its energy.

he has arrived at his diagnosis the practitioner will take you through to a treatment room. Depending on the treatment he feels is required you may be asked to lie on a couch or to sit in a specially designed structure in which you can rest your head, neck and shoulders, so that you are completely relaxed and ready for treatment.

Treatment can sometimes take the form of aquasonics, in which case it takes place in a heated pool situated in an air-conditioned building. The molecular structure of water can be altered by certain sound frequencies, making it an easier medium in which people who have mobility problems can move. People with arthritis, rheumatoid problems and physical disability are often treated in this way. Even patients who are paralysed can still experience some sense of movement because of their own dilation in the water.

The nature and length of treatment depends on the condition from which you are suffering. For example, a difficult viral condition may need to be treated with several different frequencies for 45–60 minutes, but something as straightfor-

ward as arthritis could benefit from just 30 minutes of treatment. Treatment in the heated pool may last as little as 20 minutes, because it can be so relaxing that the person in the pool just falls asleep. In all cases the sensation the treatment gives is pleasant, relaxing and slightly stimulating as the sound frequencies are transmitted through your entire body.

How many sessions do I need?
It is impossible to say. It depends on the nature of your condition, how long you have had it and your body's individual healing ability. Treatment is believed to speed up a person's healing rate by 50%. You are recommended to have treatment twice a week to begin with and then once a week until the problem is cleared or the condition starts to respond to the technique and improves. Practitioners say that you should normally start to see some positive benefits by about the third treatment session.

Which problems can it help?
The therapy reduces pain and inflammation and also helps to improve mobility of

the joints and muscles. It has been noted as a successful treatment for conditions such as arthritis, rheumatism, back pain, post-operative healing, sports injuries, soft tissue damage, bone fractures and muscular injury.

But Dr Manners states that every condition, illness or psychological state can be treated or improved by the cymatics technique because it releases stress and tension in the body system and allows the mind and body to return to a normal or balanced level.

Is it safe?
Cymatic therapy, when it is administered properly by a qualified therapist, is perfectly safe for everyone to undertake, irrespective of their age or general level of fitness. Even pregnant women, very young babies, and the very frail and elderly can all be treated safely with cymatics.

In over 30 years of practice of the technique, there have been no recorded side effects or adverse reactions that have come about from this type of sound wave treatment.

BODYWORK

Bodywork is a term used for manipulative techniques that include psycho-emotional work. Practitioners work on muscles or go deep into the connective tissues to rebalance the mind, body and emotions.

ROLFING

Rolfing originated in the United States in the 1930s when biochemist Dr Ida Rolf discovered that the connective tissue around every muscle could be manipulated to reshape a misaligned body. She also recognized that gravity has a bearing on our shape. When we are well aligned and move in harmony with gravity it can flow naturally through us, allowing us to move easily. But a poorly aligned body is pulled down by gravity and must struggle to keep its balance, weakening the structure.

The aim of the rolfer is to re-align the body's structure, restore it to balance, and improve physical and emotional health.

How does it work?

A misaligned body puts unnecessary stress on the supporting muscles so that they lose their elasticity, and knots and adhesions develop in the connective tissue.

Rolfers aim to reverse this by manipulating the connective tissue to allow the body to move more appropriately so that it returns to a state of balance. When balanced, the mind, nervous system, the organs and tissues, and the innate healing system function more efficiently.

What happens in a consultation?

You will need several treatments. It is usual to undress to your underwear for the consultation. The first session begins with the rolfer taking details about you and your medical history:

♦ *She will ask about any injuries or structural weaknesses*
♦ *She may ask you about your own aims as rolfing can support personal development*

For the treatment you will lie down on a massage couch, where the rolfer uses her fingertips, hands, knuckles and elbows to work with the connective tissue. Initially the practitioner will work to free restrictions around the ribcage and the upper body to help you to breathe more deeply. In subsequent treatments, the practitioner will work around your body. Rolfing is often described as uncomfortable and you may find some areas sensitive to treatment.

Emotional and physical problems may surface during treatment, making you feel uncomfortable before you feel better.

How many sessions do I need?

A full course involves 10 treatments, lasting 60–90 minutes, often a week apart. These sessions work gradually from the outer surface structures to the deeper ones, ending with an integration of the two. You may feel an improvement after one or two sessions, but always complete the series to reap the long-term benefits, which include being more supple to feeling more confident and energetic.

Which problems can it help?

Rolfing is not aimed at alleviating specific conditions, but many people find they gain relief from postural problems, emotional problems, aggravating back pain, neck, shoulder and joint pain as well as asthma and digestive problems.

Is it safe?

Rolfing is safe for adults and children who are not suffering from diseases such as cancer or rheumatoid arthritis. A modified rolfing technique is safe for women over three months pregnant and babies and children suffering from structural problems such as scoliosis of the spine.

HELLERWORK

Hellerwork is a derivative of rolfing and aims to re-align the body and rebalance the connection between mind and body. It was developed in the United States in 1978 by a former US aerospace engineer called Joseph Heller. He applied the principles he had learnt from engineering to the human body to help prevent illness and improve vitality.

How does it work?

Practitioners believe that every movement is stressful to a body that is structurally misaligned. Misalignment can occur because of bad postural habits or emotional stress. Physical and emotional stress affect the connective tissue which holds together all the body muscles and which also forms ligaments and tendons.

In a balanced body this tissue should be loose and moist; under stress it becomes rigid and 'knotty' setting up body tension. The Hellerworker aims to re-align the body and release the rigid physical, mental and emotional patterns causing the misalignment. To achieve this they use manipulation, movement re-education and discussion.

Manipulation stretches tightened and shortened tissue back to its normal shape. Movement re-education involves learning to move effortlessly, allowing your body to maintain perfect alignment. Through discussion the practitioner tells you how emotions can cause structural tension.

What happens in a consultation?

The complete programme consists of several sessions. You are advised not to eat for two hours before each and you will need to undress to your underwear. At the first session the therapist will talk to you about:

♦ *Your medical history and previous illnesses*
♦ *Your specific needs and how Hellerwork may help you*

The practitioner will take a photograph at the beginning and end of the programme to show postural changes over the course. The work takes place on three different levels: the superficial, the core and the integrative. Some of the deeper work can hurt slightly, but most people feel relaxed and energized after a session.

Practitioners begin by working on the superficial layers of connective tissue and the first three sessions focus on re-aligning and freeing tension in the chest area, feet and arms. Sessions four to seven are known as the core sessions because they work more deeply into the body's core. Our core muscles are usually tight, inflexible and primed for problems. The practitioner manipulates these muscles to allow freer and harmonious body movement. The third group are integrative sessions. The aim of these treatments is to integrate the work of the superficial and core sessions by improving overall balance.

How many sessions do I need?

A full course of treatment is 11 sessions. Some people return for advanced sessions. Many people claim to feel benefits after just one treatment and use the remaining sessions to make the improvements permanent.

Which problems can it help?

Hellerwork is about disease prevention rather than just treatment. The practitioner's aim is to keep mind and body in perfect balance to prevent health problems. However, it does help aches and pains, including neck ache, headaches and back pain.

Is it safe?

Hellerwork can be adapted to suit most people. Pregnant women can benefit from treatment, as can children, although many rarely need it. It is not suitable for some cancers where manipulating tissues may speed up the spread of the disease.

BIODYNAMIC THERAPY

Biodynamic therapy combines specialized massage techniques with advanced psychotherapy to bring about emotional and physical healing. It was developed by Norwegian psychologist and physiotherapist Gerda Boyesen who discovered that emotional and psychological problems registered in the body's muscles and organs, especially in the intestines, which she saw as having two functions: to digest food and digest stress. In psychotherapy sessions she noted that many patients would produce loud intestinal gurglings, particularly when releasing emotions. She also noted that massage could cause patients to be sick or have diarrhoea and that such patients improved more quickly than those with no physical release.

Boyesen devised the word 'Biodynamic' to describe the life force or energy that constantly flows through us, linking body, mind and emotions into one organic unit.

How does it work?

Through massage and counselling, biodynamic therapy works to release physical and emotional tension. For example, you may hold grief from a bereavement inside until it becomes part of you and you no longer feel the emotion. Here, the biodynamic therapist would work on your body to release this grief so that you could again experience a healthy emotional cycle. Therapists believe that as every emotion rises it causes a physical reaction in every body cell. As it subsides, emotional residue is eliminated through the intestines and through breathing, enabling body function to return to normal.

However, if you are stressed, the process becomes impaired. The energy flow becomes sluggish and the intestine muscles will no longer function correctly. Much of the residue stays in the system wreaking physical and mental havoc. Therapists use massage to wring this out of the tissues, and stimulate healing.

What happens in a consultation?

There is no set course of treatment; it depends on you, the therapist and your interaction. A session usually lasts for an hour and the first begins with a detailed interview with a consultant who will ask:

♦ *About your medical history and any problems bothering you*
♦ *About any vulnerable areas and whether you have tried previous therapies*

The consultant will then choose a suitable therapy. The therapeutic session might involve massage, discussion, or both. Because the intestinal health is so important, therapists often listen to the intestines with a stethoscope and direct treatment according to what they hear. Therapists use different massage techniques to free old emotions from clogged muscles and encourage energy flow.

How many sessions do I need?

On average, people need about a year of weekly sessions, but this varies depending on the problem. Problems from the recent past can be resolved more quickly, whereas childhood ones can take more than a year to resolve.

Which problems can it help?

The therapy is beneficial in all stress-related illnesses. This includes lower back pain, migraine, angina, MS, Parkinson's disease and rheumatoid arthritis. Therapists also claim success in helping clients overcome deep-seated negative attitudes and feelings of fear and despair.

Is it safe?

Biodynamics is safe for most people except those in advanced stages of disease. Most people who choose it are adults with problems, but children with psychological problems can also benefit from adapted techniques. Milder forms of the therapy can suit pregnant women.

ARTS THERAPIES

Painting and drawing, singing and playing musical instruments, dancing and acting are all powerful and exciting forms of self expression. It is no small wonder therefore that the arts have become a valuable therapeutic tool, especially for rehabilitating the mentally and emotionally disturbed. In the 1940s some artists working in psychiatric hospitals began to realize that exploring, discussing and sharing an artwork could form the basis of a therapeutic relationship. Consequently, art as therapy evolved into art therapy.

Similarly, other media also began to be used therapeutically and the arts therapies gradually became accepted and integrated into the healthcare system. Arts therapists are now valued and respected health professionals, but work to a holistic philosophy.

What are the arts therapies?

Arts therapies cover four different and distinct therapies – art therapy, music therapy, dramatherapy and dance movement therapy. Each can help people with psychological problems to explore how they feel about themselves and their relationships with others. The aim is to develop deeper self-awareness, allowing people to change or accept aspects of themselves that are preventing them from leading fulfilling lives. The choice of therapy is usually a personal preference, but assessment might indicate that one is particularly appropriate.

How do they work?

Arts therapies are concerned with finding a language to demonstrate what cannot be expressed verbally. All four therapies work on the principle that art is cathartic. They can be used to access the unconscious mind. Emotional problems can arise from painful experiences that have been repressed, but survive as unconscious memories that subtly influence our lives.

Because the arts therapies involve much non-verbal work, they can explore even those painful experiences that occurred before we could talk. Through the chosen medium and discussion with your therapist it is possible to bring these past issues to the conscious level to resolve them.

The feelings you experience as you paint, improvise music, move or act, reflect your unconscious mind. In each session the therapist aims to create a confident environment where you can explore, experiment and liberate your thoughts. Therapy can also involve some discussion to explore thoughts and feelings that emerge as your therapy progresses.

What happens in a consultation?

The therapy sessions can take place on a one-to-one basis or in a small group. Adult therapy sessions last for 60–90 minutes, children's about 30 minutes.

Before therapy begins, the therapist will want to meet you for an individual assessment. This gives you both the chance to decide if you could work together.

♦ *The therapist will ask you to describe your emotional problems and will want to know what you hope to gain from the therapy*
♦ *She may ask for details about your life and relationships, past and present*

This is also a good time to ask questions. Assessments sometimes include using the arts medium concerned so you can discuss how you feel about it. Some people need a second assessment before they decide whether to go ahead with the therapy.

If you both decide to proceed you will agree on when it will begin, times of sessions and the cost. You are agreeing to a contract with the therapist and will be expected to operate within their boundaries. During the therapy everything done within the group is confidential. There is no set arts therapy session. Different therapists take different approaches to their work and the course of the therapy will be determined by the individual or group needs. Sessions usually include periods of reflection and discussion.

Art therapy This therapy helps people communicate through creativity using paint, pastels, clay or other art materials. Your choice of medium can be as relevant as the work you create. For example, coloured pencils make a faint mark on paper and the person who chooses them is conveying a different message from someone who splashes paint everywhere. The former may be afraid to make their mark, while the latter may feel it is safe to let go.

You and the therapist will explore any problems you may have in approaching the work as well as the content of what you create. The therapist may invite you to share your feelings about your painting, but will not attempt to analyse it for you. Your work is confidential and is not displayed or shown outside the group. Group members can work on a single project or on a theme or may also work individually, and talk about their experience near the end of the session.

Dance movement therapy This uses movement techniques and dance to explore how a patient's emotional disturbance is linked to their bodily experiences. Everyone has an individual way of moving. The therapist observes and analyses how you express yourself through your body, she assesses your strengths and identifies areas in which you might benefit from therapy. The therapist may also work with you individually, using movements to help you build a stronger sense of your own identity. Movement can also be used to help resolve issues that may have occurred before you learnt to speak.

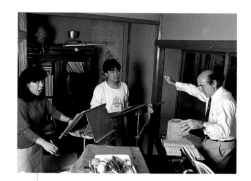

Above: Art therapy helps people to communicate using paint, pastels or clay. The work and discussions are confidential.

Movement should not be underestimated in developing the often neglected qualities of playfulness and creativity. In group work the therapist notes how members share emotional expression and judges when to intervene. As the session develops the therapist may notice a theme emerging and may encourage the group to develop it.

Music therapy Group members use their voices or musical instruments for expression. The way people communicate musically with others reflects their emotional problems. Music can form a link between people. It can also be used to symbolize feelings, for example, you may learn to control unmanageable feelings in an acceptable way by challenging someone musically or by contradicting their style.

The therapist's role is to offer support, either through music or discussion, perhaps by engaging in a playful musical 'fight' or by playing along with you. By meeting you on a level where you feel you can communicate safely the therapist can help you work through your feelings so you emerge feeling more confident.

Music is usually improvised by the group although composed pieces are sometimes used. Group members can choose from simple, usually percussion, instruments to produce music that is a source of satisfaction.

Dramatherapy This therapy uses various forms of drama to develop creativity, imagination, learning, insight and growth. The different forms can involve awareness, exploration and reflection of feelings and relationships. The group can act out different ways of thinking, feeling and behaving. Role play can explore social situations where group members feel inadequate. Sessions can also involve exploring group feelings and areas of personal growth through myth or metaphor. Sessions may focus on creating drama, working as part of a team, building self-confidence and awareness and having fun.

The therapist can introduce one or all of these forms of exploration into a session, depending on the individual or group needs. Central to all activity is the belief that drama provides a safe place for you to examine your inner feelings and experiment with new ways of being in the world.

Throughout the session the therapist encourages you to release your memories and anxieties, express your emotions and develop a better understanding of yourself and others. In other sessions all the work is contained in the metaphor or symbolism.

How many sessions do I need?
It is impossible to say how many sessions are needed, but be committed to at least six months. Sessions are usually weekly.

Which problems can they help?
The arts therapies can benefit people with many types of psychological and emotional problems. In private practice therapists may see patients who feel they are not fulfilling their potential, perhaps because of anxiety or poor self-esteem. It can also benefit people with physical illnesses that are exacerbated by stress. Therapists who work in hospitals, day centres or institutions focus more on people who have been isolated by learning disorders, dementia or severe psychiatric disorders such as schizophrenia. Patients

with speech or hearing impairment can also communicate through non-verbal aspects. All the therapies are effective with children. Certain aspects of the therapies make each one suitable in specific cases. For example, art therapy is valuable for people who feel threatened by close relationships as it lets them express their feelings. Music therapy is a traditional form of adolescent expression. It can be appropriate for hyperactive children, or people suffering from Alzheimer's disease. Dramatherapy can be used to improve relationships between couples, family or individuals within a group. Dance movement therapy is effective with young children and can benefit the mother/baby relationship. Patients with advanced dementia may still be reached through movement therapy.

Are they safe?
It is more appropriate to talk in terms of the suitability of the therapies rather than their safety. However, you should see a qualified therapist, who can deal with all psychological disturbance.

PLAY THERAPY
◆

Play therapy is suitable for children from the age of three upwards. The therapist does not usually try to direct the child, although if a child is suffering with post-traumatic stress disorder therapists may be more directive if they feel it is necessary.

Like arts therapies, play therapy deals indirectly with the child's unconscious by using play for communication. It is based on the principle that the child has an inherent capacity to heal and address their emotional life through play.

REIKI

Reiki, which means 'universal life force energy' is an ancient holistic hands-on healing technique that was revived in the mid-19th century by Dr Mikao Usui in Japan and is still popular today.

Dr Usui, a convert to Christianity, lived in Kyoto and taught at a small Christian university. During a lesson one day his students asked him whether he believed in the healing miracles of Christ. When he replied yes, they then requested him to teach them this ability. He replied that he could not and felt that he had failed his students and reluctantly resigned his post. Still intrigued by the question he began a quest to find out about the healing powers. His travels took him to America but it was not until he was back in Japan in a Zen monastery that he studied Buddhism and started to make some progress.

He studied many scriptures and scrolls and learnt Chinese and Sanskrit to read more and found some answers. Finally, he decided to seek enlightenment by going on a 21-day retreat in the mountains outside Kyoto. It was here on the 21st day that in a moment of revelation he received what are now known as the reiki symbols. Rushing back down the mountain to tell the abbot at his monastery of this experience he tripped and cut his toe. Bending down he held his toe with his hands and found in a few minutes that the bleeding had stopped and the pain gone – he had acquired the ability to heal with his hands.

For some time Dr Usui used his healing skill to treat beggars in Kyoto but found that although he healed them physically he had not healed their spirit and they returned to begging. He began to understand that an exchange of energy was essential for the healing received.

So he went on to teach healing throughout Japan and developed the five spiritual principles to complement the physical healing. He started to train other men as Reiki masters, and one of these, Dr Chujiro Hayashi helped him to create the teaching system. He later chose him to be his successor.

Dr Hayashi founded a Reiki clinic in Japan and it was here in 1935 that Mrs Hawayo Takata, a Japanese-American, came to be treated for depression and physical disorders. After several months of treatment she was cured and eventually convinced Dr Hayashi, who was reluctant to train a woman, to initiate her in First and Second degree Reiki. She returned home to Hawaii to practise Reiki and in 1938 Dr Hayashi made her a master. Shortly afterwards with war looming between Japan and the United States, Dr Hayashi an ex-naval officer became fearful of conscription and named Mrs Takata as his successor so that the Reiki tradition would not be lost. However, he died before he could be called up, just before the start of the war.

In the following 40 years after the war Mrs Takata brought Reiki to the United States, but it was not until the last 10 years of her life that she started to train other Reiki masters. When she died in 1980 she had initiated 22 masters. Shortly after her death, the Reiki Alliance was formed and Mrs Takata's granddaughter, who had been promoting the Usui system of Reiki, was asked to be the Grand Master. This is a position she still holds today.

What is Reiki?
Reiki is a safe healing energy which is channelled by the healer who places her hands on different parts of the body during treatment. The energy is channelled from the universal life force and everybody can benefit from the treatment. The healing, life force energy is not directed by the practitioner but goes where it is needed, stimulating the the body's own innate healing mechanism. It is a holistic healing system that can treat many chronic and acute conditions and aims to cleanse the body of emotional and physical blockages to bring about spiritual, mental and physical harmony.

How does it work?
When a Reiki treatment is given the energy goes deep into the body where physical illness begins, helping to create balance by releasing blockages and getting rid of any toxins and wastes that have accumulated there. It also works on an emotional and mental basis helping the recipient to make changes in their outlook and lifestyle so that they can lead a more fulfilled life.

The healing energy works on both the organs and the endocrine system which controls the secretion of the body's hormones. It also works on the seven main chakras – the body's spiritual centres. In Reiki and other healing methods, the endocrine and chakra systems are believed to be linked with an ongoing energy flowing between them. Medical science is sceptical of this process, although the relationship between energy and matter has always been well documented.

Reiki healing can also be given to the terminally ill. It generally will not bring about a cure, although miracles can happen, but it can help the recipient to come to terms with their illness, make peace with their life and say goodbye to their friends and relatives.

A practitioner who has second degree Reiki can also send distant healing incorporating the Reiki symbols to sick friends or relatives anywhere in the world. This process can also be used to send healing energy back to a troubled childhood or forward to a forthcoming event.

What happens in a consultation?
Healing takes place on an individual basis. The room used is normally warm, often

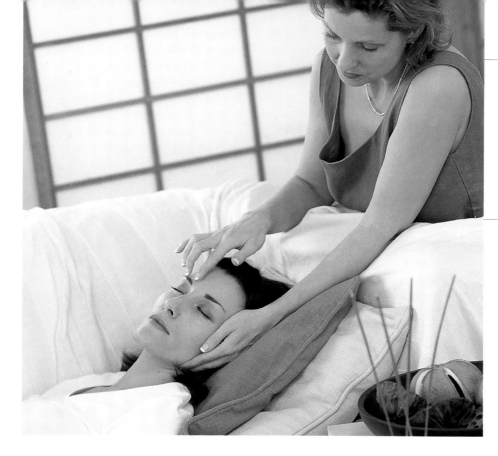

Left: In Reiki, safe energy is channelled through the healer's hands to stimulate the body's own healing mechanism.

has essential oils burning, and soft relaxing music playing in the background. A case history is not taken by a Reiki healer but they will note down basic details about yourself and write down any medication you are taking. They will also ask:

♦ *What problem you are suffering from, or whether you are looking for general stress relief*

♦ *If you have a pacemaker fitted as Reiki can affect its functioning or if you suffer from diabetes as the insulin levels may have to be adapted*

After this brief discussion you will lie on your back, fully clothed, on the massage couch for the hour-long session. The healer will first scan your body to find any energy imbalances or blockages in the body. She may ask you to set an intent on where you want the energy to go. She will then start on the first four head positions sitting behind you. To do the other four positions on your front she will stand, moving her hands down your body. Great heat, tingling or throbbing, or sometimes coldness may be felt from the hands when a lot of energy is being pulled into an area.

If this is not felt it does not mean that the healing is not working. She may briefly work on your knees as emotion from the past can be stored here, and then move the energy down to your feet.

You may well be in a peaceful Reiki slumber by this time but will normally wake up sufficiently as the healer finishes your feet to turn over.

Lying on your front a further four positions are treated on your shoulders and back, and then the healer again takes the energy down to your feet. She then normally brings it up to your head to ground you for the journey home, and will often clear your aura of any negativity. Sometimes as the treatment progresses there may be an emotional release and you may burst into tears. This is quite normal and the healer will normally have some tissues to hand.

After the treatment you will probably be given a glass of water to help with the detoxifying process and be told to drink more water over the next few days, and to avoid alcohol for 24 hours. Most people feel very relaxed after the session and may want to talk about what they experienced before their journey home.

How many sessions do I need?

It is generally recommended to have an initial course of three to four treatments as the healing effects are accumulative. For a chronic condition it is best to have five treatments in one week, then four, then three, then two getting down to one a week for several weeks so that they can have maximum exposure to the energy. If this is not possible, start off with three a week going down to one a week as there is improvement. For stress relief, benefits will be felt after one session.

Which problems can it help?

Reiki is particularly good for stress-related problems and can often cure or greatly relieve acute conditions such as colds, flu, viral infections and headaches. It also helps chronic conditions such as ME, asthma, migraine, eczema, arthritis and rheumatism. Reiki can also be given as first aid for minor problems such as toothache, burns, cuts and bruises, backache, chest problems and ear ache.

Is it safe?

Reiki is a safe healing treatment for everyone, and the elderly can certainly benefit from treatment. Children need a shorter treatment of about 20 minutes. Pets and even plants will also respond to the positive energy. It can soothe terminal patients, and is a very positive treatment for pregnant women, helping to alleviate some of the pregnancy symptoms, aiding pain relief in child birth and promoting faster healing of a normal birth or a Caesarean section. It is not advisable to give Reiki to anyone under anaesthesia but it can help relieve the after-effects of radiotherapy and chemotherapy.

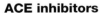

DRUG GLOSSARY

This glossary explains the more important or common types of drugs referred to in this book.

ACE inhibitors

Angiotensin-converting enzyme inhibitors. Angiotensin is a hormone involved in blood pressure. By blocking its action, ACE inhibitors reduce blood pressure and treat heart failure. Examples are captopril, lisinopril and enalapril.

Anaesthetics

Medication that reduces pain during surgery. Local anaesthetics, given by injection, deaden pain in a small area. General anaesthetics, in the form of injection or gas, make the patient unconscious.

Antacids

Substances that neutralize stomach acids. Many proprietary brands contain aluminium or magnesium hydroxide.

Antibiotics

Drugs that kill or damage microscopic organisms, especially bacteria, by affecting some vital part of their metabolism. Types include penicillin (amoxycillin and ampicillin), cephalosporins (cephalexin and cefaclor), tetracyclines (minocycline and oxytetracycline), 4-quinolones (ciprofloxacin), macrolides (erythromycin) and many others. Different infections respond to different antibiotics. Antifungal antibiotics include nystatin and clotrimazole. Viruses do not respond to conventional antibiotics (see antivirals).

Anticonvulsants

Drugs that reduce the chances of an epileptic fit. Examples are phenytoin, carbamazepine and vigabatrin.

Antidepressants

Mood-altering drugs that affect brain chemistry to relieve depression. The most widely used are tricyclics (amitryptiline, dothiepin and imipramine) and selective serotonin reuptake inhibitors, SSRIs, (fluoxetine and paroxetine), and mixed types (venlafaxine).

Antihistamines

These block histamine, a biochemical involved in allergic reactions, itch and hay fever. Examples are chlorpheniramine, loratadine and cetirizine.

Antihypertensives

Medication to reduce blood pressure. Common types are diuretics, beta-blockers, calcium-channel blockers and ACE inhibitors (see entries).

Antiemetics

Drugs that reduce sickness and giddiness by sedating the organs of balance in the ear or the 'nausea centre' within the brain. Types include prochlorperazine and domperidone.

Antipsychotics

Sedatives (see entry) for the agitation, aggression or disordered thought of serious mental illness such as schizophrenia or manic depression. Examples are haloperidol and risperidone.

Antivirals

Fairly recently developed antibiotics effective against viruses. Not many are available and only for a few infections, for example aciclovir for herpes. Zidovudine (also called AZT) fights AIDS.

Aspirin

Aspirin reduces pain and fever; in a low dose it makes blood less likely to clot. It works via the prostaglandin system, biochemical substances involved in many basic body functions. Aspirin must not be taken by children under the age of 12, nor by people with severe indigestion or previous peptic ulcer.

Beta-blockers

Adrenaline is a substance produced by the body in response to stress. Beta receptors are nerves that respond to adrenaline in the heart, lungs, brain and blood vessels. By blocking these nerves, beta-blockers reduce heart rate and palpitations, ease anxiety, lower blood pressure and control migraine. They include atenolol, propranolol and labetolol.

Bronchodilators

Medication to make airways widen within the lungs, to treat asthma and chronic bronchitis. Available as aerosol sprays, tablets and injections. Examples are salbutamol and terbutaline or long-acting ones, e.g. salmeterol.

Calcium-channel blockers

By affecting calcium metabolism in the muscles around arteries, these drugs make blood vessels dilate. A treatment for high blood pressure and angina. Common examples are nifedipine, amlodipine and diltiazem.

Clot busters

Drugs that dissolve blood clots within arteries or veins after pulmonary embolus, deep vein thrombosis or heart attack, allowing blood flow to recommence. Their use has greatly improved the outlook of these conditions. Examples are streptokinase and urokinase.

Contraceptives
Means of controlling fertility using hormones. Their actions include stopping the release of an egg each month and altering conditions at the cervix to prevent sperm from penetrating. The combined Pill is a mixture of oestrogen and progestogen (see entries); the minipill contains progestogen only.

Cough mixtures
Liquids that loosen mucus, often with a sedative to improve sleep as well.

COX-2 inhibitors
Recently available anti-inflammatory drugs that relieve arthritic pain without causing stomach irritation, e.g. rofecoxib.

Cytotoxics
Treatments for cancer that destroy cancer cells. They need specialist monitoring to minimize side effects. Examples are methotrexate, cyclophosphamide and fluorouracil.

Decongestants
Medication to reduce the flow of mucus by constricting blood vessels in the nose and sinuses during colds or sinusitis. They are advisable for a few days only. Examples are pseudoephedrine and xylometazoline.

Diuretics
Drugs that make the kidneys pass more urine. Useful in treating high blood pressure, heart failure and severely swollen legs. Types include bendrofluazide and frusemide.

H2 blockers
Substances that block histamine receptors in the stomach involved in acid production. They have revolutionized the treatment of chronic indigestion and peptic ulcers. Examples are cimetidine and ranitidine.

Hormones
Natural proteins, produced by glands, that circulate in the blood stream, having effects around the body. Examples are insulin, thyroid hormone and oestrogen.

Immunosuppressants
Drugs that reduce the immune response, important in transplant surgery. Examples are azathioprine and cyclosporin.

Laxatives
Substances that relieve constipation. Some (senna) stimulate the bowels to pass out material, while others (lactulose) hold fluid within the bowel.

Non-steroidal anti-inflammatory drugs (NSAIDs)
Drugs related to aspirin (see entry) that work similarly; especially useful for joint pain and minor injuries. They can cause indigestion and must not be taken by anyone with a peptic ulcer. Names include ibuprofen, diclofenac, naproxen.

Oestrogens
Hormones produced mainly in the ovaries, which cause female sexual characteristics and regulate the menstrual cycle. Oestrogens are used for contraception, menstrual disorders and hormone replacement therapy (HRT).

Opioids
Powerful painkilling drugs such as morphine, diamorphine (heroin), pethidine and codeine. They affect parts of the brain which normally respond to the body's natural painkillers. They are potentially addictive but, if properly used, are immensely helpful for relieving pain.

Paracetamol
A painkilling, fever-reducing substance, safe at all ages. In excess it causes liver damage so do not exceed the safe dose.

Progestogens
Hormones involved in pregnancy, which can regulate periods, act as contraceptives and are included in most HRT preparations.

Proton pump inhibitors
Highly effective drugs that work on molecular pumps in cells involved in acid production, greatly reducing acid in the stomach. They are more powerful than H2 blockers (see entry). Examples are omeprazole and lansoprazole.

Sedatives
Drugs that reduce brain activity, relieving anxiety, agitation or major psychiatric disturbances such as mania. They include diazepam, chlorpromazine, chloral and certain antihistamines.

Sleeping tablets
Sedatives with a powerful, rapid action that induces sleep. Generally recommended only for short-term use. A common example is temazepam.

Steroids
Biochemicals that, by affecting cell activity, have many powerful actions on the body. They reduce inflammation in arthritis and skin disorders, dampen the immune response in asthma, are used in transplant surgery and to restore blood pressure after severe blood loss and collapse. Side effects after prolonged use at high doses include high blood pressure, weight gain and thinning of the skin. However, steroids, properly used, have transformed the management of many serious or chronic conditions such as asthma and eczema. Examples are prednisolone, dexamethasone, betamethasone and hydrocortisone.

DIRECTORY

◆

CIRCULATORY SYSTEM

◆

British Heart Foundation (BHF)
14 Fitzhardinge Street
London W1H 6DH   Tel: 020 7935 0185

Coronary Prevention Group (CPG)
2 Taviton Street
London WC1H 0BT   Tel: 020 7927 2125

Raynaud's and Scleroderma Association
112 Crewe Road
Alsager
Cheshire ST7 2JA   Tel: 01270 872 776
Fax: 01270 883 556
www.raynauds.demon.co.uk

RESPIRATORY SYSTEM

◆

Action Against Allergy
PO Box 278
Twickenham
Middlesex TW1 4QQ   Tel: 020 8892 2711

Action on Smoking and Health (ASH)
102 Clifton Street
East London EC2A 4HW   Tel: 020 7739 5902
Helpline: 0800 169 0169
Fax: 020 76130531
www.ash.org.uk

Cancer Information Service (BACUP)
3 Bath Place
London EC2A 3DR   Tel: 020 7613 2121
Freephone: 0808 800 1234
www.cancerbacup.org.uk

Macmillan CR
89 Albert Embankment
London
SE1 7UQ   Tel: 020 7840 7840
Info Line: 0845 601 6161

National Asthma Campaign
Providence House
Providence Place
London N1 0NT   Tel: 020 7226 2260
Helpline: 08457 010 203
(Mon–Fri 9am–7pm)

MIND, BRAIN & NERVOUS SYSTEM

◆

Alcohol Concern
Waterbridge House
32–6 Loman Street
London SE1 0EE   Tel: 020 7928 7377
Fax: 020 7928 4644
www.alcoholconcern.org.uk

Alzheimer's Disease Society
Gordon House
10 Greencoat Place
London SW1P 1PH   Freephone: 0800 727 2627

British Epilepsy Association
New Anstey House
Gateway Drive
Yeadon
Leeds LS19 7XY   Tel: 0113 210 8800
Helpline: 0808 800 5050

Cruse, Bereavement Care
Cruse House
126 Sheen Road
Richmond
Surrey TW9 1UR   Tel: 020 8940 4818

Encephalitis Support Group
44a Market Place
Malton
North Yorks
YO17 7LW   Tel: 01653 699 599

Migraine Action
(formerly British Migraine Association)
178a High Road
Byfleet
Surrey KT14 7ED   Tel: 01932 352 468
Website: www.migraine.org.uk

MIND (National Association for Mental Health)
Granta House
15–19 Broadway
London E15 4BQ   Tel: 020 8519 2122
Helpline: 0808 800 8000
(Mon–Fri 9.15am–5.15pm)

MS Counselling Line
     Tel: 020 8422 2144
MS Society
MS National Centre
372 Edgware Road
London NW2 6ND   Tel: 020 8438 0700
www.mssociety.org.uk

National Meningitis Trust
Fern House
Bath Road
Stroud
Gloucester GL5 3TJ   Tel: 01453 768 000
24-hour supportline: 0845 6000 800

Parkinson's Disease Society
215 Vauxhall Bridge Road
London SW1V 1EJ   *Helpline: 020 7233 5373*

Schizophrenia – A National Emergency (SANE)
1st Floor
Cityside House
40 Adler Street
London E1 1EE   Tel: 020 7375 1002
Helpline: 0845 767 8000
(12pm–2am)

The Stroke Association
Stroke House
123–7 Whitecross Street
London EC1Y 8JJ   Tel: 020 7490 7999
Stroke info line: 0845 303 3100

ENDOCRINE SYSTEM & METABOLISM

◆

Diabetes UK
(formerly British Diabetic Association)
10 Queen Anne Street
London W1G 9LH   Tel: 020 7323 1531
Careline: 020 7636 6112
Fax: 020 7637 3644
www.diabetes.org.uk

URINARY SYSTEM

◆

Association for Continence Advice (ACA)
Winchester House, Kennington Park
Cranmer Road
London SW9 6EJ   Tel: 020 7820 8113

British Kidney Patient Association (BKPA)
Bordon
Hampshire GU35 9JZ   Tel: 01420 472 021

National Kidney Federation
6 Stanley Street
Worksop
Nottinghamshire S81 7HX
     Helpline: 0845 601 02 09
www.kidney.org.uk

MALE REPRODUCTIVE SYSTEM

◆

The Herpes Viruses Association (HVA)
41 North Toad
London N7 9DP   *Helpline: 020 7609 9061*

ISSUE: The National Fertility Association
114 Lichfield Street
Walsall WS1 1SZ   Tel: 01922 722 888

FEMALE REPRODUCTIVE SYSTEM

◆

The Amarant Trust
Gainsborough Clinic
22 Barkham Terrace
London SE1 7PW   Tel: 020 7401 3855
(Mon–Fri 11am–6pm)

Association of Breastfeeding Mothers
PO Box 207
Bridgewater
Somerset TA6 7YT   Tel: 020 7813 1481

Association for Postnatal Illness
25 Jerdan Place
London SW6 1BE   Tel: 020 7386 0868

Breast Cancer Care
Kiln House
210 New Kings Road
London SW6 4NZ   Tel: 020 7384 2984
                        Fax: 020 7384 3387
              Helpline: 0808 800 6000
              www.breastcancercare.org.uk

British Pregnancy Advisory Service (BPAS)
Austy Manor
Wootton Wawen
Solihull
West Midlands B95 6BX   Tel: 01564 793 225
              Helpline: 08457 304 030

Family Planning Association (FPA)
2–12 Pentonville Road
London N1 9FP   Tel: 020 7837 5432
              Helpline: 020 7837 4044

Foresight (Pre-Conceptual Care)
28 The Paddock
Godalming
Surrey GU7 1XD   Tel: 01483 427 839

Miscarriage Association
c/o Clayton Hospital
Northgate
Wakefield
West Yorks WF1 3JS   Admin: 01924 200 795
                        Fax: 01924 298 834
                     www.the-ma.org.uk

National Childbirth Trust (NCT)
Alexandra House
Oldham Terrace
London W3 6NH
                        Tel: 020 8992 8637
                        Fax: 020 8992 5929
                     www.nct-online.org

National Endometriosis Society
50 Westminster Palace Gardens
Artillery Row
London SW1P 1RL   Tel: 020 7222 2781
                        Tel: 020 7222 2786
              Helpline: 020 7222 2776
                     www.endo.org.uk

Women's Nationwide Cancer Control Campaign
Suna House
128–130 Curtain Road
London EC2A 3AQ   Tel: 020 7729 4688

DIGESTIVE SYSTEM
◆

Coeliac Society
PO Box 220
High Wycombe
Buckinghamshire HP11 2HY   Tel: 01494 437 278

Digestive Disorders Foundation
(formerly British Digestive Foundation)
3 St Andrew's Place
London NW1 4LB   Tel: 020 7486 0341
                        Fax: 020 7224 2012
              www.digestivedisorders.org.uk
                     (Send SAE for info)

National Association for Colitis and Crohn's Disease
4 Beaumont House
Sutton Road
St Albans
Hertfordshire AL1 5HH   Tel: 01727 844 296
           (10am–1pm Monday–Friday except Tuesday)

EYES
◆

Royal National Institute for the Blind (RNIB)
224 Great Portland Street
London W1N 6AA   Tel: 0845 766 99 99
                   (UK Helpline callers only)
                        Fax: 020 7388 2034
Textphone users call via Typetalk 0800 51 51 52

EAR, NOSE & THROAT
◆

British Dental Association (BDA)
64 Wimpole Street
London W1G 8YS   Tel: 020 7935 0875

Defeating Deafness (Hearing Research Trust)
330–2 Gray's Inn Road
London WC1X 8EE   Tel: 020 7833 1733

Ménière's Society
98 Maybury Road
Woking
Surrey GU21 5HX   Tel: 01483 740 597

The Royal National Institute for Deaf People (RNID)
PO Box 16464
London EC1Y 8TT By voice phone: 0808 808 0123
                 By textphone: 0808 808 9000
                      By fax: 020 7296 8199
                        www.rnid.org.uk

SKIN & HAIR
◆

Acne Support Group
PO Box 230
Hayes
Middlesex UB4 0UT   Tel: 020 8561 6868
                   (Send large SAE for info)
                        www.m2w3.com

Hairline International
The Alopecia Patients' Society
Lyons Court
1668 Highstreet
Knowle
West Midlands B93 0LY   Tel: 01564 775 281

National Eczema Society
163 Eversholt Street
London NW1 1BU   Tel: 020 7388 4097
              Helpline: 0870 241 3604
                   (1–4pm Mon–Fri)
                   Fax 020 7388 5882
                     www.eczema.org

Psoriasis Association
Milton House
7 Milton Street
Northampton NN2 7JG   Tel: 01604 711 129

MUSCULO-SKELETAL SYSTEM
◆

Arthritis Research Campaign
St Mary's Court
St Mary's Gate
Chesterfield S41 7TD   Tel: 01246 558 033
                        Fax: 01246 558 007
                     www.arc.org.uk

Brittle Bone Society
30 Guthrie Street
Dundee DD1 5BS   Tel: 01382 204 446
              Freephone: 0800 0282 459

Muscular Dystrophy Campaign Group of Great Britain and Northern Ireland
7–11 Prescott Place
Clapham
London SW4 6BS   Tel: 020 7720 8055

National Back Pain Association
Backcare
16 Elmtree Road
Teddington
Middlesex TW11 8ST   Tel: 020 8977 5474
                        Fax: 020 8943 5318
                     www.backpain.org

National Osteoporosis Society (NOS)
PO Box 10
Radstock
Bath BA3 3YB   Tel: 01761 471 771
              Helpline: 01761 472 721
                        Fax: 01761 471 104
                     www.nos.org.uk

BLOOD, GLANDS & THE IMMUNE SYSTEM
◆

The Leukaemia Care Society
2 Shrubbery Avenue
Barbourne
Worcester
WR1 1QH   Tel: 0345 767 3203 & 01905 330 003
                        Fax: 01905 330 090
         24-hour support line: 0800 169 6680
                   www.leukaemiacare.org

Lupus UK
St James's House
1 Eastern Road
Romford
Essex RM1 3NH   Tel: 01708 731 251
                        Fax: 01708 731 252
                     www.geocities.com

Lymphoma Association
PO Box 386
Aylesbury
Buckinghamshire HP20 2GA   Tel: 01296 619 400
              Freephone: 0808 808 5555

Myalgic Encephalomyelitis (ME) Association
4 Corringham Road
Stanford-le-Hope
Essex SS17 0AH   Tel: 01375 642 466
              Info line: 01375 361 013

National Blood Service
                        Tel: 0345 711 711

Sickle Cell Society
54 Station Road
London NW10 4UA
Tel: 020 8961 4006

INFECTIOUS DISEASE

◆

Children with AIDS Charity
9 Denbigh Street
London SW1V 2HF
Tel: 020 7233 5966
Fax: 020 7233 5866
www.cwac.org

Malaria Information Line
Tel: 09065 508 908

National AIDS Helpline
Tel: 0800 567 123

Terrence Higgins Trust
52–4 Gray's Inn Road
London WC1X 8JU
Tel: 020 7831 0330
Helpline: 020 7242 1010
www.tht.org.uk

CHILDREN

◆

Association for Spina Bifida and Hydrocephalus (ASBAH)
42 Park Road
Peterborough PE1 2UQ
Tel: 01733 555988
Fax: 01733 555 985
www.asbah.org

Cerebral Palsy Helpline
Tel: 0808 800 3333

Community Hygiene Concern
(Information on headlice and other parasitic diseases)
160 Inderwick Road
London N8 9JT
Tel: 020 8341 7167

Down's Syndrome Association
155 Mitcham Road
London SW17 9PG
Tel: 020 8682 4001

Foundation for the Study of Infant Death
Artillery House
11–19 Artillery Row
London SW1P 1RT
Tel: 020 7222 8001
24-hour helpline: 020 7233 2090
Fax: 020 7222 8002
www.sids.org.uk

Hyperactive Children's Support Group
71 Whyke Lane
Chichester
West Sussex PO19 2LD
Tel: 01903 725 182

SCOPE (formerly the Spastics Society)
6 Market Road
London N7 9PW
Tel: 020 7619 7100
Helpline: 0808 800 3333

Helpline address:
PO Box 833
Milton Keynes
MK12 5NY
www.scope.org.uk

COMPLEMENTARY THERAPIES

◆

British Complementary Medicine Association
Kensington House
33 Imperial Square
Cheltenham
Gloucestershire
GL50 1QZ
Tel: 01242 519 911

Institute for Complementary Medicine
PO Box 194
London SE16 7QZ
Tel: 020 7237 5165

ACUPUNCTURE

British Acupuncture Council
63 Jeddo Road
London W12 9QH
Tel: 020 8735 0400

ALEXANDER TECHNIQUE

The Society of Teachers of the Alexander Technique
129 Camden Mews
London NW1 9AH
Tel: 020 7284 3338
Website: www.stat.org.uk

AROMATHERAPY

Aromatherapy Organisations Council
PO Box 19834
London SE25 6WF   Tel: 020 8251 7912 (10am–2pm)
Fax: 020 8251 7942

International Federation of Aromatherapists
Stamford House
182 Chiswick High Road
London W4 1PP
Tel: 020 8742 2605
(For a list of practitioners, send an A5 SAE and a cheque for £2)

ARTS THERAPIES

Association for Dance Movement Therapy
Quaker House
Wedmore Vale
Bedminster
Bristol BS3 5HX
Tel: 020 8672 9911

Association of Professional Music Therapists
26 Hamlyn Road
Glastonbury
Somerset BA6 8HT
Tel: 01458 834 919

British Association of Art Therapists
5 Tavistock Place
London WC1
Tel: 020 7383 3774

British Association of Dramatherapists
Tel: 020 7383 3774
membership enquiries only: 01929 555017

AUTOGENIC TRAINING

British Association for Autogenic Training and Therapy (BAFATT)
The Administrator
British Autogenic Society
The Royal London Homoeopathic Hospital
Great Ormond Street
London WC1N 3HR
Tel: 020 7713 6336

AYURVEDIC MEDICINE

Ayurvedic Medical Association UK
17 Bromham Mill
Giffard Park
Milton Keynes MK14 5QP
Tel: 01908 617 089

BACH FLOWER REMEDIES

The Edward Bach Centre
Mount Vernon
Bakers Lane
Brightwell cum Sotwell
Wallingford
Oxon OX10 0PZ
Tel: 01491 834 678

BIODYNAMIC THERAPY

The Gerda Boyesen Centre
15 The Ridgeway
London W3 8LW (for correspondence only)
Tel: 020 8993 5777

CHINESE HERBALISM

Chinese Herbal Medicine
73 High Street
Hounslow
London TW3 1RG
Tel: 020 8814 2654

CHIROPRACTIC

The British Chiropractic Association
Blagrave House
17 Blagrave Street
Reading RG1 1QB
Tel: 0118 950 5950

CYMATICS

Dr Sir Peter Guy Manners
Bretforton Medical and Scientific Academy
Bretforton Hall
Bretforton
Vale of Evesham
Worcestershire WR11 5JH
Tel: 01386 830537

HELLERWORK

The European Hellerwork Association
c/o Roger Golten
The Macintyre Gallery
29 Crawford Street
London W1H 1PL
Tel: 020 7723 5676

HOMOEOPATHY

The British Homoeopathic Association
15 Clerkenwell Close
London EC1R 0AA   Tel: 020 7566 7800

The Society of Homoeopaths
2 Artizan Road
Northampton NN1 4HU   Tel: 01604 621 400
(Send large SAE for list of practitioners)

HYPNOTHERAPY

The Central Register of Advanced Hypnotherapists (CRAH)
PO Box 14526
London N4 2WG   Tel: 020 7354 9938
www.users.globalnet.co.uk/~enneauk/crah.htm

The National Register of Hypnotherapists and Psychotherapists
12 Cross Street
Nelson, Lancashire BB9 7EN   Tel: 01282 699 378
(Send SAE for register of practitioners)

MACROBIOTICS

The Macrobiotics Association of Great Britain
377 Edgware Road
London W2 1BT   Tel: 07050 138 419

MASSAGE

Massage Therapy Institute of Great Britain
PO Box 27/26
London NW2 3NR   Tel: 020 7724 4105
(Send SAE for register of practitioners)

NATUROPATHY

The General Council and Register of Naturopaths
Goswell House
2 Goswell Road
Street
Somerset BA16 0JG   Tel: 01458 840 072

NUTRITIONAL THERAPY

Society for the Promotion of Nutritional Therapy
PO Box 85
St Albans
Hertfordshire AL3 7ZQ
freespace.virgin.net/nutrition.therapy

Dietary Therapy Society
33 Priory Gardens
London N6 5QU   Tel: 020 8348 8242

OSTEOPATHY

General Council and Register of Osteopaths
176 Tower Bridge Road
London SE1 3LU   Tel: 0118 957 6585

PILATES

The PILATES foundation ® UK Limited
80 Camden Road
London E17 7NF   Tel: 07071 781 859
Fax: 020 8281 508
www.pilatesfoundation.com

REFLEXOLOGY

The Association of Reflexologists
27 Old Gloucester Street
London WC1N 3XX   Tel: 0870 567 3320

The British Reflexology Association
Monks Orchard
Whitbourne
Worcester WR6 5RB   Tel: 01886 821207

REIKI (HEALERS)
A Robertshaw BA, M.B.R.A (Reiki therapist offering a natural, hands-on method of healing)
Manor House
20 High Street
Albrighton
Wolverhampton
West Midlands WV7 3JB   Tel: 01902 374697
or
John Scott-Cameron
Crowborough Clinic of Osteopathy and Complementary Therapies
3a London Road
Crowborough
East Sussex TN6 2TT
Tel: 01892 662935
Mobile Phone: 0831 742341

ROLFING

(ask for) Alan Richardson
Neal's Yard Therapy Rooms
2 Neal's Yard
Covent Garden
London WC2H 9DP   Tel: 020 7379 7662

SHIATSU

Shiatsu Society UK
Eastlands Court
St Peter's Road
Rugby
Warwickshire CV21 3QP   Tel: 01788 555 051

SPIRITUAL HEALING

The National Federation of Spiritual Healers
Old Manor Farm Studio
Church Street
Sunbury-on-Thames
Middlesex TW16 6RG   Tel: 01932 783164

WESTERN HERBALISM

The National Institute of Medical Herbalists
56 Longbrook Street
Exeter EX4 6AH   Tel: 01392 426 022

YOGA

British Wheel of Yoga
1 Hamilton Place
Boston Road
Sleaford
Lincolnshire NG34 7ES   Tel: 01529 306 851

The Iyengar Yoga Institute
233a Randolph Avenue
London W9 1NL   Tel: 020 7624 3080
Website: www.iyi.org.uk

The Yoga Therapy Centre
Homoeopathic Hospital
60 Great Ormond Street
London WC1N 3HR   Tel: 020 7419 7195
(For therapists who can treat specific medical problems)

AUSTRALIA

Allergy Information Network
Suite 14
370 Victoria Avenue
Chatswood
NSW 2067   Tel: 02 419 7731

Association of Massage Therapists
18a Spit Road
Mosman
NSW 1088

Asthma Australia
(Asthma Victoria)
Tel:03 9326 7088
Fax:03 9326 7055
Email: afv@asthma.org.au
www.asthma.org.au

Australian Acupuncture Association
Suite 2
77 Vulture Street
West End
QLD 4551   Tel: 07 3846 5866

Australian Federation of Aids Organizations
Level 8
33 Bligh Street
Sydney
NSW 2000   Tel: 02 9231 2111

Australian Institute of Homoeopathy
Box 122
Roseville
NSW 2069   Tel: 02 9415 3928

Australian Medical Association
42 Macquarie Street
Barton
ACT 2600   Tel: 02 9231 2092

Australian National Association for Mental Health
PO Box 146
Kippax
ACT 2615   Tel: 02 6278 3148

Australian Nutrition Foundation
1–3 Derwent Street
Glebe
NSW 2037   Tel: 02 9552 3081

Australian Osteopathic Association
PO Box 699
Turramurra
NSW 2074   Tel: 02 499 4799

Cancer Information and Support Society
6/81 Alexander Street
Crows Nest
NSW 2065   Tel: 02 9906 2189

Children's Medical Research Institute
214 Hawkesbury Road
Westmead
NSW 2145   Tel: 02 9687 2800

Chiropractors' Association of Australia
319 Victoria Road
Brunswick
VIC 3056   Tel: 03 9387 9377

Heart Support – Australia
PO Box 3940
Weston Creek
ACT 2611   Tel: 02 6285 2557

National Heart Foundation
cnr Denison Street and Geils Ct
Deakin
ACT 2600   Tel: 1300 36 2787

NEW ZEALAND

Allergy Awareness Association
PO Box 12701
Penrose   Tel: 09 303 22024

Auckland Asthma Society
581 Mt Eden Road
Auckland   Tel: 09 630 2293

Community Alcohol Drug Service
Grafton Road
Auckland   Tel: 09 377 0370

Karori Acupuncturist
92a Karori Road
Wellington   Tel: 04 426 2765

National Child Health Research Council
297 Rosebank Road
Avondale   Tel: 09 828 5155

New Zealand Homoeopathic Association
PO Box 2929
Auckland   Tel: 09 630 5458

New Zealand Nutrition Foundation
12-14 Northcroft Street
Takapuna
Auckland   Tel: 09 486 2036

New Zealand Psychological Society
Level 2 Fogel Building
22 Garret Street
Wellington   Tel: 04 801 5414

South Pacific Association of Natural Therapy
28 Willow Avenue
Birkenhead
Auckland 10

CANADA

Acupuncture Foundation of Canada
21-31 Laurence Avenue East
Suite 204
Scarborough
Ontario M1R 5G4   Tel: 416 752 3988

Canadian AIDS Society
130 Albert Street
Suite 90
Ottawa
Ontario K1P 5G4   Tel: 1-800-499-1986
Ontario 1-800-668-2437 (English)
1-800-267-7432 (French)

Canadian Cancer Society
20 Holly Street, Suite 101
Toronto
Ontario M4S 3B1   Tel: 416-485-0222
Fax: 416-485-0223
www.cancer.ca

Canadian Chiropractic Association
1396 Eglinton Avenue West
Toronto
Ontario M6C 2E4   Tel: 416 781 5656

Canadian Institute of Stress
P.O. Box 665, Station 'U'
Toronto
Ontario M8Z 5Y9   Tel: (416) 237-1828
www.stresscanada.org

Canadian Society of Homeopathy
87 Meadowlands Drive West
Nepean
Ontario K2G 2R9

College of Massage Therapists
1867 Yonge Street
Toronto
Ontario M4S 1Y5   Tel: 416 489 2626

Heart and Stroke Foundation of Canada
222 Queens Street
Suite 1402
Ottawa
Ontario K1P 5V9   Tel: 613 569 4361

Migraine Foundation
365 Bloor Street East
Toronto
Ontario M4V 3L4   Tel: 416 920 4916

National Institute of Nutrition
265 Carling Ave
Suite 302
Ottawa
Ontario K1S 2E1   Tel: 613 235 3355
Fax: (613) 235-7032
www.nin.ca

National Cancer Institute
Suite 200
10 Alcorn Avenue
Toronto
Ontario M4V 3B1   Tel: 416 961 7223

Ontario Herbalists Association
7 Alpine Avenue
Port Burwell
Ontario
N0J 1T0   Tel: (416) 536-1509
www.herbalists.on.ca

USA

American Art Therapy Association
Illinois 60060-3808   Tel: 888 290 0878/847 949 6064
Fax: 847 566 4580
www.arttherapy.org

American Association of Acupuncture
433 Front Street
Catasanqua PA 18032   Tel: 610 266 1433
Toll free: 888 500 7999
Fax: 610 264 2768
www.aaom.org

American Association of Naturopathic Physicians
8201 Greensboro Drive
Suite 300
McLean, Virginia   Tel: 703 610 9037
Fax: 703 610 9005

American Chiropractic Association
1701 Clarendon Blvd
Arlington
Virginia 22209   Tel: 800 986 4636
Fax 703/243-2593
www.amerchiro.org

American Heart Association
7272 Greenville Avenue
Dallas
Texas 75231

American Herbalist Guild
1931 Gaddis Road
Canton GA 30115

American Institute of Hypnotherapy
16842 Von Karmen Ave
Ste 475
Irvine
California 92606   Tel: 949 261 6400

American Massage Therapy Association
Evanston, IL 60201-4444   Tel: 847/864-0123
Fax: 847/864-1178
www.amtamassage.org

American Osteopathic Association
142 East Ontario Street
Chicago
Illinois 60611   Tel: (800) 621-1773 l
Fax: (312) 202-8200
E-mail: info@aoa-net.org

American Psychiatric Association
1400 K Street NW
Washington DC 20005   Tel: (888) 357-7924
Fax: 202-682-6850
apa@psych.org

American Shiatsu Association
Po Box 718
Jamaica Plain
Maryland 01230

American Society for the Alexander Technique
P.O. Box 60008
Florence, MA 01062

Tel: (800) 473-0620-413-584-2359
Website: www.alexandertech.org

The Ayurvedic Institute
11311 Menaul NE
Albuquerque,
New Mexico 87112 USA   Tel: (1) 505-291-9698
Fax: 505-294-7572
www.ayurveda.com

Hellerwork International
3435 M Street
Eureka, CA, USA, 95503
Tel: 1-800-392-3900 or 707-441-4949
www.hellerwork.com

International Institute of Reflexology Inc.
PO Box 12642
St Petersburg FL 33733-2642   Tel: (727) 343-4811
Fax: (727) 381-2807
www.reflexology-usa.net

National Cancer Institute
Public Inquiries Office: Building, 31, Room 10A03
31 Center Drive
MSC 2580, Bethesda, Maryland 20892-2580
Tel: (301) 435-3848
www.nci.nih.gov

National Center for Homeopathy
801 North Fairfax Street
Suite 306
Alexandria
Virginia 22314   Tel: (877) 624-0613 (703) 548-7790
fax: (703) 548-7792
www.homeopathic.org

Nelson Bach USA Ltd
Wilmington Technology Park
100 Research Drive
Wilmington
Massachusetts 01887 4406
Tel: 1-800-319-9151/1-978-988-3833
Fax: 1-978-988-0233

Pacific Institute of Aromatherapy
PO Box 6842
San Raphael
California 94903   Tel: 415 479 9129

Rolf Institute
205 Canyon Blvd
Boulder
Colorado 80302
Tel: 303.449.5903 or 800.530.8875
Fax: 303.449.5978
guide.boulder.net/Rolf

Spiritual Healing Common Boundary Inc
7005 Florida Street
Chevy Chase
Maryland 20815

Traditional Acupuncture Institute
American City Building
Suite 108
Columbia
Maryland 21044   Tel: 410 997 3770

SOUTH AFRICA
◆

The Cancer Association of South Africa
PO Box 2121, BEDFORDVIEW, 2008
Tel: (011) 616-7662
www.cansa.org.za

**Confederation of Complementary Health
Associations of South Africa**
PO Box 2471
Clareinch 7740   Tel: 021 58 8709

Heart Foundation of South Africa
Postal Address:
PO Box 15139, VLAEBERG, 8018
Street Address:
Health Park, Anzio Road
Groote Schuur Hospital
Observatory 7925   Tel: (021) 447 4222
Telefax: (021) 4470322
www.heartfoundation.co.za

**Holistic Massage Practitioners Association South
Africa**
42 Emerald Road
Fish Hoek 7975   Tel: 021 782 5909

South African Federation for Mental Health
PO Box 2587
Johannesburg 2000   Tel: 011 725 5800

**South African Naturopaths and Herbalists
Association**
PO Box 18663
Wynberg 7824   Tel: 021 797 8629

Stroke Aid Society
PO Box 51283
Raedene 2124   Tel: 011 882 1612

Western Cape Su Jok Acupuncture Institute
3 Periwinkle Close
Kommetjie 7975   Tel: 021 783 3460

INDEX

◆

ACKNOWLEDGEMENTS

◆

ACKNOWLEDGEMENTS IN SOURCE ORDER

Bach Remedies 420 Top

Bridgeman Art Library, London/New York/"Sweet Dreams" by Thomas Brooks/Phillips, The International Fine Art Auctioneers, UK 375 Main Picture, /"Pierre Quthe, apothecary, 1562" by Francois Clouet/Louvre, Paris, France/Giraudon 405 Main Picture, /"The Physician's Visit" (oil on panel) by Jan Havicksz Steen/Noortman, Maastricht, Netherlands 347 Main Picture, /"The Surgeon", by Jan Sanders van Hemessen/Cheltenham Art Galleries and Museums, Gloucestershire 361 Main Picture, /"A barber surgeon tending a peasant's foot", c.1650, by Issac Koedyck/Johnny van Haeften Gallery, London 389 Main Picture, /detail from "Cataracts III" by Bridget Riley, 1967, emulsion PVA on linen canvas, 88"x87½", collection: British Council 189 Centre Right, /"Cat in a Rainbow" by Louis Wain/Bonhams, London 84 Bottom Left

Bubbles 16 Top, 24 Top Right, 26 Top Centre ,59 Top Left, 86 Main Picture, 87 Bottom, 88 Top Right, 89 Bottom Left, 130 Top Right, 136 Main Picture, 141 Top Left, 141 Top Right, 155 Top Centre, 199 Top, 204 Top, 219 Top, 223 Top, 227 Top, 256 Top Left, 259 Top, 273 Top, 275 Bottom, 277 Centre, 283 Centre Right, 285 Top, 297 Top, 298 Top, 301 Top, 303 Top, 326 Top, 335 Top, 339 Top Centre, 344 Top, 379 Top, 380 Top

Collections 72 Top Centre, 343 Top

Format 453 Top

Angela Hampton/Family Life 11 Top, 12 Top, 13 Bottom, 14 Top, 18 Top, 25 Top Centre, 63 Centre Left, 88 Bottom Left, 93 right, 229 Bottom, 273 Bottom, 278 Bottom, 280 Bottom, 283 Top Right, 287 Bottom Right, 292 Bottom, 310 Centre, 316 Bottom, 317 Top, 317 Bottom, 318 Top, 322 Top, 345 Top, 378 Bottom Right, 384 Top, 385 Bottom /29.113 11 Top

Robert Harding Picture Library 89 Centre Left, 407 Top, 459 Top
Trevor Hill Photos 183 Top

Hulton Getty Picture Collection 260 Top, 363 Top

The Hutchison Library 450 Top

Image Bank 15 Top, 21 Top Left, 60 Main Picture, 78 Centre Right, 88 Centre Right, 89 Top Left, 91 Bottom Left, 91 Bottom Centre, 103 Top Left, 130 Centre Right, 206 Top, 226 Main Picture, 296 Centre, 302 Top, 314 Top, 319 Top, 323 Top, 327 Top, 351 Top Centre

Kobal Collection 288 Bottom

Niall McInerney 291 Top

Oxford Scientific Films 64 Top Right

Octopus Publishing Group Ltd. 425 Bottom, 428 Top, 442 Top, 461 Top /HECH p76 408 Top, /HECH p79 409 Top

Science Photo Library 9 Main Picture, 27 Top Left, 42 Top Right, 44 Main Picture, 45 Top Centre Right, 47 Centre Left, 49 Top Right, 54 Top Centre, 54 Centre Right, 63 Top Left, 83 Top Right, 90 Top, 92 Top, 102 Top Right, 103 Bottom Left, 104 Top, 105 Bottom, 109 Bottom, 111 Top, 121 Top, 122 Top Centre, 122 Centre, 126 Main Picture, 127 Top, 132 Top, 133 Top, 139 Centre Left, 155 Top Left, 161 Centre, 173 Top, 176 Top, 178 Top, 180 Top Centre, 180 Top Right, 188 Main Picture, 189 Top, 192 Top, 194 Top, 195 Bottom, 197 Top, 202 Top, 215 Top, 220 Top, 224 Top, 230 Top, 230 Top Centre Right, 230 Top Right, 230 Centre Centre Right, 231 Top, 238 Top Centre, 238 Top Right, 242 Top, 243 Bottom, 245 Bottom, 250 Top, 254 Top, 255 Bottom, 256 Top Right, 256 Centre Left, 256 Centre Right, 256 Bottom Left, 256 Bottom Right, 268 Bottom Centre, 275 Top, 306 Bottom, 309 Top, 348 Top, 350 Top, 351 Top Right, 352-353 Top, 353 Top Centre, 354 Top, 355 Top, 357 Top, 358 Top, 359 Top, 362 Top Right, 364 Top, 365 Top, 366 Top Centre, 367 Top, 368 Top, 370 Top, 372 Top, 378 Bottom, 411 Top, 412 Bottom, 416 Top, 419 Top, 423 Top, 426 Top, 430 Bottom, 433 Top, 435 Top, 444 Bottom, 448 Top, 455 Top

British School of Shiatsu-Do 447 Bottom

Still Pictures 438 Top

Stone 17 Top, 19 Top, 20 Bottom Centre, 22 Top Centre, 23 Top Left, 39 Top Left, 45 Centre Right, 49 Centre Right, 59 Centre, 61 Top Left, 62 Right, 74 Top Centre, 74 Centre Right, 75 Bottom Left, 76 Top Right, 85 right, 87 Centre Left, 89 Top Centre, 91 Left Centre Top, 98 Centre Right, 100 Main Picture, 101 Top Right, 102 Bottom Left, 103 Centre Left, 131 Main Picture, 142 Top, 151 Top, 184 Bottom, 191 right, 191 Top Left, 191 Centre Left, 214 Top, 216 Top, 229 Top, 235 Top, 251 Bottom, 268 Bottom Left, 270 Main Picture, 276 Centre, 287 Top, 289 Top, 290 Centre, 294 Top, 295 Bottom, 302 Bottom, 304 Bottom, 308 Bottom, 313 Bottom, 324 Bottom, 349 Top, 362 Top Centre, 366 Top Right, 376 Bottom, 377 Top, 386 Top, 387 Top, 415 Top, 436 Top, 445 Top

John Walmsley 441 Top

Wellcome Institute Library, London 51 Top Right, 163 Top, 218 Bottom, 253 Top, 339 Top Left

◆

Editors: Mary Lambert, Joanna Smith and Anne Crane
Creative Director: Keith Martin
Excecutive Art Editor: Geoff Fennell
Designer: Martin Topping
Production Controller: Lee Sargent
Picture research: Joanne Beardwell